A Handbook on Stuttering

A Handbook on Stuttering

Fifth edition

Oliver Bloodstein
Brooklyn College of the City University of New York

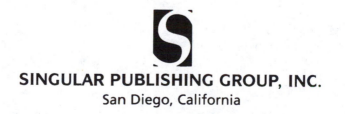

SINGULAR PUBLISHING GROUP, INC.
San Diego, California

Singular Publishing Group, Inc.
4284 41st Street
San Diego, California 92105-1197

Fifth edition 1995

©1995 by Singular Publishing Group, Inc.

Typeset in 10/12 Palatino by So Cal Graphics
Printed in the Untied States of America by BookCrafters

Library of Congress Cataloging-in-Publication data
Bloodstein, Oliver.
   A handbook on stuttering / Oliver Bloodstein. — 5th ed.
      p.   cm.
   Includes bibliographical references and index.
   ISBN 1-56593-395-8
   1. Stuttering.   I. Title.
   [DNLM: 1. Stuttering.   WM 475 B655ha 1995]
RC424.B54   1995
616.85'54—dc20
DNLM/DLC
for Library of Congress   94-36577
                                              CIP

CONTENTS

PREFACE

In the eight years that have passed since the last revision of *A Handbook on Stuttering*, some 400 new studies of stuttering have been reported. Among various areas that have been explored, by far the most prominent has been the subject of speech motor control in stutterers. Prompted by expanding knowledge about normal motor control and the availability of computerized instrumentation for investigating it, a large number of workers, including an active group in the Netherlands, have applied themselves in this effort. The principal objects of this investigation have been the neuromotor aspects of stutterings, the control of the stutterer's oral structures in nonspeech activities, and above all the stutterer's speech motor control during what are judged to be fluent utterances. To date, the outcome of this research has been somewhat murky at best. One reason is the high frequency of conflicting findings that has perennially frustrated virtually all comparative studies of groups of stutterers and nonstutterers. In this regard, Martin A. Young's paper on the limitations of the group difference research design has provided a valuable insight. Another reason for the ambiguity of the results is that questions have been raised about the interpretation of the abnormalities that have often been observed in stutterers' ostensibly fluent speech. Note especially the discussion of the subject by Armson and Kalinowski.

Nevertheless, this eight-year interval has not been without its harvest of new findings and developments. For example, it appears increasingly certain that acquired (neurogenic) stuttering has features that clearly differentiate it from developmental stuttering. There is now convincing evidence that essentially any change in the way stutterers hear themselves speak results in greater fluency. From conflicting findings on stutterers' manual reaction times, it now seems clear that they will not exhibit the consistent and unambiguous lag that characterizes stutterers' vocal reaction times. There has been a notable increase in research on early stuttering by a considerable number of workers, and studies of parent-child interactions have raised questions about some of the advice that is frequently given to parents. The self-help and consumer advocacy movement among stutterers has burgeoned rapidly, and this is bound to affect the way therapy is administered.

Twenty-five years have elapsed since the National Easter Seal Society agreed to expand a booklet by the author to a textbook for students and a resource for speech-language pathologists. We must now bid a grateful farewell to the National Society, which ably saw *A Handbook on Stuttering* through four editions, despite the fact that book publishing was not part of its mission. Although the *Handbook* now has a new home, it has not changed its theme and purpose. As in previous editions, the book's endeavor is to guide the reader to the edge of our knowledge about stuttering and, where the edge is not well defined, to point out where the footing is insecure and where we stand on solid ground.

—*Oliver Bloodstein*

To the memory of

WENDELL JOHNSON
ROBERT WEST
BRYNG BRYNGELSON
JOSEPH G. SHEEHAN
LEE EDWARD TRAVIS
DEAN E. WILLIAMS
CHARLES VAN RIPER

1
SYMPTOMATOLOGY

DEFINING STUTTERING

Most of us believe we know what stuttering is; yet a great deal of disagreement generally results when we try to define it. Some of the disagreement stems from conflicting inferences about the underlying nature of the disorder that reveal themselves in our definitions. When we try to avoid this problem by adhering strictly to the description of behavior, other difficulties present themselves. Traditionally, stuttering has been viewed as a disorder in which the "rhythm" or fluency of speech is impaired by interruptions, or blockages. For many ordinary purposes such a definition is adequate, and in this chapter we will discuss at some length those moments of interruption or blockage that are a dominant feature of the disorder. Yet it cannot be denied that what we identify as stuttering is sometimes evident not only in the intermittent impairment of fluency, but also in the rate, pitch, loudness, inflectional patterns, articulation, facial expression, and postural adjustments of the speaker and that there are stutterers for whom its features are not always confined in an easily identifiable manner to discrete "moments."

Furthermore, when, with our definition in hand we stride to the task of specifying just where or when a "block" has taken place, we find that it is not so simple. Research has shown that the most highly expert observers may have considerable difficulty in agreeing on whether an instance of stuttering has occurred on a given occasion, as we will see in Chapter 9.

It is particularly important to point out in addition that conventional definitions of stuttering, even when considerably elaborated, do not adequately serve to differentiate it objectively from various other forms of disfluency that are regarded as distinct from the familiar clinical entity under discussion here. They are of notably little help in clarifying the relationship between stuttering and "normal" disfluency and so ride roughshod over some of the most critical questions of stuttering theory. Johnson (1959, Chap. 8; 1961a) demonstrated that there is little the stutterer does, of a sort that can be conveyed by available descriptions of nonfluent speech behavior, that the nonstutterer does not also do to some extent and in some instances in equivalent measure. We will discuss this problem at some length in Chapter 9.

THE MEASUREMENT OF STUTTERING BEHAVIOR

From a scientific standpoint the problem of defining a phenomenon is intimately bound up with the question of the operations we use to measure it. Consequently, it will be useful to explore the measurable dimensions of stuttering. How does one express quantitatively such a concept as the degree, amount, or severity of stuttering behavior? In Investigations of this problem so far essentially five ways have been found for doing this.

Frequency of Stuttering

The frequency of stuttering, expressed as a number or percentage of moments of stuttering or of stuttered words or syllables, is one of the most familiar of such measures and has been extensively used in research on the variability of the disorder beginning with studies by Johnson and his associates at the University of Iowa in the 1930s. We may impart a rough notion of the frequency with which people who stutter block by saying that on the average about 10 percent of words are stuttered in oral reading, but the variability of this measure, both from person to person and under different conditions, is quite high. To cite some representative data, thirty adult stutterers, reading "average factual prose" to two listeners, stuttered on a mean of 10.8 percent of the words and ranged from 0.0 percent to 47.0 percent of words stuttered (Bloodstein, 1944). In clinical experience it is not unusual to find both stutterers who have difficulty on a large majority of words in ordinary speaking situations and those who so rarely appear to block at all, most of their trouble consisting of the anticipation of difficulty, that Freund (1934a) referred to their problem as "inneres Stottern" (interiorized stuttering).[1] Variations in the frequency of stuttering from situation to situation are equally striking and will be discussed in Chapters 7 and 8.

---

[1]See also Douglass and Quarrington (1952) on the subject of interiorized stuttering.

The distribution of stutterers with respect to frequency of stuttering is skewed, as Soderberg (1962b) and Johnson, Darley, and Spriestersbach (1963, p. 252) pointed out. That is, there are more "mild" than "severe" stutterers if the mean frequency of stuttering is arbitrarily taken as the line of demarcation for making such a judgment. To put it more succinctly, the median stutterer blocks less frequently than the average stutterer.

Special techniques that have been discussed for measuring the frequency of stuttering include electronic counters (Norcross and Andrews, 1973) and time-expanded speech (Manning, Lee, and Lass, 1978; O'Keefe and Kroll, 1980; Kroll and O'Keefe, 1985).

Agreement among different observers on the frequency of stuttering is not high. Kully and Boberg (1988) found poor agreement among clinicians at nine treatment centers on counts of stutterings in the same recorded speech samples. Ingham and Cordes (1992) noted substantial differences between trained judges at both the same and different speech clinics. Ingham and his co-workers have reported improved agreement in counts of time intervals containing stuttering.[2]

Mean Duration of Stutterings

The average duration of a stuttering block as judged by laboratory observers is about one second. Blocks tend to vary in duration only within a few seconds, although some appear to be extremely fleeting and those of severe stutters may occasionally be observed to continue for longer than a minute. Johnson and Colley (1945) found that the combined mean of the ten longest blocks was 0.41 second.

If measures of the duration of individual moments of stuttering vary so little, then, as might be expected, the *mean duration of stutterings*, employed as a measure of amount of difficulty on a given reading or speaking task, varies still less. In a study referred to above (Bloodstein, 1944) thirty subjects ranged in mean duration of stutterings from less than .05 second to 3.7 seconds in oral reading, the median subject having a mean duration of 0.9 second. Only 25 percent of the subjects had a mean duration of more than 1.4 seconds.

As Table 1 shows, mean duration of stutterings does not appear to be related in any notable degree to other measures of severity of stuttering. The chief reason for this is its restricted range of variability. In general, one stutterer does not differ very much from another in the mean duration of blockages. This characteristic somewhat limits its usefulness as a measure of severity of stuttering.

---

[2]Cordes, Ingham, Frank, and Costello Ingham (1992), Ingham, Cordes, and Gow (1993), Ingham, Cordes, and Finn (1993).

Table 1. Coefficients of Correlation Between Measures of Severity of Stuttering

	Reading	Speaking
Judges' Rating vs. Frequency of Stuttering		
Sherman, Young, and Gough (1958)	.87	
Aron (1967)	.57	
Judges' Rating vs. Rate or Time*		
Sherman, Young, and Gough (1958)	.76	
Minifie and Cooker (1964)	−.69	
Aron (1967)	−.89	
Young (1961)**		.68
Young (1961)**		.67
Prosek, Walden, et al (1979)	−.80	
Frequency of Stuttering vs. Rate or Time*		
Bloodstein (1944)	−.88	
Dixon (1955)	.89	
Sherman, Young, and Gough (1958)	.76	
Aron (1967)	−.72	
Andrews and Cutler (1974)		.81
Prins, Mandelkorn, and Cerf (1980)		−.69
Judges' Rating vs. Frequency of Specified Disfluencies		
Young (1961)**		.87
Young (1961)**		.85
Frequency of Specified Disfluencies vs. Rate or Time		
Sander (1961)***	.86	.81
Young (1961)**		.59
Mean Duration of Stutterings vs. Frequency of Stuttering		
Bloodstein (1944)	.17	
Johnson and Colley (1945)	.54	
Mean Duration of Stutterings vs. Rate or Time*		
Bloodstein (1944)	−.46	

*Correlation coefficients are positive or negative depending on whether time or rate in words or syllables per minute was used.
**Disfluencies included part-word repetition, sound prolongation, broken utterance, and unusual stress.
***Disfluencies included Johnson's eight categories.

Frequency of Specified Disfluency Types

Speech as produced on most occasions contains a considerable variety of interruptions or hesitancies. This is true whether the speaker is regarded as a stutterer or a normal speaker, as Johnson and his students have abundantly demonstrated, or is a "clutterer," or repeats syllables in a manner characteristic of certain types of neurological impairment. Convenient broad generic terms for the phenomenon of interruption in the smooth flow of speech are "disfluency" or "dysfluency." It is clear, and of basic importance, that not every instance of disfluency is to be regarded as an example of the specific type of disorder to which we refer as stuttering.

Unfortunately, we have no satisfactory *objective* means of differen-tiating moments of stuttering from other instances of disfluency. Consequently, the identification of moments of stuttering always involves the judgment of a listener. This means that any measure of severity of stuttering that requires the identification of stutterings is based upon an evaluative process subject to such troublesome uncon-trolled variables as the standards, definitions, or criteria of the person who is doing the identifying. It should be clear that the measures already discussed, frequency of stuttering and mean duration of stut-terings, belong in this category.

This raises the question whether there is any type of serviceable index that is free of the process of identification of stuttering. The problem is essentially one of finding an objectively measurable fea-ture of speech that is highly related to subjective judgments of amount or severity of stuttering. One obvious possibility is that there are certain particular *aspects or kinds of disfluency* that might fulfill these requirements. We therefore turn briefly to some investigations that have been carried out on the subject of disfluency and its rela-tionship to judgments of stuttering.

Johnson (1959, Chap. 8; 1961a), with the help of his students and co-workers, gathered normative data on the disfluencies of stuttering and nonstuttering adults and young children through analysis of tape-recorded speech samples. For this purpose he devised a system of class-ification of disfluent types of speech behavior consisting of eight categories: *1) interjections* ("uh," "er," "well"), 2) *part-word repetitions* (repetitions of sounds or syllables of words), 3) *word repetitions, 4) phrase repetitions* ("I was I was going"), 5) *revisions* ("I was—I am going"), 6) *incomplete phrases* ("She was—and after she got there he came"), 7) *broken words* ("I was g— (pause) —oing home"), 8) *pro-longed sounds.*

This scheme is usable in obtaining such measures of a speaker's disfluency as the total number of instances per hundred words read or spoken.[3] Similar normative data have been gathered on school-age children by F. H. Silverman (1974). In conjunction with the normative data these measures afford a basis for judging how usual or unusual the speaker's disfluencies may be. It should be clear, however, that they are not concerned with anyone's "stuttering." In varying degrees, of course, the counting of "broken words" or of "prolonged sounds" also depends upon the perceptions and judgments of a lis-tener.[4] But these are relatively descriptive terms compared with which

---

[3]For a more complete description of procedures for obtaining such measures see Darley and Spriestersbach (1978, Chap. 9). Pauses were omitted for lack of a precise way of distinguishing hesitant pauses from meaningful ones.

[4]In fact, judges did not agree well in applying Johnson's categories to the disfluencies of young children in a study by Onslow, Gardner, Bryant, Stuckings, and Knight (1992).

"stuttering" is a highly inferential construct usually embodying the evaluational notion of failure or abnormality.

The question is, can any useful *relationship* be found between the counting of types of disfluencies and the identification of stutterings? As is to be expected, Johnson's classification of disfluencies appears to contain certain types that would probably not fit most listeners' definitions of stuttering and, conversely, there are aspects of stuttering not described by any of the features of disfluency in his list. Yet, on the whole, Johnson's stutterers proved to have much more disfluency than his normal-speaking subjects. While with respect to certain categories (e.g., revisions, incomplete phrases, and interjections such as "uh") the differences were small or nonexistent and the distributions markedly overlapping, with respect to others (notably, part-word repetitions and prolonged sounds) there were large differences between the two groups with little overlapping of distributions.

Johnson's findings suggest, in other words, that within his classification there are certain descriptions that are distinctly typical of disfluencies likely to be considered stuttering. This view is strengthened by other research findings showing that listeners are likely to classify sound or syllable repetitions and prolonged sounds as stuttering and revisions and interjections as normal disfluency (Boehmler, 1958; Williams and Kent, 1958; Schiavetti, 1975). A measure that attempts to separate "stutter-type" disfluencies from others is the index of disfluency used by Sander (1961), which has found some application in research. It is a count of disfluent words for which a disfluency is defined as a sound, syllable, or word repetition; a sound prolongation; a broken word; or an interjection within a word.

The basic question of the relationship between stuttering and disfluency was attacked directly by Young (1961), who set out to determine whether judges' ratings of severity of stuttering in recorded speech samples could be adequately predicted from selected measures of disfluency and speaking time. Young found a relatively high degree of association (*see Table 1*) between severity of stuttering as rated and the frequency of occurrence of a category of disfluencies made up of syllable or sound repetitions, sound prolongations, broken words, and words involving "apparent undue stress or tension."

Despite this relationship for his speech samples as a whole, Young found that his measures did not permit the prediction of individual ratings of severity with a satisfactory degree of precision. When he examined the ten speech samples that had resulted in the largest discrepancies between predicted and obtained ratings, Young made some interesting observations. In all ten cases the predictions had underestimated the actual ratings made by the judges. Each of the ten samples appeared to be "characterized by some unusual and distinctive pattern" that had not been adequately represented in the frequency count of disfluencies. In particular, these patterns tended to include drawn-out repetitions of syllables, or "audible manifestations of excessive tension." Among other features evident in isolated cases were severe harshness and a rapidly rising pitch level during syllable repetitions.

Young's findings implied that much more work remains to be done on our descriptions of disfluency. At the same time, they offered the hope that as these descriptions become more refined they will lend themselves to the development of useful measures of stuttering. The problem is apparently not that stuttering is indistinguishable from any other kind of disfluency, but that some of the differences are easily obscured by our rough-and-ready verbal classifications. The findings of Kalotkin, Manschreck, and O'Brien (1979) suggested that electromyographic measures of masseter muscle tension during speech may be a useful indicator of severity of stuttering. Suter, Hutchinson, and Mallard (1979) identified visible concomitants of stuttering that appear to influence judgments of severity. Studies by Manning, Emal, and Jamison (1975) and Curran and Hood (1977b) made a beginning in the investigation of the number of repeated units per speech repetition as related to judgments of severity of stuttering.

We have been discussing the features of disfluencies that must be taken into account when we attempt to measure the frequency of "stuttering" as opposed to other kinds of disfluency. Note that our main concern here is with the measurement of stuttering in its developed form. The differentiation of stuttering from normal disfluency in early childhood is a question with special implications and difficulties which we will take up in Chapter 9.

Speech Rate

Our discussion of disfluency counts in the preceding paragraphs was prompted by the question of whether there are any measures of severity of stuttering that are independent of a listener's judgment of the occurrence of stuttering. Another type of objective measure is rate of speech production—for example, oral reading rate in words or syllables per minute, or speaking time in the utterance of a given number of words. Stuttering, of course, tends to retard the speaker's speed of verbal output. In a study of oral reading rates of adult stutterers (Bloodstein, 1944), a mean rate of 123 words per minute was found in the reading of factual prose of average word length, and a range among thirty subjects of 42 to 191 words per minute. By contrast, the same material was read by normal speakers in a previous study (Darley, 1940) at a mean rate of 167 words per minute, with a range of 129 to 222 words per minute. Extensive normative data presented by

Johnson (1961a) for both reading and speaking show comparable differences and overlapping between stutterers and nonstutterers.

From a practical standpoint, measures of rate have the advantage of being convenient to use. They take into account both frequency and duration of stutterings and tend to be fairly highly correlated (see Table 1) with frequency. They are also influenced, however, by various factors that presumably do not enter into listeners' criteria for the occurrence of stuttering and are insensitive to any aspects of symptomatology that do not waste time, and so have usually been found to be only moderately related to judges' ratings of severity of stuttering. Young, in the study cited above, found that speaking time did not contribute as much to the prediction of ratings of severity as did his count of specified disfluencies, except in the case of the more severe stutterers. On the other hand, Prosek, Walden, et al (1979) found reading rate, as well as frequency of pauses within sentences, to be more closely related to judged severity of stuttering than were other measures including frequency of stuttering.

From these observations and the data in Table 1 we may infer that speech rate is not so highly correlated with any other measure of severity as to be considered merely its equivalent and yet is sufficiently related to other measures as to suggest that it may be reflecting an aspect of severity that they do not adequately take into account. For this reason there has been a tendency to use it in conjunction with other measures in which the amount or severity of stuttering has been a variable. For the same reason it lends itself to use in composite indices such as that of Minifie and Cooker (1964).

Ratings of Severity

Listeners' ratings of severity of stuttering constitute a frankly subjective measure giving full play to the judgmental nature of the criteria that we use to define stuttering, and there is perhaps no better evidence of that judgmental nature than the common practice of validating other measures of severity by comparing them with the results obtained on the same subjects by means of listeners' ratings of severity. Of all measures, in short, this one has the highest "face" validity.

It is also by far the oldest and most familiar type of measurement in general use, in the sense that we employ it on every occasion on which we characterize stuttering as "mild," "moderate," or "severe." In the 1950s this method underwent a major development with the introduction of tape-recorded speech samples, multiple judges, and refined psychological scaling techniques by Sherman and others, and a considerable amount of work was done in an effort to find the most advantageous ways of obtaining severity ratings for clinical and research purposes.

These investigations resulted in reliable methods for scaling the severity of stuttering of continuous speech, of short samples, or of individual moments.[5] Studies have shown that by and large, the reliability of the measures is not critically affected by such factors as the type of scale used, the number of scale points, the definition of scale points, the addition of visual or "live" cues, the number of judges, their sophistication, or the kinds of instructions they receive.[6] In addition, work has been done on the measurement and improvement of observer agreement and on the control of observer bias in judging severity of stuttering.[7]

The scale of severity of stuttering constructed by Lewis and Sherman (1951) by the method of equal-appearing intervals consists of a series of tape-recorded speech samples representing the whole range of severity from very mild to very severe. These samples form touchstones, as it were, with which the speech of a given subject may be compared. The scale affords a precise method of rating severity, though a study by Berry and Silverman (1972) suggests that the scale has ordinal rather than interval properties—that is, the intervals are not subjectively equal.

An alternative rating method is known as direct magnitude estimation. In place of a scale, raters use a single stimulus as a standard for comparison. Assigning any number (e.g., ten) to that standard, they then estimate the numerical magnitude of other stimuli as proportions of the magnitude of the standard. Martin (1965) showed that the severity of stuttering could be rated reliably in this way. Results of a more recent study by Schiavetti, Sacco, Metz, and Sitler (1983) suggested that direct magnitude estimation is a more valid method of rating the severity of stuttering than interval scaling.

Summary Remarks

The foregoing discussion has served to raise several fundamental questions. How is stuttering to be defined? What are its measurable dimensions? How is it to be differentiated from other kinds of disfluent behavior including that of normal speech? We have seen that, except for the evaluation of a listener that stuttering has occurred, we as yet have no operational definition serving to characterize the stuttering response in a wholly satisfactory way. On the other hand, we can identify certain features of speech, notably sound or syllable repe-

---

[5]Lewis and Sherman (1951), Sherman (1952), Sherman (1955), Sherman and Trotter (1956), Sherman and McDermott (1958).

[6]Young and Prather (1962), Cullinan, Prather, and Williams (1963), Williams, Wark, and Minifie (1963), Martin (1965), Cullinan and Prather (1968).

[7]Young and Downs (1968), Young (1969a, 1969b, 1970).

titions, broken words, prolonged sounds, and signs of unusual effort or tension that are more closely related than others to what most listeners judge to be stuttering. There are thus hints that with further description we may eventually be able to define stuttering more adequately in terms of its observable features.

We can summarize the import of essentially all we have said so far in this chapter by suggesting that for investigators who are anxious to define carefully what they mean by stuttering the best definition we appear to be able to offer at present is: whatever is perceived as stuttering by a reliable observer who has relatively good agreement with others. If we want to be guided by a more "objective" definition we must not ask questions about "stuttering," but about repetitions, prolongations, broken words, speech rate, and the like, and must be content with answers that are not about stuttering, but about repetitions, prolongations, and so forth.

In any consideration of the problem of defining stuttering it is, of course, vitally necessary to keep distinct a number of different meanings with which the term may be used. For example, the question of whether a person "is a stutterer" (i.e., stutters habitually) is one on which it is generally fairly easy to obtain agreement, except with respect to young children, on the basis of observed speech behavior on a series of occasions, as well as the speech history, the conditions under which the behavior varies, the person's self-concepts, speech attitudes, and methods of coping with the problem, and the like. Agreement that the person "is a stutterer," however, does not help much to answer the question of whether he or she has spoken in a stuttering manner in a given speech situation. That question, in turn, is not as difficult to answer as the question of whether the speaker has stuttered on a given word. The use of the term stuttering in each of these cases must not be allowed to become a source of confusion. If we are unable to define the moment of stuttering so as to differentiate it easily from other instances of speech interruption, this is a curious and by no means trivial fact. But it does not rule out an operationally meaningful definition of stuttering as a disorder.

It is, of course, within the realm of possibility that not only stutterings or stuttered speech, but even individuals who stutter, may prove impossible to characterize in every case with absolute unambiguity. If so, the prospect need not alarm us unduly. There is, as we shall see, more than one conceptual scheme available to stuttering theory that is compatible with the assumption that the population of "stutterers" is not separable from the normal-speaking population in a sharply dichotomous way.

PHYSIOLOGICAL AND ACOUSTIC DESCRIPTIONS OF STUTTERING

The instruments and methods of the speech laboratory have been put to greatly increased use in the study of stuttering symptomatology. After a period of many decades during which such research was largely confined to the investigation of the stutterer's breathing patterns by means of the kymograph or pneumograph, we now have considerable electromyographic, spectrographic, fiberoptic, radiographic, aerodynamic, and other kinds of data about the stuttering block.

Respiration

Disordered breathing is associated with stuttering so often and so conspicuously that it was one of the earliest factors to be investigated as a possible cause of stuttering. Pneumographic research has consequently been conducted over a long period of time. Breathing curves during stuttering show a series of abnormalities, some of which are obviously parallel to audible or visible aspects of symptomatology. These include antagonisms between abdominal and thoracic breathing, irregularity of consecutive respiratory cycles, prolonged expirations or inspirations, complete cessation of breathing, interruption of expiration by inspiration, and attempts to speak on intake of air.[8]

Phonation

Breath-holding, glottal fry, and stutterers' reports that their "throat closes tightly" are common clinical observations that point to the larynx as a site of abnormal activity during stuttering. As with the respiratory mechanism, various attempts have been made since the nineteenth century to identify the larynx as the primary source of difficulty for those who stutter. Such speculation has become intensified as a result of a series of laboratory investigations.

In 1963 Chevrie-Muller reported a study of the vocal folds during stuttering by the technique of glottography. The method employed by Chevrie-Muller provided a continuous record of the size of the glottal opening by measuring the amount of light permitted to pass through it. She found many abnormalities including "breaks in the rhythm of

---

[8]Halle (1900), Ten Cate (1902), Gutzmann (1908), Fletcher (1914), Lambeck (1925), Hansen (1927), Travis (1927a), Fossler (1930), Steer (1935), Henrikson (1936), V. Travis (1936), Steer (1937), Morley (1937), Starbuck and Steer (1954), Umeda (1962b), Brankel (1961, 1963).

vocal fold vibration and a clonic fluttering of the folds in some but not all of her stutterers" (cited by Van Riper, 1971, p. 150).

More recently, Janssen, Wieneke, and Vaane (1983) used glotto-graphic recording to test the assumption that stuttering blocks are associated with slowness in initiating phonation, relative to the start of articulatory activity. Among five subjects this proved to be true of only two. Weiner (1984a) produced a series of glottograms corre-sponding to various types of stuttering by using a technique that measured the impedance of the glottis to an electrical current passing over it. Using the same technique, Borden, Baer, and Kenney (1985) found that after a stuttering block on initial /t/ in the word "two," almost all subjects tended to build up voicing gradually instead of abruptly as in fluent utterances of the word. They speculated that the subjects used this as a means of releasing themselves from the block. Borden, Baer, and Kenney also noted evidence of rigidity of the vocal folds during stuttering, as well as tremors that coincided with visible tremors of the lip.

Electromyography, the recording of electrical potentials from the muscles, was first used to observe a stutterer's laryngeal activity by Bar, Singer, and Feldman (1969). They reported an increase in the action potentials just before and during stuttering. Freeman and Ushijima (1975, 1978) took electromyographic recordings simultane-ously from six separate intrinsic laryngeal muscles of four subjects. Their results showed high levels of muscular activity during stutter-ing, as well as simultaneous contractions of adductor and abductor muscles *(see Figure 1)*. These observations—excessive muscular activ-ity and poor coordination of antagonistic laryngeal muscles—were confirmed by Shapiro (1980) with four additional subjects. Laryngeal hyperactivity was also reported by Thürmer, Thumfart, and Kittel (1983) in an electromyographic study of forty-two stutterers. Metz, Conture, and Colton (1976) found a delay in laryngeal activity prior to disfluencies as measured electromyographically in two stutterers.

Conture, McCall, and Brewer (1977) used a fiberoptic technique to make direct visual observations of the glottis during stuttering in ten subjects. In 60 percent of the part-word repetitions the vocal folds were in a state of abduction throughout the block, regardless of whether the repeated speech segment was voiced or unvoiced. In the remaining cases the vocal folds were either adducted or alternately adducted and abducted. During prolongations of sounds the position of the folds was always appropriate to the voicing characteristics of the sound. In a later fiberoptic study, Conture, Schwartz, and Brewer (1985) found that during voiced prolongations the vocal folds were usually appropriately adducted, but that during sound or syllable

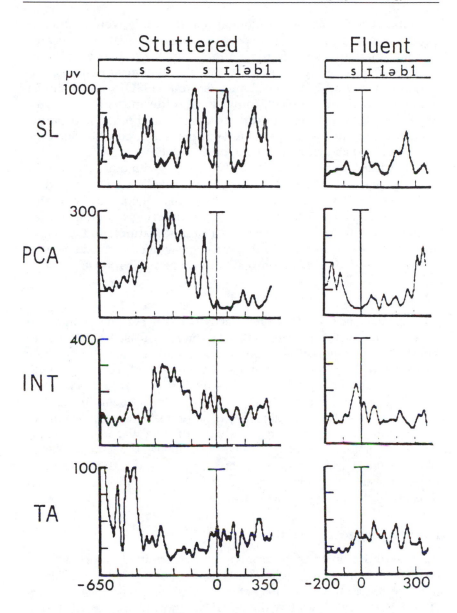

Figure 1. Comparison of muscle activity—superior longitudinal (SL), posterior cricoarytenoid (PCA), interarytenoid (INT), and thyroarytenoid (TA)—for one subject's stuttered and fluent utterances of the word *syllable*. Note the simultaneous contraction
of the PCA (abductor) and INT (adductor) muscles during stuttering, as well as the
increased muscular activity. Reproduced from "Laryngeal muscle activity during
stuttering," by Freeman and Ushijima, *J. Speech Hearing Res., 21,* 538–62.
Copyright 1978 by the American Speech-Language-Hearing Association. Reprinted
by permission.

repetitions and voiceless prolongations the folds were adducted, abducted, or in an intermediate position. Their observations appeared to show that stutterers do not "simply 'squeeze' their vocal folds together during all instances of stuttering"; the vocal folds may be inappropriately adducted or abducted. Wolk (1981), using a similar technique with one subject, found a "shuddering" of the larynx, asymmetry of the arytenoid cartilages and vocal folds, and partial adduction of the folds, seeming to represent a conflict between adductory and abductory behavior, during all types of stuttering.

It is clear that the larynx is involved, along with other parts of the vocal apparatus, in the abnormality of stuttering. Whether the deviant activity of the larynx is "primary" in any sense is not a question that can be answered by descriptive studies of stuttering symptomatology. Such studies fail to distinguish among causes, features, and effects of stuttering. We will return to this question when we consider other types of investigations of laryngeal functioning in Chapter 4.

Articulation

Research has been done on the activity of the peripheral organs of articulation during stuttering, as well as on certain aspects of the stutterer's speech sounds. The earliest of these studies were kymographic investigations by Robbins (1935) and Cords (1936), concerned with durational aspects of speech sounds during stuttering blocks or in stuttered speech. Shaffer (1940) measured jaw movement during stuttered and nonstuttered productions of stop-plosive consonants in initial position in words. He found that stuttering was characterized, among other abnormalities, by longer time intervals between onset of jaw movement and onset of phonation, by more directional changes in jaw movement, and by longer intervals between initiation and first directional change of jaw movement.

Electromyographic Studies

The development of electromyography permitted observations to be made of individual muscles of articulation during stuttering. Electromyographic studies of the masseter muscles by Travis (1934), Morley (1937), Steer (1937), and Williams (1955) showed that in stuttering there is frequent evidence of defective synchronization, as well as other abnormalities of the action potentials of the paired musculatures. In a different type of investigation Sheehan and Voas (1954) used unilateral masseter action potentials to show that muscular tension appears to build up during stuttering, reaching its peak near the termination of the block.

Further studies were done on the orbicularis muscle by Tatham (1973) and Belyakova (1973) and on the masseter and geniohyoid muscles by Brankel (1963). In each case the occurrence of stuttering was found to be recognizable in some manner in the electromyographic recordings. In a study by Shapiro (1980), four subjects with electrodes at the lip and tongue showed excessive muscular activity on stuttered words, poor coordination of muscles, and inappropriate bursts of activity during silence *(see Figure 2)*. Craig and Cleary (1982) observed high levels of activity in the orbicularis oris in their three subjects during stuttering, while Thürmer, Thumfart, and Kittel (1983) found excessive activity in the orbicularis oris and tongue in forty-two subjects.

A frequent observation, in studies of both the articulatory and laryngeal muscles, is that the same electromyographic phenomena that characterize overt stuttering may sometimes appear in the absence of any noticeable blocks (see especially Shapiro, 1980; Freeman, 1984). The reverse—stuttering without evidence of increased muscular tension—was reported by McClean, Goldsmith, and Cerf (1984). In an electromyographic and strain-gauge study of the depressor labii inferior and mentalis muscles (antagonists in the elevation and depression of the lower lip) during stuttering on bilabial consonants by five subjects, the investigators failed to find simultaneous contraction of antagonistic muscles or increased levels of electromyographic activity.

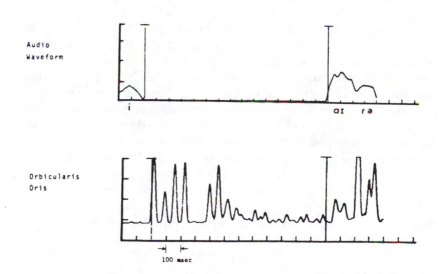

Figure 2. Abnormal supraglottal muscular activity during stuttering on "Ira." Reproduced by permission of the publisher from "An electromyographic analysis of the fluent and dysfluent utterances of several types of stutterers," by Arnold Shapiro, *Journal of Fluency Disorders, 5,* 203–231. Copyright 1980 by Elsevier Science Publishing Co., Inc.

Smith (1989) correlated the activity of neck, jaw, and lip muscles during stuttering. She found little indication that the coordination of these muscles differed from that of normal speaking control subjects, but unlike any of the nonstutterers, 6 of 10 stutterers exhibited large rhythmic oscillations in muscle activity during stuttering. These occurred at the same frequency in all of the muscle groups, suggesting that they had a common source. In the same muscles Smith, Denny, and Wood (1991) observed tremorlike oscillations and increased activity which were not timed precisely with perceived stutterings, but occurred in their "neighborhood." Denny and Smith (1992) reported that neither the oscillations nor the high electromyographic amplitudes always occurred with stuttering, but appeared in varying degrees in different subjects.

Two lip muscles were the subject of a study of three stutterers and three control subjects by Guitar, Guitar, Neilson, O'Dwyer, and Andrews (1988). In articulating the initial *p* of the words *peek, puck*, and *pack*, the normal speakers typically activated the depressor anguli oris before the depressor labii inferior. The stutterers reversed this sequence most of the time when stuttering and half the time when not. The authors hypothesized that the stutterers were deliberately stiffening their lips in the expectation of stuttering. If so, this demonstrated what Van Riper (1937d) described as one of the stutterer's "preparatory sets," namely the tendency to establish a focus of tension in the articulators in advance of the attempt on a difficult word (see p. 66).

Van Riper (1982, pp. 123–126) remarked on the occurrence of tremors in the speech muscles during stuttering and the role of strenuous postures of the articulators in precipitating them. Through the use of electromyographic recordings Platt and Basili (1973) discovered that such tremors appear to be similar to those that are commonly produced by isometric contractions of muscles (i.e., co-contractions of antagonists). They found three stutterers who exhibited jaw tremors during stuttering and instructed the stutterers to produce contractions of the jaw muscles by opening and closing the jaw simultaneously without dental contact. The resulting tremors were compared with the stuttering tremors and found to be alike in frequency and amplitude. This lends support to Platt and Basili's parsimonious explanation that tremors in stuttering may result from isometric muscle status due to struggle.

Aerodynamic Studies

Another approach to the description of stuttering has made use of devices for measuring intraoral air pressure and the rate of airflow from the oral cavity during speech. In a study of the stutterings of 8 subjects, Hutchinson (1975) identified 7 distinctive aerodynamic patterns. Repeated peaks in intraoral air pressure were associated with syllable repetitions. A gradual elevation of intraoral air pressure occurred with prolongation of a sound, especially a stop consonant. Multiple elevations of intraoral pressure without airflow were associated with a silent block on a stop consonant. Prolonged airflow terminating in an excessive peak of airflow corresponded to a breathy articulation of a sound such as /w/ with an aspirated release. A sudden drop in air pressure and flow rate accompanied a brief silent interval. A prolonged peak of intraoral air pressure and absence of airflow signified the silent prolongation of an articulatory posture. Intraoral pressure elevations of low magnitude without airflow were observed on a prolonged pause between syllables.

These aerodynamic findings correspond in a predictable way to the repetitions, prolongations, and other types of stuttering as they are conventionally described. But they also reflect a feature of stuttering to which our unaided clinical observations are unable to penetrate—the underlying tension that appears to pervade the vocal organs during the block. Although we sometimes speak of tension among the features of stuttering as though we were employing a description, the tense state of muscles is something we must infer rather than anything we can observe directly. The electromyographic findings we have reviewed give us the most direct evidence of this state. Hutchinson's aerodynamic patterns do so less directly, but they graphically reveal the source of that tension to be the attempt stutterers make to speak through an airway they have constricted at some point.

Spectrographic Studies

Acoustic investigation of stuttering done with the aid of the spectrograph has centered mainly around the transitions between speech sounds during part-word repetition. Van Riper (1971, pp. 23-25) speculated that the stutterer's difficulty is not with sounds but with the transitions between them. He suggested that in stutterers' part-word repetitions, as distinguished from those of nonstutterers, the neutral vowel is almost universally heard (e.g., *suh-suh-sandwich*) in place of the intended vowel that would be required by normal coarticulation. Neither perceptual judgments of trained observers nor spectrograms have wholly borne out this observation, however. In a perceptual and acoustic analysis, Montgomery and Cooke (1976) found that stutterers' part-word repetitions do not ordinarily contain the neutral vowel, but a vowel that often approximates that of the word being pronounced. Van Wyk (1978) reported an absence of formant transitions in the repetitions of eighteen stuttering children and adults, but perceptual and spectrographic analysis showed that the neutral vowel was not being used. Similar observations have been made by others.[9] Howell and his co-workers showed that what often strikes the ear as a neutralization of the vowel in stutterers' repetitions actually is occasioned by a decrease in the duration and amplitude of the vowel.[10]

Nevertheless, Stromsta and Fibiger (1981) produced evidence suggesting reduction of normal coarticulation during stutterers' sound repetitions. Spectrograms and electromyographic recordings were made from the upper lip of stutterers while reading a passage weighted with syllables revealing anticipatory coarticulation by labial movement (e.g., Europe, screw). The spectrograms showed less coarticulatory labial activity during repetitions than on stutterers' fluent utterances or normal speakers' utterances of the same words.

Other Studies

Another technique applied in the study of articulatory dynamics is the strain-gauge transducer, a device for converting mechanical movement into electrical signals. Hutchinson and Watkin (1976) used it to study the jaw movements of four stutterers at the terminations of blocks. In confirmation of clinical observations, they found that the articulatory movement was abnormally rapid at the moment of release from the stuttering block. In addition, in a number of instances the movement of the jaw was not coordinated with the onset of vocalization, sometimes preceding and sometimes lagging behind it.

Zimmermann (1980a) used x-ray motion picture photography to observe movements of the lower lip and jaw during stuttering in two subjects and of the tongue as well in two others. His main finding was that there is a repositioning of the articulators preceding the release of a stuttering block. This usually takes the form of a lowering of the jaw and lower lip and a reshaping of the tongue toward its resting position.

In summary, instrumented laboratory studies to date have served mainly to confirm a number of significant clinical impressions. During stuttering there is abnormal functioning of essentially the whole speech system including the larynx. A notable aspect of that abnormal functioning is excessive muscular tension. Judging from the way in which stuttering is reflected in elevations of intraoral breath pressure, at least part of that tension must result from efforts to force the outgoing breath stream past heightened resistance.

---

[9]Hutchinson and Watkin (1974), Freeman, Borden, and Dorman (cited by Freeman, 1979), Harrington (1987).

[10]Howell and Vause (1986), Howell, Williams, and Vause (1987), Howell and Williams (1988), Howell, Williams, and Young (1991), Howell and Williams (1992).

ASSOCIATED SYMPTOMS

There is more to stuttering than repetitions, prolongations, or pauses. We must include in our description any number of associated features, often referred to as "secondary" symptoms. The concomitant features of stuttering are many and extremely varied. Their precise specification is difficult since it depends to a large extent on what is meant by the essential or integral features of stuttering. The term *associated* may be applied to aspects, attributes, or correlates of speech blockages or to clearly independent behaviors. We will use the term broadly and somewhat loosely here to stand for 1) visible or audible reactions accompanying or interspersed among stutterers' speech interruptions, 2) visceral or physiological correlates of stuttering, and 3) changes in stutterers' perceptions of their environment and in their subjective states when experiencing difficulty with speech.

Overt Concomitants

The observable concomitants of stuttering consist of a number of different kinds of reactions, chief among them being movements and interjections.

Associated Movements

Stutterers often display visible tensions of the face or such movements as a jerk of the head. These reactions may be simple and brief or complicated and bizarre. Most often, the mannerisms accompanying stuttering involve parts of the speech mechanism or related structures. Among the most frequent are eye-blink, wrinkling of the forehead, and sudden exhaustion of breath. Also common are frowning, distortions of the mouth, quivering of the nostrils, and movements of the eyes, head, tongue, and muscles of respiration. It is difficult to catalog all of the acts or tensions that may become associated with stuttering; any part of the voluntary musculature of the body may participate, including that of the hands, arms, legs, feet, and torso. Although these concomitants are usually closely associated with a stuttering block, they may appear independently of any readily observable interruption in speech.

A systematic classification of these visible concomitants of stuttering was made by Prins and Lohr (1972) on the basis of a motion picture study. Riley (1972) devised a test of severity of stuttering in which ratings of such overt concomitants contribute to the total measure, along with frequency of stuttering and duration of the longest blocks.

Kraaimaat and Janssen (1985) and Janssen and Kraaimaat (1986) studied the temporal relationship of associated facial movements to the primary symptoms of stuttering. Jaw and mouth movements almost always occurred during moments of stuttering, while eye-blinking generally did not. Kraaimaat and Janssen speculated that jaw and mouth movements resulted from tension or struggle, whereas eyeblinks were avoidance reactions.

Interjected Speech Fragments

Interjections take the form of sounds, syllables, words, or phrases, and, like the associated movements, they usually, but, not necessarily, occur in immediate conjunction with observable stutterings. Typical examples are "um," "er," "well," "now," "you see." They tend to be superfluous, as in "I'm g—er, well you see, I'm going home now," and they may be inappropriate as well (e.g., "I live at—in other words—19 Cadwallader Place").

In a factor analysis of stuttering symptoms by Lewis (1991), inter-jections, word and phrase repetitions, and revisions separated them-selves from other features, a division that Lewis interpreted as one between stuttering and its avoidance.

Vocal Abnormalities

Stuttering is often accompanied by a variety of abnormal features of voice and speech. These may include rapid or slow rate, changes in vocal quality, odd inflections or sharp shifts in pitch level, and monot-one. Quarrington and Douglass (1960) commented provocatively on the habitual tendency of some stutterers to suspend phonation, apparently in order to avoid audibility while stuttering.

Phonatory disturbances in the speech of stutterers, especially a frequent lack of normal pitch variation, were demonstrated by photo-phonographic techniques in early studies by Travis (1927b), Bryngelson (1932), and Adams (1955), and were studied spectro-graphically and oscillographically by Schilling and Göler (1961), and Luchsinger and Dubois (1963). Other intonational deviations besides monotony were found by Stock (1966). Largely conflicting results were reported by Lechner (1979), however. She found that stutterers did not differ from nonstutterers in extent of pitch shifts and inflec-tions or in rate of inflectional variations during speech. They differed from nonstutterers only in having more downward and therefore total inflections. Schäfersküpper (1982) also found more falling inflec-tions in stutterers' conversational speech and fewer rising inflections. His subjects, 10- to 12-year-old children, accented the first word of a sentence more than twice as often as nonstutterers. Neither Adams (1955), Schmitt and Cooper (1978), nor Lechner (1979) observed any deviation in average pitch level or any unequivocal deviations in pitch range. A tendency toward higher pitch levels approaching statistical significance in 10- to 12-year-old stutterers' spontaneous speech was reported by Schäferskúpper and Simon (1983).

Skin Reactions

In severe stuttering, flushing, pallor, or perspiration may be visible as accompanying reactions.

The Meaning of the Overt Concomitants of Stuttering

Some stutterers seem to have few of the associated symptoms so far enumerated. Others have a great many and may exhibit them in highly individual combinations or patterns (Barr, 1940). They tend to be performed relatively automatically and unconsciously, particularly when they have persisted for some length of time. Most of them appear to be first adopted as devices for minimizing stuttering. In the effort to avoid or terminate blocks, the stutterer may discover by trial and error that blinking the eyes or taking a deep breath can be helpful expedients.

Since the effectiveness of such devices appears to lie in their ability to distract attention momentarily from the act of speaking, the eye-blink is no longer effective once it has lost its novelty, and the stutterer must then cast about for another contrivance. In this process, however, the outworn eye-blink often remains as a habitual part of the stuttering reaction. It appears to be in this way that the complex symptom patterns of some stutterers develop. In a study of such patterns Van Riper (1937a) found that in many cases most of the overt abnormality of stuttering consists of devices for concealing it.

Van Riper (1963) suggested a useful five-fold classification of such devices. The first category consists of symptoms of *avoidance*, by means of which feared words are evaded altogether. The most common examples are word substitution and circumlocution, which may become so awkward and extreme as to interfere with communication. A second category, symptoms of *postponement*, consists of maneuvers to delay the attempt on the feared word in the hope that the fear will subside sufficiently for the stutterer to say it normally. The speaker may pause strategically, repeat preceding words or phrases, or interject such expressions as "you see" or "well" in a pretense at thought. Third are symptoms of *starting*, tricks enabling the stutterer to say the feared word by making it easier to produce the difficult first sound. Adroitly timed grimaces or other associated movements may serve this purpose. A particularly common starter is an easy sound or syllable—for example "uh," prefixed to the feared word. Fourth are symptoms of *escape*. These embrace all of the stutterer's struggles to terminate the block. The person may attempt to "break" the block by means of a head-jerk, gasp, or interjection; exhaust all breath and finish the word on residual air; or "back up and get a running start" on the word. The fifth category, symptoms of *antiexpectancy*, includes expedients the stutterer uses for preventing the anticipation of difficulty from arising. For example, the person may speak in a rapid monotone so that no particular word stands out to be feared or may attempt to distract attention from fear of stuttering by the use of almost any other unnatural speech pattern.

Van Riper's classification of concealment devices anticipates later discussions by virtue of the role it assigns to expectancy in stuttering behavior. It is cited here, however, because it exposes with particular clarity a valid sense in which many of the overt symptoms of stuttering may be regarded as "secondary" to or overlaid upon certain essential or "primary" symptoms.

Physiological Concomitants

Stuttering is accompanied by a variety of covert, internal bodily phenomena which must be observed indirectly by the use of suitable instruments for physiological investigation.

Eye Movements

Unusual eye movements, associated mainly with the stuttering block, have been found during both the oral reading and spontaneous speech of stutterers (Jasper and Murray, 1932; Moser, 1938; Kopp, 1963). Some of the outstanding phenomena described are vertical "twitches" of the eyes, prolonged fixations, slow continuous or rapid "aimless" horizontal movements, and binocular incoordination exemplified by independent horizontal movements of the two eyes (temporary strabismus), or fixation of one eye and simultaneous vertical twitching of the other.

Cardiovascular Phenomena

During speech, and just prior to speech under conditions likely to produce stuttering, there is often an acceleration of the heart and pulse rate.[11] Robbins (1920) also observed changes in blood distribution associated with stuttering in a plethysmographic study of a single stutterer, and this has been confirmed by Kurshev (1968a) and Ickes and Pierce (1973) with groups of subjects. Such changes become

---

[11]Fletcher (1914), Travis, Tuttle, and Cowan (1936), Moore (1959), and Brunner and Frank (1975). See Golub (1953), however, for contradictory evidence.

overt in severe instances as the pallor and flushing referred to earlier. In two stutterers Wood et al (1980) found lower blood flow during stuttering in Broca's area in the left cerebral hemisphere than in the corresponding area of the right hemisphere.

Uenishi et al (1973) reported changes in maximum blood pressure in stutterers during speaking and reading. Curiously enough, however, Dabul and Perkins (1973) found that when systolic blood pressure had been elevated by electric shock stuttering served to decrease it.

Tremors

Herren (1932) found that normal hand tremors of a rate of 8 to 12 per second were depressed during stuttering. A more rapid type of hand tremor (40 to 75 per second) tended to become more pronounced. Movement was recorded by means of a photographic procedure designed by Travis.

Brain Waves

Although the findings of electroencephalographic research on stuttering are difficult to interpret, there appears to be evidence from studies by Travis and Knott (1936), Travis and Malamud (1937), and Freestone (1942) that alpha wave activity is intensified during the stuttering block. Fox (1966) found that stuttering produced more disruption in the regularity and interhemispheric synchronization of the waves than did nonstutterers' imitations of stuttering and thought it possible that this was due to a difference in emotional arousal. Sayles (1971), concerned with clinically abnormal wave patterns in stutterers, found a considerable number, but observed no tendency for the patterns to be related to moments of stuttering or speech activity in oral reading.

Of interest are some electroencephalographic findings of Boberg, Yeudall, Schopflocher, and Bo-Lassen (1983). During verbal tasks, normal speakers showed a suppression of alpha waves in the left cerebral hemisphere a phenomenon evidently related to the greater role of the left hemisphere in speech processing in most individuals. Boberg and his co-workers failed to observe the expected interhemispheric difference in stuttering subjects during speech tasks in which stuttering presumably took place. However, the normal alpha relationship appeared after a three-week program of therapy in which the subjects' stuttering was markedly reduced through the use of a slow speaking rate and easy vocal onsets.

Biochemical Changes

Moore (1959) reported that with increases in stuttering there was a decrease in blood sugar and total protein. Edgren, Leanderson, and Levi (1970) found a greater increase in urinary excretion of adrenaline in stutterers than in nonstutterers after a period of public speaking. Following a speech situation, Chmelová, Kujalová, Sedláčková, and Zelený (1975) observed a rise in adrenaline, noradrenaline, dopamine, and 5-hydroxyindolacetic acid.

Electrodermal Response

Berlinsky (1955) failed to find a consistent relationship between stuttering symptoms and electrical conductance of the skin (GSR). Kurshev (1969) studied GSR responses just prior to subjects' attempts on words and found them to occur in advance of stuttering in many instances. Brutten (1963), using a photometric technique to measure palmar sweating, found that this reaction decreased concomitantly with decreases in the amount of stuttering, but contradictory results were obtained in subsequent research (Gray and Brutten, 1965; Adams and Moore, 1972).

Other Reflex Activity

During the stuttering block there appears to be an inhibition of the eye-blink (Amirov, 1962), an augmentation of the Achilles and patellar reflexes (Travis and Fagan, 1928), and a change in the impedance of the middle ear (Shearer, 1966). Gardner (1937) also reported a greater dilation of the pupils among stutterers than among normal speakers during speech and increases in dilated diameter during stuttering. On the other hand, a contraction of the pupils at the onset of speech was noted by Luchsinger (1943). Stuttering has been found to be accompanied by abnormal solar and oculocardiac reflexes (Sedláček, 1948) and by increased monosynaptic spinal cord reflex activity (Lastovka, 1970, 1979a, 1979b). Langová, Morávek, Siroký, and Šváb (1975) reported an increase in the frequency and amplitude of the electronystagmographic response in stutterers during speech. In nystagmographic records of stutterers, Siroký, Langová, Morávek, and Šváb (1978) observed many saddle-formed nystagmic jerks which increased significantly during speech.

The Meaning of the Physiological Concomitants

Although many of the changes just described were originally believed to be clues to an underlying physiological etiology of stuttering, they are now widely regarded simply as inward aspects of the symptomatology. In the first place, these manifestations are confined to the moment of stuttering and to a brief period just prior to it. Generally speaking, they are not present when the stutterer is silent or appears to be speaking normally. Furthermore, there is little evidence to suggest that any of these symptoms is a universal concomitant of all stutterings. Some systematic checking of this last point was done by Strother (1937).

Finally, many of these same bodily changes have been observed to occur in normal speakers under conditions of excitement or tension, while others may be produced in normal speakers while responding in ways that simulate stuttering. For example, the deep tendon reflexes increase with effort. Ainsworth (1939) found breathing abnormalities similar to those of the stutterer in normal speakers while they were listening to stuttering. Williams (1955) showed that the abnormal action potentials of the jaw muscles that occur during stuttering can be produced in nonstutterers by instructing them to imitate stuttering or merely to perform certain movements of the jaw.

In short, as a result of laboratory studies over several decades, the physiological symptoms are now generally understood to be the visceral correlates of tension, exertion, or emotional arousal or to represent other indirect effects of stuttering or of some of its overt concomitants.[12] Some of these studies were focussed in whole or in part on the period immediately preceding the stuttering block. We will therefore have occasion to refer to them again in somewhat more detail when we take up the question of fear and anticipation in relation to stuttering.

Introspective Concomitants

The subjective evaluations the stutterer makes while experiencing speech interruptions are from certain points of view an exceedingly important part of the accompanying symptomatology of stuttering. These evaluations, as they are known to us for the most part through the introspections of older stutterers, are chiefly of three types: 1) a sense of being frustrated in the attempt to speak, 2) feelings of muscular tension, and 3) emotional or affective reactions.

Feelings of Frustration in the Effort to Speak

Stutterers in a block tend to experience the feeling of being physically halted in their attempt to speak. For a time they are literally unable, by any ordinary definition of that word, to move or to control

---

[12]Furthermore, the observations of Golub (1953) and McCroskey (1957) suggest that at least a few of these symptoms are to be found as accompaniments of speech in normal speakers and may therefore be "symptoms" of vocal expression rather than of stuttering.

their speech organs for the purpose of articulating the intended word. Those having a more detailed awareness of the experience may report that their lips involuntarily "come together hard," that their tongue "sticks" to the roof of their mouth, that their "throat closes tightly," and the like. It is noteworthy that stutterers generally appear to know precisely what word they want to say, but simply cannot say it.

This failure of the speech organs to do the speaker's bidding is often as baffling and disturbing to stutterers as an inexplicable spasm or paralysis might be. They can, however, interrupt the stuttering reaction at short notice to perform some other activity, such as a protrusion of the abdomen, as Van Riper (1938) has shown. In fact, they often appear to be able to interrupt the "spasm" to produce a fluent utterance of an alternative word.

Feelings of Muscular Tension

For most stutterers the act of blocking is associated with some feeling of strain or tension. This is usually localized in the speech musculature (i.e., the muscles of articulation, phonation, or respiration), but in some cases may also be felt elsewhere in the body—for example, the arms, legs, or shoulders. In a group of adult stutterers Snidecor (1955) found that tension was reported primarily in the jaws, the front of the mouth, the front of the throat, the chest, and the abdomen, with subsidiary foci often perceived in the inside or back of the throat and the front of the tongue.

Affective Reactions

These vary widely in intensity and are of several types, depending upon whether they occur before, during, or after the stuttering block.

Prior to the block there is often an apprehension of impending difficulty, varying in severity from mild uneasiness to extreme panic, which is well known as anticipation or expectancy. It is typically one of the most unpleasant aspects of the disorder for stutterers and often the one that interferes most with communication. Anticipation may also occur independently of blocks, and it is not unusual for stutterers to experience the repeated threat of stuttering even in situations in which they have little or no overt speech difficulty. Conversely, some blocks seemingly occur with little or no overt speech difficulty. Conversely, some blocks seemingly occur with little if any prior awareness of their imminence on the part of the stutterer. By and large, however, older stutterers are able to predict the occurrence of their blocks with striking accuracy. An assumption long shared by a considerable number of workers is that the prediction itself frequently serves to precipitate the stuttering block. From this point of view anticipation is among the phenomena lying at the heart of the stuttering problem. We will need to discuss this question in some detail in a later chapter.

During the stuttering block the affective reactions, especially in severe stuttering, tend to be reported predominantly as confusion or mental "blankness." In extreme cases stutterers may feel what they describe as a kind of momentary loss of "contact." Subjective reports such as these are illuminated by certain objective research findings. Herren (1931) found that voluntary movements of the hands (alternately flexing and extending the fingers about a rubber ball) tended to cease or become reduced in extent during stuttering blocks. Dewar, Dewar, and Anthony (1976) happened on the same phenomenon when they instructed stutterers to turn on a masking noise the moment they began to stutter; the stuttering caused delays in the operation of the hand-actuated device. Similarly, stutterers' finger-tapping rates appeared to be slowed down by stuttering in a study by Greiner, Fitzgerald, and Cooke (1986). In a related observation Ringel and Minifie (1966) demonstrated that stuttering tends to impair the ability to estimate the passage of time. Froeschels and Rieber (1963) reported that during the block stutterers gave evidence of a considerable inability to perceive auditory and visual stimuli—for example, the banging of a fist on a desk or the waving of a hand, as signals to stop speaking. This was not confirmed in studies by Perkins (1969) or Hugo (1972), however; it may be that auditory and visual imperceptivity is one of the more extreme symptoms of stuttering. Kamhi and McOsker (1982) found evidence that stuttering during oral reading of a passage may interfere with subjects' comprehension of the material read.

Following the block, affective reactions frequently verbalized by stutterers are frustration, exasperation, embarrassment, and feelings of anxiety about further stuttering. That there may also be some measure of relief or tension reduction immediately after a block was suggested by the results of a study by Wischner (1952a) in which subjects used projective drawings to depict their behavior before, during, and after the moment of stuttering. Using a similar method, Sheehan, Cortese, and Hadley (1962), on the other hand, found evidence of shame and guilt following stuttering. Bar and Jakab (1969) found both types of reactions, with relief more characteristic of the drawings done by adults than of those done by children.

"Real," Forced, and Faked Blocks

Frankly introspective studies of the stuttering block have rarely been done because of their obvious limitations, but a sidelight was thrown on this aspect of the problem in a study of stutterers' ability to throw themselves into blocks. Curious about Van Riper's observation that tense articulatory postures often seem to trigger involuntary tremors of the stutterer's jaw, tongue, or lips, Bloodstein and Shogan (1972) instructed subjects to try to force themselves into blocks by exerting articulatory pressure on the initial sounds of isolated words. After each attempt the subjects were asked whether the block they produced was real or fake and how they knew. Of twenty subjects all but three were able in at least a few instances to force themselves into what they regarded as real blocks. In general, however, articulatory pressure was not enough. In most cases they were able to do this only on a word that began with a difficult or feared sound or by "thinking" of the word as difficult. None had notable difficulty distinguishing real stuttering from faked or imitated blocks. The two essential features of real stuttering referred to repeatedly were its tension and its involuntary quality. The following are a few of the comments the subjects offered to explain how they knew when blocks were real: "It's like a rock inside." "I could have stopped the others at any time, but not this one." "There's tension and heaviness." "When it's real it's like being drunk or like having your foot on the gas with no control—you can't control the speech. If I control the word it has weight. If not, it's like a balloon."

Kelly and Conture (1988) could find nothing in the spectrographic record to differentiate stutterers' imitated from their actual stuttering. In a study by Moore and Perkins (1990), listeners were unable to distinguish a stutterer's real from her simulated stuttering with an accuracy much greater than chance. The stutterer herself was not much better at it when listening to the tape recording only an hour afterward.

THE "FLUENT" SPEECH OF STUTTERERS

Researchers have become increasingly concerned about the possible existence of abnormality in the intervals of speech that are presumed to be free from stuttering. The studies that have resulted have differed somewhat in their purposes as well as in some of their basic assumptions.

Is Stuttering Confined to Discrete Instances?

The first question raised was whether listeners could distinguish the recorded speech of stutterers from that of nonstutterers if all identifiable instances of disfluency were removed. Wendahl and Cole (1961) reported that they could and that listeners judged the stutterers' edited samples of oral reading to contain more force and strain and to be less normal in rate and rhythm than samples of nonstutterers' speech. In a replication of this study using a different type of analysis, however, Young (1964) found that listeners were not able to pick out the stutterers reliably. Young also pointed out that the outcome of such research must depend to a large degree on such factors as the severity of the stuttering of the subjects and the experimenter's definition of disfluency.

Subsequently Love and Jeffress (1971) used an electronic speech-pause counting device to study the occurrence of brief pauses in the oral reading of stutterers who were ostensibly fluent in reading aloud. The stutterers were discovered to have significantly more brief pauses in the 150- to 250-millisecond range than did a group of normal speakers, although a trained listener was unable to differentiate the stutterers from the nonstutterers.

Few and Lingwall (1972) obtained somewhat inconclusive results in a study of stutterers' 10-second spontaneous speech samples, all of which were judged to be fluent by three trained observers. There was a consistent tendency for the stutterers to be rated slower in speaking rate by listeners, to articulate more slowly in terms of number of phonemes per second, and to have more pause time than nonstutterers, but none of these differences reached statistical significance. Few and Lingwall also reported that listeners could not distinguish the stutterers' samples from those of the nonstutterers. Applying an alternative type of analysis of their data, however, Young (1984) showed that the listeners were able to make the differentiation to an extent exceeding chance.

Krikorian and Runyan (1983) used perceptually fluent samples of young children aged four to six years. They found that sophisticated judges did not correctly identify stutterers and nonstutterers often enough to rule out chance with confidence. Again, with young children aged 4 to 9 years, Colcord and Gregory (1987) found that listeners had considerable difficulty identifying stutterers from the children's perceptually fluent speech. By contrast, when the speech samples were produced by adolescents aged 12 to 16 years, judges discriminated well between stutterers and normal speakers in most cases (Brown and Colcord, 1987).

Phonation During "Fluency"

The first few efforts to examine the fluent speech of stutterers had been prompted by the question whether stuttering is confined to discrete "moments," as has commonly been assumed, or whether it is a broader abnormality in a person's way of speaking of which the discernible moments are only a part. In the mid-1970s a somewhat different reason arose for conducting such investigations. As we have seen, it became apparent that the laryngeal musculature functions abnormally during stuttering. Some workers believed that this abnormal functioning might be the immediate cause of the stuttering block, and they thought that this possibility could be verified by observing the activity of the stutterer's larynx during intervals of nonstuttered speech.

Raising the question whether the larynx is "responsible for the dysfluencies observed in stuttering," Gautheron, Liorzou, Even, and Vallancien (1973) studied samples of the conversational speech of four stutterers by glottography. They came to the conclusion that the stutterer does not use the larynx correctly even when not stuttering. In producing sequences such as "sha," in which a voiceless consonant is followed by a vowel, the subjects in many cases appeared to preset the laryngeal musculature with so much tension that phonation was possible only with strong airflow; consequently, the transition to the vowel was often delayed and initiated with a glottal catch.

Agnello (1975) reported that spectrograms of stutterers' fluent utterances of nonsense syllables such as /pa/ and /ap/ showed that stutterers tend to take longer than nonstutterers in both initiating and terminating phonation.[13] This observation was confirmed by Hillman and Gilbert (1977), who found that during what was perceived as fluent oral reading, stutterers' voice onset times following voiceless stop consonants were on the average 9 milliseconds longer than those of their controls.

Subsequent findings on stutterers' voice onsets during fluent speech have been conflicting. No differences between stutterers and nonstutterers were reported by Watson and Alfonso (1982), Borden, Baer, and Kenney (1985), Borden, Kim, and Spiegler (1987), and Jäncke (1994). Metz, Conture, and Caruso (1979), observing longer voice onset times for stutterers on about one-third of the sounds they studied, considered their findings equivocal. Healey and Gutkin (1984) studied subjects' fluent utterances of words and syllables beginning with stop consonants and found that stutterers had longer voice onset times than nonstutterers for voiced stops. Healey and Ramig (1986) found longer voice onset times for stutterers and reported as a major result of their study that the difference was greater for utterances extracted from a reading passage than for a short nonsense phrase. All of these observations were made on adults. Two studies of school-age subjects both produced negative findings (McKnight and Cullinan, 1987; De Nil and Brutten, 1991b). In preschool subjects, there have been positive findings by Seebach and Caruso (1979) and Adams (1987) and negative findings by Zebrowski, Conture, and Cudahy (1985) and Molt (1991).

---

[13]One offshoot of this finding—a long series of studies of voice initiation time—has involved stutterers saying words, nonsense syllables, or simple phonations such as /a/ as quickly as possible on signal. Almost without exception the findings have agreed that stutterers on the average have longer voice initiation times than nonstutterers, even when no stuttering is perceived. These investigations are reviewed in Chapter 4 in the discussion of stutterers' reaction times.

Stutterers' pitch levels have not been found to differ from non-stutterers' during fluent speech.[14] Healey (1982) reported a more limited range of pitch variation in stutterers' fluent production of sentences. In subsequent studies of pitch variation during fluency, however, Healey (1984), Healey and Gutkin (1984), and Sacco and Metz (1989) obtained largely negative results. Likewise, Ramig, Krieger, and Adams (1982) failed to find any difference between stutterers and nonstutterers in pitch variation or vocal intensity during fluent speech.

Newman, Harris, and Hilton (1989) observed more shimmer (cycle-to-cycle variations in amplitude) in stutterers than nonstutterers when subjects were instructed to sustain a vowel and they suggested that stutterers had "less stable neuromuscular control" of phonation. Hall and Yairi (1992) reported the same observation with regard to vowels selected from the spontaneous speech of preschool subjects.

In an electroglottographic study of preschool subjects, Conture, Rothenberg, and Molitar (1986) measured the proportion of the vibratory cycle in which the vocal folds were in contact during fluent utterances. During consonant-vowel and vowel-consonant transitions all eight stutterers, as compared with four of the eight nonstutterers, showed what the experimenters defined as atypical patterns of glottal activity. Electroglottographic observations by Peters and Boves (1988) showed abrupt voice onsets to occur more often in stutterers than controls in perceptually fluent utterances of single words.

By means of a transducer inserted in the trachea through the nose and glottis, Peters and Boves (1987, 1988) observed patterns of subglottal air pressure build-up during subjects' fluent utterances of single words. Stutterers more frequently exhibited disruptions in the smooth and continuous increase in pressure and more often began phonation at least 100 msec after pressure had reached a maximum. Peters and Boves interpreted these findings to mean that "covert stuttering" can occur in perceptually fluent speech.

Articulatory Rate and Coordination During Fluency

Various other abnormal characteristics have been observed in what is judged to be the fluent speech of stutterers, especially with regard to aspects of duration and rate. Di Simoni (1974) found longer durations of both consonants and vowels in nonsense words. Colcord and Adams (1979) found longer voicing durations in oral reading. Starkweather and Myers (1979) reported longer vowel-consonant-vowel segments in connected speech, the lengthening usually occur-

---

[14]Ramig, Krieger, and Adams (1982), Healey (1984), Healey and Gutkin (1984), Bergmann (1986), Hall and Yairi (1992).

ring in the transitional segments rather than the steady-state portions. On the other hand, during a study in which both school-age and adult subjects produced consecutive fluent utterances of the same sentences, Healey and Adams (1981) observed no consistent differences between stutterers and nonstutterers with respect to duration of consonants, vowels, pauses, or utterances. Healey and Adams speculated that the repetitions of the utterances may have had a "normalizing effect" on the stutterers' speech.

McMillan and Pindzola (1986) measured the duration of the first vowel in a vowel-consonant-vowel nonsense word embedded in a carrier phrase. Stutterers and subjects with articulation defects both produced longer steady-state portions of the vowel than control subjects. The stutterers also had shorter vowel-to-consonant transitions than the controls. (See also Pindzola, 1987.) In fluent utterances of "two" in a series of numbers, Borden, Kim, and Spiegler (1987) found that the stop gap and vowel durations of severe stutterers were longer than those of controls. Jäncke (1994) had subjects continuously repeat a three-syllable nonsense word. Stutterers did not differ from normal speakers in the duration of the first vowel, but had more intrasubject variability.

Similar studies of younger subjects have yielded more equivocal results. Reimann (1976) found shorter vowels in the speech of 3 adolescent stutterers than in that of 3 normal speakers. Neither Winkler and Ramig (1986) nor McKnight and Cullinan (1987) found differences in vowel or consonant durations of school-age stutterers and nonstutterers. Adams (1987) recorded longer vowel and consonant durations of preschool stutterers and interpreted these lags as "inherent features of their speech-timing control." This was in sharp contrast to the findings of Zebrowski, Conture, and Cudahy (1985), who found no differences between 3-to-6-year-old stutterers and nonstutterers in either vowel and consonant duration or duration of transitions between sounds in fluent utterances.

In keeping with most of the reports on the duration of the stutterer's speech sounds has been the repeated finding that stutterers tend to have slower rates of fluent speech. In an early study Bloodstein (1944) found that stutterers had a slower average rate of oral reading in words per minute even when the total duration of observed stuttering was subtracted from the total reading time. Slower rates of fluent utterances have been reported in a series of more recent studies of adult stutterers.[15] Meyers and Freeman (1985c)

---

[15]Adams, Runyan, and Mallard (1975), Ramig, Krieger, and Adams (1982), Borden (1983), Schäfersküpper and Dames (1987), Bosshardt and Nandyal (1988), Van Lieshout, Hulstijn, and Peters (1991). In conflict was a report by Gronhovd (1977). Pindzola (1986) found no difference between stutterers and nonstutterers in the velocity of transitions from vowel to consonant and consonant to vowel in nonsense words.

found slower rates of fluent speech in preschool stutterers. In addition, considerable evidence of articulatory slowness in stutterers has come from a computer analysis of a cinefluorographic film of movements of the lip and jaw of six stutterers and seven normal speakers by Zimmerman (1980b). In what were judged to be fluent utterances of the syllables /bab/, /pap/, and /mam/, the stutterers had longer transitions, longer steady state positions, longer time intervals between the onset and peak velocity of movement, and longer latency of onset of movement. Zimmermann also found less coordination between lip and jaw movements in the case of the stutterers.

At variance with these findings were the results of an investigation by Caruso, Abbs, and Gracco (1988). In fluent productions of the utterance "sapapple," they found that stutterers were not deficient in the range and velocities of lip and jaw movements. Instead, the stutterers deviated from the usual order of onset of speech movements: upper lip, then lower lip, then jaw. This sequence was followed by all of the 6 control subjects, but only 1 of the 6 stutterers. McClean, Kroll, and Loftus (1990) reported a further replication of this study with the addition of a group of stutterers who had recently undergone speech therapy, chiefly of the rate reduction kind. This group exhibited abnormal movement durations. There was little difference between the other stutterers and the normal speakers. As for the sequence of activation of the lips and jaw, 7 of the 10 no-therapy stutterers used the supposedly normal sequence and 4 of the 10 nonstutterers did not. In a later analysis of their results, McClean, Kroll, and Loftus (1991) found that the more severe stutterers had a slower lip closure on the first "p" in "sapapple."

Further Studies

The subject of the stutterer's speech during perceptually fluent intervals has lent itself to an almost endless variety of further investigative approaches, as the following will show.

In an early study Shaffer (1940) found that the interval between initiation of jaw movement and phonation was longer for stutterers than for nonstutterers. On the other hand, in fluent utterances of single words, Janssen, Wieneke, and Vaane (1983) found that the time interval between voice onset and electromyographic activity in the articulatory muscles was the same for stutterers and nonstutterers.

Klich and May (1982) reported that formant frequencies were more centralized in the spectrograms of stutterers' vowels than in those of nonstutterers and interpreted the finding to mean that stutterers "use restricted articulatory adjustments to control their speech." Prosek, Montgomery, Walden, and Hawkins (1987) failed to find any greater vowel centralization in stutterers' than nonstutterers' fluent speech, but they observed a trend for the second formant frequencies of stutterers' front vowels to be lower than those of nonstutterers.

In the supraglottal musculatures of stutterers during "acoustically fluent" utterances of words, Shapiro (1980) observed the same abnormally high levels of electromyographic activity usually present in the recordings of stuttered words. (See Figure 3.)

Wingate (1982) noted that whereas amplitude tracings of normal speakers' stress patterns showed distinct peaks corresponding to stressed syllables, in stutterers' fluent speech the stressed syllables were less clearly identifiable.

Metz, Samar, and Sacco (1983) found a significant positive relationship between frequency of a subject's stuttering and the amount of silence in the voiced stop consonant intervocalic interval during fluent speech. In a later study Samar, Metz, and Sacco (1986) found a positive correlation between release of the consonant and peak air flow.

Janssen, Wieneke, and Vaane (1983) found that in successive fluent repetitions of a word, the durations of the stutterers' words varied more than those of nonstutterers. The same within-subject variability was found with regard to repeated sentences by Janssen and Wieneke (1987) and Wieneke and Janssen (1987, 1991). Cooper and Allen (1977) found

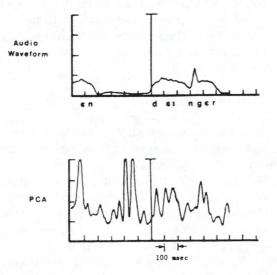

Figure 3. Abnormal abductor (posterior cricoarytenoid muscle) activity before and during a perceptually fluent utterance. Because the word "danger" is voiced throughout, there should be no abductor activity. Reproduced by permission of the publisher from "An electromyographic analysis of the fluent and dysfluent utterances of several types of stutterers," by Arnold Shapiro, *Journal of Fluency Disorders*, 5, 203–231. Copyright 1980 by Elsevier Science Publishing Co., Inc.

stutterers more irregular than nonstutterers in the duration of repeated fluent utterances of the same sentence, paragraph, or nursery rhyme.

In a study by Guitar, Guitar, Nelson, O'Dwyer, and Andrews (1988), stutterers repeated the words "peek," "puck," and "pack" until their utterances were fluent. Activation of two lips muscles for the initial "p" was studied. In 50 percent of the fluent utterances the depressor labii inferior was activated before the depressor anguli oris. This was the reverse of the nonstutterers' pattern, but was similar to 82 percent of the stuttered utterances.

Molt (1991) found that the timing of velopharyngeal movement for nasal consonant production in the fluent speech of 5 stutterers aged 5 to 6 years was very similar to that of 5 nonstuttering children.

Van Lieshout, Peters, Starkweather, and Hulstijn (1993) recorded electromyographic potentials during lip rounding for Dutch /o/ in initial position in stutterers' fluent syllables, words, and sentences. The stutterers had higher levels of activity than their controls and a longer delay between the beginning of electromyographic rise and the onset of speech.

Normal speech presents certain regulatories in the timing of articulatory events. (For example, the latency of onset of the stop consonant in a vowel-consonant-vowel sequence is always a constant fraction of the interval between the onset of the two vowels.) Prosek, Montgomery, and Walden (1988) studied four such ratios in the fluent reading of 15 stutterers and found them comparable to those of 15 normal speakers.

Howell and Wingfield (1990) extracted perceptually fluent segments from the speech of stutterers. They found that listeners could reliably distinguish segments that were adjacent to stuttered words from those that were not. Spectrographic examination showed a decrease in rate and intensity in segments judged to be near stutterings.

Conture, Colton, and Gleason (1988) recorded the onsets, offsets, and durations of activity of the rib cage, abdomen, larynx, and lips during utterances of words by preschool subjects. They concluded that there was no appreciable difference between the speech coordinations of stutterers and nonstutterers during fluent speech.

In a study by Viswanath (1989, 1991), stutterers read a passage aloud 5 times. Analysis showed that words stuttered in the first reading were significantly lengthened when they were uttered without perceptible stuttering in subsequent readings. Viswanath also observed a lengthening of words preceding stutterings and a lengthening of the last word in a clause preceding one in which stuttering occurred.

Summary Remarks

In summary, the weight of evidence strongly suggests that what observers consider to be the fluent speech of stutterers frequently reveals features on careful study that are not to be found, at least in the same degree, in the speech of nonstutterers. Although the precise extent of these differences is not yet fully clear, most of them appear to entail aspects of slowness or limitation of movement, lateness of response, or incoordination of the vocal apparatus. Many of the abnormal features of stutterers' "fluency" appear to bear a broad resemblance to those of overt stuttering. And there are hints in the literature we have cited that these disturbances may be more likely to occur in the near vicinity of overt stuttering than when subjects are free from any tendency to stutter.

What these observations mean involves difficulties of interpretation not often recognized. If we discover that stutterers exhibit a mismanagement of their speech during what we take to be intervals of fluency, one possible inference is that this mismanagement is a reason why they stutter. An alternative interpretation is that it reflects the reduced spontaneity and excessive caution of a person who expects to have difficulty with speech. The abnormalities in the stutterer's fluent speech, then, may be a cause or a result of the stuttering. There is, however, yet another possibility. It would be just as reasonable to conclude that we were mistaken about the fluency. What appeared to us to be fluent intervals of speech may perhaps have contained instances of stuttering so minimal that we only perceive them, with the aid of refined techniques of measurement, as subtle forms of slowness, incoordination, and the like. It is not, after all, so farfetched to suppose that, just as identifiable stutterings may range from very severe to extremely mild, the mild ones may merge by fine degrees with many more that are imperceptible. This view was aptly expressed by Adams and Runyan (1981) when they suggested that stuttering and fluency are "events along a continuum, so that as speech flows forward there is a drift, sometimes gradual, sometimes rapid, toward stuttering."

We have not yet arrived at the main difficulty, however. At first glance the question of whether such imperceptible disfluencies as brief pauses or delayed voice onsets are stuttering may seem to be a sensible question. But further reflection will show that there are no logically imaginable observations that will serve to answer it. Observation will reveal only that the delayed voice onsets and other deviations are there. What we ought to call them is only a question of definition of terms. We can define stuttering in any way that we agree on, but the question of whether anything is "really" stuttering or "really" fluency is unanswerable. Who is to say that slowness, uncoordination, and brief pauses are not stuttering, whether they result from anticipation of difficulty in speaking, from neurological impairment, or from anything else? We must conclude that many of the questions raised about the so-called fluent speech of stutterers are not meaningful questions. There are, however, certain meaningful questions we can ask about the *nonspeech* activities of the stutterer's vocal organs which relate to the issue of whether some of the abnormalities we have been discussing are symptoms or causes of stuttering. We will consider these questions in Chapter 4.

ATTITUDES AND ADAPTATIONS

In addition to what is ordinarily considered stuttering behavior, there is a pattern of attitudes, assumptions, and habitual methods of attempting to cope with stuttering that tends to characterize the disorder in its fully developed forms. These aspects are advantageously considered in connection with symptomatology since they often constitute a major part of the problem of stuttering.

At the most basic level are the attitudes that stuttering is shameful, that speech is unpleasant and threatening, and that people who stutter are for some unaccountable reason innately unable to speak in any other way. From these primary beliefs there is likely to develop in time a systematic and detailed ideology. Specific words, sounds, and speaking situations may become "difficult" and eventually feared. Listeners may be perceived as critical, impatient, embarrassed, pitying, or amused to a degree that often seems to distort reality. The conviction of basic inability to speak normally may become elaborated in subtle ways until it amounts to what Williams (1957) referred to as stutterers' magical belief in a "something" inside that strives to prevent them from speaking. An increasingly rigid self-concept as a stutterer—first, last, and always—may be reinforced by an equally unrealistic concept of nonstutterers as people who are almost totally without speech hesitancy or anxiety.

Motivated by attitudes such as these, stutterers tend to acquire a variety of exaggerated and inefficient adaptations to their problem. They are likely to form the habit of avoiding difficult words by using synonyms or circumlocutions, and some become extremely adept at this. They may anticipate difficult speech situations long in advance, may frequently avoid feared situations, and, in general, may severely restrict their verbal output and the range of their social relationships. Some stutterers attempt to avoid stuttering through behavior contrived to inhibit expectancy, as Van Riper (1963) pointed out—for example, by artificiality of manner, bravado, or clowning. Still other adaptations stem from a desire to alleviate what stutterers see as the social penalty for stuttering. For example, they may habitually avoid eye contact with the listener, avoid mentioning their stuttering or discussing it with others, or attempt to compensate for speech inadequacy by maladjustive efforts to gain approval in other ways.

Research on the Reactive Aspects of Stuttering

Although much of our knowledge of the reactive aspects of the problem is derived from clinical experience, an increasing amount of research has been devoted to the subject. In early studies Johnson (1932, 1934a, 1934b) and Kimmell (1938) found evidence that college stutterers' attitudes toward stuttering tended to influence their personal, social, heterosexual, home, and school behavior and adjustment and even their choice of a vocation. Knott (1935) investigated stutterers' ratings of the unpleasantness of their stuttering experiences. A study by Frasier (1955) was concerned in part with certain of the assumptions held by stutterers about the nature of their stuttering and the factors that cause their difficulty to come and go. Bloodstein and Bloodstein (1955) and Wingate and Hamre (1967) reported data on stutterers' conflicting interpretations of listeners' facial reactions. Nutall and Scheidel (1965) showed that stutterers frequently fail to appreciate the extent to which the nonstutterer, as well as the stutterer, may experience anxiety in speaking situations.

In more recent years investigators have continued to find evidence of stutterers' reactions to stuttering in unusual and varied ways. Yovetich, Booth, and Tyler (1977) gave stutterers the task of uttering a continuous reproduction of speech heard at one ear while hearing a competing message at the other ear. When the competing message contained stuttering, the subjects made more errors than nonstutterers, though they were more accurate than their controls when the competing message was fluent. Brutten and Janssen (1979) studied the eye movements of stutterers during the silent reading of a passage they were about to read aloud. The stutterers exhibited more regressions and long forward jumps than nonstutterers, evidently related to the habit of looking ahead in search of danger.

Leith and Mims (1975) found that white stutterers generally tended to have overt speech repetitions and prolongations, while black stutterers were more likely to have few of these features and more devices for avoiding, terminating, or concealing them. Leith and Mims related this finding to a difference between the groups in the social stigma they attached to stuttering. In a survey of the experiences of male and female stutterers by Silverman and Zimmer (1982), most subjects reported that they took little part in classroom activities, tended to avoid speaking privately with instructors, took jobs for which they were overqualified, and expected limited vocational success. There was some evidence of a tendency for stuttering to be a more serious problem for males. Manning, Dailey, and Wallace (1984) investigated the attitudes of older stutterers, chiefly members of self-help groups, between 52 and 82 years of age. Most perceived their speech difficulty to be less severe and handicapping than it had been in early childhood, although their performance on tests of attitude did not differ from that of younger subjects. Leith and Timmons (1983) reported a study concerned specifically with stutterers' attitudes toward use of the telephone. The earliest age at which negative reactions to the telephone was recalled was approximately ten.

Martens and Engel (1986) obtained objective evidence that many stutterers avoid words beginning with certain sounds. In a questionnaire study, Hohmeier (1987) gathered information about the problems that stuttering created for subjects in their vocations. Black (1987) was concerned with subjects' perceptions of the barriers that stuttering created to the enjoyment of leisure activities. Craig (1990) showed that stutterers' self-reported anxiety during a phone call to a stranger was greater than that of nonstutterers. Resnick and Tureen (1990) found that stutterers rated their stuttering more severe than did a group of unsophisticated listeners.

Nonverbal Behavior in Dyadic Communication

Krause (1978, 1982) conducted a unique study of the nonverbal behavior of stutterers filmed in conversation with normal-speaking partners, a group of normal-speaking dyads serving as a control. He reported several thought-provoking findings. Whereas the normal-speaking dyads shared the floor equally, the stutterers used more floor time than their partners; this was also true of a subgroup of some ten subjects who were judged by observers not to have stuttered on the film. The stutterers displayed relatively little of the "back-channel" behavior (smiling, nodding, and the like) so usual in nonstutterers while being spoken to. In general, the stutterers tended to keep their faces immobile. Compared with the nonstutterer dyads, the stutterers and their partners exhibited fewer of the simultaneous utterances that frequently occur in ordinary conversation. There were also fewer of the turn-taking speaker switches that tend to accompany simultaneous interruptive speech. While these observations may be open to various interpretations, they clearly point to a disruption of the spontaneous interactive behavior that characterizes a normal conversational relationship.

Jensen, Markel, and Beverung (1986) also found some evidence of aberrant turn-taking behavior on the part of stutterers involving eye contact, body movement, and latency of response.

Reactions of Children

Some special attention has been given to the reactive aspects of stuttering in children, chiefly of school age. In a study of grade school stutterers' oral recitation problems, Knudsen (1939) found that about half of their group had attempted to avoid stuttering by giving the wrong answer or saying "I don't know" in response to questions in the classroom and that some had played truant in order to avoid recitation. Furthermore, large numbers believed they had concealed their stuttering from some of their teachers by remaining in the background. More recently Pukacová (1974) found similar evidence of social speech fears in children. Silverman (1976a) found that by the time stutterers reached grades 4 to 6 they tended to speak fewer words than nonstutterers when asked to tell a story. Silverman and Williams (1973) observed that stuttering children stopped to correct only half the number of oral reading errors that normal speakers did, although the number of errors was about the same for the two groups. Similar findings were reported by Janssen, Kraaimaat, and van der Meulen (1983). Although unclear, the reason may reflect anxiety about stuttering or the diffident behavior of a reader who has no pretensions about doing well and is bent on completing the task as inconspicuously as possible. In a study of the eye movements of schoolchildren during silent reading, Brutten, Bakker, Janssen, and van der Meulen (1984) noted that stutterers had more fixations and regressions. They related the observation to "searching and sorting" arising from concern about words and sounds. In a comparison of stutterers and nonstutterers aged 7 to 14 years, De Nil and Brutten (1991a) found more negative attitudes toward speech among the stutterers at all ages.

The reactions of schoolchildren to their stuttering should not be exaggerated, however. Many of them, and some adults as well, do not seem to be highly concerned. Silverman (1970a) asked a group of stuttering children to make three wishes. Of sixty-two children in grades 2 to 5 only four made wishes that had anything to do with speech, and of these one wished that he could go on with speech class as long as he lived. These observations were corroborated by Culatta, Bader, McCaslin, and Thomason (1985). Woods (1974) discovered that while grade school stutterers tended to rate themselves as relatively poor speakers, this had little effect on their own estimation of their social position among their classmates. Bloodstein (1960a) and McLelland and Cooper (1978) found that, as might be expected, there appears to be an increase with age in reactive features in stuttering such as word substitutions, avoidance of speaking, self-perception as a stutterer, and communication fear.

Reactions of Listeners

Since the attitudes and adaptations of stutterers must be due in large measure to the reactions which they receive from others, it is relevant that a good amount of research has been done on the behavior of people listening to stuttered speech, on prevalent attitudes toward stutterers, and on the effect of stuttering on listeners' perception of a message.[16] For the most part, negative stereotypes of stutterers as nervous, fearful, and insecure have been found to be common. Krause (1978, 1982) noted that listeners tend to increase their head-nodding behavior in conversation with stutterers, engage in more "compulsive" smiling, and as a correlate of this behavior use fewer words expressing anger than when speaking with nonstutterers.

Measuring the Reactive Aspects

Inasmuch as speech therapy for the stutterer has often been concerned in part with the removal of unfavorable attitudes and reactions, there has been some interest in the development of devices for their identification and measurement.

Attitude Scales and Rating Sheets

The measuring devices have consisted chiefly of self-administered scales for the rating of attitudes or reactions to stuttering and speaking situations. Initially, some use was made of the Knower Speech Attitude Scale and the Knower Speech Experience Inventory,[17] neither of them designed specifically for administration to persons with speech impairments. These tests were employed in research on stutterers by Brown and Hull (1942), who found that their subjects were less "confident and enthusiastic in their use of speech" than nonstutterers and had made less use of speech in social situations. Naylor (1953) used the Knower tests for studying the relationship between stutterers' attitudes toward speech and various measures of severity of stuttering.

Of several early attempts to devise a specific measure of attitudes concerning stuttering the only one to come into significant use was the Iowa Scale of Attitude Toward Stuttering devised by Ammons and Johnson (1944). This Likert-type scale consists of a series of state-

---

[16]Rosenberg and Curtiss (1944), McDonald and Frick (1954), Yairi and Williams (1970), Woods and Williams (1971, 1976), Woods (1974), Duffy, Hunt, and Giolas (1975), Andrews and Smith (1976), Hulit (1976), Krause (1978), Phillips and Myers (1978), Turnbaugh, Guitar, and Hoffman (1979), Crowe and Walton (1981), Maxwell (1981), Turnbaugh, Guitar, and Hoffman (1981), Ragsdale and Ashby (1982), Silverman (1982), Hurst, M. A. and Cooper (1983), Hurst, M. I. and Cooper (1984), Tatchell, van den Berg, and Lerman (1983), Cyprus, Hezel, Rossi, and Adams (1984), White and Collins (1984), McKinnon, Hess, and Landry (1986). Burley and Rinaldi (1986), Well and Terrell (1986), Yeakle and Cooper (1986), Horsely and FitzGibbon (1987), Kalinowski, Lerman, and Watt (1987), Atkins (1988), Lass, Ruscello, and Pannbacker (1989), Collins and Blood (1990), Ham (1990a), Ham (1990c), Silverman (1990), Silverman and Paynter (1990), Patterson and Pring (1991), Bebout and Bradford (1992), Doody, Kalinowski, Armson, and Stuart (1993).

[17]See Knower (1938).

ments (e.g., "A stutterer should not plan to be a lawyer") with which the subject may indicate "moderate" or "strong" agreement or disagreement. A defect of many attitude inventories is that the approved or desirable choices are so obvious, but Robey (1976) found that scores on the Iowa Scale of Attitude were not correlated with measures of a response set toward acquiescent or socially desirable behavior.

Shumak (1955) reported normative data on a scale for measuring stutterers' reactions to speech situations, originally prepared for clinical use by Johnson in 1943.[18] The test consists of a list of forty common speech situations each of which the stutterer rates on a five-point scale with respect to 1) tendency to avoid the situation, 2) enjoyment of dislike of the situation, 3) the severity of stuttering in the situation, and 4) the frequency with which the situation is encountered. Further data on both stutterers and nonstutterers were obtained with this scale by Trotter and Bergmann (1957).

Lanyon (1967) described the construction of the Stuttering Severity Scale, a self-report inventory consisting of sixty-four true-false items for measuring the severity of stuttering, including behaviors such as avoidance, effort, and breathing difficulty as well as attitudes of worry, dissatisfaction, sensitivity, and the like. A factor analysis of stutterers' responses to the scale by Lanyon, Goldsworthy, and Lanyon (1978) showed that the behavioral and attitudinal items represented two distinct dimensions.

Woolf (1967) devised the Perceptions of Stuttering Inventory consisting of 60 items representing struggle, avoidance, or expectancy. Stutterers judge whether the item is characteristic of their stuttering. Examples are: Running out of breath while speaking, Making your voice louder or softer when stuttering is expected, Avoiding asking for information. St. Louis and Atkins (1988) administered the inventory to normal speaking college students in order to gather comparison data for use with stutterers.

Erickson (1969) contributed an empirically derived S-scale for assessing the attitudes of stutterers toward verbal communication. Constructed with attention to factors of reliability and validity, the scale consists of thirty-nine true-false items that were found to differentiate stutterers from nonstutterers—for example, "I usually feel that I am making a favorable impression when I talk," and "I dislike introducing one person to another." To facilitate comparison with nonstutterers' attitudes, the items make no mention of stuttering. Andrews and Cutler (1974) suggested a revision of the scale which they found to be more valid and reliable in repeated administrations to stutterers

---

[18]Shumak's speech situation rating sheet for stutterers is reproduced, with instructions for its use and interpretation, in Darley and Spriestersbach (1978, Chap. 10).

undergoing speech therapy. Quesal and Shank (1978) found that while persons with voice or articulation difficulties tended to have poorer communication attitudes as measured by the Erickson scale, stutterers' attitudes were poorer still. In a study by Cox, Seider, and Kidd (1984), stutterers scored lower than recovered stutterers, non-stuttering relatives, and controls. E.-M. Silverman (1980) reported that a group of women who stuttered exhibited poorer attitudes on the Erickson scale than women who did not, but that they showed signifi-cantly more favorable attitudes than a group of male stutterers. An item analysis of the scale was reported by Jehle, Kühn, and Renner (1989), who administered it to a group of German stutterers and non-stutterers. Members of a national stutterers' self-help organization (the National Stuttering Project) showed poorer speech attitudes than nonstutterers on the Erickson scale, but active members had more favorable scores than inactive ones (Miller and Watson, 1992).

The Stuttering Problem Profile of F. H. Silverman (1980b) aims to identify behaviors to be modified and is based on the statements of 108 stutterers who were asked to tell how their problem had improved in therapy. The instructions ask stutterers to identify those statements that they would like to be able to make at the end of treat-ment. Sample items are: I no longer have a great deal of difficulty speaking in school, I am usually willing to use the phone, I don't usu-ally feel a great deal of tension and panic before speaking.

Brutten (1975) and Brutten and Janssen (1981) reported on the use of a Speech Situation Checklist consisting of fifty-one situations that subjects rate on a five-point scale for the amount of anxiety experi-enced in them. A shortened version was developed by Hanson, Gronhovd, and Rice (1981).

On a Self-Efficacy Scale for Adult Stutterers devised by Ornstein and Manning (1985), subjects rate each of 50 situations both for the confidence that they would enter and the confidence that they would maintain a level of fluency in the situation.

An Inventory of Communications Attitudes for adult stutterers was developed by Watson (1987, 1988) and Watson, Gregory, and Kistler (1987). Subjects rate 39 situations with respect to their enjoyment of the situation, their speech skills in the situation, how they believe others feel in the situation, their perception of other people's speech skills in the sit-uation, and how frequently they meet the situation.

Guitar and Grims (1979) reported preliminary work on a ques-tionnaire on communication attitudes for children. Five stutterers, aged 5 to 10 years, did not differ from their controls on this scale in a study by Devore, Nandur, and Manning. Brutten's Communication Attitude Test for children did elicit unfavorable attitudes when administered to 6-to-14-year old stutterers in both English and Dutch versions (De Nil and Brutten, 1986; Brutten and Dunham, 1989; Vanryckeghem and Brutten, 1992).

Speaking-Time Log

The amount of time stutterers spend in speaking may frequently be taken as a basic measure of the extent to which the speech difficulty is handicapping. For clinical purposes, therefore, Johnson suggested the use of a personal log, kept by stutterers for varying periods of time to record each situation in which they spoke, together with an estimate of the time in which they spoke. Detailed suggestions for the use of such a log were given by Darley and Spriestersbach (1978, Chap. 9). Trotter and Brown (1958) made use of this technique to demonstrate that there were often considerable increases in stutterers' verbal output after a period of therapy.

Measures of Anxiety

There has been some interest in the objective measurement of speech-related anxiety under varying conditions. Brutten (1959) developed a useful photometric technique for measuring the palmar sweat response for this purpose and applied it in a number of research investigations on stuttering (Brutten, 1963; Gray and Brutten, 1965). Haywood (1963) showed that this method is apparently more sensitive to speech-related anxiety than are measures of heart rate or pulse pressure. Using a very different kind of approach, Lerman and Shames (1965) attempted to measure stutterers' level of anxiety in relation to a given speech situation by analyzing certain aspects of their language content as they talked about the situation.

DEVELOPMENTAL CHANGES IN STUTTERING

In our discussion so far we have been concerned chiefly with the features of stuttering as a fully developed disorder. Many of these features, however, appear to be acquired through a process of development that typically begins in early childhood, and stuttering in its earliest forms therefore tends to differ in certain respects from stuttering as we find it in older children and adults. Comprehensive studies of the development of all of the various features of stuttering are almost nonexistent. The information presented here is taken mainly from a report by Bloodstein (1960a) based on the author's clinical examination of 418 stutterers aged 2 to 16 years at the Brooklyn College Speech and Hearing Center from 1950 to 1956 (see Table 2).

Table 2. Percentage of Subjects Exhibiting Each of Various Features
of Stuttering Behavior at Age Levels from Two to Sixteen*

	Age Level						
	2-3 N=30 %	4-5 N=74 %	6-7 N=79 %	8-9 N=60 %	10-11 N=79 %	12-13 N=47 %	14-15-16 N=49 %
Slow, easy repetitions	30	34	28	37	30	9	8
Easy repetition or prolongation as sole symptoms of stuttering	43	32	18	18	11	4	4
Hard contacts	40	32	44	45	53	51	53
Associated symptoms	33	39	57	58	57	64	65
Fluent periods	47	45	27	10	10	9	00
Difficult situations			27 (15)	67 (27)	71 (56)	75 (40)	72 (39)
Difficult words or sounds				82 (17)	62 (45)	72 (32)	73 (33)
Anticipation				38 (26)	45 (51)	62 (37)	71 (41)
Word substitution				48 (23)	65 (48)	66 (32)	83 (36)
Avoidance of speech	0	5	11	17	28	40	45

*Numbers in parentheses indicate the number of subjects on which the percentage was based where this differs from the total number (N) in the age group. From Bloodstein (1960a). Copyright 1960 by the American Speech-Language-Hearing Association. Reprinted by permission.

Repetitions and Prolongations

As might be expected, repetitions and prolongations were observed at every age level. Before the age of 6 or 7 years, repetitions were a conspicuous feature of the child's stuttering and often involved whole words such as *he, I, but, and, in,* or *so.* Table 2 shows a steady decline in easy repetitions and prolongations as the sole symptoms of stuttering, but even at ages 2 and 3 years they were the sole symptom in only 43 percent of the cases. Even at that early age, repetitions of words or sounds were by no means always slow and easy, and were often accompanied by additional features.

Hard Contacts

Tense and forceful attacks on words or syllables were very commonly observed during the interview at every age level. Table 2 shows only a slight tendency for these struggle reactions to increase with age. A striking fact was that they appeared in the Brooklyn group at the earliest ages. Of the nine 2-year-olds in the group, 5 exhibited signs of effort and strain and one had been observed to do so by the mother. To be sure, these may not have been typical cases; 2-year-olds are perhaps not likely to be taken to a speech clinic unless their stuttering is severe. They are, however, representative of what may be found in a clinical setting.

Although the child's stuttering was most often said to have begun with repetitions, in some instances the earliest symptoms were described as strenuous forcings. This was true in 8 instances among 34 cases of children aged 2, 3, and 4 years in which parents gave "seemingly unequivocal descriptions . . . of the symptoms at onset." The records contained such reports as "Onset a few weeks ago. Forcing from the start. Mother is certain of that," or "Child taken for injection a month ago. Was very frightened. The next day he began to stutter with forcing, eye-blink, fist-clenching." Similar reports of severe stuttering at "onset" have been cited by Yairi and Ambrose (1992b).

Associated Symptoms

As shown in Table 2, the Brooklyn children who were observed to show the concomitant features of stuttering during the clinical interview rose steadily from 33 percent at ages 2 and 3 years to 65 percent at ages 14 to 16 years. The large percentage at the earliest age level is notable, even more so considering that stutterers may not exhibit secondary symptoms on all occasions.

> Among the symptoms noted in some cases at age two and three were eye blinking, head jerking, violent gasping, clenching of the fists, exaggerated pausing, and "doubling up" of the body. The great majority of the secondary symptoms commonly seen in adults were to be observed in these subjects by age five (Bloodstein, 1960a).

Tensions of the respiratory muscles (gasping or rapid expulsions of breath) were observed in 13 percent of the 2- and 3-year-olds. Yairi, Ambrose, and Niermann (1993) noted frequent facial and head movements in the same age range. Schwartz, Zebrowski, and Conture (1990) observed associated symptoms (especially opening, closing, and movements of the eyes) in each of 10 children within 12 months of reported onset of stuttering. Conture and Kelly (1991) recorded facial, hand, arm, and head movements during the stuttering of thirty 3- to 7-year-olds.

Occurring as they do at all stages in the development of stuttering, associated symptoms may appear in conjunction with virtually any other feature of the problem. In the Brooklyn group they sometimes accompanied the relatively simple repetitions of syllables or whole words of the youngest children. In many cases conspicuous secondary mannerisms were observed in the speech of children who were highly communicative and showed no outward sign of fear or shame because of their stuttering.

> A typical example was a boy of eleven whose symptoms included dilation of the eyes, frowning, repetition of "oh" before certain words, and speaking on residual air. In spite of his fairly severe stuttering, he spoke freely in all situations and resented the fact that his teacher did not call on him to recite in class (Bloodstein, 1960a).

Another boy, aged 6 years, exhibited pausing, gasping, or rapid expulsions of breath before speech attempts, but evinced so little emotional reaction that both his mother and a speech clinician who had worked with the child thought that he was not aware of his speech difficulty. Secondary symptoms do not necessarily mean anxiety or embarrassment, or even a self-concept as a defective speaker. It is no doubt frustrating to children to be interrupted in their speech attempts, and so they can easily become conditioned to employ devices that temporarily help them to avoid or terminate blocks. As for how much "awareness" this process requires, awareness has so many levels, and the word has so many meanings, that the question can have no simple answer.

Fluent Periods

As can be seen in Table 2, reports of intervals of normal speech decreased markedly past age 7 years and were nonexistent in the 14 to 16 age range. In the preschool children they were very common and lasted for days, weeks, months, or even years. Here are two typical examples:

> L. A. exhibited only phrase repetitions when he was interviewed at age 5–7. His first stuttering symptoms, consisting of rapid sound repetitions, were said to have appeared at age three for only about a week or two. At age five stuttering recurred in the form of sound repetition accompanied by severe eye blinking. It became progressively more severe for several months but had become much milder again by the time the child was examined.

> A. F. stuttered, blocking and repeating, at age three for two or three months, and then again at age four-and-a-half for a week. When seen again at age six he had been stuttering again, so badly that his teacher at school found it difficult to understand him, but there was no stuttering when he came for the interview.

In follow-up studies of preschool stutterers, Yairi and Ambrose (1922a) and Yairi, Ambrose, and Niermann (1993) found a distinct tendency for stuttering to disappear or decline markedly in severity several months after the initial contact. Even children with severe stuttering accompanied by facial and head movements seemed to have recovered after 6 months.

These fluent periods mark much early stuttering as an ephemeral phenomenon with a tendency toward spontaneous recovery as episodes come and go and often fail to develop into persistent cases.

Difficult Situations

The data in Table 2 relating to difficult speaking situations are based upon the children's own reports. At age 7 years, the earliest age at which any children were questioned about this, about one-fourth spoke about specific situations, and the proportion remains at over two-thirds at all later ages. The outstanding situations are much the same at all age levels: recitation in the classroom, especially oral reading; going to the store; talking at home in the presence of company; and asking directions of strangers.

The remaining one-third of the group had nothing to say about specific occasions when they stuttered. At younger age levels many of these children said that they stuttered whenever they "talked fast." Older children or teenagers in this category often spoke of stuttering when they were "nervous," "excited," or "talking fast."

Parents of children younger than 7 years were regularly asked about the conditions under which the children stuttered. They most often reported difficulty when the child was excited, enthusiastic, tense, upset, or "nervous," as when wanting something badly, being scolded, arguing with a sibling, or being "bothered" by other children. Another frequent report was about communicative urgency, as when the child had a lot to say, seemed to be trying to talk too fast, was telling a long story, or was fearful of being interrupted. Fatigue was also mentioned quite often.

Difficult Words or Sounds

As many as 82 percent of these children already regarded certain sounds or words as difficult to say by the earliest age at which they were questioned about this aspect, that is to say by age 8 years, suggesting that it often develops earlier. In preschool children parents sometimes reported noticing difficulty with particular words, in a few cases in children as young as 2.5 years. From age 8 years on, children commented that long words, words difficult to pronounce, their first or last names, or words with certain initial sounds or "letters" gave them particular trouble.

At every age level at which the children were questioned, there were many who seemed to have no awareness of any words or sounds as especially difficult.

Anticipation

In response to the question, "Can you sometimes tell even before you say a word that you're going to stutter on it?" the answer "yes" rose steadily from 38 percent at ages 8 and 9 years to 71 percent in the 14 to 16 age group. One 13-year-old boy said, "I know when I'm going to stutter by my mouth becoming tense just before the word I'm going to block on."

On their face, a notable implication of the numbers in Table 2 is that at every age level there were numerous individuals who said they did not anticipate any of their stutterings, and this is in accord with a report of Silverman and Williams (1972b), who found that about one-fourth of school-age children were unable to predict the occurrence of any of their blocks by saying "yes" or "no" before their attempt on each word of a list. Because the relationship between the anticipation and occurrence of stuttering has certain theoretical implications (see Chapter 7), some workers have argued that children may in some sense anticipate their stutterings even when they are unable to signal their occurrence in advance. Bloodstein (1960a) found that each of 14 preschool children in the Brooklyn group exhibited the so-called consistency effect, blocking on the same words in repeated utterances of the same sentence, and inferred that even young children may anticipate their stutterings on a low level of awareness.

Word Substitution

The children who used synonyms to avoid difficult words increased from 48 percent to 83 percent between ages 8 and 16 years. It can be presumed that many children substitute words before the age of 8 years. One mother noticed her 6-year-old doing this, and two parents reported the use of circumlocutions by a 4-year-old and a 3-year-old.

A distinction must be made between many of the substitutions of children and those of older stutterers. The majority of the school-aged children who were questioned said that they used substitutions only occasionally after the attempt on a word failed. For the most part, this was not the continual search for synonyms in response to anticipation of stuttering that characterizes so many fully developed cases. That development was not evident in the Brooklyn group before the age of 15 years. For most of the children, word substitution did not seem to be a reliable indicator of fear or shame; it appeared to be merely a reaction to speech frustration.

Avoidance of Speech and Other Signs
of Emotional Reaction to Stuttering

Of all the items in Table 2, perhaps the only one that can be taken at face value as an indication of strong emotional reaction to stuttering is habitual avoidance of speaking. This was already manifest in a few children by age 5 years and increased steadily to 45 percent of subjects in the oldest age group. Occasional avoidance of speech occurred in a few children even younger than 5 years. Two 2-year-olds were said to have stopped talking for a few days after their first experience of stuttering. One child of 3 years sometimes gave up speech attempts; another sometimes asked his mother to speak for him; and a third at times refused to speak to adults when his stuttering was severe. But fairly consistent avoidance of speech was first reported at age 5 years, in most cases at school. At every age level children avoided classroom recitation more often than any other situation, usually by not volunteering to speak, saying that they didn't know the answer, or pretending to be unprepared. Other situations that were avoided increasingly with age were errands requiring speech, talking to adult strangers, and using the telephone. Only a few children showed any tendency to withdraw from social contacts with others of their own age, but many said that at times they let their friends do the talking.

As is evident from Table 2, large numbers of these subjects did not systematically avoid any speech situations. The assertion that this was so came from both the subjects themselves and their parents. An 8-year-old girl who stuttered severely was said to talk "constantly," to be "popular," and to have been elected president of her class. A 10-year-old boy with severe stuttering had a reputation as a "talker" and frequently volunteered to speak in class, as did a 15-year-old with conspicuous secondary symptoms. It was not that these children were contented with the way they spoke. Given a choice, they would rather not have stuttered. But they were in sharp contrast to those of their age mates who were panicked and tormented by their stuttering and sought every avenue of escape from speaking in class.

The emotional reaction to stuttering that avoidance of speaking expresses was often confirmed by vivid indications of other kinds. Many of the preschool children were said to have reacted to some of their severe stuttering blocks by hitting themselves on the mouth, crying, laughing, looking down and blushing, placing their hands in front of their face, hitting the wall with their hands, or saying "I can't talk," "Why can't I talk?" "Help me talk," "My goodness," "I'm doing it again," or "I'll tell you later." At age 3 years about half the children had exhibited some such behavior.

These early reactions of very young children had two distinctive characteristics. First, they usually occurred sporadically; in the main the child talked freely and happily even while stuttering. And second, the behavior occurred in response to a specific occasion of stuttering, usually of some severity. The children were not complaining about being afflicted with defective speech. Rather, they were simply upset by the frustration of being blocked in their efforts to communicate. In other words, there was as yet no evidence of a clear self-concept as a stutterer. Expressions of such a self-concept first began to appear in a few of these children at age 4 years, when one child said, "Mommy, why can't I talk like other children"; another asserted that he "talked funny"; and a third on leaving the speech clinic was heard to say, "Is my talking fixed now?" From age 4 years on, increasing numbers of children asked "Why do I talk this way?" "When am I going to stop doing this?" and "Why was I born this way?" By age 7 years a few children were beginning to ask to be taken to a doctor and one 7-year-old girl asked, "Will I stutter after I get married too?"

From age 9 to 16 years the verbal reactions were essentially similar to those that accompany fully developed stuttering. Subjects more and more frequently admitted that they were frustrated, concerned, or embarrassed by their stuttering, that they mentally rehearsed speaking situations, that they were resentful of the unfavorable reactions of some of their listeners, and that they found it difficult to discuss their stuttering with others.

THE QUESTION OF DEVELOPMENTAL PHASES

In view of the observable changes that come about in so many aspects of stuttering with time, a question that naturally arises is whether it is possible to demonstrate that the problem, when persistent, follows a predictable course from its inception in childhood to its full-blown development in adolescents and adults. Are there identifiable stages of stuttering? No conceptual scheme of this sort has yet been generally accepted, and in fact only a few have been proposed.

"Primary" and "Secondary" Stages

An early view that was given wide currency by Froeschels, Bluemel, and others and which undoubtedly reflects an important core of accurate observation is that much of the stuttering of young children consists of simple repetitions of sounds, syllables, or words unaccompanied by signs of effort or emotion. Froeschels (1921) depicted the development of stuttering as a process in which simple repetitions by progressive stages became more rapid, irregular, forced, and finally "inhibited" under the pressure of social penalty. Bluemel (1932) termed the incipient stage of the disorder "primary" stuttering. He noted that it often consisted of the repetition of the first word or syllable of the sentence and that it frequently had a tendency to disappear and return repeatedly over a period of months or years. He observed that a "secondary" stage of stuttering began after a "lapse of several years" or much sooner in cases in which the child is "made conscious of his stammering as a social defect." He described secondary stuttering as characterized by the child's consciousness of the impediment, physical effort, the use of starters, synonyms, and other attempts to control or conceal stuttering, anticipation and above all fear—of letters, words, people, and speech situations.

Van Riper (1954, Chapter 9) sought to refine Bluemel's concept of primary and secondary stuttering by adding a "transitional" stage. Later, he proposed an additional modification of the scheme in which simple, effortless repetitions and prolongations at normal tempo (primary stuttering) are followed by a stage of faster, longer, and less regular repetitions and prolongations with occasional reactions of surprise, then by struggle reactions accompanied by feelings of frustration, and finally by secondary stuttering characterized by fear and avoidance (Van Riper, 1963, p. 327ff.).

Although Bluemel's two-stage concept has had a far-reaching influence on modern thinking about the development of stuttering, it has long been apparent that the concept represents the process in an over-simplified way. It is at odds with the following observations:

The presence of secondary symptoms in stutterers' speech is not sufficient evidence that they are habitually fearful of speaking. In reality, fear, in any stable, chronic sense, seems to be one of the last features of the problem to develop in most cases, while a large variety of associated symptoms may often be observed— apparently as reactions to the momentary frustration of the impulse to speak—at the earliest age levels and in children who appear to talk willingly and with enjoyment almost all the time.

It is difficult to find a stuttering child, no matter how young, whose speaking behavior does not seem to contain some element of tension, hurry, caution, anticipatory preparation, or reduced spontaneity symptomatic in some small measure of "awareness" of interruptions in his or her speech.

Finally, to the extent that such a child does sometimes come to our attention as a "stutterer," it would appear to some workers to raise the question of how that child is to be distinguished from any ordinary child with "normal" disfluencies in speech.

Four Phases in the Development of Stuttering

A developmental framework for stuttering proposed by the present author (Bloodstein, 1960b) emerged from a survey of the clinical case histories of a series of 418 stutterers, ranging in age from 2 to 16 years, whom he had examined at the Brooklyn College Speech and Hearing Center over a 6-year period. When these 418 stuttering problems were viewed with attention to all of their elements—observable symptoms, reactions, adaptations, and conditions under which stuttering occurred—the great majority seemed to adhere to at least an approximate degree to one of four recurring patterns. Each of the four was a familiar type of clinical case. Each had a distinctly different typical age of occurrence, despite extreme overlapping of the age ranges represented, so that they were clearly in a sequential relationship to each other. It was thus possible to discern a broad trend conveniently described in terms of four major phases. These are summarized below.

It must be cautioned that the process of development as outlined here appears to be typical, not universal. It is, moreover, a continual and gradual process. The four descriptions to follow are best seen as descriptions of reference points along a continuum. Many stutterers correspond in an approximate way to one of these four "phases"; others are more accurately described as being in transition between one phase and the next.

Phase One

The preschool period, roughly between the ages of two and six years, is one in which a large number of stutterers are to be seen. During this early period there are some six characteristics that may be said to typify most stuttering cases.

1. *The difficulty has a distinct tendency to be episodic.* One of the best indications that stuttering is still in its most rudimentary form is that it appears for periods of weeks or months between long interludes of normal speech. During this phase there is apparently a high percentage of spontaneous recoveries from stuttering that consist essentially of cases in which episodes of stuttering have failed to recur. How high this percentage is would be very difficult to determine. It is not improbable that single episodes of stuttering so mild and brief that they are overlooked or soon forgotten are exceedingly common during these years.
2. *The child stutters most when excited or upset, when seeming to have a great deal to say, or under other conditions of communicative pressure.*
3. *The dominant symptom is repetition.* This must be hastily qualified. Practically any of the integral or associated symptoms of stuttering may be seen in some of the youngest stutterers, and in some cases there seems to be little or no repetition. For the most part, however, the more severe symptoms appear briefly and intermittently in these children, and relatively simple repetition is far more common. In some cases repetition is practically the only symptom to be observed. While much of it consists of repetition of initial syllables, as it does

in older stutterers, there is also usually a conspicuous tendency to repeat whole words.

4. *There is a marked tendency for stutterings to occur at the beginning of the sentence, clause, or phrase.* In some of the youngest children stuttering seems to be limited almost entirely to the first word of the sentence.

5. *In contrast to more advanced stuttering, the interruptions occur not only on content words, but also on the function words of speech—the pronouns, conjunctions, articles, and prepositions.* Stuttering on such words often tends to consist of whole-word repetitions. In short, there is frequent repetition of such words as "like," "but," "and," "so," "he," "I," and "with."

6. *Most of the time children in the first phase of stuttering show little evidence of concern about the interruptions in their speech.* This is not to say that they are completely unconscious of them. It is commonplace for children as young as two or three to show acute frustration when they stutter by refusing to speak, crying, beating the wall with their hands, or saying, "Why can't I talk?" Such reactions are usually brief and sporadic, however, in contrast to the chronic fear and embarrassment of many older stutterers. Furthermore, the characteristic reaction of the Phase 1 stutterer may be epitomized by saying that when there is any reaction at all it is apparently in response to the immediate experience of being thwarted in efforts to communicate rather than to the ramified implications of the knowledge on the part of the child that he or she "is a stutterer."

Phase Two

The second phase in the development of stuttering is marked by the following:

1. *The disorder is essentially chronic.* There are few if any intervals of normal speech.

2. *The child has a self-concept as a stutterer.*

3. *The stutterings occur chiefly on the major parts of speech—nouns, verbs, adjectives, and adverbs.* There is much less tendency to stutter only on the initial words of sentences and phrases, and whole-word repetitions are no longer quite as common.

4. *Despite a self-concept as a stutterer, the child usually evinces little or no concern about the speech difficulty.* There is an absence of such features of more advanced stuttering as conscious anticipations of stuttering, substitution, circumlocution, avoidance of speaking, and word, sound, and situation fears.

5. *The stuttering is said to increase chiefly under conditions of excitement or when the child is speaking rapidly.*

This description of Phase 2 is, of course, an abstraction that fits few stutterers perfectly. The developmental process being continual, many children whom one would be inclined to classify in this or any other "phase" of stuttering exhibit some of the attributes of later or earlier forms of the disorder. Perhaps the single outstanding characteristic by which Phase 2 may be recognized as a familiar clinical entity is the tendency of children, by their own reports and that of others, to stutter chiefly when they "talk fast and get excited," even though they may long since have passed the age limits of Phase 1.

Phase 2 stutterers are to be found for the most part among children of elementary school age. The age limits of this stage are very broad, however, and there are individuals who exhibit its principal characteristics as early as age four and as late as adulthood.

Phase Three

The third phase of stuttering has these typical features:

1. *The stuttering comes and goes largely in response to specific situations.* Among the situations the person often reports to be especially difficult are classroom recitation, speaking to strangers, making purchases in stores, and using the telephone.
2. *Certain words or sounds are regarded as more difficult than others.*
3. *In varying degrees, use is made of word substitutions and circumlocutions.* This tends to be done only occasionally and more often as a reaction to frustration, or its imminence, than in actual fear of stuttering.
4. *There is essentially no avoidance of speech situations and little or no evidence of fear or embarrassment.*

In addition, anticipation of stuttering as a highly conscious process sometimes begins to develop while the disorder is still in this form. The distinguishing feature of this phase of stuttering is the tendency to speak freely in virtually all situations despite the fact that the person may exhibit all of the other attributes of fully developed stuttering and may even stutter quite severely. When there is a reaction to the speech difficulty, it is likely to be a reaction of irritation rather than of shame or anxiety.

Phase 3 stuttering is encountered at all ages from about eight to adulthood. It appears to be most common in late childhood and early adolescence.

Phase Four

At the apex of its development stuttering is marked by:

1. *Vivid, fearful anticipations of stuttering.*
2. *Feared words, sounds, and situations.*
3. *Very frequent word substitutions and circumlocution.*

4. *Avoidance of speech situations, and other evidence of fear and embarrassment.*

Phase 4 stuttering is typically seen in later adolescence and adulthood, although it may be recognized in children as young as ten years of age. Its distinctive aspect is the emotional reactions by virtue of which it tends to become a serious personal problem. Stutterers in this phase may become acutely conscious of the reactions of others to their speech, and they may be victimized by a tendency to exaggerate and misinterpret these reactions. They are likely to be unusually sensitive to the stigma involved in being regarded as a stutterer, to shrink from discussing their speech difficulty with others, and to go to extreme lengths to maintain a pretense as a normal speaker. All of this, together with avoidance of speaking, tends to impair their capacity for spontaneous and constructive social relationships and in some cases may even serve to isolate them to some extent from others.

Van Riper's Four Tracks

Whatever regularities exist in the development of stuttering, there are also differences among stutterers in the manner in which the problem undergoes changes. Van Riper (1982, Chapter 5) offered a descriptive scheme which placed particular stress on the developmental variability of stuttering. In his own cases, including forty-four that he was able to observe longitudinally, he discerned four alternate paths or "tracks" along which the disorder appeared to develop.

Track I

In by far the largest group of children, Van Riper found the symptoms to consist initially of effortless, unhurried repetitions of syllables and words, marked by extreme fluctuations and long remissions. Onset was gradual. As the disorder progressed the repetitions became more rapid and irregular, and there appeared in sequence prolongations, tension and forcing with intermittent evidence of concern on the part of the child, associated movements, word and situation fears, and avoidance.

Track II

In a second large group, consisting chiefly of children who were late in beginning to talk, the stuttering was said to take the form of rapid, irregular syllable and word repetition from the beginning. Later, silent intervals, revisions, and interjections appeared, and the pattern took on many of the aspects of cluttering. Thereafter the pattern changed relatively little. Word and sound fears were generally mild and tended to develop late.

Track III

A third group was made up of a small number of children who were said to have begun to stutter with sudden inability to speak, or complete blockage. Very soon this was followed by severe forcing and struggle, breathing abnormalities, signs of frustration, associated facial and other tensions, fear, and avoidance. In most cases the severe struggle reactions abated after a while and were followed first by prolongation and then by syllable repetition.

Track IV

Van Riper assigned a final track to a few children who were reported to have begun to stutter rather suddenly with repetition of phrases, words, and later syllables. They tended to stutter openly with few avoidances and showed little change in their stuttering over the years.

Suggested Readings

Adams, M. R. Freeman, F. J., and Conture, E. G., Laryngeal dynamics of stutterers. In Curlee, R. F., and Perkins, W. H. (eds.), *Nature and Treatment of Stuttering: New Directions*, San Diego: College-Hill Press (1984).

Adams, M. R., and Runyan, C. M., Stuttering and fluency: Exclusive events of points on a continuum? *J. Fluency Dis.*, 6, 197–218 (1981).

Armson, J., and Kalinowski, J., Interpreting results of the fluent speech paradigm in stuttering research: difficulty separating cause from effect. *J. Speech Hearing Res.*, 37, 69–82 (1994).

Bloodstein, O., The development of stuttering, Parts I, II, and III. *J. Speech Hearing Dis.*, 25, 219–37, 366–76 (1960); 26, 67–82 (1961).

Bloodstein, O., and Shogan, R. L., Some clinical notes on forced stuttering. *J. Speech Hearing Dis.*, 37, 177–86 (1972).

Caruso, A. J., Abbs, J. H., and Gracco, V. L., Kinematic analysis of multiple movement coordination during speech in stutterers. *Brain*, 111, 439–55 (1988).

Conture, E. G., McCall, G. N., and Brewer, D. W., Laryngeal behavior during stuttering. *J. Speech Hearing Res.*, 20, 661–68 (1977).

Darley, F. L., and Spriestersbach, D. C., *Diagnostic Methods in Speech Pathology*, 2n ed., New York: Harper & Row (1978), Chaps. 9, 10.

Freeman, F. J., and Ushijima, T., Laryngeal muscle activity during stuttering. J. *Speech Hearing Res.*, 21, 538–62 (1978).

Hutchinson, J. M., Aerodynamic patterns of stuttered speech. In Webster, L. M., and Furst, L. C. (eds.), *Vocal Tract Dynamics and Dysfluency*, New York: Speech and Hearing Inst. (1975).

Johnson, W. (ed.), Studies of speech disfluency and rate of stutterers and nonstutterers. *J. Speech Hearing Dis.*, Monogr. Suppl. 7 (1961), pp. 1–54.

McClean, M. D., Kroll, R. M., and Loftus, N. S., Kinematic analysis of lip closure in stutterers' fluent speech. *J. Speech Hearing Res.*, 33, 755–60 (1990).

Shapiro, A. I., An electromyographic analysis of the fluent and dysfluent utterances of several types of stutterers. *J. Fluency Dis.*, 5, 203–31 (1980).

Starkweather, C. W., Armson, J. M., and Amster, B. J., An approach to the study of motor speech mechanisms in stuttering. In Rustin, L., Purser, H., and Rowley, D., (eds.), *Progress in the Treatment of Fluency Disorders*. London: Taylor and Francis; San Diego, Singular Publishing Group (1987).

Van Riper, C., *The Nature of Stuttering*, 2nd ed., Englewood Cliffs, N.J.: Prentice-Hall (1982), Chap. 6.

Viswanath, N. S., Global and local-temporal effects of a stuttering event in the context of a clausal utterance. *J. Fluency Dis., 14*, 245–69 (1989).

Zimmermann, G., Articulatory behaviors associated with stuttering: A cine-fluorographic analysis. *J. Speech Hearing Res., 23*, 108–21 (1980a).

Zimmerman, G., Articulatory dynamics of fluent utterances of stutterers and nonstutterers. *J. Speech Hearing Res., 23*, 95–107 (1980b).

2

THEORIES OF STUTTERING

THEORIES OF ETIOLOGY VERSUS CONCEPTS
OF THE MOMENT OF STUTTERING

For a proper understanding of the array of formulations that have
been elaborated about stuttering, it is important to keep in mind that
they are not all theories in the same sense of the word. Some, like
Johnson's view that stuttering is caused by its own diagnosis, offer an
account of the *etiology*, or so-called onset of stuttering. That is, they
attempt to generalize about the conditions under which the disorder
comes about. A second type of theory is concerned primarily with the
nature of discrete instances of stuttering behavior. Like Coriat's theory that stuttering is a symbolic sucking activity, its emphasis is on a
conceptual model of the individual *moment* of stuttering. Needless to
say, some theorists have dealt with both the moment of stuttering and
the etiology of stuttering in systematic detail. But this is not always
so. And it is clarifying in any case to keep the two aspects of their theoretical formulations distinct.

There is still a third type of theory whose basic contribution lies in
a reformulation of a previous theory, either of the etiology or of the
moment of stuttering, in terms of a new frame of reference. Much of
the interest in the application of learning theory to stuttering has been
of this type. It is only by keeping these three kinds of theories clearly
separated that we will be able to appreciate the important connections
existing among them and the contributions each of them has to make
to our understanding of stuttering.

CONCEPTS OF THE MOMENT OF STUTTERING

We shall begin by putting aside the matter of the etiology of stuttering for the moment to consider the nature of the discrete stuttering response itself. When we ask what the response consists of we find that we have several hypotheses from which to choose. Almost all contemporary points of view about stuttering behavior are represented by three major conceptions. These we may term the *breakdown*, *repressed need*, and *anticipatory struggle* hypotheses.[1]

The Breakdown Hypothesis

Some theories appear to view the stuttering block as a momentary failure of the complicated coordinations involved in speech. In the context of such theories, the words *breakdown, disorganization, disintegration*, and *disruption* are often used to describe what is believed to be happening when the person stutters.

It might be objected that this is less an explanation than a description, and a rather figurative one at that. That is, regardless of the reasons for which it occurs, it is no more than self-evident that the stuttering block entails a breakdown of the speech function. The hypothesis, however, contains an additional element by virtue of which it is more than mere description. This is the element of environmental pressure as a precipitating agent. The breakdown is usually considered to be the effect of emotional or psychosocial stress, including speech anxiety, on the rapid, smooth, complex neuromuscular adjustments required for normal speech. It would be more accurate, perhaps, to call it the breakdown under-stress hypothesis. Such a model calls for assisting stutterers in some way to cope with the external pressures that are viewed as the precipitants of their speech disruptions, and it is perhaps in terms of this type of clinical rationale that the hypothesis is to be distinguished pragmatically from others.

Those who adhere to this point of view have had much to say about the possible reasons for which a child's speech originally becomes inclined to "fall apart," as it were, and we shall develop some of the implications of this hypothesis at greater length when we consider various theories of the etiology of stuttering in which the breakdown concept is embedded.

---

[1]All of these have their roots in a long history of thought about stuttering in the course of which counterparts of many modern views have reappeared many times. A valuable account of the extensive earlier developments in Europe and the United States was contributed by Freund (1966, pp. 1–47).

The simple notion of the moment of stuttering as a physical breakdown has often been elaborated in unique ways. Some well-known examples are the theories that the block is an expression of cerebral interhemispheric conflict (Travis, 1931), a miniscule convulsion (West, 1958), or a perseverative response similar to the perseverative motor behavior of some brain-injured patients (Eisenson, 1958, 1975). Van Riper (1971, Chap. 15), Adams (1974), and Perkins et al (1976) viewed stuttering as a failure of coordination of respiration, phonation, and articulation. Zimmermann (1980c) suggested that brainstem reflexes affecting the speech structures may become abnormally facilitated or inhibited when the movement of these structures exceeds certain ranges of velocity, displacement, or positioning. Moore and Haynes (1980) theorized that stuttering is a linguistic segmentation dysfunction due to right-hemisphere processing of language. A variety of other conceptions of the stuttering block as a breakdown in speech coordinations have recently emerged, due in part to a renewal of interest in organic factors in stuttering.[2]

The Repressed Need Hypothesis

Since the advent of psychoanalysis various attempts have been made to account for the stuttering act as a neurotic symptom rooted deeply in unconscious needs and treated most appropriately by psychotherapy. Far from being viewed primarily as a type of failure, stuttering is seen in this frame of reference as an integrated, purposeful activity that a person performs because of an unconscious wish to do so. Over several decades such writers as Brill (1923), Coriat (1928, 1943), Fenichel (1945, Chap. 15), Glauber (1958), and others advanced psychoanalytic concepts of the moment of stuttering differing somewhat in their emphases. A fairly comprehensive notion of this thinking may be given by enumerating the various needs that stuttering has been said to satisfy.

First, it has been said to satisfy an infantile need for oral erotic gratification. In stuttering the immature sexual pleasure of nursing, biting, and oral incorporation of objects that the person enjoyed as an infant is unconsciously perpetuated, according to this theory, and, concomitantly, the pleasure of complete dependence upon and identification with the mother.

Second, the act of stuttering has been regarded as an attempt to satisfy anal erotic needs. The function of the anal sphincter is symbolically

---

[2]See Zimmermann, Smith, and Hanley (1981), Andrews, Craig, Feyer, Hoddinott, Howie, and Neilson (1982), Kent (1984), MacKay and MacDonald (1984), Yeudall (1985) Stromsta (1986), Harrington (1988), Nudelman, Herbrich, Hoyt, and Rosenfield (1989), Perkins, Kent, and Curlee (1991).

"displaced upward," according to this view, and in stuttering the person seeks again those anal gratifications the need for which is said to characterize the infantile libido in a certain phase of its development.

Third, stuttering has been viewed as a covert expression of hostile or aggressive impulses that the person fears to express openly. Stuttering may be considered aggression in the sense that it is painful to the listener. It may also be regarded as aggression in the less obvious sense that stutterers, in "chewing up" their words, are symbolically attempting a cannibalistic destruction of their parents. Above all, stuttering is frequently seen as the persistence of a peculiarly anal kind of aggression characteristic of infantile levels of personality development. In this last sense the stutterer's forcing out and holding back of words may represent a hostile expulsion and retention of feces.

Fourth, stuttering may represent the unconscious desire to suppress speech. It is in this form that the need hypothesis has perhaps been most extensively developed (Fenichel, 1945, Chapter 15). According to this reasoning, the stoppages result from a conflict between all of the conscious pressures and needs that force stutterers to speak and their unconscious wish to be silent. For what reason do they need to be silent? A number of different answers are possible. To begin with, children may unconsciously fear that in speaking they will reveal certain forbidden wishes or feelings. For example, they may block in order to prevent themselves from saying obscene, anal words. In the main, however, they are thought to want to suppress speech because of what the act of speaking means to them. Speaking may represent oral gratification about which they may feel guilt. Speaking may also be seen as an aggressive act for which stutterers may fear retaliation. Such aggression may be predominantly oral or anal. In the Oedipal phase of psychosexual development, speech may be seen by the boy as an exhibitionistic kind of behavior and as an act of competition with the father. To the girl speech may symbolize a usurpation of the male role. In all of these cases the impulse to speak may be intermittently thwarted by guilt and anxiety.

This brief account does not do justice to the great subtlety with which psychoanalytic ideas about stuttering have been elaborated. The possible shades of meaning of stuttering to the psychoanalyst have not been exhausted here. Nor must it be assumed that the various unconscious needs that have been mentioned are mutually exclusive. Stuttering is frequently seen as satisfying a number of such needs simultaneously (Glauber, 1958). Writers differ chiefly in the amount of emphasis they give to different factors of unconscious motivation. Although the basic needs of classical Freudian theory, sex and aggression, predominate in most systematic psychoanalytic discussions of stuttering, there is also abundant reference to other unconscious uses of stuttering—for example, to gain attention, sympathy, or isolation; to provide an excuse for failures; or to avoid the necessity for coping with life's problems. Barbara (1954) contributed an extended analysis of the stutterer's personality employing the concepts of Horney and Adler, and Murphy and FitzSimons (1960) suggested some interpretations influenced by Sullivan. More recently Gemelli (1982a, 1982b) reiterated and extended the psychoanalytic theory of stuttering as a childhood neurosis along classical Freudian lines. For a detailed history of psychoanalytic thinking about stuttering, see Bloom (1978).

Repressed need theories found support chiefly in the clinical observations and case findings of psychoanalysts. Objective scientific corroboration of any of these theories of the moment of stuttering is largely lacking and is made extremely difficult by the very nature of the process by which psychoanalysis obtains its data. The studies that have been done on the stutterer's personality have not shown that stutterers are likely to be emotionally disturbed or markedly neurotic people, as we will see in Chapter 5. Neither have the end results of psychoanalytic treatment of stutterers afforded conclusive evidence for the repressed need hypothesis. It may be said that neither psychoanalysis nor various other forms of psychotherapy have as yet proved outstandingly effective in modifying stuttering behavior. Psychoanalysts, however, tend to attribute this to an unusual amount of resistance to therapy on the part of the stutterer. Stuttering has sometimes been compared to obsessive-compulsive neurosis in this respect.

The Anticipatory Struggle Hypothesis

Although there remain a number of other ways of conceiving of the moment of stuttering, they all appear to be so similar that they may be placed under a single general heading. The underlying idea common to all of them is that *stutterers interfere in some manner with the way they are talking because of their belief in the difficulty of speech*. This idea, termed here the anticipatory struggle hypothesis, has been, in one or another of its forms, one of the most widely employed explanations of the moment of stuttering and has exerted a strong influence on theory, treatment, and research.

As long as any serious professional concern about the problem of stuttering has existed, there appear to have been many workers to whom a very significant feature of the disorder was the tendency of stutterers to have difficulty whenever they expect to stutter and to speak fluently when not"thinking" about their speech. In this respect, stuttering is similar to the mistakes that may occur in typing or playing a musical instrument in an audience situation, or to the stiffness that may hamper some graduates' walking while crossing the stage to receive their diploma. The central thesis, succinctly stated, is that it is the anticipation of stuttering that leads to stuttering. But why should this be?

An analogy will serve to amplify this hypothesis. Most people are likely to have little difficulty keeping their balance while walking the length of a narrow plank lying upon the ground. Place the same plank twenty feet in the air, however, and the task assumes an entirely different character. We may describe what happens to the manner in which people walk under such conditions by saying that they now anticipate falling off the plank, try hard to avoid this, and ultimately may come to be in real danger of falling off as a result of their struggle to stay on.

In the course of its long history the anticipatory struggle hypothesis has been reiterated many times in a variety of ways. It will be helpful to examine carefully various alternative statements of the hypothesis.

Early Formulations

The early literature on speech disorders contains numerous references to stuttering as stemming from "fear," "doubt," or anticipation of speech difficulty. This simple and somewhat empty kind of statement became more elaborate as workers in modern times began to grope for formulations that explained more fully how a belief in the inability to speak normally might lead to stuttering. Boome and Richardson (1931, p. 99) and Gifford (1940, p. 30) inferred that stuttering was due to faulty autosuggestion. Freund developed a conception of stuttering as an "expectancy neurosis," analogous to disturbances such as male sexual impotence that tend to be made more severe by the fear that they will occur.[3] Others referred to it as an anxiety neurosis, or speech "phobia."

Failure of Automaticity

A distinctive form of the hypothesis was one stating that stuttering resulted from the attempt to exercise conscious control over the automatic processes of speech. The idea occurs widely in earlier writings on stuttering, where it is often accompanied by the analogy of the centipede who was crippled by the injunction to explain how it walked. The notion has come down through the years. West offered it in more refined form when he stated that stutterers tend to create difficulty for themselves by voluntarily producing individual speech

---

[3]Freund (1966) has summarized much of his earlier thinking, as well as that of others, on the relationship between expectancy and stuttering.

movements rather than by initiating "automatic serial responses." Later, he contributed a more extended discussion of stuttering as articulatory "dysautomaticity," postulating its relationship to genetic factors, however, rather than to the learning of fear or anticipation.[4] Mysak (1960) made use of the concept of "deautomaticity" in a servo theory context, as will be seen.

This general version of the anticipatory struggle hypothesis is an important one, since it calls attention to the interesting fact that both stuttering and what appear to be other stutterlike phenomena are likely to occur in serially ordered activities (such as speech, walking, typing, or playing musical instruments) consisting of integrated patterns or series of acts that by some mechanism appear to be evoked as wholes rather than as chains of individual responses. To put it in another way, interruptions produced by fear or anticipation seem to take place readily in the course of behavior demanding extensive motor planning (Frick, 1965). Perhaps the most pertinent example is the stutterlike difficulty reported to occur in some cases in the manual communication of the deaf (Silverman and Silverman, 1971; Montgomery and Fitch, 1988). Cases of stutterlike difficulty in the playing of musical instruments have been documented by Silverman and Bohlman (1988) and Meltzer (1992).

Anticipatory Avoidance

The anticipatory struggle concept is perhaps best known in the special form in which Johnson developed it in a series of writings spanning three decades.[5] In accordance with this view, the very things stutterers do in order not to stutter are their stuttering. Stuttering is, then, little more than the effort to avoid stuttering. Stated somewhat more elaborately, it is an "anticipatory, apprehensive, hypertonic avoidance reaction." That is, it is what happens when a person anticipates stuttering, dreads it, and becomes tense in the attempt to avoid it. In a phrase, stuttering is "what the speaker does while trying not to stutter again." From this point of view, stuttering is not a symptom of a constitutional abnormality or an emotional disorder, but a consequence of certain inappropriate perceptual and evaluative reactions with regard to speech that a speaker has learned from the social environment. Considerable research has been done on the moment of stuttering with Johnson's anticipatory avoidance theory as the primary impetus, and we shall therefore refer to it again in Chapter 7.

---

[4]See West, Ansberry, and Carr (1957, p. 255), and West and Ansberry (1968, Chapter 5).

[5]ee especially Johnson and Knott (1936), Johnson (1938), Johnson et al. (1956, pp. 216, 217), Johnson et al. (1967, p. 240).

Approach-Avoidance Conflict

Stuttering may be represented as the resultant of a conflict between opposing wishes to speak and to keep silent. This view was developed extensively by Sheehan (1953, 1958a) in a learning theory context to be considered further on. At this point it will be sufficient to indicate how the conflict idea is related to certain others already mentioned.

From a practical standpoint the conflict hypothesis may be reduced to the statement that stuttering results from the desire to avoid speech. (The conflicting desire to speak may be regarded as implicit, since without it there would merely be silence.) In contrast to Johnson's view of stuttering as the avoidance of stuttering, then, the conflict theory depicts it as the avoidance of speaking. This is quite a different notion, and we may be inclined to raise the question whether it belongs logically among anticipatory struggle concepts at all. The answer seems to be yes and no, depending on what reason is given for the avoidance of speaking. If it is because of the wish to avoid expected stuttering or any other real or imagined difficulty or failure in speech, we are clearly dealing with a form of anticipatory struggle hypothesis. But if, like Fenichel, we believe that stutterers wish to avoid speech because they unconsciously regard it as a hostile act, or if, like Glauber, we see stuttering as a kind of mutism or articulatory spasm designed to block unconscious expressions of biting or sucking, the conflict motif is more reasonably regarded as belonging to the repressed need hypothesis.

Preparatory Set

Van Riper (1937d; 1954, pp. 429–43) developed his concept of the role of the preparatory set in stuttering primarily as a therapeutic tool (*see Chapter 11*) and has not appeared to place much emphasis on its theoretical implications. Yet, when seen in the proper light, it proves to be a highly descriptive statement of the anticipatory struggle hypothesis. Van Riper pointed out that, in advance of the attempt on a word perceived as difficult or feared, stutterers tend to place themselves in a characteristic muscular and psychological "set" which determines the form of the subsequent stuttering block. This set has essentially three identifiable features. First, stutterers establish an abnormal focus of tension in their speech organs. Second, they prepare themselves to say the first sound of the difficult word as a fixed articulatory posture rather than as a normal movement blending with the rest of the word. That is, in their lack of conviction that they will be able to say the feared initial sound, they may prepare themselves to say "b" rather than "boy." This can only result, however, in failure to produce the word in a normal way. Third, they may adopt this unnatural posture of the speech organs appreciably before initiating voice or airflow, resulting in a silent "preformation" of the sound. Having done all of these things because of their anticipation of difficulty on the word, it is apparent that they have effectively destroyed their chances of saying it normally. Conversely, it may be hypothesized that if they did none of these things they would not stutter on the word.

Tension and Fragmentation

Finally, we may note that practically all of the integral features of stuttering behavior are reducible to the surface effects of two underlying forms of behavior—tension and fragmentation. Whenever we are faced with the threat of failure in the performance of a complex activity demanding accuracy or skill we are likely to make use of abnormal muscular tension. We are also apt to produce a portion of the act separately and sometimes repeatedly before we complete it. In stuttering the underlying tension produces prolongations and hard attacks. The repetitions of stuttering may be interpreted as a fragmentation of speech units somewhat analogous to the behavior of dart-throwers rehearsing the initial part of their throw. Such an interpretation is useful in explaining why it is almost always the first sound of the word that the stutterer repeats, as well as certain other puzzling features of its distribution in the speech sequence. We will develop this model more fully later.

Compatibility of Alternative Statements of the Anticipatory Struggle Hypothesis

We have examined a number of different ways in which essentially a single general conception of the moment of stuttering has been expressed. Some of them are undoubtedly to be preferred to others for various reasons. But it will in all probability have occurred to many readers that some of these statements differ from others only in their concern with different temporal phases of the hypothetical anticipatory struggle act. We might say that there occurs in sequence 1) a suggestion, in the form of some outside stimulus, of imminent difficulty in speech, 2) an anticipation of failure, 3) a feeling of need to avoid it, 4) abnormal motor planning for the voluntary articulation of the speech activity, 5) the mustering of certain preparatory sets for this purpose, and 6) the production of tensions and fragmentations which interfere with the normal process of speech.[6]

---

[6]It is interesting that to virtually each step in this sequence there corresponds at least one unique therapy which has been used with stutterers.

THEORIES OF THE ETIOLOGY OF STUTTERING

So far we have been concerned only with the moment of stuttering. In the light of what has been surmised about it, we may now go on to examine various inferences about the conditions under which this behavior first arises. Various schemes have been proposed for classifying theories of the etiology of stuttering. None of them is completely satisfactory; the thinking that has been done on the subject of stuttering tends to defy the simple logic of mutually exclusive categories. It may not be difficult to see, however, that in the foregoing review of concepts of the moment of stuttering we have been afforded a convenient means of making such a classification. Any satisfactory theory of the etiology of stuttering carries with it, either explicitly or by implication, an assumption about the nature of the individual stutterings. Taking our three major hypotheses about the moment of stuttering as a basis, therefore, we may classify virtually all etiological theories as breakdown, repressed need, or anticipatory struggle theories.

Breakdown Theories: The Dysphemic Viewpoint

At present most theories that regard stuttering behavior as a breakdown of the speech function under some type of pressure are associated with the view that constitutional or organic factors are involved in its etiology. The reason for this is not difficult to see. There was a time in the history of modern thinking about stuttering when it was believed by many that a child's speech might begin to go to pieces for no reason other than environmental stress. That is, it was often suggested that stuttering resulted simply from the impact of shock, fright, illness, injury, or the like. Even today, expressions of this type are heard occasionally, with *emotional pressures* or *insecurity* used in place of terms such as shock or fright. To most serious workers on the problem of stuttering, however, it is now clear that the vast majority of children who have pneumonia or fall off bicycles even repeatedly do not stutter as a result. It is equally apparent that most children with emotional difficulties do not stutter. This difficulty may be glossed over by saying that some people have a "weakness" in the "area of speech" that causes them to react to such stresses by stuttering, but this is after all only a figure of speech and serves chiefly to raise questions about the form in which such a weakness might manifest itself.

For this reason, more recent breakdown theories have gone to considerable pains to show why speech disintegrates under stress in some cases and not in others. For the most part they have done so by asserting that children must be predisposed in some way to breakdown before their speech can give way under stress, and the more satisfactory of these theories attempt to explain both the nature of this predisposition and the reason for which its effects appear to be confined to speech. While it is possible to assume, as did Bluemel (1957), that children are made prone to disorganized speech by the nature of their personality, on the whole the predisposition is believed to take a genetic, or constitutional, form.

The hypothesis that stuttering is basically an organic disorder is at least as old as Aristotle, who speculated that there was something wrong with the stutterer's tongue. It is now well known that stuttering cannot be attributed to any gross structural abnormality of the speech organs, but it is interesting that as recently as 1841 the Prussian surgeon Johann Dieffenbach was performing tongue operations for stuttering. Dieffenbach believed that by removing a wedge-shaped section of the base of the tongue he could stop the muscular spasms of the glottis that he thought were the cause of stuttering. His operation at first appeared to be a sensational success, evidently because of the powerful suggestion it produced, but the improvement in his patients proved to be temporary.[7]

The point to be emphasized is that present-day constitutional theories of stuttering differ in certain fundamental respects from the naive speculations of Aristotle and Dieffenbach. The first and most important difference is that today's theories are *predisposition* theories. They adopt the assumption familiar to medical science that a disorder may be a joint product of a hereditary predisposition and environmental precipitating factors.

According to this point of view, which was developed in detail by West and some of his students, there exists in certain persons an inherited predisposition to breakdown of the speech function. This predisposition takes the form of a pervasive constitutional abnormality, sometimes termed "dysphemia," whose exact nature has not yet been established. Dysphemia is, then, considered to be an inner condition of which stuttering is an outward symptom. Given a sufficient amount of dysphemia, the stuttering symptom may be precipitated by illness, emotional disturbance, or the stress of other accidental environmental circumstances during childhood. A child who is heavily predisposed to stutter, as indicated by an extensive family history of the disorder, may never become a stutterer in a favorable environment. On the other hand, a child who is subjected to many serious environmental pressures may stutter even though lightly predisposed by heredity to do so. Clearly, it is not difficult to explain on the basis of this type of reasoning why so many persons with a family background of stuttering have no speech difficulty and why those who stutter often have no known stuttering relatives or ancestors.

---

[7]See Rieber and Wollock (1977).

Research has so far produced no conclusive evidence regarding the precise description of dysphemia, if such a thing exists, or the manner in which it predisposes a person to stutter. In the past it was common to look for organic causes in easily identifiable organs such as the tongue, the breathing apparatus, the larynx, or the thymus gland. Interest in the larynx as a source of stuttering, in fact, enjoyed a revival in the 1970s. For the most part, however, the predisposing cause of the stutterer's difficulty is now sought—and this is a second important distinction of present-day constitutional theories—not in the peripheral organs of speech, but in subtle aspects of the neuro-muscular organization of the body or in other features of the stutterer's physiology whose effects on speech are indirect. It is at this point that the dysphemic point of view about stuttering becomes divided into many different theories. A number of these are noteworthy because they have had a wide influence on modern thinking or have provided an impetus for research.

Theory of Cerebral Dominance

Few theories of stuttering are as well known as the theory that children are predisposed to stutter by a conflict between the two halves of the cerebrum for control of the activity of the speech organs.[8] Sometimes known as the "handedness theory," it was put forward in an attempt to account for some assumptions about stutterers' lateral dominance that have since been largely rejected. In the late 1920s it was widely believed that an unusual number of stutterers were left-handed or ambidextrous or had been shifted to right-handedness in childhood, and there had been some convincing clinical reports of onset of stuttering after enforced change of handedness.

The great virtue of the cerebral dominance theory was that it offered a single, clear explanation for all of these alleged facts. Its authors, Dr. Samuel T. Orton and Prof. Lee Edward Travis, took note of the fact that the right and left halves of the tongue, jaw, and other "midline" speech structures received their motor nerve impulses from separate sources in the two cerebral hemispheres. They reasoned that for purposes of smooth, fluent speech these two streams of impulses needed to be accurately synchronized. What mechanism was responsible for this synchronization? They hypothesized that one cerebral hemisphere was "dominant" over the other for the purpose of timing the nerve impulses. The nondominant hemisphere, they argued, accepted the temporal rhythm of innervation established by the dominant one. If, however, one hemisphere were not sufficiently dominant over the other, they would tend to function independently, actions of the two halves of the speech musculature would be poorly synchronized, and a predisposition to speech breakdown would exist.

---

[8]See Travis (1931).

Cerebral dominance had long been a familiar concept in a different connection. The belief had become established that in cases of symbolic language disorder due to brain damage the injury was usually to be found in the left half of the brain in right-handed persons, while there was speculation that in left-handed aphasics the injury was in the right half of the brain. From this had grown the belief that one cerebral hemisphere tends to become specially developed for the formulation and comprehension of language and for the purpose of establishing lateral preference.

According to the Orton-Travis theory it was this very same side of the cerebrum that was dominant for the purpose of "motor lead control." This was an essential element of the theory because it made it possible to explain how handedness was related to stuttering. In the first place, children who were innately ambidextrous were lacking by heredity in a safe margin of cerebral dominance. In the second place, training "naturally" left-handed children to use the right hand meant reducing their margin of cortical dominance by exercising their minor hemisphere at the expense of the major one. And in the third place, left-handed persons might become predisposed to stutter even when not deliberately shifted because they were subject to so many pressures exerted by a right-handed society to use the right hand.

The Orton-Travis theory met with one of the most favorable receptions ever accorded a theory of stuttering, and the literature in such fields as medicine, psychology, and education still makes scattered references to it as a current point of view about stuttering. The great vogue it enjoyed in the '30s, however, has long since passed. A considerable amount of laterality research done since then has failed to show to the satisfaction of most workers that stutterers are particularly distinguished either by left-handedness or ambidexterity, as was once thought. Also, evidence eventually accumulated that the vast majority of children whose handedness is changed by parents or teachers do not stutter. Finally, there have been the disappointing results of therapy. The cerebral dominance theory had some obvious clinical implications. Strict unilaterality was to be enforced in all of the stutterer's activities. Furthermore, if right-handed stutterers seemed to be natively left-sided as determined from case history or by certain types of laterality tests, they would need to learn to exercise their natural dominance by changing to the use of the left hand. At the time that the popularity of the theory was at its height, a great many apparently right-handed stutterers were judged to be innately left-handed and rigorously trained in sinistrality. At first the results seemed to be good and were sometimes reported in enthusiastic terms. The initial promise of this therapy was not fulfilled, however, and it fell into disuse.

Biochemical Theory

A second conception of the nature of dysphemia that had considerable influence was developed over a period of years by West. According to this theory the source of stuttering is to be found in a basic difference between stutterers and nonstutterers in metabolic factors and tissue chemistry. The speech interruptions are triggered by social and emotional pressures, but the stutterer's neurophysiological mechanism for speech is rendered vulnerable to the disruptive effects of such pressures by a biochemical imbalance.

West regarded dysphemia as genetically bound up with a predisposition to certain other conditions, notably allergy, left-handedness, late development of speech, twinning, and respiratory disease. He eventually formulated a concept of stuttering as a convulsive disorder related to epilepsy and particularly akin to an epileptiform disorder of childhood known as pyknolepsy (West, 1958). According to this concept the stutterer is a basically seizure-prone person in whom outright convulsions are held in check by a relatively large amount of blood sugar. The convulsive tendency is, however, reflected in stuttering. As noted earlier, West's theory in one of its later forms viewed the moment of stuttering as a kind of miniature seizure that principally affects the speech musculatures and is precipitated by emotional stress. This theory was supported by a number of observations purporting to show an elevated blood sugar in stutterers, a high incidence of stuttering among persons with epilepsy, and a rareness of stuttering among those with diabetes. There are conflicting research findings on all of these points, however, and none of them has thus far been generally accepted as fact.

Perseverative Theory

Another viewpoint that may be considered advantageously in the context of dysphemia was suggested by Eisenson (1958, 1975). Eisenson believes that in the majority of cases stuttering is based upon a constitutional predisposition to motor and sensory perseveration. His investigations reported in 1936 and 1938 showed that on the average stutterers were inclined to perseverate more than nonstutterers in performing certain psychomotor tasks. Subsequent research by other investigators, including two studies by King (1961) and Martin (1962), produced inconsistent results.

Hormonal Theory

Cerebral dominance has made its appearance again in a theory proposed by Norman Geschwind.[9] On the strength of some evidence,

---

[9] See Geschwind and Galaburda (1985).

Geschwind hypothesized that the male sex hormone testosterone tends to retard neuronal development in the fetal brain. Because the right hemisphere develops earlier than the left, the effect is more pronounced in the left hemisphere. The male fetus is exposed to higher levels of testosterone than the female, so excessive delays in the development of the left hemisphere will be more common in males. As a result, according to Geschwind's theory, males will be more prone to developmental disturbances of left-hemisphere functions, including those of speech and language. On this basis Geschwind saw relationships among maleness, left-handedness, and such disorders as dyslexia, delayed speech, and stuttering.

As a theory of stuttering this is somewhat incomplete, since it says nothing about why some children stutter while others have dyslexia or delayed speech but do not stutter. Moreover, there is an absence of convincing evidence that stutterers differ from others in handedness.[10] The theory accounts for the preponderance of males who stutter, however, as well as for the high incidence of delayed speech and language among stutterers (see Chapter 6), and it fits well with research reports suggesting that many stutterers process speech with the right cerebral hemisphere (see Chapter 4).

The Demands and Capacities Model

Starkweather (1987) has elaborated the point of view that stuttering results when demands for fluency from the child's social environmer exceed the child's cognitive, linguistic, motor, or emotional capacities for fluent speech. According to this formulation, either low innate capacity of excessive speech and language pressures may cause fluency to disintegrate. Unlike most breakdown theories, it does not assume that organic deficits are a necessary condition for stuttering. The concept invokes environmental factors that have more often been considered in connection with anticipatory struggle theories, but the failure of the child's capacity for fluency to meet demands imposed upon it is assumed to lead directly to disorganization or breakdown of speech. (See also Adams, 1990, and Starkweather and Gottwald, 1990.)

Repressed Need Theories

We have considered the psychoanalytic assumption that the moment of stuttering represents an attempt to fulfill some type of unconscious neurotic need. On this assumption, the question of how stuttering originally develops becomes the question of how children acquire such needs and under what conditions they first try to satisfy them by stuttering. The answer we are given within the framework of

---

[10]See Chapter 4. Geschwind and Behan (1982) found dyslexia and stuttering more common among highly left-handed than among highly right-handed subjects.

classical Freudian theory is that these are essentially the same needs that underlie any other symptoms of psychosexual fixation and are brought about by the same conditions. Broadly speaking, the fixations are thought to stem from early conflicts over the satisfaction of the special psychic needs of infancy—chiefly oral and anal eroticism, dependence, aggressiveness, and self-assertion. Such conflicts are generally considered to grow out of disturbed parent-child relationships and to be related to abnormal feeding or nursing behavior of the mother, excessively harsh or early weaning or toilet training, parental domination, overprotection or overanxiety, or other traumatic features of the family environment that frequently go back to the parents' own neurotic conflicts.

Psychoanalytic writers for the most part have not been concerned with the special antecedent conditions leading to stuttering, as opposed to those leading to other forms of neurotic behavior, although a notable attempt to describe a specific family "constellation" for stuttering was made by Glauber (1958). From this point of view there as yet appears to be little in the way of a unique psychoanalytic theory of the etiology of stuttering, to say nothing of competing theories of this kind. The important contributions of psychoanalysis have been the conceptual models of the moment of stuttering considered earlier in this chapter.

Anticipatory Struggle Theories

In our earlier discussion of the anticipatory struggle hypothesis, we reviewed a series of statements about the moment of stuttering which said in effect that stutterers interfere with the way they speak because of their belief in the difficulty of speech and their anticipation of speech failure. The question of the etiology of anticipatory struggle reactions is, then, the question of how children acquire such beliefs and anticipations. The explanations that have been called on to account for this are essentially three in number and differ in the respect that they consider the causative factor of central importance to be 1) the child's excessive hesitations and repetitions (primary stuttering), 2) the parents' high standards of fluency (diagnosogenic theory), or 3) communicative failures or pressures, broadly viewed.

Theory of Primary and Secondary Stuttering

In Chapter 1 we had occasion to refer to an early view that stuttering as a developed disorder arises as a reaction to unusual but relatively simple repetitions in a child's speech, termed *primary stuttering*. In accordance with this view, first advanced in somewhat different forms by Froeschels and Bluemel, stuttering first appears in the form of speech repetitions that occur without effort or awareness on the part of the child. This stage of the disorder was held to be essentially a phenomenon of early childhood and one which tends to disappear of its own accord if the child is prevented from learning that he or she is speaking differently. Sooner or later, however, it was argued, many primary stutterers are urged to "think" before they speak, to take a deep breath or to "stop and start over" so often that they become guilty and apprehensive about their mild speech interruptions. The more serious form of the disorder was then believed to develop from the child's efforts to avoid primary stuttering. This advanced form, marked by strenuous blockages, fear, embarrassment, and various concomitant symptoms of effort and emotion, was characterized as *secondary stuttering*.

According to this theory of the development of stuttering, then, it is only some time after its onset, in a so-called secondary stage, that it becomes an anticipatory struggle behavior as children begin to react with anticipation, fear, and avoidance to their primary stuttering. In its incipient stage it was considered to be something quite different. Primary stuttering was usually held to be a type of disintegration or breakdown, and both genetic and environmental factors were suggested as its chief cause. Van Riper, once its principal exponent, stated that in some instances the etiology was primarily constitutional, in others neurotic, and in still others stemmed from a home environment marked by frequent interruption, unresponsive listeners, demands to confess guilt orally, or other "fluency disruptors."

The theory of Weiss (1964) regarding the relationship between stuttering and cluttering is also of interest here, in view of Weiss's identification of cluttering with primary stuttering. Cluttering, as it is usually described, is a disorder of fluency marked by monotonous, rapid, jerky, repetitive, indistinct utterance with frequent telescoping of words, unaccompanied by fear, anticipation, any sense of difficulty with specific words or sounds or even a detailed awareness of speaking abnormally. It has long been noted (e.g., Freund, 1934b) that stuttering and cluttering not infrequently appear in the same person. In 1934 Weiss advanced the hypothesis that stuttering essentially always has its onset as a reaction of effort or struggle for the purpose of overcoming cluttering. Later, Weiss (1964, p. 71), perhaps employing a broader definition of cluttering than is usual, reflected that the difference between cluttering and Bluemel's primary stuttering was largely one of nomenclature.

As we noted in Chapter 1, knowledge of the early development of the symptoms of stuttering on the basis of scientific observation is as yet meager. There is little doubt that relatively simple repetitions with little *consistent* emotional reaction is a frequently observed feature of the speech of young children who are regarded as stutterers. Whether these features are invariably present as a distinguishable initial stage; how they are to be differentiated from developed stuttering, cluttering, or normal childhood speech hesitancy; and whether stuttering in its developed form is always, or ever, precipitated by penalties incurred because of them are questions concerning which we as yet have very incomplete evidence.

Diagnosogenic Theory

An alternative theory about the manner in which children learn to have anticipatory struggle reactions in their speech was offered by Johnson in 1942. This is the theory that the disorder is usually caused by a parent's diagnosis of normal disfluencies in the child's speech as stuttering. As we have seen, Bluemel, Froeschels, and others have already identified developed stuttering, whether correctly or not, as a reaction to the relatively simple repetitions often noticeable in the speech of young stutterers. Froeschels, among others, had noted the similarity of these repetitions to those of many normal children during the early years of speech development. It remained for Johnson to make a final leap. Primary stuttering was not merely similar to normal childhood nonfluency nor was it late-persisting or excessive normal nonfluency. The two were simply one and the same. According to Johnson's theory, it was not excessive hesitancy that usually caused a child to develop anticipatory reactions of struggle or avoidance, but abnormal parental reactions to this hesitancy. What others had termed primary stuttering was not a disorder to be treated. It was a normal attribute of speech that was to be prevented from giving rise to stuttering by altering the parents' evaluations of it.

Johnson was led to his conclusions while assisting in a study of young stuttering and nonstuttering children conducted under the direction of Lee E. Travis at the University of Iowa between 1934 and 1939. In the course of this investigation he was struck by the fact that it was not always easy to distinguish the stutterers from the nonstutterers by listening to their speech. This led him to question the parents of the stutterers systematically about the nature of the speech interruptions they had originally diagnosed as stuttering. Johnson found that the great majority of the descriptions offered were confined to brief, "effortless" repetitions of syllables, words, and phrases of which the child was apparently "unaware," and he inferred that these descriptions were essentially similar to those that might have been made of the speech hesitations of most ordinary children.[11]

---

[11]The findings of this study (Johnson et al, 1942) were presented in more detail in a subsequent publication (Johnson, 1955a) and also form the basis for Study I in his later and more extensive report of investigations of the onset of stuttering (Johnson and Associates, 1959).

Johnson's findings, as he summarized them some time later, may stand as a formal statement of his theory:

1. Practically every case of stuttering was originally diagnosed as such, not by a speech expert, but by a layman—usually one, or both, of the child's parents.
2. What these laymen had diagnosed as stuttering was, by and large, indistinguishable from the hesitations and repetitions known to be characteristic of the normal speech of young children . . .
3. Stuttering . . . as a definite disorder was found to occur, not before being diagnosed, but after being diagnosed (Johnson, 1944).

Having been evaluated as a stutterer, in Johnson's view, the child was indeed likely to begin speaking differently in response to the parental anxieties, pressures, help, criticism, and correction that tended to go along with such a diagnosis.

As Johnson put it, stuttering generally began "not in the child's mouth but in the parent's ear." This was not, however, because the parents were necessarily as aberrant in their perceptions of reality as this might seem to imply. Johnson believed that in most cases they were essentially ordinary people whose concern about their child's speech hesitations, though exaggerated, was simply a reflection of rather unrealistic standards of speech and somewhat anxious, perfectionistic parental attitudes and child training policies broadly characteristic of our culture.

This is one of the best known of modern theories of stuttering, and various attempts have been made by research workers to verify it. So far evidence has accumulated that most young children are relatively disfluent and that parents of stutterers often tend to be dominating, overanxious, or perfectionistic. But Johnson's basic premise that "on the date of original diagnosis, stuttering children may speak in a manner that is not always to be clearly differentiated from that of other children of like age who have not been diagnosed as stutterers" is exceedingly difficult to verify by means of an objective scientific test. Attempts to confirm it, based upon intensive interviewing of parents in cases of recent onset of the problem, have yielded results that must be regarded as highly equivocal at best. We will return to this question in Chapter 9.

Theory of Communicative Pressure

So far we have considered two ways in which anticipatory struggle reactions have been theorized to develop—chiefly through fear and avoidance of so-called primary stuttering and chiefly through fear and avoidance of "normal" disfluency. If stuttering is based upon the child's belief in the difficulty of speech, however, there would appear on the surface to be no clearly visible reason for supposing that there might not be other sources of such convictions from which stuttering might stem, and scattered references in the literature on stuttering for many years have hinted strongly of such sources. An approach of this kind to the problem of the onset of stuttering was made by Bloodstein (1958, 1975) on the basis of a clinical study of 108 stuttering children. In essence, this viewpoint states that what is first identified as stuttering usually begins as a response of tension and fragmentation in speech, not sharply different from certain types of normal disfluency, and is brought about largely by the provocation of continued or severe communicative failure in the presence of communicative pressure.

This hypothesis finds its most significant elaboration with reference to the variety of factors that may contribute to a child's conviction that speech demands unusual effort or precautions. On the basis of clinical evidence it appears possible that retarded language development, articulatory errors, reading difficulty, cluttering, difficulties of phonation, or practically any other kind of verbal ineptness or obstacle to communication may render children more or less chronically subject to the threat of speech failure to the degree that their attempts at speech may become more tense and fragmented than those of ordinary children who experience such difficulties in mild and intermittent form.

Such provocations may be assumed to be particularly likely to take effect if the children are subject, to a greater degree than average, to unrealistically high parental standards of speech or to other speech pressures such as competition with siblings more advanced in speech development, excessive praise for good speech, or identification with an adult having a reputation for superior speech. Finally, the likelihood cannot be ignored that there are certain personality traits (e.g., the tendency to be unusually sensitive, fearful, dependent, perfectionistic, easily frustrated, or too anxious for approval) that render a child more vulnerable to the provocations and pressures that may lead to anticipatory struggle behavior.

Such a theory may perhaps be summarized most succinctly by the statement that stuttering is caused by communicative failure as perceived by the child. From certain standpoints it may be seen as a generalization of the two anticipatory struggle theories previously described. It differs from them, however, in denying that either a diagnosis of stuttering or the occurrence of excessive repetitions in a child's speech is necessary in order for anticipatory struggle reactions to develop. Furthermore, it holds that incipient stuttering in its clinical form differs only in degree from anticipatory struggle reactions to be found in the speech of most children and so does not draw the sharp line between stuttering and normal disfluency that is required by the assumption that the one is the avoidance of the other. We will consider these issues further in Chapter 10.

THEORIES THAT SHIFT THE FRAME OF REFERENCE

A useful approach to the problem of stuttering is represented by the kind of theory that reformulates an existing concept about the disorder in terms of some new theoretical framework of scientific thinking. Such approaches to stuttering frequently present earlier theories in new relationships to other viewpoints and observations or reword them in new language with a desirable gain in verifiability.

Learning Theory Interpretations

Chief among such frames of reference that have held considerable appeal for theorists in the area of stuttering have been the stimulus response theories of learning that behavior scientists have developed through several decades of laboratory experimentation with animals. These learning theories have lent themselves to a number of systematic statements about stuttering. In general, the aim of such statements has been to make use of the relatively precise language of behavior science in order to try to define the process by which stuttering is learned and maintained by identifying the motivational factors, stimulus variables, and reinforcing conditions.

Stuttering as an Instrumental Avoidance Act

Much of the initial interest in the learning approach to stuttering was stimulated by the work of Wischner (1947, 1950, 1952b) within the framework of Clark L. Hull's theory of learning. Wischner based his formulations chiefly on two observations that had been the subject of considerable earlier research. One of these was the adaptation effect and the other was the phenomenon of expectancy or anticipation, which he equated with anxiety.[12] Drawing an analogy between the tendency for stuttering to decrease with successive readings of the same passage (adaptation) and the experimental extinction of a learned response, he performed further adaptation studies that demonstrated what appeared to be analogues of such conditioning phenomena as spontaneous recovery, disinhibition, and conditioned inhibition.

One of the central problems in the application of learning principles to stuttering is to explain the nature of the reinforcement that

---

[12]Adaptation and expectancy are discussed in Chapters 7 and 8.

causes it to persist in the face of repeated punishment. Wischner posited that this reinforcement consisted chiefly of a reduction in the stutterer's anxiety following the block. Prior to the moment of stuttering there was a building up of expectancy, or fear. The immediate effect of stuttering was a reduction of this tension. Although the block obviously had punishing consequences, Wischner pointed out that these did not follow as immediately on the termination of the block as did the anxiety reduction. Consequently, the stuttering behavior was reinforced rather than extinguished.[13]

In general, Wischner likened stuttering to the so-called instrumental avoidance act, of which animal learning research has afforded many examples. A guinea pig may be placed in a cage constructed so that it will revolve when the animal runs and may be given an electric shock intermittently through the grillwork of the cage, preceded each time by the sound of a buzzer. If the apparatus is wired so that the electric current is shut off whenever the cage is in motion, the animal will quickly learn to escape the shock by running in response to the sound of the buzzer. This type of learned avoidance response has a peculiar feature distinguishing it from ordinary instrumental acts, such as learning to secure a pellet of food by depressing a bar. *It is unusually difficult to extinguish.* The bar-depressing act may be eradicated simply by withholding the food pellets. No such effect on the guinea pig's running response is produced by eliminating the shock, however, unless the animal accidentally fails to run and thereby "discovers" that the grill is no longer charged. Wischner stated that from this point of view there appeared to be a significant parallel between stuttering and the running behavior of the guinea pig. What is generally termed stuttering behavior, as Johnson had pointed out, may consist of little or nothing but stutterers' efforts to avoid stuttering. If stutterers could bring themselves to attempt their feared words without such efforts they would be able to say them fluently. Like the guinea pig, however, they do not stop running long enough or often enough to acquire the conviction that the grill is not "hot."

Wischner's main analysis clearly consisted in part of a reformulation of Johnson's concept of the moment of stuttering as an anxiety-motivated avoidance reaction. In discussing the origin of the disorder, Wischner suggested that it was to be found in some kind of painful, anxiety producing stimulation. He referred to Johnson's diagnosogenic theory as a tenable hypothesis from this standpoint, suggesting that the original instigators to anxiety in the stutterer might be found in parental disapproval of normal disfluency.

---

[13]See Wischner (1952a), Sheehan and Voas (1954), Luper (1956), and Sheehan, Cortese, and Hadley (1962) for experimental findings relating to the fear-reduction hypothesis regarding the reinforcement of stuttering.

Stuttering as Approach-Avoidance Conflict

Sheehan (1953, 1958a) viewed stuttering primarily as the resultant of a conflict between opposing drives to speak and to hold back from speaking and has developed an interpretation of the moment of stuttering based on Neal E. Miller's research and theoretical formulations on approach-avoidance conflict in animals. Miller (1944) showed that as a hungry rat approaches a food trough at the end of a runway its motivation to reach the food steadily increases. It is possible to measure the strength of its approach drive and to show by means of a sloping line precisely how it increases with nearness to the goal. If electric shock is substituted for the food the rat flees. The farther it gets from the feared object, however, the weaker becomes its motivation to avoid it, and this declining avoidance drive may also be represented by a sloping line, or gradient. If electric shock and food are now combined, together with the appropriate cue-stimuli by which the rat may recognize their presence, the element of conflict is introduced. In such a situation the approach and avoidance drives are present together, and it is possible to represent this by showing both gradients superimposed on the same field *(Figure 4)*. Since the gradients slope in the same direction (both approach and avoidance increasing with nearness to the goal) they would appear as close parallel lines or the same line, except for one all-important fact. *The gradient of avoidance is steeper than the gradient of approach*.[14] As a result, if the opposing drives are of about the same average strength, at a certain distance from the goal the two gradients will intersect. This fact has some rather significant implications. Before the point of intersection is reached, the approach gradient is higher than the avoidance gradient, and the rat could be expected to run toward the goal. Once the animal had passed the intersection, however, it would find itself in a zone in which the strength of avoidance exceeded the strength of approach, and it could therefore be expected to turn and run the other way until approach exceeded avoidance again. This is precisely how Miller's rats behaved. They ran back and forth, vacillating within progressively narrower limits until they came to rest where the gradients apparently crossed, unable to go forward or back.

In Miller's description of the oscillatory behavior and fixations of these animals, Sheehan found a paradigm of the speech hesitations of stutterers. He stated that stuttering was basically an approach-avoidance conflict. Whenever stutterers' urge to speak was distinctly stronger than their desire to avoid speech, they spoke fluently. When

---

[14]This simply means that, within any given unit of distance from the goal or feared object the amount of change in the strength of avoidance is greater than the amount of change in the strength of approach.

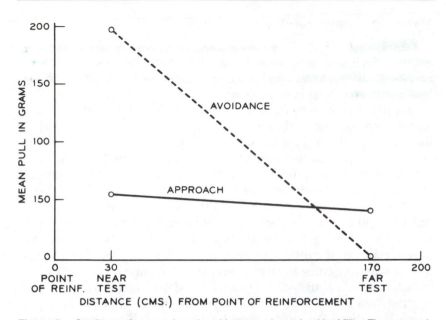

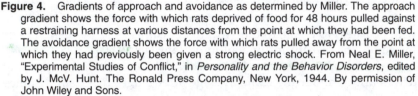

Figure 4.   Gradients of approach and avoidance as determined by Miller. The approach gradient shows the force with which rats deprived of food for 48 hours pulled against a restraining harness at various distances from the point at which they had been fed. The avoidance gradient shows the force with which rats pulled away from the point at which they had previously been given a strong electric shock. From Neal E. Miller, "Experimental Studies of Conflict," in *Personality and the Behavior Disorders*, edited by J. McV. Hunt. The Ronald Press Company, New York, 1944. By permission of John Wiley and Sons.

avoidance of speaking was the clearly dominant drive, they were silent. But when their approach and avoidance drives were in relative equilibrium, so that the gradients crossed, they stuttered. Unlike the rat, however, the stutterer does not remain fixated for an indefinite time. How could the termination of the block be accounted for? Sheehan offered the hypothesis that once the blocking had begun to take place the fear that had elicited it became reduced, the avoidance drive was consequently decreased, and so the conflict was temporarily resolved. Sheehan theorized further that the stutterer's conflicting feelings of approach and avoidance toward speech tended to be complicated by similar attitudes toward silence, and he pointed out that this, too, had its counterpart in the laboratory in the condition which Miller termed "double approach-avoidance conflict."

As we have already said, in a conflict analysis of stuttering behavior the fundamental question of why the act of stuttering occurs finally reduces itself to the question of the reasons for which a person might wish to avoid speech. Sheehan postulated five distinct "levels" on which speech avoidance drives might operate. He stated that these drives might emanate from 1) reactions to specific words, resulting principally from past conditioning to phonetic factors, 2) reactions to threatening speech situations, 3) guilt and anxiety concerning the emotional content of speech, 4) feelings of anxiety in the stutterer's relationships with listeners, especially when these are seen as authority figures, and 5) the ego-defensive need to avoid competitive endeavors posing "threat of failure or threat of success."

This clearly suggests that stuttering may have its origin both in the learning of speech anxieties and in unconscious factors of personality. Sheehan's formulations make little explicit reference to events surrounding the onset of stuttering. The essence of their contribution to stuttering theory is in the development of Miller's approach-avoidance conflict structure as a model of the moment of stuttering. The unique feature of this model, which Sheehan fully exploited, lies in its ability to adapt itself to both the repressed need and anticipatory struggle concepts of stuttering behavior and so by implication to admit a very broad array of logically possible etiologies. Sheehan (1970, 1975) later extended his theory still further by viewing the stutterer's difficulty as an approach-avoidance conflict between alternate roles assumed as a stutterer and as a normal speaker.

Perkins (1953) pointed out that the logical implication of the conflict hypothesis was that the stuttering block itself was not learned behavior. Since it was the involuntary resultant of the learned avoidance and approach drives, he believed that the block itself was not dependent on reinforcement and should not be subject to extinction by nonreinforcement. Both Sheehan (1951) and Perkins (1953) attempted to determine the effect on stuttering of nonreinforcement, which they defined by a procedure in which the subjects repeated each stuttered word until they could say it normally, and obtained somewhat conflicting results.

Stuttering as Operant Behavior

In 1958 Flanagan, Goldiamond, and Azrin announced that they had been able to reduce the stuttering of three laboratory subjects very markedly by presenting a 105 dB blast of tone immediately after each occasion on which the subjects blocked and to increase the frequency of stuttering by briefly turning off a continuous tone each time they stuttered. Not long afterward they reported that they had produced speech blockages at a high rate in a normal speaker by similar use of continuous electric shock (Flanagan, Goldiamond, and Azrin, 1959). These reports suggesting that stuttering and normal disfluency could be brought under "operant control" did much to arouse interest in investigating these behaviors by applying the conditioning principles of B. F. Skinner.

In Skinner's system of behavioral analysis, a central role is played by the kind of response, termed an operant, that is capable of being increased or decreased through its consequences as they affect the organism. In terms of a reference experiment, such as that in which a rat learns to press a lever when the response produces a pellet of food, operant conditioning is identical with what other workers termed instrumental conditioning, or instrumental act learning, but Skinner developed a distinctive conceptual scheme for its laboratory investigation. An outstanding feature distinguishing this scheme from theories of learning such as that of Hull is its strict renunciation of terms referring to hypothetical states inside the organism, such as *drive* or *anxiety*. In such a context the analysis of a given behavior consists essentially of a specification of the contingent consequences serving to reinforce and maintain it as a response to certain occasioning stimuli. This reinforcement is described as "positive" when it consists of such a stimulus as a pellet of food or as "negative" when it consists of the termination of an aversive stimulus such as shock. An important aspect of its laboratory description is the precise schedule on which it is administered.

It is such an analysis that Shames and Sherrick (1963) attempted to make of stuttering behavior in the light both of the diagnosogenic theory and of certain psychodynamic inferences about stuttering. Asserting that there is "no single, simple contingency for stuttering," they suggested that it is maintained by both positive and negative reinforcements on complex, multiple schedules. In large part, the paradigms they proposed as worthy of investigation were suggested by Johnson's theory of the etiology of stuttering.

They hypothesized that when a child's nonfluent responses are punished the child may respond by changing the form of nonfluency to struggle or silence. This change is reinforced by the termination of the aversive stimuli of nonfluency (negative reinforcement), but may occasion new punishment. Further cycles of change in the response may then take place, reinforced in each case by the termination of aversive stimuli emanating from the listener, and are also occasioned by the fact that stutterers tend to become their own listeners. In the process the original simple repetition degenerates through negative reinforcement into the abnormal response forms characteristic of stuttering. At the same time, however, there are certain positive reinforcements for stuttering. The child may gain attention or may use stuttering as an excuse for failure or inadequacy. Shames and Sherrick speculated that the cycles of change cease when a "dynamic equilibrium" evolves in which the positive reinforcements for a particular pattern of stuttering are stronger than its aversive consequences or the negative reinforcements for further change.

Approaching the problem from a somewhat different point of view, Shames and Sherrick posited that normal disfluency is also operant behavior and that stuttering and normal disfluency are in certain respects similar and continuous rather than completely separate classes of responses. On this assumption, any contingencies observed to influence the emission of disfluencies in children may be similar to those that control stuttering as a clinical disorder. Shames and Sherrick called attention to several ways in which disfluency may come to be reinforced by its contingent consequences.

For example, in a group situation speech repetitions have been found to occur frequently when the normal-speaking child tries to gain attention, to direct the activities of another child, to obtain an object possessed by someone else or is criticizing another child, being coerced into changing an activity, or the like (Davis, 1940). These examples belong for the most part to a type of verbal behavior that Skinner termed *manding*. They tend to occur on occasions of aversive stimulation or in states of deprivation, and as a consequence the listener frequently does something for or gives something to the child. In this way, not only the verbalization, but the repetition as well, is reinforced. This reinforcement is likely to be particularly strong because of the variable schedule on which it is usually given, responses intermittently reinforced being particularly resistant to extinction. Furthermore, if an unresponsive listener delays the reinforcement until the child has repeated the "manding" verbal behavior several times, the child is in effect being taught to repeat. Shames and Sherrick offered similar operant analyses of the increased repetition that may often be observed in children when confessing guilt, speaking to interrupting listeners, competing with other speakers, or attempting to hold the listener's attention during pauses.

Various other workers have made use of the operant model in connection with stuttering. For the most part, however, they have been less concerned with etiological theories than with experimental demonstrations of the operant nature of stuttering and disfluency. The result has been a considerable amount of research on punishment in relation to stuttering, which we will review in Chapter 8.

Stuttering as Conditioned Disintegration

In sharp contrast to the operant position is that of Brutten and Shoemaker (1967). They theorized that stuttering in its integral aspects is a failure or disruption of fluency resulting from emotional arousal that has become associated with speech and speech-related stimuli through a process of classical conditioning. From this point of view the stuttering block represents not operant, but respondent, behavior.

Most investigators of the learning process recognize at least a rough distinction between two kinds of learning, one based on operant or instrumental conditioning and the other on respondent or classical conditioning. Classical conditioning is represented by the well-known Pavlovian experiment in which a dog learns to salivate in response to a bell after several contiguous presentations of the bell with food. The fundamental point of contrast with operant learning is that the salivation is not instrumental in securing a reward. The dog gets the food whether performing the response or not, unlike the rat who is learning to operate a lever in a Skinner box. From the standpoint of the method used to bring learning about, in instrumental conditioning the basic contingency is between a response and a consequence. In classical conditioning, it is between two stimuli, one (e.g., food) having the power to elicit the response as an unlearned organismic reaction and the other a "neutral" stimulus having no such power until it is associated with the first.

How broad a role is played in human behavior by classical conditioning is a matter of theory. It appears to be widely agreed, however, that it plays an important part in the learning of anxiety reactions or other motivational states of autonomic arousal. Through classical conditioning, for example, a child who has once or twice responded autonomically to the doctor's needle may show a similar response to the doctor, or (by "higher-order" classical conditioning) to the doctor's driveway, and (by stimulus generalization) to white-coated persons anywhere.

This is the significance that classical conditioning has for stuttering from the point of view of Brutten and Shoemaker. They based their theory on the observation that in normal speakers stress may produce autonomic reactions capable of disrupting speech fluency. If a child repeatedly encounters stress in a given situation the negative emotion aroused may become a conditioned response to neutral stimuli in the situation. This marks the onset of the initial stage of stuttering. The child now regularly experiences emotional arousal with its attendant fluency failure each time the situational cues are present, instead of infrequently and sporadically as is usually the case. Furthermore, these cues, still chiefly situational in nature, increase in number through higher-order conditioning and stimulus generalization. Brutten and Shoemaker suggested that a further, or "advanced," stage of stuttering comes into being through penalties the child receives for abnormal speech behavior. As a result of such punishment, the act of speaking itself, or the words employed, come to elicit conditioned negative emotion, and in time the conditioned stimuli for fluency failure may for this reason consist increasingly of speech associated cues (i.e., words, listeners, and the like).

In support of their basic premise that stress, occasioned by the threat of painful stimulation, tends to increase disfluency, Brutten and Shoemaker pointed to observations by Hill (1954), Stassi (1961), and others. Perhaps the most direct experimental support for their theory comes from the work of Hill. In a study of normal-speaking subjects, Hill found that, when a red light that served as a signal for speech had been paired with electric shock on several occasions, the light by itself produced disorganized speech responses often "indistinguishable from what is generally termed stuttering."

It should be noted that Brutten and Shoemaker regard the so-called secondary features of stuttering as instrumental escape or avoidance mechanisms for coping with fluency failures or the noxious states resulting from them. This, however, is the only role they assign to operant conditioning. Their theory therefore presents us with a useful and relatively clear-cut issue, whether the integral symptoms of stuttering represent classically or instrumentally conditioned behavior, assuming that they represent one or the other. Brutten and Shoemaker actually referred to their conception of stuttering as a two-factor theory since it holds that the integral and associated symptoms are learned through two different kinds of conditioning. There does seem to be some evidence that the distinction between the two types of symptoms is not one of outward appearance alone,[15] but there is as yet no satisfactory answer to the question whether they represent two different types of conditioning.

Finally, it is of interest that it is clearly a breakdown concept of the moment of stuttering that is expressed in this theory, and, unlike other learning-oriented viewpoints, it owes less to Johnson's thinking than to that of West. The development of stuttering is ascribed, not to speech anxiety, but to stress in essentially any form, and constitutional predisposition, in the form of innate conditionability and autonomic reactivity, is considered to play a part.

It was an observation of West's that in time speech anxiety came to be a major source of the stress that precipitated moments of breakdown in speech. This, too, has its counterpart in Brutten and Shoemaker's observation that as stuttering develops the autonomic reactions disruptive of fluency become increasingly conditioned to speech-associated stimuli as a result of speech-related punishment. A difference of major importance is in the role assigned to learning. The dysphemic viewpoint

---

[15]The integral and secondary features of stuttering have been reported to load differently in a factor analysis of stuttering phenomena (Prins and Lohr, 1972), to vary in frequency differently in the course of repeated readings of the same material (Sakata and Adams, 1972; Webster and Brutten, 1972), and to respond differently to contingent stimuli and instructions to avoid stuttering (see Chapter 8).

that was widely influential some years ago contained a notable gap. It never explained convincingly how the chronic tendency to breakdown in speech that was postulated to underlie the stutterer's blocks could have been initiated by a single original episode of breakdown in early childhood, as though speech were a strut that, once broken, remained irreparably weak. In transferring the breakdown concept to a learning frame of reference, Brutten and Shoemaker bridged the gap effectively through the medium of stimulus substitution by classical conditioning.

Cybernetic Models of Stuttering

As we all learned as schoolchildren, the widespread replacement of hand tools with power-driven machines that began in the nineteenth century is commonly regarded as an industrial "revolution." It is interesting, therefore, that less than a century later there has been a second development in the use of mechanical devices that qualified observers view as no less revolutionary than the first. This is the introduction of machines that regulate themselves by automatic control systems or servomechanisms.

Automatic Control Systems

The basic principle of a servomechanism is that of *feedback.* An ordinary machine consists of an effector unit producing output in the form of some type of work and a device for regulating or controlling it. In a servosystem the essential added feature is a means for feeding back part of the output of the machine and allowing it to play on the control mechanism in such a way that what the machine does is regulated by its performance. A simple example of a servomechanism is the one that regulates the usual type of home heating system. The heating unit is controlled by a temperature-sensitive device, or thermostat, which automatically turns on or shuts off the unit when its output, the temperature of the room, differs by a certain amount from a desired output as represented by the setting on the thermostat. A system of this sort obviously depends upon its ability to perform a simple internal handling of information. The invention in this century of highly successful information-processing devices known as electronic computers has made possible the development of a large variety of complex servomechanisms for such purposes as automatic control of industrial processes and automatic guidance of space vehicles.

The major components of an automatic control system may be described in general terms. The system contains a *sensor,* through which part of the output of the machine is converted to a form in which it can be fed back as information to the *controller* unit. The controller unit contains a *comparator,* which compares the actual output with some intended performance in the form of instructions that have been stored in the controller as a unit of input. The difference between these two sets of data emerges from the comparator as an error signal. This is mixed with the input signal to produce an effective driving signal, which modifies the action of the *effector* unit so that its output more nearly equals the intended output.

Cybernetic Theory of Speech

An exceedingly interesting fact about the principle of feedback is that its signiflcance appears to extend substantially beyond the realm of mechanical devices. Wiener (1948) coined the term cybernetics to cover the broad application of automatic control principles and a related development known as information theory to engineering, biology, and the behavioral sciences. Some notable examples of biological systems that are illuminated by servo theory are the kinesthetic and proprioceptive mechanisms for automatic control of motor activity and the various internal homeostatic mechanisms for regulating body temperature, blood pressure, water balance, and the chemical contents of the blood and alveolar air.

The normal production of speech is an automatic process whose dependence on feedback has long been taken for granted. Although the extent of this dependence is no longer accepted without question, it should come as no surprise that cybernetic models of speech have been proposed and thoughtfully worked out. A basic schematic of the speech mechanism as a servosystem was drawn by Fairbanks (1954). In Fairbanks' model (*Figure 5*) the effector unit corresponds to the vocal organs and their motor innervation. The major sensor is the ear, which senses the output of the effector unit through two channels, symbolizing air and bone conduction. The hypothetical controller unit is obviously some feature of the brain. Fairbanks deliberately refrained from speculating about its precise identity. He hypothesized that at a given moment during speech its storage contains a unit of input that corresponds to as much as we can "hold in mind" of what we intend to say. This unit of input is continually compared with feedback about the output. The error signal that results from this comparison is a measure of the amount by which the speech unit displayed in the storage device has not yet been realized. The error signal is sent to the mixer, where it contributes to the effective driving signal. Simultaneously, it is also sent to the storage, where it signals the storage to continue to display the speech unit, or, when the error signal is about to equal zero, to display the next unit. Fairbanks pointed out that the source of input to the controller was a language system, not shown in his diagram, which originates messages. His model was concerned only with the speaking system.

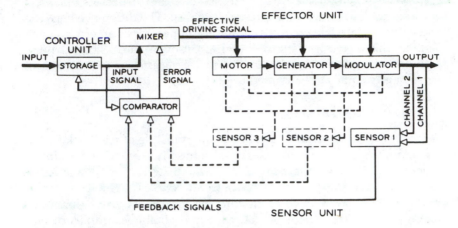

Figure 5. Fairbanks' model of an automatic control system for speaking. The respiratory, phonatory, and articulatory parts of the speech mechanism are represented as motor, generator, and modulator, respectively. Part of their audible output is conducted to the speaker's ear (sensor 1) by means of two channels (air and bone conduction). A hypothetical comparator unit compares the feedback signals from the sensor with an input signal (from a language system, not shown) representing an intended message unit. The difference, representing the amount by which the intended unit of message has not yet been completed, is fed to the mixer where it is combined with the input signal and serves to modify the operation of the effector so that its output more closely approximates the intended message unit. The portions of the model represented by broken lines represent tactile and proprioceptive feedback mechanisms providing information about the operation of the effector, but not about its output. From Fairbanks (1954). Copyright 1954 by the American Speech-Language-Hearing Association. Reprinted by permission.

Delayed Auditory Feedback (DAF) and "Stuttering" in Normal Speakers

At about the same time that Fairbanks offered his feedback theory of speech, attention was being drawn to the possibility that a link existed between feedback and stuttering. This came about principally as the result of an observation that was first made by Lee (1950a, 1950b, 1951) and that has been confirmed by a large number of further investigations by others. It is possible, by means of a magnetic-tape recording and reproducing device suitably designed, to return a subject's vocal output to the subject via earphones with a brief delay in transmission. The basic observation with which we are concerned is that when normal speakers' air-conducted auditory feedback is retarded in this way by a time interval of the order of 0.2 seconds and amplified sufficiently to compete with their normal bone-conducted feedback, there tends to be a disintegrative effect on their verbal output. This disintegration takes the form of a slow speaking rate, articulatory inaccuracy, and disturbances of fluency, including, in some cases, blockings and repetition of syllables that may offer a realistic imitation of clinical stuttering. In addition, there is usually an increase in loudness and pitch which Fairbanks (1955) inferred to result from the subjects' struggle to resist the interference with their response.

It is, of course, in the repetitions that we are most interested. Fairbanks and Guttman (1958) found that there was a relatively small number of subjects for whom frequent repetition was a characteristic response and that the repetition consisted almost entirely of simple double articulations. Several explanations of them have been offered. Lee (1950a) initially compared them with the behavior of an unstable electronic circuit oscillating with feedback which the first chance disturbance has set off. More generally, they are regarded as a direct effect of the misinformation that DAF gives to subjects about their speech output. Lee (1950b) conjectured that the "unsatisfied monitor" of the speech circuit causes the loop to "continue for an extra turn or two" until the missing feedback returns. In short, if you say it and you don't hear it, you think you haven't said it, so you say it again. Fairbanks and Guttman offered a somewhat different explanation. They inferred that in a rapid sequence of serial speech responses each response cannot be evoked individually. It must therefore be cued automatically by feedback from the preceding response. This being so, if delayed feedback from the first response dominates the feedback complex during a second response, it will trigger a repetition of the second response.[16]

Speech Behavior Under DAF as an Analogue of Stuttering

Lee referred to his effect as "artificial stutter" and expressed the view that it might have significant implications for speech therapy. Soon afterward Fairbanks (1955) and other investigators of the DAF phenomenon were similarly intrigued by its hypothetical relationship to stuttering as a clinical disorder of speech. Chase (1958) discovered that most subjects could repeat a speech sound faster under DAF than with nor-

---

consistency and adaptation effects are discussed in Chapters 7 and 8.
[16]Fairbanks and Guttman showed that, given certain assumptions, this explanation implies that a single repetition will temporarily restore the normal phase relationship between response and feedback. The explanation is therefore consistent with their observation that the repetitions of normal speakers under DAF generally consist of simple double articulations except in rare instances that "give the impression of wild and uncontrolled oscillation of the vocal mechanism." It should be noted, incidentally, that the syllable repetitions of stutterers consist largely of double and triple articulations that appear with about equal frequency (see the normative data gathered by Johnson, 1961a).

mal feedback and suggested that the factors responsible for this might also be at work in some types of stuttering. In the meantime experiments had shown that many stutterers speak fluently under conditions of loud white noise (*see Chapter 8*), and it was tempting to speculate that the noise served to mask out the stutterer's innately deviant auditory feedback.

Clearly, the interest which developed in the Lee effect as an analogue of stuttering rests on what may be nothing more than a chance resemblance between two unrelated kinds of behavior. Attempting to gauge the extent of this similarity, Neelley (1961) found that listeners were usually able to distinguish the speech of normal speakers under DAF from the speech of stutterers and that stutterers for the most part felt that their habitual stuttering and their speech behavior under DAF were different kinds of experiences. Neelley also tried to determine whether normal speakers' errors under DAF tended to occur consistently on the same words and to decrease in frequency with successive readings of the same material in a manner characteristic of stuttering.[17] He found far less consistency and adaptation in the normal speakers under DAF than in his stuttering subjects in an ordinary reading situation. Neelley concluded that his findings as a whole tended to discredit the hypothesis that stuttering is related to delayed auditory feedback. This conclusion has been countered by Yates (1963), Beech and Fransella (1968, p. 169), and others with the argument that behavior that has been subject to change and development over many years is bound to differ in many respects from similar behavior when it is exhibited by laboratory subjects for the first time.

Brandt and Wilde (1977) found that, like stuttering, the disfluency of normal speakers under DAF was reduced when the subjects read in unison with another voice and when they timed their speech to the beat of a metronome. Borden, Dorman, Freeman, and Raphael (1977) observed both similarities and differences between normal speakers under DAF and stutterers in the electromyographic recordings from laryngeal and articulatory muscles. Venkatagiri (1980, 1982a) found that, like stutterings, the DAF disfluencies of normal speakers showed a distinct adaptation effect over successive readings and occurred more often on content words than on function words and on long words than on short words. Unlike stutterings, they did not occur preponderantly on the first syllables of words or the first words of sentences.[18] Although the consistency effect was present, it was considerably smaller than it is in the case of stuttering.

---

[18]See Chapter 7. Venkatagiri comments, "These differences, however, are not unexpected . . . In order to delay the feedback, the speech must be produced in the first place." How stutterings can occur on initial syllables poses a problem for the delayed auditory feedback theory.

Stuttering as "Verbalizing Deautomaticity"

Whether or not stuttering is related to delayed auditory feedback is not crucial to a theory of stuttering based on automatic control principles. Mysak (1960, 1966) brought a wide range of concepts about stuttering within the scope of servo theory by a cybernetic interpretation of the view that stuttering is basically a failure of the automaticity of speech. Mysak proposed the hypothesis that a disturbance in essentially any of the feedback circuits of the servosystem that maintains the automatic flow of verbal communication may result in stuttering. Extending Fairbanks' model to include language as well as speech, he discussed the various parts of the system in which the disturbances may occur:

1. They may occur in a hypothetical integrator unit in which thought and language connections are made. For example, unconscious guilt about verbal expressions of hostility may cause blocks or hesitations as the speaker "feels the need to guard against the automatic processing of his thoughts into words." Mysak refers to psychoanalytic concepts of stuttering and to Sheehan's conflict theory in this connection.

2. Disturbance may occur in that part of the speech controller (transmitter, in Mysak's terminology) in which word patterns are formulated internally as commands to the effector unit. As examples, Mysak cites the repetitive speech disruptions that have been observed to accompany such disorders as parkinsonism and pseudobulbar palsy and the interference with speech that Penfield and Roberts noted on electrical stimulation of certain areas of the brain in their well-known studies. West's theory of stuttering as an epileptiform disorder of speech is also noted here.

3. Reformulating Johnson's views in terms of servo theory, Mysak suggests that the overmonitoring of fluency by "another communication system" may cause the development of a predicted fluency error signal in a child's speech comparator. As a result, the child's system may engage in an intentional scanning of its output for nonexistent error signals in a manner that interferes with speech automaticity.

4. Stuttering may originate in the sensor unit, as indicated by the effects on speech of disturbances in auditory feedback.

5. Finally, speech automaticity may be affected by disturbances in a feedback loop involving the listener. That is, if children repeatedly receive listener reactions indicating that their message has not been understood, they may come to anticipate such feedback and to "habitually re-formulate or repeat" their utterances.

It is clear that in Mysak's theoretical formulations stuttering is defined very broadly. The possibility must be considered, however, that such a broad definition is inherent in the servo model. That is, if stuttering results from the breakdown of an interdependent circuitry that functions as a whole, then from the standpoint of the model there may be little justification for making sharp distinctions based on the cause or locus of the disturbance.

CONCLUDING OBSERVATIONS

Types of Theories Reviewed

We may conclude this chapter by calling attention once more to two distinctions we have made. First, there is the very fundamental one that exists between conceptual models of the stuttering moment and theories about the conditions under which the disorder develops. With regard to the moment of stuttering, there appear, broadly speaking, to be three major hypotheses, which view it respectively as a breakdown under stress, the fulfillment of a neurotic need, and an anticipatory reaction of struggle or avoidance. These three descriptions subsume a large variety of interpretations of the act of stuttering. In the effort to find the most accurate model, analogues of stuttering have been discerned in, to mention a few examples, the convulsive seizure, the perseverative reactions of the brain-injured, the compulsive act of the emotionally disturbed, sexual impotence, writer's cramp, the posture of runners on their mark, the behavior of golfers rehearsing the start of a swing, the bodily tremors of rage or fear, the oscillatory breakdown of a mechanical device pushed beyond its capacity by internal damage or external stress, and the behavior of a rat as it runs from danger, is caught immobilized between two feared goals, or presses a bar to gain a pellet of food.

Theories of the etiology of stuttering are conveniently classified as breakdown, repressed need, or anticipatory struggle theories, depending upon the model of the moment of stuttering adopted. Breakdown theories of onset attribute the disorder to the effects of early environmental stress and usually assign an important role to constitutional predisposing factors. The principal issues they serve to raise concern the precise nature of these organic factors and the extent to which the incidence of stuttering is influenced by heredity. Repressed need theories about the etiology of stuttering tend to merge with theories of the etiology of neurotic behavior generally. They raise the question of whether stutterers typically possess a neurotic type of personality and why they choose stuttering as a symptom. Current theories of the etiology of stuttering as anticipatory struggle behavior ascribe it to parental penalties for normal disfluency or to pressures extending to a broader range of possible speech failures. Among the issues they raise, perhaps the most fundamental is the specific nature of the relationship, if any, that exists between stuttering and normal disfluency.

Having made a distinction between theories of the moment of stuttering and theories of etiology, we may say that any adequate theoretical formulation about stuttering provides both. Above all, a theory of the etiology of stuttering tends to make a marked impression of incompleteness unless it is accompanied at least implicitly by a consistent conceptual model of the stuttering act to bridge the gap between the conditions under which the disorder is said to develop and the precipitation, at any later point, of a discrete example of the behavior. Lacking this particular kind of elaboration, the mere statement that stuttering is "due to" insecurity or "caused by" an enlarged thymus gland, delayed myelinization of cortical areas, or the like, is somewhat like the representation of a body without a visible connection between head and torso.

The converse of this, a theory that is incomplete because it is wholly concerned with the stuttering moment, perhaps does not strike us quite so unfavorably. It will be recalled, for example, that some of the systematic discussions of stuttering in terms of learning theory that we have reviewed have given scant attention to the etiology of the disorder. Perhaps the reason for the greater acceptability of such theories is that with a proper understanding of the moment of stuttering it would be possible, in principle, to devise effective therapeutic measures in the absence of essentially any notion of its etiology.

The second distinction we have made is between theories that are indigenous to their frame of reference and those representing old theories shifted to a new conceptual orientation. The new frameworks have been provided chiefly by theories of learning and to a lesser extent by cybernetic theory. Learning interpretations of stuttering have represented it as an instrumental avoidance response reinforced by anxiety reduction, as an approach-avoidance conflict, as positively and negatively reinforced operant behavior, and as classically conditioned disintegrative emotional arousal. They have drawn chiefly upon Johnson's diagnosogenic theory, upon psychoanalytic concepts of stuttering, and upon dysphemic breakdown theories. The basic research issue that the conflicting formulations have served to raise concerns the nature of the reinforcement by which stuttering is maintained.

A frequent advantage in the use of new frames of reference is the gain in verifiability that a reformulation in more rigorous terms may bring about. A theory may be poor not because it is untrue, but because it is logically incapable of verification as stated. For example, the conceptions that stuttering is due to "habit," to "nervousness," or to children's attempts to talk faster than they can think—or to think faster than they can talk—are so ambiguous in their terminology that it is possible neither to prove them nor to dispose of them. In its proper frame of reference, however, the meaningless question of whether stuttering is a "habit" becomes the question of whether it is a conditioned operant, a formulation that suggests certain observations that might be employed to answer it.

Multicausality

To some workers the complexity of the stuttering problem has appeared to justify the question whether stuttering has not one but many causes. When we consider the varied meanings with which the term *multicausal* may be used in connection with stuttering, however, it becomes evident that such a question needs considerable refinement before it can be answered. Perhaps some clarification may be gained by noting that the concept of multicausality appears in discussions of stuttering in three general forms which may be referred to for convenience as the *no-model*, *single-model*, and *multimodel* forms.

No-Model Multicausality

The impressive accumulation of plausible theories about the etiology of stuttering sometimes evokes the reaction that there must be "some truth" in all of them. Those who find this an easy solution to the problem must be prepared to answer the objection that we as yet have essentially no conclusive evidence to show that *any* of the current theories of stuttering is wholly or partially valid, let alone to support the somewhat improbable conclusion that they all are. There is, however, an even more basic deficiency inherent in such casual appeals to the concept of multicausality. Let us take as a fabricated example the simple assertion that stuttering may be caused in some cases by an organic predisposition, in others by a parental misdiagnosis of stuttering, and in still others by neurotic insecurity fostered by disturbed family relationships. As it stands, such a proposal is essentially empty because it offers no model of the *moment* of stuttering to make the assumption of a multiplicity of causes necessary or plausible. Hence, it is open to the same criticism that may be made of any theory of the etiology of stuttering that fails to erect a bridge between the cause of the disorder and the precipitation of the individual instance of speech interruption. We are left to wonder how all these things eventually result in repetitions or prolongations of speech sounds.

Single-Model Multicausality

The term *multicausal* has sometimes been used to characterize theories of somewhat broad scope that offer a single model of the moment of stuttering. Examples are Sheehan's conflict theory, Mysak's deautomaticity theory, Eisenson's perseverative theory, and various others. Through their single concept of the stuttering moment, such theories often seek to unite several viewpoints or various observations on the etiology of stuttering by showing how they all add up to conflict, or to deautomaticity, or whatever. Despite this fact, we have grounds for questioning whether the term *multicausal* has unambiguous meaning as applied to such theories.

In the first place, it is obvious that multicausality may refer either to the interaction of multiple factors that contribute jointly to the etiology in a given case or to the notion of different etiologies in different cases. We pass over this ambiguity, however, to deal with a more serious one. In the case in which we assume a single model of stuttering behavior, *the extent to which stuttering is a multicausal phenomenon appears to be merely an artifact of the level of abstraction on which we happen to be discussing its causation.*

An analogy will suffice to make this clear. Does the motor disorder known as athetosis have one or more than one cause, and if several, how many? Ignoring certain areas of doubt or controversy, we could obviously set down a fairly long but not endless list of "textbook" causes, including birth injury, anoxia, maternal disease, and the like. But each of these causes has causes, and if we pursued these branching pathways for any distance we would soon have to admit that athetosis has a practically limitless number of "causes," or, to put it somewhat differently, it is highly improbable that any set of causal circumstances will ever exactly duplicate themselves from case to case.

Instead of being more specific, however, we can, if we choose, be more abstract and reduce our original list of causes to a smaller number of more general ones in almost any way we please. In fact, if we are willing to be abstract enough we can say that athetosis has just one possible cause—damage to certain parts of the extrapyramidal motor tract of the central nervous system. Clearly, any question about the number of "causes" of athetosis is meaningless unless we can somehow specify the level of generality or abstractness on which we are asking it.[19] Similarly, hoarseness has a great variety of causes; yet it also has just one cause: aperiodic vibration of the vocal folds.

This is not to say that it is not useful to describe differences in the factors or sets of circumstances that may lead to athetosis or hoarseness. In this book we shall, in fact, place considerable emphasis on different circumstances as they relate to the etiology of stuttering. The point we are making here is simply that when they are seen in their

---

[19]Korzybski (1941, p. 433) expressed this succinctly by saying that "cause" is a multiordinal term (i.e., a term that has different meanings on different levels of abstraction).

proper light essentially all theories that imply a single, unique model of the stuttering block must in some sense be both unicausal and multicausal. To say that stuttering has multiple causes with this type of concept in view is to add relatively little to our understanding. What we need to know in addition is the nature of the immediate *single* cause of stuttering and precisely how it is related to the numerous more remote causes.

Multimodel Theories

Finally, it is possible to suppose that stuttering in one person represents an act of oral gratification, in another the effort to keep from stuttering again, and in still a third a disruption due to internal delayed auditory feedback. In other words, we may say that stuttering has multiple causes because what appears to be a single type of speech difficulty actually represents several basically different forms of abnormal speech behavior having little or no relationship to each other beyond their superficial similarity. In one sense, whether or not this is true may depend on how broadly we define the term *stuttering*. To most workers it seems unlikely that any and all types of speech interruption are symptoms of a single underlying disorder. Freund (1966, Chapter 17) distinguished "common" stuttering systematically from certain hysterical symptoms resembling it, from the "stuttering" that appears to be associated with certain types of brain damage, and from the disfluencies belonging to the symptomatology of cluttering.[20] Few would be inclined to quarrel with the mutual differentiation of these phenomena. Not all would use the term *stuttering* for all of them at the present time, but that is a matter of definition. We will return to this subject shortly.

A more controversial issue arises when the multimodel hypothesis is invoked in connection with "common" stuttering in an attempt to account for some of its obscurities. The idea that what we ordinarily call stuttering represents two or more separate and unrelated disorders can hardly be dismissed as impossible and must always be kept in view. As a theory, however, it is far from ideal from the standpoint of parsimony, and requires the assumption that a number of totally separate underlying causes produce symptoms which quite by chance strongly resemble each other. Before we advance such a theory we should be sure that it does not merely reflect a failure to generalize far enough about our "separate and unrelated" disorders to unite them with reference to one ultimate concept of the moment of stuttering.

---

[20]See also Johnson et al. (1967, p. 241) for a similar differentiation.

In addition, it cannot be insisted too strongly that a theory stating that we have in stuttering not one but several distinct clinical entities is meaningless unless it provides hypotheses about the procedures or observations for their differential diagnosis on the basis of differences in the symptomatology, in the conditions under which the difficulty varies, in the pattern of distribution of stutterings in the speech sequence, or in some other observable features of the behavior. In short, if the hypothesis is that different etiologies give rise to different forms of stuttering, then one must attempt to theorize about the respects in which the forms are actually different. Without such operational definitions of the separate clinical entities which we are postulating, we do not have a multimodel theory, but only the surmise that it might be possible to advance one. This surmise has been made rather frequently, but theories of this type are as yet essentially lacking.

The Search for Subtypes of Stutterers

In place of multimodel theories, all we have are a few widely scattered research efforts to identify etiological subtypes of stutterers. Berlin (1955) and Andrews and Harris (1964, Chap. 6) tried to do it largely on the basis of features of subjects' case histories, while Prins and Lohr (1972) based their attempt on visible and audible features of their stuttering. Two of these studies employed factor analysis. In each instance little difficulty was found in isolating clusters of characteristics that seemed to belong together, but their etiological significance is an open question. Belyakova (1973) reported quantitative differences in the electromyographic recordings from the orbicularis oris muscle during stuttering in patients who exhibited signs of "diffuse organic lesions of the central nervous system" and patients whose stuttering represented "neurotic reactions." Riley and Riley (1980) factor analyzed the performance of stuttering children on tests of motor coordination, psycholinguistic abilities, and severity of stuttering. The analysis yielded factors that could be presumed to be related to the development of stuttering, notably oral motor ability, language skills, and auditory perceptual ability. Subgroups of stutterers were not identified, however (Riley and Riley, 1984).

Preus (1981) made a comprehensive search for subgroups among 100 stutterers using seventy variables related to symptomatology, reactive aspects, language development, frequency of stuttering under various conditions, intellect, signs of brain damage, general anxiety, and emotional adjustment. He could find no evidence that stuttering is an "aggregation of separate disorders." In a subsequent study Preus (1983) reported some success in distinguishing a "neurogenic" and a "psychogenic" subgroup as defined by Halstead's Impairment Index (suggesting cerebral dysfunction) and the Minnesota Multiphasic Personality Inventory.

Schwartz and Conture (1988) subgrouped 43 young stutterers on the basis of disfluency types and the number and variety associated behaviors. They found a number of clusters and partial support for differentiating between a predominantly "clonic" and a predominantly "tonic" type of stutterer.

Poulos and Webster (1991) used family history of stuttering as a basis for subgrouping 169 stutterers. Like West, Nelson, and Berry (1939), they found that those without such a history were considerably more likely to have suffered birth injuries or other early conditions suggesting possible brain damage. Janssen, Kraaimaat, and Brutten (1990) noted some possible differences in type of stuttering between subject with and without a family background of stuttering.

Acquired Stuttering

It is possible to work the other way. One can choose groups of subjects among whom there are good grounds to suspect a representation of different etiologies and try to find features that differentiate them. The attempt to differentiate so-called *acquired stuttering* from ordinary developmental stuttering is an outstanding example. Aquired stuttering is a relatively uncommon phenomenon having sudden onset in adulthood. Although adults have been reported to acquire stuttering as a result of combat fatigue or other types of emotional stress,[21] adult-onset stuttering is generally a symptom of brain injury and is often referred to as neurogenic or cortical stuttering.[22] It may be transient or persistent. It has been observed in cases of traumatic head injury, stroke, degenerative disease of the central nervous system, brain tumor, brain surgery, and drug-induced brain dysfunction. The frontal, parietal, or temporal lobes may be involved. The injury is usually reported in the left hemisphere of the brain, but sometimes in the right in right-handed individuals. Neurogenic stuttering is often associated with aphasia, apraxia of speech, or dysarthria, but may occur in the absence of any other speech or language difficulties. The majority of cases reported have been male.

---

[21]See Peacher and Harris (1946), Dempsey and Granich (1978), Deal (1982), Roth, Aronson, and Davis (1989),Tippett and Siebens (1991), Mahr and Leith (1992).

[22]Schiller (1947), Arend, Handzel, and Weiss (1962), Shtremel (1963), Canter (1971) Caplan (1972), Rosenfield (1972), Helm and Butler (1977), Quinn and Andrews (1977) Helm, Butler, and Benson (1978) Rosenbek, Messert, Collins, and Wertz (1978), Donnan (1979), Inglis (1979), Helm, Butler, and Canter (1980), Rosenfield Miller, and Feltovich (1980), Baratz and Mesulam (1981), Mazzucchi, Moretti, Carpeggiani, Parma, and Paini (1981), Homer and Massey (1983), Koller (1983), Lebrun, Leleux, Rousseau, and Devreaux (1983), Lebrun, Rétif, and Kaiser (1983), Rentschler, Driver, and Callaway (1984), Lebrun and Leleux (1985), McClean and McLean (1985), Ardila and Lopez (1986), Nagafuchi and Saso (1986), Rousey, Arjunan, and Rousey (1986), Marshall and Neuburger (1987), Nowack and Stone (1987), Lebrun, Bijleveld, and Rousseau (1990), Market, Montague, Buffalo, and Drummond (1990), Meyers, Hall, and Aram (1990), Rosenfield, Viswanath, Callis-Landrum, Di Danato, and Nudelman (1991).

In most instances the symptoms of neurogenic stuttering are described as repetitions or prolongations of initial sounds, syllables, or words without effort, secondary symptoms, or signs of anxiety. However, exceptions to this description are not uncommon. Pauses, hesitations, and "blocks" are sometimes said to occur. In a case described by Baratz and Mesulam (1981) stuttering was accompanied by grimacing, and Rosenbek et al (1978) cited three cases in which signs of effort, hurry, grimacing, and eye-blinking were evident. Koller (1983) noted mild annoyance or frustration as reactions to stuttering in three of six patients, though none had the ability that most stutterers possess to predict the occurrence of their blockages.

There is frequent mention of more stuttering on function words than on content words. In contrast, developmental stuttering occurs more often on content words (*see Chapter 7*), although difficulty on function words does occur and is very common in its early forms. Canter (1971), however, heard repetitions and prolongations on the final consonants of words in most of his cases of neurogenic stuttering—an observation rarely noted in ordinary stuttering. This was not so in any of the seven cases of Rosenbek et al (1978), but in the single case described by Lebrun and Leleux (1985) a few repetitions occurred "in medial or final positions," and Ardila and Lopez (1986) noted repetitions in final positions in their case. In eight cases described by Rosenfield, Viswanath, Callis-Landrum, Di Danato, and Nudelman (1991), all were said to stutter in all positions in words, including the final.

Canter (1971) suggested on the basis of his clinical observations that failure to diminish in frequency with repeated readings of the same passage (adaptation) was one of the features by which neurogenic stuttering could be differentiated from developmental stuttering. In confirmation, others have reported the absence of an adaptation effect.[23] The adaptation effect was evident, however, in the sixteen cases studied by Mazzucchi et al (1981) and in the six of Koller (1983). One of the two neurogenic stutterers presented by Quinn and Andrews (1977) exhibited both adaptation and the consistency effect. The five cases of Caplan (1972) adapted in repeated answers to questions, but not in reading sentence material. From a questionnaire survey of 81 cases, Market, Montague, Buffalo, and Drummond (1990) concluded that about 46 percent did not exhibit the adapation effect.

In the case of ordinary developmental stuttering, individuals who do not show the adaptation effect are not uncommon, nor are those

---

[23]Helm and Butler (1977), Helm, Butler, and Benson (1978), Ardila and Lopez (1986), Nagafuchi and Saso (1986), Nowack and Stone (1987), Rosenfield, Viswanath, Callis-Landrum, Di Danato, and Nudelman (1991).

who fail to exhibit secondary symptoms or clear signs of anxiety. Very rare, however, is the person who stutters when singing, speaking in time to rhythm, speaking at a reduced rate, or when subjected to various other fluency-inducing conditions (see Chapters 7 and 8) Rosenfield (1972) reported on a patient with neurogenic stuttering whose speech difficulty did not decrease in singing or in speaking rhythmically or in unison with another person. Of the two cases described in detail by Quinn and Andrews (1977), one showed improvement with masking noise, delayed auditory feedback, and the use of a slow speaking rate, but the other did not. The patient cited by Helm and Butler (1977) stuttered more rather than less when speaking syllable by syllable with the aid of a pacing board. Koller (1983) mentioned two individuals with neurogenic stuttering who stuttered when singing. In contrast, Horner and Massey (1983) described a sixty-two-year-old stroke patient who sang without stuttering. However, the writers preferred a diagnosis of palilalia, rather than neurogenic stuttering, for this patient inasmuch as his speech pattern was dominated by rapid rate, monotony, and more word and phrase than sound or syllable repetition. A further counterexample was a forty-two-year-old man who began to stutter after being put on Dilantin for the control of seizures due to an accidental head injury (McClean and McLean, 1985); his stuttering was reduced in unison reading and when speaking at a decreased rate under delayed auditory feedback. However, the stroke patient cited by Ardila and Lopez (1986) stuttered in unison reading and metronome-timed speech. One of the two patients described by Nowack and Stone (1987) stuttered when whispering. And the eight patients of Rosenfield, Viswanath, Callis-Landrum, Di Danato, and Nudelman (1991) for the most part stuttered when singing, speaking at a slow rate, and speaking in masking noise.

In sum, it has become increasing clear that the stutter of many adults with brain damage has features that distinguish it from the developmental variety of stuttering. It appears that we are dealing, not with multiple causation of one speech disorder, but with a case of different causes producing different disorders.

Cluttering

The hasty, repetitive, hesitant pattern of speech known as cluttering is another type of disfluency believed to differ in etiology from the common variety of stuttering it often resembles. A number of efforts have been made to differentiate it objectively from stuttering. Langová and Morávek (1964) found differences between stutterers and clutterers in brain waves and in the effects of drugs on their speech. They also observed that delayed auditory feedback had a more deleterious effect on the speech of those regarded as clutterers, as did Hutchinson and Burk (1973). Rieber, Breskin, and Jaffe (1972) found higher mean pause times in stutterers than clutterers during oral reading, and Rieber (1975) reported lower reading rates in stutterers. Five clutterers studied by Dewar, Dewar, and Barnes (1976) were aided far less by masking noise than were a group of stutterers. Rieber, Smith, and Harris (1976) found that word length and word position in the sentence influenced stuttering and cluttering similarly, but that stuttering was more closely associated with the initial sound of the word. St. Louis, Hinzman, and Hull (1985) found less complex and complete utterances in the speech of "possible clutterers," whom they defined as children judged to be disfluent in articulation, but not stutterers.

Summary

We may sum up this discussion of the concept of multicausality in stuttering by saying that our chief concern has been to show, not that the concept is erroneous, but that it is all too easy to adopt it without proper regard for its implications. Multicausality has so many possible meanings that we simply are not conveying very much information about stuttering when we say, without extensive further qualification, that it has "multiple causes." Furthermore, when we do make the appropriate qualifications we find that, depending on the kind of multicausality we are talking about, the extent to which it applies to stuttering is partly a matter of the level of abstraction that we choose or of how broadly we define "stuttering." It is possible to define a type of multicausality in stuttering that is neither meaningless nor trivial. The differentiation of acquired stuttering, cluttering, and "common" stuttering is an example. But theories of common developmental stuttering that are multicausal by this multimodel definition have not yet been advanced.

Suggested Readings

Adams, M. R., The demands and capacities model: I. Theoretical elaborations. *J. Fluency Dis., 15,* 135–41, (1990).

Bloom, L., Notes for a history of speech pathology. *Psychoanal. Rev., 65,* 433–463 (1978).

Brutten, E. J., and Shoemaker, D. J., *The Modification of Stuttering.* Englewood Cliffs, NJ.: Prentice-Hall (1967), Chaps. 1, 2.

Eisenson, J. (ed.), *Stuttering: A Second Symposium.* New York: Harper & Row (1975).

Fenichel, O., *The Psychoanalytic Theory of Neurosis.* New York: W. W. Norton (1945), Chap. 15.

Geschwind, N., and Galaburda, A. M., Cerebral lateralization: Biological mechanisms, associations, and pathology: I. A hypothesis and a program for research. *Arch. Neurol., 42,* 429–459 (1985).

Johnson, W., et al, *Speech Handicapped School Children*, 3rd ed., New York: Harper & Row (1967), pp. 277–85.

Mysak, E. D., *Speech Pathology and Feedback Theory.* Springfield, Ill.: Charles C Thomas (1966), Chaps. 1, 2, 7.

Rosenbek, J. C., Stuttering secondary to nervous system damage. In Curlee, R. F., and Perkins, W. H. (eds.), *Nature and Treatment of Stuttering: New Directions.* San Diego: College-Hill Press (1984).

Shames, G. H., and Rubin, H., *Stuttering Then and Now, Part II.* Columbus: Merrill (1986).

Shames, G. H., and Sherrick, C. E., Jr., A discussion of nonfluency and stuttering as operant behavior. *J. Speech Hearing Dis., 28,* 3–18 (1963). (Reprinted as Chap. 4 in Barbara, D. A. [ed.], *New Directions in Stuttering.* Springfield, Ill.: Charles C Thomas [1965].)

Sheehan, J. G., Theory and treatment of stuttering as an approach-avoidance conflict. *J. Psychol., 36,* 27–49 (1953).

Starkweather, C. W., *Fluency and Stuttering.* Englewood Cliffs, N. J.: Prentice-Hall (1987).

Wischner, G. J., Stuttering behavior and learning: a preliminary theoretical formulation. *J. Speech Hearing Dis., 15,* 324–35 (1950).

Wischner, G. J:, An experimental approach to expectancy and anxiety in stuttering behavior. *J. Speech Hearing Dis., 17,* 139–54 (1952).

3

PREVALENCE AND INCIDENCE

In the last chapter we reviewed theories of stuttering. The next seven chapters will be devoted to a survey of the research on stuttering in which we will be concerned with what we can infer about the validity of these theories.

There are a number of important questions about stuttering for which answers are to be sought chiefly by the operation of counting heads of persons who stutter. Such surveys have constituted a significant portion of the research on stuttering. Surveys of populations selected in various ways have resulted in information about the relationship between stuttering and such variables as age, sex, familial background of stuttering, and factors of social and cultural environment. Perhaps the major interest of this research derives from the fact that most of it has been focused on the broad question of the relative influence of heredity and environment in relation to stuttering.

We may establish a basic point of reference by first raising the question of how prevalent stuttering is in a population generally representative of our culture at a randomly selected moment in our time. A precise answer to such a question presents considerable obstacles. Almost all attempts to achieve a reasonable approximation of it have dealt with the question of the number of stutterers to be found in populations of children attending school. Tables 3 and 4 present the findings of surveys of this kind done chiefly in the United States and Europe. Whatever variations are to be seen in these findings must be evaluated in the light of all of the factors by which such data may be influenced. In addition to any inherent differences in the nature of the populations sampled, the studies shown differed with respect to the size of the sample, the methods by which it was surveyed, and,

105

Table 3. Prevalence and Sex Ratio of Stuttering Among American Schoolchildren

	N	Population and Grades Sampled	Percentage of Stutterers	Sex Ratio
Hartwell (1893)	129,060	Boston, K-12	0.77	3.0-1
Conradi (1904)	87,440	Six American Cities,[a] 1-12	0.87	3.0-1
Blanton (1916)	4,862	Madison, Wis., 1-8	0.72	3.4-1
Wallin (1916)	89,057	St. Louis, Mo., K-12	0.77	2.6-1
Root (1926)	14,072	S. Dakota, 1-8	1.20	2.2-1
McDowell (1928)	7,138	New York City, 1-8	0.87	2.9-1
Louttit and Halls (1936)	199,839	Indiana, 1-12	0.77	3.1-1
Burdin (1940)	3,602	Indianapolis, 1-4	0.53	
Mills and Streit (1942)	4,685	Holyoke, Mass., 1-6	1.47	5.3-1
Schindler (1955)	22,976	Iowa,[b] 1-12	0.55	2.8-1
Hull (1969)	6,287	Rocky Mountain Region, 1-12	0.30	6-1
Gillespie and Cooper (1973)	5,054	Tuscaloosa, Ala., 7-12	2.12	2.7-1
Leavitt (1974)	10,445	New York City, 1-6[c]	0.84	6.3-1
Leavitt (1974)	10,449	San Juan, P.R., 1-6	1.50	2.9-1
Brady and Hall (1976)	187,420	Illinois, Pennsylvania, K-12[d]	0.35	3.9-1
Hull et al (1976)[e]	38,802	U.S., Nationwide, 1-12	0.80	3.0-1
Leske (1981)	7,119	U.S., 1-6[f]	2.00	2.6-1

[a]Milwaukee, Cleveland, Louisville, Albany, Kansas City, and Springfield, Mass.
[b]Analysis of data from survey of urban and rural schools of five counties conducted from 1939 to 1942.
[c]Puerto Rican children.
[d]Included were 3,514 pupils with mental retardation.
[e]Cited by Leske (1981).
[f]Health examination surveys, 1963-1970. National Center for Health Statistics.

Table 4. Prevalence of Stuttering Among Schoolchildren
in Other Countries

	N	Population	Percentage of Stutterers
Westergaard (1898)*	34,000	Denmark	0.61
Lindberg (1900)*	212,000	Denmark, Rural	0.90
Lindberg (1900)*	85,000	Denmark, Urban	0.74
Von Sarbo (1901)*	231,468	Hungary	1.02
Rouma (1906)	14,235	Belgium	1.40
Ballard (1912)	13,189	London	1.20
Watzl (1924)**	136,000	Vienna	0.60
Parker (1932)	32,123	Tasmania, Australia	1.27
McAllister (1937)	5,705	Glasgow	1.00
McAllister (1937)	38,736	Ayrshire	0.94
McAllister (1937)	21,452	Dunbartonshire	1.00
Wohl (1951)	20,101	Dunbartonshire	1.30
Morgenstern (1956)	29,499	Scotland	1.20
Seeman (1959)**	26,000	Prague	0.55
Petkov and Iosifov (1960)	45,068	Bulgaria	1.70
Aron (1962)	6,581	Johannesburg Bantu	1.26
Andrews and Harris (1964)	7,358	Newcastle upon Tyne	1.20
Okasha, Bishry, et al (1974)	8,494	Egypt	0.93
Glogowski (1976)	875,384	Poland	1.82, 1.72***
Ralston (1981)	1,999	British West Indies	4.70

*Cited by Conradi (1904).
**Cited by Van Riper (1971, p. 39).
***Two studies, the first in 1964 and the second in 1970-71.

inevitably, the criteria on the basis of which perceptual judgments of stuttering were made. The fact that these surveys were carried out in different eras during a span of about eighty years introduces still a further possible source of variation about which little is known. All these things considered, the data are in general quite consistent. They point to a prevalence of stuttering of approximately 1 percent or somewhat more in the European populations studied and to somewhat less than 1 percent in the United States. The unexpected difference between the American and European findings is notable.

AGE VARIABLES

Prevalence with Grade Level

Having established a general estimate of the prevalence of stuttering as about 1 percent or less, we may now raise the question whether it

changes in any significant fashion with age. Again we must depend
for an answer upon surveys of school populations. The results of several surveys that have compared the percentages of stutterers to be
found on various grade levels are shown graphically in Figure 6. It is
clear that the prevalence of stuttering does not vary appreciably from
grade to grade, with the possible exception of a gradual decline as the
high school years are reached. A more recent survey by Brady and
Hall (1976) produced a similar graph, including the same decline in
the upper grades.

Stuttering, then, seems to differ markedly from infantile articulatory
difficulties, which drop very sharply in prevalence during the first few
grades of elementary school. At first glance this is puzzling. We have
long had evidence that many children "outgrow" stuttering, just as they
do articulatory difficulties, after episodes of brief duration. Why, then, is
there no drop in the figures? A reasonable hypothesis is that additional
instances of stuttering develop for a considerable period of time during
childhood. In other words, the stability in the prevalence of stuttering
depicted in Figure 6 in all probability hides the fact that throughout the
early years the disorder is passed about to an extent, new cases arising to
take the place of those that disappear. In order to verify this, there are evidently two processes we must explore further. One is the reported onset
of stuttering as it relates to the age of the child. The other is the process of
spontaneous recovery from stuttering.

Reported Age at Onset

Most of our information about the ages at which children are said
to begin to stutter comes from systematically gathered reports of parents, usually made many weeks or months afterward. Those who
have gathered this information generally tend to emphasize that in
the majority of cases the parent has perceived the onset of stuttering
as gradual and is frequently vague and uncertain about the date of its

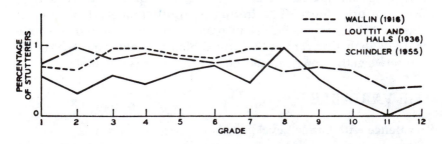

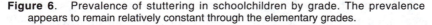

Figure 6.   Prevalence of stuttering in schoolchildren by grade. The prevalence
appears to remain relatively constant through the elementary grades.

occurrence. The data summarized in Table 5 must be examined with this in view. Above all we must keep in mind that any unqualified statement we make about the date of onset of stuttering begs some controversial questions about the identification of stuttering in young children and how it is to be differentiated from normal disfluency. Consequently, we need to face the fact that all we can be sure we are talking about here is the age at which the onset of stuttering was first perceived or reported by a parent.

It is apparent from Table 5 that the earliest age of onset of stuttering is quite consistently recalled as about eighteen months, apparently with the beginning of speech in sentences. Of particular interest are the reports of the latest age of onset, which vary from age seven to thirteen. Such information must be evaluated in the light of the age range of the subjects in each study since this obviously places a limit on the latest as well as the average age at which onset is observed. Nevertheless, there is clearly a decline in the frequency of new cases as we approach the upper age limit of the children investigated in these studies. It is also significant that the average age at onset as usually recalled is distinctly closer to the earliest than to the latest age. Year for year, onset is reported more frequently in the earlier than in the later years of childhood. A large proportion of cases begin with the beginning of speech, according to several investigators. Thereafter, the decline in frequency of reported onset with age takes place at a decreasing rate, following a negatively accelerated growth curve, as Andrews and Harris (1964, p. 113) pointed out, and new cases may therefore continue to appear for a considerable time.

Of exceptional interest are some findings reported by Andrews and Harris (1964, p. 31) since they were based, not on parents' recollections, but on direct observation of 1,000 children in the city of Newcastle upon Tyne, England, who were followed from birth to age 16 years in a longitudinal study of childhood disorders conducted by the University of Durham and the city Health Services.[1] By the conclusion of the study a total of forty-three cases of stuttering had been identified *(see Figure 7)* Sixteen represented transient episodes (less than 6 months' duration), occurring between ages 2 and 4 years. Of the remaining 27 cases, 5 were first observed at age 3 years, half had begun by age 5 years and the last appeared at age 11 years. There was a progressive decrease in frequency of onset with age.

---

[1]This study should not be confused with one cited in Table 5 (Andrews and Harris, 1964 p. 113). The 1,000-family survey referred to here has also been reported by Morley (1957, pp. 13–56) and others. Ingham (1976) has pointed out that there was an attrition of subjects and a reduced frequency of contacts during the later years of this study. It remains, however virtually the only long-term longitudinal study of stuttering onset and recovery available.

Table 5.   Age at Reported Onset of Stuttering

	N	Age Range of Subjects in Years	Mean or Median[a] Age on Onset in Years	Range and Distribution of Ages at Onset
Meltzer (1935)	50	8-16		"Onset of speech" to 13 years. Onset after 8 years in more than one-third of cases.
Milisen and Johnson (1936)	56	3-22	3	From 18 months to 8 years. Onset by age 3 years in 70 percent of cases.
Berry (1938c)	430	9-10	4.86	Latest age at onset was 9 years.
Johnson (1955a)	46	2-9	3	From 2 to 9 years. Seventy-fifth percentile 3 years, 2 months.
Darley (1955)	50	2-14	3.87[b]	From 15 months to 9 years.
Johnson and Associates (1959)	150	2-8	3.53[b]	From 18 months to 7 years. Ninetieth percentile 5.33 years.
Andrews and Harris (1964)	80	9-11	5	From 2 to 9 years. Seventy-fifth percentile 6 years.
Dickson (1971)	369	[c]	3	From 18 months to 10 years. Onset by age 3 in almost half the cases.
Preus (1981)	98	16-21	4-5	More than a third began at age 2 or 3, another third by age 5, four after age 10.
Seider, Gladstien, and Kidd (1983)	437[d]	—	5.17	From 1:5 to 43, 50% by age 4:5, 90% by age 8.

[a]Ages without decimal places are medians, except for Dickson's which is the mode.
[b]As reported by the mothers. The mean age at onset reported by fathers was six months later in Darley's study, but comparable to that of the mothers in the study by Johnson and Associates.
[c]Kindergarten through 9th grade.
[d]Subjects were 305 stutterers and their recovered and persistent first-degree stuttering relatives.

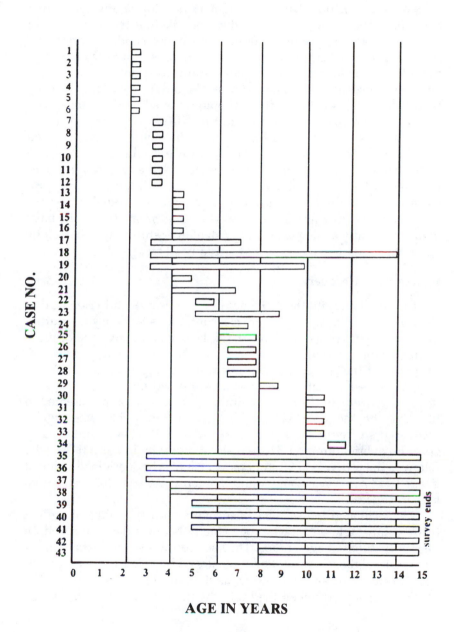

Figure 7. Onset and duration of stuttering of forty-three children identified as stutterers in a longitudinal survey of 1,000 children, all those born within the city limits of Newcastle upon Tyne, England, during May and June of 1947, who were followed from birth to age sixteen years. Redrawn from Andrews, G., Epidemiology of stuttering. In Curlee, E. F., and Perkins, W. H. (eds.), *Nature and Treatment of Stuttering; New Directions.* Copyright© 1984 by Allyn and Bacon. Reprinted by permission.

We may conclude that stuttering may develop at any age during childhood. The younger the child the more likely is the occurrence of an identifiable episode of stuttering, and many children apparently stutter with their first attempts to say sentences. But new cases continue to appear in considerable numbers up to about 9 years of age, and some arise later. In a few instances the onset of stuttering is even reported in adolescents or adults, although not all workers are agreed that this is basically the same kind of difficulty as is ordinarily referred to as stuttering.[2] Although it has sometimes been asserted that there are "peaks" in the frequency of onset of stuttering at certain ages, this does not appear to be borne out by the research findings. Following the preschool years there is little evidence of any pronounced vulnerability to stuttering at one age or another; the curve seems to be all downward. Andrews (1984a) estimated, "On the basis of data presently available, half the risk of ever stuttering is passed by age 4, three-quarters by age 6, and virtually all by age 12."

Spontaneous Recovery

Concomitant with the incidence of new cases of stuttering during childhood, and offsetting it, there is a continuous tendency for stuttering to disappear of its own accord. Of those who at any time begin to stutter, a large proportion will stop by the time they reach adulthood. Estimates of the percentage who recover, varying from 36 to 79 percent, are shown in Table 6. Almost all are based on subjects' recollections of recovery. In the only longitudinal investigation represented in the table, the one reported by Andrews and Harris, the percentage of recovered stutterers by age 16 years was 79.1. This includes early episodes of brief duration. There is also a report by Fritzell (1976), who followed the progress of 90 stutterers, most of whom originally ranged in age from 7 to 9 years, and found that ten years later 46.7 percent no longer stuttered.

The estimated percentages of recovery shown in Table 6 are not really comparable with each other, chiefly because they are based on markedly different age groups. They suggest, however, that at almost any age level those who stutter are matched by at least an equal number who recall or are reported as having stuttered at one time. The older the group surveyed the higher is the proportion of recovered

---

[2]At least some cases of adult-onset stuttering appear to have an abrupt psychogenic origin different from those that develop during childhood. For example, Deal (1982) studied the case of a depressed twenty-eight-year-old who was addicted to heroin and who began to stutter after a suicide attempt. He stuttered in singing, unison reading, and even in miming speech movements. Another ambiguity about stuttering that appears to begin in adulthood is the uncertainty of determining whether it is not a recurrence of a forgotten early episode of stuttering.

Table 6. Incidence of Stuttering (Percentage of Those Who Have Stuttered at Any Time) and Rate of Recovery.

	N	Population	Percentage of Lifetime Incidence	Percentage Rate of Recovery
Quinan (1921)	100	Male Adults, Over Age 44	5.0	
Milisen and Johnson (1936)	8,000	Council Bluffs, Iowa, Kindergarten Through High School	2.5	42.3
Voelker (1942)	96	Nonstuttering University of Iowa Students	10.4	
Villarreal (1945)	271	Nonstuttering University of Texas Students	14.0	
Hertzman (1948)	4,213	Cincinnati Junior and Senior High School Students	5.8	
Glasner and Rosenthal (1957)	996	Anne Arundel County, Md., First Grade Entrants	15.4	54.2
Andrews and Harris (1964)	1,000	Newcastle upon Tyne Children Followed from Birth to Age 16	4.9[a]	79.1
Andrews and Harris (1964)	206	Newcastle upon Tyne Adults	4.8	
Sheehan and Martyn (1970)[b]	5,138	Berkeley and UCLA Entering Freshmen and Graduate Students	2.9	78.9
Dickson (1971)	3,923	Buffalo, Kindergarten Through Junior High School	9.4	54.4
Cooper (1972)	5,054	Tuscaloosa, Alabama, Junior and Senior High School Students	3.7	36.3
Porfert and Rosenfield (1978)	2,107	University of Massachusetts Students	5.5	61.7
Seider, Gladstien, and Kidd (1983)	1,857	First-Degree Relatives of Adult Stutterers	13.9	51.0
Culton (1986)[c]	30,586	University of Alabama Freshmen 1971-1983	0.7	58.8

[a]Based on an N of 875, the median number in the study as attrition took place (Andrews, 1984a).
[b]Includes data of previous surveys by Sheehan and Martyn (1966) and Martyn and Sheehan (1968).
[c]Includes data of Cooper, Parris, and Wells (1974).

stutterers likely to be found, as Dickson (1971) and Cooper (1972) showed, and by adulthood the percentage of recovered stutterers may be as high as 80 percent. Some workers are skeptical about a figure so high when based upon subjects' diagnoses of themselves as recovered stutterers. Young (1975c) suggested that some of these subjects may not be distinguishing adequately between stuttering and normal disfluency, and such doubts are given some substance by the finding of Lankford and Cooper (1974) that two-thirds of the parents of 68 self-diagnosed, recovered stutterers of junior and senior high school age said, when interviewed by telephone, that they did not believe their child had ever stuttered. Although these inconsistencies suggest the need for more research, it is quite possible that we are dealing here with the kind of question that can have no exact answer. If, as is possible, mild episodes of troublesome disfluency are commonplace during childhood, the question of precisely how many children recover from "stuttering" ultimately becomes a matter of what we are willing to define as stuttering. There are likewise ambiguities about the term "spontaneous recovery." Shall we apply it to a person who still stutters occasionally under stress? Does it exclude someone who has received speech therapy at some time?

At what age does spontaneous recovery take place? Studies of recovered adults by Wingate (1964), Shearer and Williams (1965), and Martyn and Sheehan (1968) showed that the age varied within a very broad range, although there was a considerable tendency to recall recovery between about ages 13 and 20 years. In one of these studies the earliest age at which recovery was reported by these adult subjects was 9 years. In another it was 5. When parents are the informants, however, the age is pushed back considerably. In his study of schoolchildren Dickson (1971) found the peak age of spontaneous recovery to be 3.5 years, with the great majority of former stutterers having recovered by age 6. In most cases the stuttering had lasted no more than two years, often no more than a few months. Moreover, Glasner and Rosenthal (1957) found that as many as 8.3 percent of 996 children about to enter first grade in Anne Arundel County, Maryland, were said to have already recovered from stuttering, and over a third of the stutterers identified during the Newcastle upon Type 1,000-family survey had recovered from transient episodes by age 4 years (see Figure 7).[3] Evidently, a very large group of children who recover from stuttering in the early years will have no knowledge of it in later life. Inferences based on the recollections of older subjects about the ages at which recovery takes place must therefore be viewed with caution.

---

[3]Furthermore, in a study of 8,000 elementary and high school children in Council Bluffs, Iowa, Milisen and Johnson (1936) found that practically all of the former stutterers were reported to have recovered by age 8 years.

It appears from all available findings that recovery may occur at any age. Seider, Gladstien, and Kidd (1983) reported that among 132 stutterers' relatives who had recovered from stuttering, the ages of recovery ranged from 3 to 38 years. Shames and Beams (1956) gathered evidence indicating that stuttering may continue to become less prevalent even in older age groups. As we might expect, however, the younger the person, the better the chances of recovery. The data of Seider, Gladstien, and Kidd show a decreasing probability of recovery with age. In an analysis of findings from several studies, Andrews, Craig, Feyer, Hoddinott, Howie, and Neilson (1983) estimated that at age 16 years 75 percent of those stuttering at age 4 years, 50 percent of those stuttering at age 6 years, and 25 percent of those stuttering at age 10 years will have recovered.

Although a very large proportion of stutterers recover at some time, it is noteworthy that among adults who regard themselves as recovered, at least half report a slight, occasional tendency to stutter, particularly when the recovery has been relatively late (Wingate, 1964; Shearer and Williams, 1965). Dickson (1971) also found this to be true of some children. In addition, clinical observation suggests that recovered stutterers may bear a certain risk of developing stuttering again in later life.[4]

A few attempts have been made to learn something about the conditions under which stuttering disappears, chiefly by gaining the viewpoints of the subjects themselves and by examining their histories.[5] Among the factors to which recovery is frequently attributed by subjects in the more recent studies are speaking more slowly, relaxing, acquiring new attitudes toward self or speech problem, speaking more, and speech therapy. Subjects studied by Milisen and Johnson (1936) more frequently gave such reasons as enforced left-handedness, removal of tonsils, clipping of the lingual frenum, treatment by a chiropractor, and parental admonitions to repeat stuttered words or to "stop and start over." Both then and more recently, many were unable to offer any explanation at all. Almost all tended to recall their recovery as having been gradual. From the standpoint of sex ratio, familial incidence, reaction to their difficulty at the time they were experiencing it, and other basic features of the problem, they did not seem easily distinguishable as a group from those whose stuttering fails to disappear. The one factor that seemed to make a difference is severity of

---

[4]The German speech pathologis Erwin Richter (1982) relates that he stuttered as a young man, then spoke fluently for 28 years and all but forgot about his speech difficulty until the age of 57 years when he stuttered again for 9 or 10 months.

[5]Milisen and Johnson (1936), Wingate (1964), Shearer and Williams (1965), Sheehan and Martyn (1966, 1970), Lankford and Cooper (1974), Fritzell (1976).

stuttering; the more severe cases tended to be more persistent (Sheehan and Martyn, 1970; Dickson, 1971). Presumably because recovered stutterers had less severe problems, Sheehan and Martyn found that they had less often received formal speech therapy.

Cox and Kidd (1983) could find no evidence from familial data for supposing that persistent and recovered stuttering are transmitted differently as two genetic subtypes of differing severity.

Lifetime Incidence

We have been examining the hypothesis that the essentially constant level which the prevalence of stuttering maintains through the school years represents an equilibrium resulting from two opposing processes in which stuttering develops in some children while it simultaneously ceases in others. We may make a final check on this. If it is true, then the lifetime incidence of stuttering (i.e., the percentage of the population who have stuttered at any time in their lives) should be appreciably higher than the prevalence of stuttering—the percentage who are stutterers at a given time. Estimates of the lifetime incidence of stuttering are summarized in Table 6. Although they vary widely, they are all well above the prevalence of stuttering, which is roughly 1 percent of the population. It should be noted that almost all the estimates are based on subjects' recollections and that most of the data were obtained from college or university populations.

The disparity among some of the entries under "percentage of incidence" in Table 6 is quite large. The Voelker and Villarreal studies, which used exactly the same procedure, found a far higher incidence than did other comparable investigations. Most of the other comparable reports shown in Table 6 are in fair agreement, five of them clustering closely at about 5 percent. The 15 percent incidence given by Glasner and Rosenthal needs to be viewed separately. It represents the percentage of 5- and 6-year-old children whose parents said they were stuttering or had stuttered at some time, and apparently reflects the unusual tendency for brief outbreaks of stuttering to occur in preschool children. About half of this 15 percent had already recovered. As we have seen, this early, transient stuttering tends to be forgotten by those who did it. It is therefore a reasonable hypothesis that at least half the incidence found by Glasner and Rosenthal must be added to the incidence found in other studies to give a complete picture.

Thus it would seem that a plausible figure for the lifetime incidence of all those who at some time either consider themselves or are considered by their parents to be stutterers is at least as high as 10 percent, which is approximately the figure that Dickson was given by parents. One difficulty with this guess is that it must be reconciled with the 4.9 percent finding of the Newcastle upon Tyne 1,000-family survey in which subjects were studied by direct observation beginning at birth. This unique study made use of periodic checks by health visitors, following which all reports of speech difficulty were confirmed through examinations by speech therapists. A series of early, mild, and transient cases was identified (*see Figure 7*). It seems possible, however, that a considerable number of early episodes of stuttering are so slight and of such brief duration that they might not be confirmed by such a procedure. Glasner and Rosenthal simply questioned the parents. Which method is preferable may be solely a matter of whether there is any interest in stuttering that is mild and short-lived. From this standpoint, the question of the exact size of the longitudinal incidence of stuttering, like that of the exact percentage of spontaneous recovery, may have no absolute answer. As we shall see later, it may be a tenable hypothesis that very minor experiences of stuttering in young children are so widespread that they blend imperceptibly with what is generally regarded as normal disfluency.

Summary

We may now summarize the major facts we have established about the manner in which the prevalence of stuttering varies with age. Stuttering is found on all age levels beginning with the onset of speech. It is almost always reported to begin at some time before adolescence, most commonly in the early years. The older the child, the less likely the development of stuttering. Throughout childhood there is a fluidity in the prevalence of stuttering such that the occurrence of new cases is balanced by a remission of old ones. There is a marked tendency for children to recover spontaneously after periods of stuttering of extremely variable duration, and this process continues at a decreasing rate from the earliest childhood through adolescence and beyond. Much of what we know about stuttering in relation to age level may be summed up succinctly by saying that from certain points of view there appears to be some justification for the inference that has sometimes been drawn that stuttering is essentially a disorder of childhood.

THE SEX RATIO

Few facts about stuttering are as thoroughly documented as its unequal sex distribution. The data in Table 3 are representative and show a consistent ratio of boys to girls among American schoolchildren of approximately 3–1. A ratio of about 3–1 has also been reported for stuttering schoolchildren in Poland by Glogowski (1976) and in Egypt by Okasha, Bishry, Kamel, and Hassan (1974). These are all prevalence figures, relating to the ratio of boys to girls at a given time. To obtain an estimate of the sex ratio in the lifetime incidence of stuttering, Kidd, Kidd, and Records (1978) investigated the first-degree relatives (fathers, mothers, sisters, and brothers) of 511 stutterers and found a ratio of 2.93–1 among those who had ever stuttered.

There is evidence that the sex ratio increases with age. Questionnaire data on schoolchildren gathered from forty-three towns and cities in the White House Conference Survey of 1930 disclosed 10,268 stutterers in a sex ratio that rose steadily from 3.1–1 in grade 1 to 5.5–1 in grades 11 and 12.[6] Glasner and Rosenthal (1957) found a ratio of only 1.4–1 among preschool stutterers. In principle, such a change in ratio might be caused either by an increasing preponderance of boys with age among new cases or by a tendency for girls to recover from stuttering with relatively greater frequency than boys. West (1931) showed that the change in sex ratio in the White House Conference data was due chiefly to a progressive increase in the proportion of new cases among males.

The question of why there is a sex ratio in stuttering has been subject to almost as varied speculation as the cause of stuttering itself. At a relatively early date some workers regarded it as evidence of a sex-limited genetic predisposition to stuttering (West, 1958; Berry and Eisenson, 1956, Chap. 11). It was frequently pointed out in this connection that there is more infant mortality, more birth injury, and greater susceptibility to most childhood diseases among males than females and that the sex ratio in stuttering may be viewed as directly or indirectly reflecting the broad congenital vulnerability of the male constitution.

Others, particularly Johnson and his students, stressed environmental explanations. Schuell (1946, 1947) found what appeared to be relevant differences in parental attitudes and reactions to boys and girls. She gathered evidence appearing to show that boys tend to compare unfavorably with girls in physical, social, and language development and that they are less sheltered than girls and encounter more unequal competition, insecurity, and frustration, especially in relation to language situations. She speculated that these factors tended to result in speech that was more hesitant and therefore more frequently lent itself to a diagnosis of stuttering by parents. Little sex difference appeared in the normal speech hesitancy of children in an extensive normative investigation by Johnson and Associates (1959, Chapter 8).[7] Consequently, Johnson even-

---

[6]Louttit and Halls' (1936) breakdown by grade and sex of 1,519 stutterers in the public schools of Indiana does not show this systematic variation in sex ratio with age. An analysis by Schuell (1946) of over a thousand stutterers' records in the files of the University of Iowa Speech Clinic does show it very clearly, but the nature of such data as Schuell's does not permit separation of factors that influence the incidence of stuttering from those influencing referrals to a clinic.

[7]Similarly, Brutten and Miller (1988) found no difference between normal speaking male and female first graders in frequency of disfluency.

tually surmised that it was not a difference in the fluency of boys and girls that accounted for the sex ratio in stuttering, but a difference in the manner in which parents perceived, evaluated, and reacted to the hesitancies of boys as opposed to those of girls (Johnson and Associates, 1959, p. 240).

There is little adequate evidence with regard to this hypothesis. Bloodstein and Smith (1954) found that, when listeners were presented with recorded speech samples previously judged to be ambiguous with respect to the sex of the child, they did not classify significantly more of the children as stutterers when told they were listening to boys than when told they were listening to girls. Unfortunately, this procedure leaves much to be desired as an analogue of the diagnosis of stuttering in actual children by their parents.

Of possible relevance to Johnson's theory are some observations relating to differing social attitudes toward the stuttering of males as compared with females. E.-M. Silverman and Van Opens (1980) presented grade school teachers with anecdotes about children with various speech and language difficulties. When the anecdote concerned a child with disfluency, the teachers were more likely to recommend referral for remediation if the child had a boy's name than if the child had a girl's name. No such difference appeared in the case of lisping, hoarseness, or language disorders. E.-M. Silverman (1982) also found that university students had stronger negative stereotypes of male stutterers than female stutterers, and an interview study of adult stutterers by E.-M. Silverman and Zimmer (1982) revealed a tendency for stuttering to be a somewhat more serious problem for men than for women.

Outside the context of the diagnosogenic theory, attempts have been made to relate the sex ratio to slower early language development in the boy and to his greater proneness to articulatory errors, reading problems, and most other difficulties of speech and communication (West and Ansberry, 1968, p. 126, and Bloodstein, 1958, p. 38). Clarice Tatman, in a personal communication to the author, made the interesting suggestion that the sex ratio is due in part to the difference between masculine and feminine roles with regard to speech. In general, the girl is not expected to be as outspoken and self-assertive as the boy. Consequently, in many situations of anxiety, guilt, or tension the girl may be permitted to take refuge in silence while the boy is more likely to feel compelled to speak under pressure.

Goldman (1967) reported some evidence in support of the hypothesis that the sex ratio is related to greater environmental pressures on the male. Reasoning on the assumption that as a lingering consequence of slavery the lower socioeconomic segment of southern Afro-American society possesses a matriarchal structure that often tends to impose less responsibility on the male than on the female, he studied the sex ratio in a sample of 694 stutterers identified in a statewide survey of school-age children in Tennessee. There was a sex ratio of only 2.4–1 among the black children, as opposed to 4.9–1 among the white children. Goldman then compared the sex ratio in stuttering among black children from "matriarchal" and "patriarchal" home environments, which he differentiated on the basis of the presence or absence of a "stable and consistent male figure in the home." Among 77 stutterers from "patriarchal" home environments he found a sex ratio of 3.5–1, while among 38 from a "matriarchal" environment it was 1.1–1.

Eisenson (1966) attempted to refute the environmental hypothesis by pointing out that the sex ratio appears to exist even among stuttering children to be found in Israeli *kibbutzim*, communal institutions where, at the date of Eisenson's observations, children generally saw their parents for only three hours a day and received "relatively objective upbringing" by nurses and teachers with "no conscious differences in the treatment of the children along sex lines." In the *kibbutz* visited by Eisenson the stutterers consisted of 12 boys and 3 girls.

On the basis of a genetic study of 2,524 first-degree relatives of stutterers, Kidd, Kidd, and Records (1978) concluded that the sex ratio is best explained by some type of sex-modified inheritance. They proposed a model in which both genes and environment contribute to the liability to stutter and in which males have a lower threshold of susceptibility than females. The difference in threshold might be either biological or social. MacFarlane, Hanson, Walton, and Mellon (1991) studied a five-generation family with a high incidence of stuttering and found that the data met all criteria for sex-modified genetic transmission.

Of recent date is Geschwind's theory that the sex ratio in stuttering is due to higher levels of testosterone in the male fetus than in the female (see Geschwind and Galaburda, 1985). As noted in Chapter 2, Geschwind suggested that testosterone retards the development of the left cerebral hemisphere, thus increasing the risk of speech and language disturbances including stuttering.

The meaning of the sex ratio has intrigued experts since the beginning of modern scientific curiosity about speech disorders. With the differences between boys and girls extending to so many factors of physiology, development, and social environment, however, all too many explanations of the sex ratio are possible, and it would unfortunately be difficult to think of a theory of stuttering that could not be reconciled with it.

THE INFLUENCE OF HEREDITY

There are several areas of research on the incidence of stuttering in which the focus of interest is on the question of whether heredity plays an important role in the disorder. They include the incidence of stuttering in the families of stutterers, in twins, and in the families that adopt stutterers.

Familial Incidence in Stuttering

The tendency for stuttering to appear in successive generations of the same family has served to provoke speculation about a genetic basis of stuttering for many years. In clinical practice cases are occasionally encountered in which a large number of the person's relatives on the maternal or paternal side have been stutterers for several generations. The literature contains an abundance of reports of large proportions of stutterers giving a history of stuttering in the family background, these proportions generally ranging from about one-third to two-thirds of cases. The findings summarized in Table 7 represent the studies that have employed control data. They show that the proportion of nonstutterers who report a family history of stuttering tends to be much smaller than that of stutterers, ranging from 5 to 18 percent. On the basis of pooled data from several studies, Andrews et al. (1983) estimated that the incidence of stuttering among first-degree relatives of stutterers is more than three times that in the general population.

Table 7. Percentage of Stutterers and Nonstutterers Reporting Familial Histories of Stuttering

	N	Stutterers	Nonstutterers
Bryngelson and Rutherford (1937)	74, 74	46.0	18.0
Wepman (1939)	250, 250	68.8	15.6
Bryngelson (1939)	78, 78	54.0	6.0
West, Nelson, and Berry (1939)	204, 204	51.0	18.1
Johnson et al (1942)	46, 46	32.6[a]	8.7[a]
Meyer (1945)	100, 246	61.0	6.5
Darley (1955)	50, 50	52.0	42.0
Johnson and Associates (1959)	150, 150	23.3	6.0[b]
Andrews and Harris (1964)	80, 80	37.5	1.3
Martyn and Sheehan (1968)	85, 277[c]	32.9	6.1
Mann (cited by Howie, 1976)	49, 49	31.9[d]	10.2[d]
Porfert and Rosenfield (1978)	44, 1,965	29.5	5.0
Accordi et al (1983)	2,802, 1,602	50.0	6.6

[a]Represents the percentage who had stuttering relatives outside the immediate family.
[b]As reported by the mothers. The percentage as reported by the fathers was 5.3.
[c]The eighty-five subjects in the experimental group consisted of both recovered and active stutterers.
[d]Represents the percentage who had stuttering offspring.

Genetic Interpretations

Many workers have for long accepted a genetic explanation of the familial incidence of stuttering as the simplest and most satisfactoy. They have had difficulty, however, in establishing the manner of transmission. The question is complicated by the fact that we are con-cemed with the transmission, not of stuttering itself, but of a trait that might or might not be expressed or manifested in stuttering by the person who possessed it, depending upon environmental circum-stances. Evidence obtained by Meyer (1945), Andrews and Harris (1964), and Kidd, Kidd, and Records (1978) from studies of the family backgrounds of stutterers appears to rule out any simple Mendelian type of inheritance, such as sex-linked, autosomal dominant, or reces-sive. None of these is compatible with the observed distribution of stuttering relatives. This does not, however, exclude the possibility of more complex types of genetic transmission.

Andrews and Harris (1964, Chapter 7), with the assistance of Roger Garside and David Kay, carried out a detailed analysis of stutterers' familial backgrounds which appeared to show that certain genetic hypotheses were tenable. From their data they determined the proba-bility of occurrence of stuttering in various categories of relatives in the immediate families of stutterers. They found that their results could be accounted for by assuming a sex-limited transmission by means of a large number of nonspecific genes. That is to say, a given amount of predisposition to stuttering might be inherited by the same type of polygenic inheritance responsible for such continuously distributed, finely graded characteristics as stature or intelligence. Accordingly, they drew the conclusion that a tendency toward stuttering might be passed down by polygenic inheritance or by a "common dominant gene with a multifactorial background." In either case it is necessary to assume the operation of sex-limitation, a mechanism by which the effects of the same genes are manifested to different degrees in males and females.

Added support for the belief that genes play a part in stuttering came subsequently from work by Kidd, Reich, and Kessler (1973, 1974) in the Department of Human Genetics at Yale University. These workers were concerned with human traits that have a high familial incidence, but show no Mendelian patterns of inheritance because they are brought about in part by environmental factors. Such traits can usually be explained genetically by either multifactorial (poly-genic) or single-gene models. Kidd and his associates had shown that when a sex ratio exists and sufficient information is at hand on the incidence of the trait in relatives of affected individuals, it is possible to test the relative adequacy of these two models statistically. Looking about for human traits to which to apply their methods, they recog-nized that stuttering fulfilled all the requirements.

By analyzing the data of Andrews and Harris combined with other available data, Kidd, Reich, and Kessler concluded that there is probably a genetic factor in stuttering with a "single major locus." They pointed out, however, that the polygenic model also gave an adequate fit to the data and that even entirely nongenetic inheritance was not totally excluded, inasmuch as unambiguous demonstration of biological transmission can only result from adoption or genetic linkage studies. Both the monogenic and polygenic models they tested assumed that an individual's total (genetic and environmental) liability to stutter is a variable trait manifested overtly in stuttering when exceeding a certain threshold value which is lower for males than females.

Further data collected by Kidd and his associates on the families of several hundred stutterers following their first study produced similar results (Kidd, 1977; Kidd, Heimbuch, and Records, 1981). Their gene-environment interaction model predicted with considerable accuracy the proportions of stuttering fathers, mothers, sisters, and brothers in these families.

Doubt has persisted over the question of single-gene versus polygenic inheritance. Contrary to the original findings, Cox, Kramer, and Kidd (1984) determined that the Multifactorial (polygenic) model offered a more satisfactory explanation for the transmission of stuttering than the monogenic model. Their results also allowed for the possibility that stuttering might be culturally transmitted in some cases. In a more recent study, Ambrose, Yairi, and Cox (1993) found that data on the extended families of 69 young stutterers were consistent with a single-gene hypothesis.

Kidd, Heimbuch, Records, Oehlert, and Webster(1980) could find no evidence that the severity of stuttering is influenced by heredity.

An interesting finding from the research of Kidd and his coworkers and the work of Andrews and Harris (but not from that of Ambrose, Yairi, and Cox) was that female stutterers tended to have more stuttering relatives than male stutterers. Puzzling as this may seem initially, it is readily explained on the assumption that a predisposition to stuttering is genetically transmitted. As Andrews and Harris (1964, p. 141) pointed out, the effect may occur for the same reason that tall women are more likely to have tall relatives than are tall men. Since men tend to be taller than women, a six-foot-tall woman is more exceptional (i.e., in a more extreme part of the distribution of females with regard to stature) than is a six-foot-tall man. Consequently she is more likely to come from a family of tall individuals. The same reasoning can be applied to stuttering if we suppose that the presumed hereditary predisposition to stutter is a continuously variable trait, like human stature, and that it takes a heavier predisposition to make a girl stutter than a boy.

Social Interpretations

Several forms of purely social inheritance have been suggested to explain the familial incidence of stuttering. The earliest of these was imitation of other stutterers in the family. Imitation is no longer regarded as an important factor by most workers. One reason for this is that stutterers who have stuttering relatives frequently have had no personal contact with them, as Nelson (1939) showed. When they do, as in the case of parents, Kidd, Kidd, and Records (1978) found that so many no longer stuttered by the time the child was born, that of 511 cases only 12 percent had a stuttering parental model to imitate. Another reason for the widespread rejection of the imitation hypothesis is that there is so often a marked dissimilarity between the features of stuttering of a young child in the earliest phase of the disorder and those of the adult whom the child might be presumed to have imitated.

The form of nongenetic inheritance of stuttering that has been accorded most serious consideration is the social transmission from one generation to the next of a family environment that for one reason or and other is conducive to the development of the disorder. Particular emphasis was given to such a concept in the thinking of Johnson and his students within the framework of his diagnosogenic theory. Johnson believed that stuttering frequently occurs in the same family because of the handing down of a "climate of anxiety" about the hesitant speech of children.

Some observations in support of this viewpoint were made by Gray (1940) in her investigation of a "stuttering" family in Iowa. Although there had been stutterers in this family for the last five generations, it appeared that there was a fairly large branch of the family living in Kansas in which there was very little stuttering. It might be argued that on the hypothesis of genetic transmission this was an improbable occurrence. Gray interviewed the living members of the Iowa branch and contacted the Kansas branch by mail. The chief result of her study was a detailed genealogy (*see Figure 8*), which showed that the last two generations of the Iowa branch stemmed from a woman whom Gray designated as III A. Not only was III A a stutterer herself, but her father and her maternal aunt and grandmother had also been stutterers. She was, moreover, the youngest of four children, all but one of whom stuttered. When these children grew up they all moved to Kansas, with the exception of III A who remained in Iowa, and there had subsequently been little contact between the two branches of the family except by occasional letter. In the last two generations of the Iowa branch (i.e., the children and grandchildren of III A) about 40 percent were stutterers, while of seventeen living Kansas members only one stuttered.

Gray offered the interpretation that the stuttering in the Iowa branch arose largely out of attitudes that were conducive to the diagnosis of more or less normal speech as stuttering. She believed that in

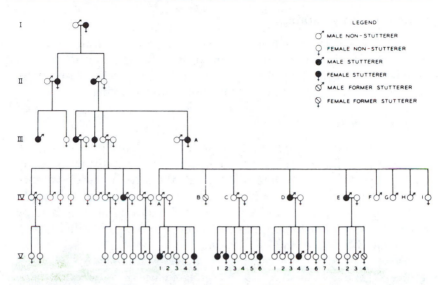

Figure 8. Five generations of a "stuttering" family. About 40 percent of the Iowa branch (the descendants of III A) were found to be or to have been stutterers. Of the seventeen living members of the Kansas branch (descendants of the siblings of III A) only one was a stutterer. These findings have been used in support of an environmental explanation of the familial incidence of stuttering. Reproduced from Gray (1940). Copyright 1940 by the American Speech-Language-Hearing Association. Reprinted by permission.

this the "tone" was set for the Iowa group by IV E, the last of III A's five biological children, by virtue of his dominant position in the family and the severity of his stuttering. Her informants made such comments as, "We wondered whether our children would stutter like IV E," or, "I couldn't stand it if I stuttered like IV E." As a group they appeared to be "stuttering conscious." They believed that the disorder was hereditary in their family and seemed to watch their children anxiously for signs of it.

At the time that Gray did her study of this family, various members of the Iowa branch received advice and information about stuttering in the context of a diagnosogenic orientation toward the problem. Twenty years later Johnson carried out a follow-up investigation of the family (Johnson, 1961b, pp. 83, 84; Johnson et al., 1967, pp. 265, 266). By now the fifth generation, children at the time of Gray's study, had grown up and many of them had children of their own. Johnson reported that of 44 people in the sixth generation only one had ever been considered a stutterer. He related this decline in the number of stutterers to indications that there had been a change in the familial assumptions about stuttering and a reduction in their tendency to make an issue of childhood lapses in fluency.

Stuttering and Twinning

The subject of twins has been of importance for stuttering, as it has been for other traits, in relation to hypotheses about the role of heredity in its causation. A number of different questions involving twins have been considered in connection with stuttering.

Prevalence in Twins

Several studies have been done on the prevalence of stuttering in the twin population. These have consistently shown unexpectedly large proportions of stutterers, although the size of the prevalence reported has varied consideration. In fairly large groups of twin pairs, stuttering has been found in 9 percent of the individual members by Berry (1938a) and in 13 percent by Nelson, Hunter, and Walter (1945), but in only 1.9 percent by Graf (1955).

In view of the large numbers of stutterers found among twins, it is reasonable to expect the converse, a high incidence of twins among stutterers. Berry (1937b) found that 4.5 percent of 461 stuttering subjects were members of a twin pair, as against only 1.2 percent among 500 nonstutterers. Later research by Johnson and Associates (1959, p. 71) showed that among 200 stutterers three were twins, while in a like number of nonstutterers one was a twin. When all of these findings are considered together the weight of evidence at present seems to favor the view that there is some relationship between stuttering and twin membership, although the extent of the relationship is still far from clear.

This finding has been subject to various interpretations. West and his students held that a tendency toward twinning and a predisposition to stuttering are genetically linked in some families (West and Ansberry, 1968, p. 127). An alternative hypothesis offered by West (1958) was that the slowness of early maturation frequently associated with multiple births may contribute to a general constitutional retardation, which he believed to underlie stuttering. Explanations stressing environmental factors are also to be considered. Schuell (1946) offered the hypothesis that when stuttering occurs in fraternal twins it is usually to be found in the physiologically less mature member and results from pressure to keep pace with the other one. It might be that in both fraternal and identical cases some part is played in producing stuttering by the competitive pressures that members of a twin pair often encounter as a result of the comparisons inevitably made between them.

Incidence in Twinning Families

While it is reasonable to consider environmental explanations for an increased incidence of stuttering in twins, it would be difficult to account in this manner for any increased stuttering to be found in twinning families, particularly those in which the twins themselves were not stutterers. It is therefore of some significance that Berry (1938a) reported that in the immediate families of a group of 250 pairs of twins she had found that 5.5 percent of the children (i.e., the twins and their siblings) were stutterers. This large percentage was due chiefly, it is true, to the abundance of stutterers among the twins themselves. When the singleton siblings of the twins are considered alone, however, as many as 2.9 percent of them prove to be stutterers.

There has yet been no definite confirmation of this finding that stuttering and twinning tend to be associated in the same families over and above their tendency to be associated in the same individuals. In a different study by Berry (1937b), the converse of the one just referred to, twins were found to be more common in the immediate families of stutterers than in the families of nonstutterers, but this difference appears to have been due essentially to the number of twins among the stutterers themselves rather than among their siblings. Johnson and his co-workers (1959, p. 72) found that of the parents of 150 stutterers, 21 mothers and 19 fathers identified twins among their relatives while of the parents of 150 nonstutterers, 28 mothers and 21 fathers reported relatives who were twins. Andrews and Harris (1964, p. 77) reported that of a group of 80 stutterers, 19 had a family history of twinning as opposed to 11 in a like number of controls, an interesting trend that was not, however, statistically significant. Unfortunately, head-counting studies are a type of research in which large numbers of subjects are often needed in order to rule out the possibility that differences are due to chance.

Concordance in Identical Twins

Because identical, or monozygotic, twins result from the cleavage of a single fertilized ovum and consequently have exactly the same heredity, they have long been of interest to scientists concerned with the relative influence of heredity and environment on human traits. It can be argued that if a trait such as stuttering is invariably found in both members of an identical twin pair and is found in both members of a fraternal pair no more often than it occurs in any two siblings, it is probably hereditary. It should be noted that this is actually quite a different question from the ones we have just discussed and would be of considerable significance even if there were no reason to believe that stuttering was rather common among twins. It is of interest, therefore, that a series of studies has been done on the concordance for stuttering in identical and fraternal twins.[8] Two conclusions appear to be warranted by the evi-

---

[8]In addition, Howie (1981b) obtained equivocal results in investigating the similarities of stuttering frequency within identical and fraternal twin pairs. She found some evidence of a genetic influence on frequency of prolongations and "blocks," but not on frequency of sound, syllable, or word repetitions.

dence from these studies (*see Table 8*). One is that there is a fairly high degree of concordance for stuttering in identical twins. The other is that there are exceptions. The exceptions do not invalidate a genetic theory of inheritance of stuttering; they only show that environment plays some part. At the same time, high monozygotic concordance is not conclusive proof of such a theory. The similarity between identical twins often extends to the most unexpected traits, and it is probable that not only their heredity, but also their environments, are more alike than those of fraternal twins. As Meyer (1945) argued, the fact that identical twins resemble each other so closely makes it more likely that they will be reacted to alike and "insures a more intimate sharing of infantile and childhood experiences and environmental influences than obtains in the case of two children whose identity is each clearly unlike the other from the start." To constitute more conclusive evidence of the biological inheritance of stuttering, its concordance would have to be demonstrable in identical twins who had been reared apart. Some information on this question has resulted from work by Farber (1981).

Farber was concerned with essentially the entire range of physical and behavioral traits of identical twins who had been reared apart. She combed the literature from 1923 to 1973 to collect all available accounts of such cases. Her book *Identical Twins Reared Apart: A Reanalysis,* is a detailed description of 95 pairs of twins about whom there was reliable information. Startling similarities of behavior emerged. The twins tended to have the same tastes in clothing, books,

Table 8. Numbers of Identical and Fraternal Twin Pairs
Concordant and Discordant for Stuttering

	Identical		Fraternal	
	Concordant	Discordant	Concordant	Discordant
Nelson, Hunter, and Walter (1945)	9	1	2	28
Graf (1955)	1	6	2	7
Luchsinger (1959)*	13	2	0	29
Godai, Tatarelli, and Bonanni (1976)	10	2	2	17
Howie (1981a)	10	6	3	10
Total	43	17	9	91

*Observations gathered by Luchsinger from his own clinical records and those of other workers: Seeman, Brankel, Gedda, and Bruno.

and music and the same mannerisms and ways of sitting, holding themselves, walking, laughing, and gesturing. In one instance they had the same nickname. The similarities extended to the twins' speech patterns and vocal characteristics, including such features as talkativeness, high pitch, and hoarseness. The only exception among speech characteristics was stuttering. Among her 95 cases Farber identified 5 with stuttering. In all 5 cases only 1 member of the pair stuttered.[9]

In a footnote, Farber mentioned an additional twin pair who were concordant for stuttering. This was a Japanese pair, reported by Yoshimasu in 1941, who had been separated at birth and reunited at age 32 years. One, Takao, had been imprisoned for theft and embezzlement and the other, Kazuo, had become a Christian minister. Both were said to stutter. They were not included in Farber's series of 95 cases, presumably because of failure to satisfy her stringent criteria for reliability.

Commenting on the twins' speech characteristics, Farber stated, "Only stuttering seems environmentally related." Most workers in the field of speech and language pathology would probably hesitate to draw so bold an inference at the present time. What Farber's cases do seem to show, if they are at all representative, is that much of the concordance for stuttering that has been observed in identical twins in the past may have been due to similarity in their environment rather than in their heredity. Take away the similarity in the environment and the high concordance seems to disappear. This is not to deny that heredity plays an important role in stuttering. The 5 nonstuttering co-twins in Farber's study may well have had a genetic predisposition to stutter, and it is even possible that some of them had recovered from early episodes of stuttering. If so, however, what would remain significant about these 5 discordant twin pairs is that it was environment, not heredity, that determined whether stuttering would manifest itself, or whether it would persist as a chronic disorder.

Stuttering in the Families of Adopted Stutterers

There is still a further stratagem by which the issue of heredity in stuttering might be resolved, and that is by studying the familial backgrounds of stutterers who have been raised as adopted children. We know as a result of past research that, because they are stutterers, approximately one-third to two-thirds of such a group are likely to have identifiable histories of stuttering in their families. But where are these histories to be found—in the biological or the adoptive families? A clear answer to this question would go far to show whether the ten-

---

[9]The relevant data in Farber's book are on page 86 and in Table A9 in the epilogue.

dency of stuttering to recur in successive generations of the same family is mainly biological or mainly social.[10]

Investigation of the biological families of adopted children unfortunately presents practical difficulties. Much might be learned, however, by limiting our study to a sufficient number of stutterers' adoptive families on the assumption that presence or absence of stuttering would indicate the reverse in the biological families. As yet, we do not have information of this kind based on an adequate sample of adopted stutterers. A small series of such cases reported by the author when there were 5 (see Bloodstein, 1961b) has grown to 13 at this writing. Among the 13 stutterers 4 have a history of stuttering in the adoptive family[11] and 9 do not. Nature is equivocating as usual. It is too soon to say that the outcome will not yet go either way. If the present ambiguous trend should continue, however, what we may be receiving is the now familiar message that both hereditary and environmental factors make their contribution to the familial incidence of stuttering—and the etiology of the disorder.

Summary Remarks

The large proportion of stutterers who have stuttering relatives and the high concordance for stuttering of identical twins have long suggested to researchers that biological inheritance plays some part in stuttering. With the discovery of models of genetic transmission that can account for observational data on the distribution of stuttering

---

[10]Children who are brought up in adoptive homes might be more likely or less likely than others to become stutterers, but this has little bearing on the question of the distribution of stutterers in their biological and adoptive families. The possibility that adults who stutter or have stuttering relatives might be more prone or less prone to give or receive children in adoption must be considered for the sake of strict logic, but this would clearly have to be a tendency of extreme dimensions in order to affect the results of such a study.

[11]One of these four cases met reasonable criteria for inclusion in a study of this type somewhat imperfectly. This was a 12-year-old boy reared from the age of 20 months by a foster mother who told the author that he "always stuttered." The foster mother's older sister as well as her only biological child, aged 4 years, were said to be stutterers. The only member of the boy's biological family known to the foster mother was his mother who was said to be a normal speaker. Two other foster children in the adoptive family, a girl 8 years of age and a boy of 11, did not stutter.

A second case was that of an 8-year-old boy, adopted at 7 months of age, who began to stutter at age 4 or 5 years. His adoptive mother had stuttered severely as a child, and her nephew, aged 18 years, was a severe stutterer.

A third case was a 7-year-old girl who had not begun to talk at age 18 months when she and her twin brother were adopted by her present mother. She was said to have stuttered from the beginning of speech at age 2 years. The adoptive mother's younger sister and brother stuttered as children.

The fourth case was a 6-year-old boy, adopted at birth, who had stuttered severely from age 1.5 years to 5 and resumed stuttering at age 6 years after the parents adopted a second child. The adoptive mother's brother and his son had also stuttered.

among stutterers' relatives, the evidence that biological inheritance plays some part in stuttering has become quite strong. It should be noted, however, that these models imply an interaction between heredity and environment. The same evidence therefore points as clearly to the importance of environmental factors. This is confirmed by the exceptions to the concordance of identical twins for stuttering. Compelling evidence of the influence of environment are the accounts that have come to light of discordance for stuttering in identical twins who were reared apart.[12] Such facts tell us little, however, about the nature of the environmental factors that play a part. For that we must turn to other types of research.

THE INFLUENCE OF ENVIRONMENT

The studies of the prevalence of stuttering that are relevant to environmental variables are chiefly those that have been concerned with stuttering in various cultures and socioeconomic groups.

Prevalence In Other Cultures

Earlier in this chapter we reviewed information on the prevalence of stuttering in the general population of the United States, England, and other countries representative of European culture. Toyoda[13] reported a prevalence of stuttering of 0.82 percent among Japanese schoolchildren, a figure that might have been found in any Western country. Nor is there any reason to expect markedly different figures from India or China, on the basis of general observation. On the other hand, there has been a steady accumulation of evidence suggesting the existence in various places in the world of societies in which the prevalence of stuttering does differ quite a bit from the amount that is usual in Western nations. In many cases it is less; in a few it seems to be more.

One of the earliest studies of the cultural incidence of stuttering was reported by Bullen (1945). For the most part, Bullen was concerned directly, not with cultures, but with anthropologists. She sent letters to such well-known workers in the field as Fortune, Mead, and Kluckhohn and simply asked them to state to what extent they recalled cases of stuttering among the primitive people with whom they were familiar. The answers were striking in their uniformity. Fortune said, "I have not met a primitive who stuttered." He esti-

---

[12]Environmental influence is revealed by still another observation. Using the pooled data of several studies, Andrews et al (1983) calculated that an ordinary same-sexed sibling of a stutterer has an 18 percent chance of being a stutterer, whereas the risk rises to 32 percent in the case of a same-sexed fraternal co-twin.

[13]Cited by Van Riper (1971, p. 39).

mated that in the course of his investigations in New Guinea he had talked with about 6,000 people among the Mundugumor, Arapesh, Tchambuli, Manus, Dobuan, New Hanover, Tabor, and Kamamentira tribes. He said he had seen leprosy, hemophilia, insanity, and "running amok," but no stuttering. Margaret Mead, referring chiefly to natives of New Guinea and parts of the South Pacific, said, "I have never seen a case of stuttering or stammering among primitive people, although I remember hearing of one among the Arapesh." Two of Bullen's informants, Warner and Birdsell, had worked extensively among the aborigines of Australia. Warner had never observed stuttering among them, while Birdsell had the impression that it was "very rare." In addition, no stutterers were reported by Ekblaw among 250 Polar Eskimos with whom he had lived continuously for four years.

The Bannock and Shoshone

Some of our knowledge about the cultural prevalence of stuttering has come from studies of American Indians. Bullen's information included several reports about the Navaho that suggested that stutterers might be rather rare among them, although they clearly indicated that cases of stuttering were to be found. Cultural contacts that have taken place between the Navaho and our own stuttering society, however, make it difficult to interpret these reports. Likewise, Clifford, Twitchell, and Hull (1965) counted thirty-two stutterers, a prevalence of 1.8 percent, among 1,799 children in several South Dakota Indian schools and believed this reflected the effects of acculturation.

This difficulty did not exist in the case of the Bannock and Shoshone, living in relative isolation on reservations in southeastern Idaho. Some years before the Bullen study it had been reported to Wendell Johnson at the University of Iowa that the Bannock and Shoshone Indians appeared to have no word for stuttering. From 1937 to 1939 one of Johnson's students, John C. Snidecor, carried out among these Indians what seems to have been the first anthropological investigation of stuttering (Johnson, 1944; Snidecor, 1947). Snidecor's mission was to find a stuttering Indian, if any existed. His first step was to gain an audience with the tribal council of chiefs. Since he knew no Bannock-Shoshone word for stuttering, he could only demonstrate what it was he was looking for. He reported that the chiefs were much amused by his behavior, but had never seen anything like it. For the next two years Snidecor pursued his investigation with the help of an indian guide to whom he had promised a reward for information leading to the discovery of a stuttering Indian. In this period, during which he personally interviewed 800 persons and obtained information on 1,000 more, he failed to find "one pureblooded Indian who stuttered."

In attempting to suggest reasons for what they believed to be the absence or low incidence of stuttering among certain tribes of American Indians, Bullen, Johnson, and Snidecor appeared to be in agreement on the importance of one factor—the absence of heavy cultural pressures, including speech pressures. In these societies the children were allowed a relatively large measure of freedom, and little was expected of them in the way of adherence to culturally approved standards of behavior until adolescence. Correspondingly, children were likely to receive little criticism of the way in which they spoke. As Snidecor observed about the Bannock and Shoshone, "Ability to speak appears to be evaluated as a normal developmental process, not to be quickened by over-anxious parents for purposes of display." Even in adulthood far less seemed to depend on the ability to speak than in our culture. There was rarely the feeling of necessity to speak under pressure. It was not obligatory to talk merely to keep a conversation going. In a tribal council an opinion could be expressed by a simple yes or no. Later, Stewart (1960) found evidence that the Ute, a people of Shoshonean stock, tended to be relatively permissive with regard to nursing, toilet training, crying, and body contact with the parent; allowed children to develop independence and language at their own rate; and placed little emphasis on conformity to standards of speech fluency.

In Johnson's mind the apparent absence of a word for stuttering among the Bannock and Shoshone was of the utmost significance in view of his theory that stuttering is caused by parental mislabeling of children as stutterers. In time, however, publication of independent observations by Sven Liljeblad, an anthropologist, and Art Frank, a speech pathologist, left little doubt that the Bannock and Shoshone possessed both stutterers and words for stuttering.[14] Both men had informants who identified individuals on the reservation who stuttered. Frank interviewed two stutterers who had been living there at the time of the Snidecor study and noted characteristic symptoms as well as word and situational avoidances. Liljeblad recorded a number of Bannock-Shoshone expressions relating to stuttering. These consisted of derivations of the stem *pybya*. Both Frank and Liljeblad stated that they had to overcome considerable reticence, embarrassment, and distrust before anyone would admit to them that they had any knowledge of stuttering on the reservation.

The Kwakiutl, Nootka, and Salish

In actuality, the notion that American Indians do not stutter was dispelled as early as 1953. In that year Edwin M. Lemert, a social anthro-

---

[14]These observations, made in the 1960s, were not published until many years later. See Zimmermann, Liljeblad, Frank, and Cleeland (1983).

pologist of the University of California at Los Angeles, reported finding numerous stutterers among the Kwakiutl, Nootka, and Salish tribes of Canada. These are the Indians who have lived from very ancient times by salmon fishing on the Pacific Northwest Coast, who carve totem poles, and who have, or had, a distinctive type of tribal organization marked by bitter interclan rivalry. They are noted for the institution of the "potlatch," a ceremonial feast at which the hosts gave away or destroyed their most treasured possessions, thereby humiliating their guests from rival clans who could then hold their heads high only by giving away or destroying even more valuable possessions at a potlatch of their own. Among these people Lemert found an abundance of stutterers. Although he made no actual count, his personal contacts with stutterers and his informants' reports of stuttering cases left little room for doubt that the disorder is rather commonplace on the Northwest Coast.

The question that immediately arises is whether stuttering is indigenous to these people or acquired through the process of acculturation they have undergone in recent times. Lemert found three pieces of evidence that speak for the antiquity of the disorder among them. First, there are native words for stuttering as well as for other speech disorders in their language. Second, their folklore contains rituals and incantations for the treatment of stuttering. Third, in some cases living members of these tribes had memories of the stuttering of their grandfathers whose childhoods must have gone back to the 1850s, or earlier, when contact with our culture was largely limited to sporadic fur trade.

To explain the prevalence of stuttering among the Northwest Coast Indians, Lemert pointed to their unique social competitiveness. It was a kind of competition in which the prestige of the family group and the clan was the prime concern and in which the failures or shortcomings of each individual might jeopardize the status of the entire group. This tended to have two consequences that may be of some importance in relation to the etiology of stuttering. In the first place, it led to exacting educational practices and the imposition of rigid standards of behavior at an early age. It may be significant, for example, that young children were often obliged to participate in solemn rituals, requiring knowledge of songs and dances of some complexity, under the scrutiny of adults of their own and rival clans. In the second place, it meant that the individual who was different in some way was a source of embarrassment to the group as a whole and did not generally strive to be conspicuous. The coastal Indians of the North Pacific exhibit attitudes of pity, condescension, amusement, and social rejection toward such differences as left-handedness, obesity, smallness, mental deficiency, and orthopedic disability, as well as toward a variety of speech impairments.

The Ibo and Idoma of West Africa

Observations on the incidence of stuttering in tribal societies have not been limited to American Indians, as we have already seen. A comprehensive cultural investigation of stuttering was reported in an unpublished dissertation by Morgenstern (1953) and summarized in some detail by Johnson et al (1967, p. 244 ff.). From 258 anthropologists working in the field, Morgenstern systematically obtained information about the prevalence of stuttering and of various cultural traits and attitudes in nonliterate groups all over the world. He found some thirteen-peoples in New Guinea, British Guiana, Borneo, Malaya, and India who reportedly had no stuttering and no word for stuttering. He also discovered that the societies in which stuttering was said to be absent tended to be societies that were rated as relatively permissive in their child-training practices and relatively tolerant of personal shortcomings and deviations from the normal.

Among the most interesting of Morgenstern's findings were those relating to the Idoma and Ibo peoples of West Africa, among whom there appeared to be an exceedingly large number of stutterers. Of the Idoma, Dr. Robert Armstrong, an American anthropologist, reported to Morgenstern, "Stammering (in the sense of spasmodic repetition of the same speech sound) is practically a mass phenomenon here. I have met many dozens of persons who stammer in some degree." Among the Ibo 2.67 percent of a group of 5,618 schoolchildren were reported to stutter on the basis of a survey conducted by teachers and headmasters. Armstrong commented further, "Ability to speak well in public is vastly admired in West Africa, and Idoma and Ibo country is no exception to this statement. People make speeches on the slightest pretext. . . . There is strong ridicule from the stammerer's age-mates. . . ."

From other sources one learns that the Ibo place great stress on the attainment of an education and that they have frequently been regarded by other tribes as the most competitive and economically aspiring people of West Africa. It would seem to be a particularly revealing kind of distinction that, of the young men who have gone from this part of Africa to study at European and American universities, an unusually large number appear to belong to the Ibo people. Interestingly enough, one such student to whom the author was introduced some years ago was a stutterer himself. In commenting on his childhood in Nigeria, he said that at age 5 years he was sent to live with his uncle's family because his parents, who hoped very much that he would acquire traits of leadership, feared that he would be excessively coddled at home. He recalled that his uncle would slap him whenever he stuttered, in a well-intentional effort to correct his speech. He remembered other children who stuttered, particularly among the boys who shared with him the good fortune of being able to go to school.

Summary Remarks

We have reviewed a number of studies of the cultural prevalence of stuttering. To these may be added several other observations. Lemert (1962) related the apparently low incidence of stuttering in Polynesian society and its relatively higher incidence in Japan to a difference in pressures for achievement and social nonconformity. Aron (1962) found a prevalence of stuttering of 1.26 percent among 6,581 Bantu schoolchildren of Johannesburg. Noting that Bantu languages contain words for stuttering that are thought to antedate the arrival of Western civilization in South Africa, she related the apparent similarity in prevalence of stuttering between European and Bantu urban societies to a similarity in basic social structure and attitudes toward acquisition of speech. Nwokah (1988) cited surveys yielding the unusually high prevalence figures of 5.5 percent for schoolchildren in Dakar (Senegal) and 3.5 percent for schoolchildren in Accra (Ghana). Kirk (1977) reported on the high frequency of a type of stuttering in Ghana among speakers of Ga, but this is said to be chiefly nonpathological in nature and is identified by speakers as a normal occurrence when it is pointed out to them. Platzky and Girson (1993) interviewed four indigenous healers of the Tsonga, South Sotho, Xhosa, and Zulu groups of South Africa. All had native names for stuttering. All cited factors consistent with their cultural beliefs, as well as heredity, as causes of stuttering. Most considered stuttering a handicap and a cause of lowered self-esteem.

Reflecting on all these observations, we may ask what our anthropological information on stuttering adds up to. That stuttering is absent from any society, as some have claimed, is a hypothesis that is essentially impossible to prove by any practical scientific investigation. So is the contrary, that stuttering is universal, as others have insisted. An easier question to answer, and a far more important one from the standpoint of our understanding of stuttering, is whether there are cultural differences in the incidence of the disorder. Fragmentary evidence suggests that this is so. There is also more than a hint in the information at hand that stuttering is a significant comment on the culture that produces it. To say that there are many stutterers in a given society is very possibly to say that it is a rather competitive society that tends to impose high standards of achievement on the individual and to regard status and prestige as unusually desirable goals, that it is sternly intolerant of deviancy, and that, as a by-product of its distinctive set of cultural values, it in all likelihood places a high premium on conformity in speech.

Prevalence in Relation to Socioeconomic Level

If stuttering actually does have these cultural implications, one might reasonably expect to find confirmation of this in the prevalence of the disorder in those subcultures of our own society known as socioeconomic levels. It is provocative from this point of view that public school speech pathologists who have had wide experience in a large metropolitan educational system frequently report that some schools seem to produce an unusually large caseload of stutterers and that these schools usually seem to be located in the "better" neighborhoods. Research findings on the question are as yet meager. The assumption that stuttering is particularly common in the middle and upper-middle classes of society has received some, though not unqualified, confirmation.

Educational Level

One useful measure of socioeconomic status is level of educational attainment. Not only must people usually be able to pay to attend college, but they also need to have acquired the social, cultural, and economic values that make a college education desirable. It is therefore of considerable interest that in speech surveys conducted in the 1930s in five American colleges and universities as reported by Bender (1939, p. 2), the prevalence of stuttering was found to be 1.87 percent at the City College of New York, 2.60 percent at Dartmouth College, 2.70 percent at the University of Minnesota, 7.80 percent at the University of Ohio, and 2.00 percent at Queens College. These percentages vary from twice as high to perhaps more than three times as high as most prevalence figures for the grade school population of the United States.

Moreover, there is indirect evidence that these figures might have been even higher if not for the operation of some selective factors. In the first place, in a series of studies college stutterers in the 1930s were consistently found to be distinctly higher, on the average, in measured intelligence than college nonstutterers.[15] By contrast, the general grade school population of stutterers, as will be seen later, is no more intelligent than the general population of nonstutterers. Evidently, stutterers who would otherwise have attended college frequently failed to do so in the past because of their speech problem, unless they had superior intellectual endowment to compensate in part for it.

To this selective factor it is very possible that we must add another. Schuell (1946) found evidence that the sex ratio was markedly higher among university students than among the nonuniversity population of like age. The difference was 7.4–1 as against 3.7–1 for the 17 to 21 year age group, and 10.0–1 as contrasted with 7.6–1 in the 22 to 30 age range. It is a reasonable inference that this difference was due to the

---

[15]See Travis (1931, p. 101), Johnson (1932), Steer (1936), and Fruewald (1936).

number of female stutterers who, not having the economic drives of the male, chose to stay away even though they had the superior intellect and the socioeconomic background that would normally have sent them to college.

It is plausible to hypothesize that, at the time the relevant information was being gathered, stuttering was particularly prevalent in those segments of American society contributing most heavily to the college population. If so, to what extent this has continued to be true is a pertinent question. The numbers receiving higher education, and the pressures to do so, have been rising in recent decades, so that both socioeconomic distinctions and stuttering have become less effective deterrents to college attendance. Perhaps it is for this reason that later prevalence figures from colleges and universities have been considerably lower than those reported in 1939 by Bender. Morley (1952), in a ten-year speech survey of students at the University of Michigan, found a prevalence of stuttering of only 0.81 percent, with the rather ordinary sex ratio of 4.3–1. Other most recent figures are: 0.6 percent among students at Berkeley and the University of California at Los Angeles (Sheehan and Martyn, 1970), 2.1 percnt at the University of Massachusetts (Porfert and Rosenfield, 1978) and 0.3 percent at the University of Alabama (Culton, 1986). In any event, educational level is not the only measure that has been used in investigating the socioeconomic status of stutterers, and there are other forms of information on the subject to which we may turn.

Occupational Class of Parent and Other Measures

The most systematic study to date of socioeconomic factors in stuttering was carried out in Scotland by Morgenstern (1956) in the course of investigations already referred to. Morgenstern was aided in his research by the fact that in 1947 the Scottish Council for Research in Education had completed a survey that showed the proportionate distribution of a large number of schoolchildren among nine socioeconomic levels. These levels were based on the occupational status of the father and ranged from unskilled salaried farm workers to members of the professional class. Using these statistics as a standard of comparison, Morgenstern conducted a speech survey of a comparable sample of Scottish schoolchildren aimed at determining whether those children who stuttered were distributed among these occupational categories any differently from the population as a whole.

The results showed a general similarity between the two distributions, particularly—interestingly enough—on the middle and upper occupational levels. There were also, however, some differences.

Disproportionately few stutterers had fathers who were on the lowest level of the scale, corresponding to unskilled industrial and agricultural workers. The outstanding finding was an unexpectedly large number of stutterers whose fathers fell into a classification, relatively low on the socioeconomic scale, which was termed "semi-skilled manual weekly wage-earner" and included such occupations as truck driver or machine-tender. What was the explanation for this? Morgenstern believed that it lay in the somewhat unique upward mobility of this particular occupational class in Scottish society. He observed that, to a greater degree than appeared to be true of members of any other class, the semiskilled workers had both the opportunity and the aspiration to rise above their origins. This being so, they could be expected to exert somewhat greater pressure on their children to improve themselves and perhaps tended to evince a somewhat finer appreciation of the advantages of such personal refinements as fluent speech in the competition for social and economic status.

The most significant implications of the Scottish data seem fairly clear. Insofar as there is any relationship between socioeconomic level and proneness to produce stutterers, it may not be primarily the amount of status that is important, but the intensity of the drive to achieve a higher status.

Morgenstern also found a definite tendency for stuttering to be related to rate of occupancy of homes. Relatively speaking, fewer stutterers came from more crowded homes (two or more persons per room, on the average). A disproportionately large number of stutterers came from homes with the relatively low average occupancy rate of one to two persons per room, and also—but to a considerably less marked degree— from homes with a rate of less than one person per room. Morgenstern did not find the prevalence of stuttering to be related to density of population in which homes were located. This is in general accord with the data of Louttit and Halls (1936), Schindler (1955), and others showing little or no difference in the percentage of stutterers in urban as compared with rural areas. On the other hand, Brady and Hall (1976) found the prevalence of stuttering among urban schoolchildren almost twice as high as among rural schoolchildren in Illinois and Pennsylvania.

Morgenstern's survey produced the most convincing evidence we have of socioeconomic variations in the prevalence of stuttering. This evidence is not clearly corroborated by the results of other studies using similar measures of socioeconomic level. In a survey of over 20,000 Iowa schoolchildren, Schindler (1955) found no significant difference in mean occupational levels of parents of stutterers and nonstutterers, although about one-third of the stutterers as opposed to only one-sixth of the nonstutterers were in the upper levels. Nor is there any more corroboration in the data of Andrews and Harris (1964, p. 51) on either social class or upward mobility of the families of eighty stutterers in Newcastle upon Tyne.[16]

Prevalence with Era

There is a widespread impression among American clinical workers of long experience that the prevalence of stuttering is considerably less than it was some decades ago. Although there is little adequate evidence on the question, a few public school surveys cited by Van Riper (1982, p. 49) do show a marked decline between the 1940s and 1960s, at least in enrollment of stutterers for speech therapy. The very low prevalence figures of 0.3 percent and 0.35 percent obtained in the surveys of school children by Hull (1969) and Brady and Hall (1976) may also be indicative. Furthermore, the conviction of many speech pathologists that stutterers in their caseloads were once both more numerous and more severe is too firm and general to dismiss.[17]

If it is true, there are various possible reasons for it. Some workers attribute it to the permissive revolution in child rearing that is often laid to Spock's popular manual on child care and appears to go back ultimately to the influence of Freud. Van Riper (1982, p. 49) believes it is due primarily to a change in the attitudes of society toward stutterers resulting from the development of speech pathology as a profession. Others ascribe it more specifically to the wide influence of Johnson's diagnosogenic theory of stuttering in the United States. It is clear that we may be able to narrow the possibilities somewhat by comparing the impressions of American workers with those of speech clinicians in other countries.

It should not be overlooked that what we seem to be observing may not be an isolated phenomenon but merely part of a continual fluctuation in the incidence of stuttering. Just as it may vary from culture to culture it may also vary from one era to the next in response to changes in cultural values, attitudes, or child training practices. On its face this would seem to be more reasonable than the egocentric view that a phenomenon that has happened only once in history has happened in our lifetime.

---

[16]In an exhaustive study of 150 stutterers by Johnson and Associates (1959, p. 75 ff.) in which subjects were matched for socioeconomic status with their controls, a relatively large proportion were found to be in the middle and upper classes on the basis of multiple criteria, but their method of selection made it difficult to be certain that the subjects could be validly compared with the general population.

[17]Figures obtained by Dean and Brown (1977) from departments of special education of nine states for the ten years from 1963 to 1973 show about the same number of stutterers annually, suggesting that the prevalence of stuttering may have stabilized by the 1960s.

At any rate, we should not ignore the most important implication of the current decline in prevalence. Whatever its cause, it constitutes one of the strongest indications that can be found of the contribution of the environment to the etiology of stuttering.

CONCLUSIONS

The prevalence of stuttering in the school population in Western society at the present time is approximately 1 percent and appears to be somewhat higher in Europe than in the United States. The incidence of those who will have stuttered at some time in their lives is substantially greater, at least 4 or 5 percent and perhaps indeterminately higher if early childhood episodes of brief duration are counted.

From certain points of view stuttering may be regarded as a disorder of childhood. It begins in childhood, typically in the early years. A very large proportion of children spontaneously recover from it. In earliest childhood mild, transient forms of stuttering appear to be very common.

Stuttering is more prevalent among males than females. The sex ratio among American schoolchildren is roughly 3–1. It is probably lower than that in preschool children and higher in adults. The sex ratio has been attributed to sex differences in constitution, physical maturation, or speech and language development or to differences in parental attitudes and expectations with regard to boys and girls.

Certain features of the incidence of stuttering strongly suggest that to a greater or lesser degree biological heredity may be a factor in the etiology of stuttering. There is a high familial incidence, as indicated by the presence of stuttering among the relatives of roughly 50 percent of stutterers. There is also a high degree of concordance of stuttering in identical twins. Neither of these findings represents conclusive evidence that genetic transmission plays any part, but genetic models of inheritance that allow for the interaction of environmental variables are capable of accounting fairly accurately for data on family backgrounds of stuttering. The possibility of such inheritance raises the challenging question of specifically what might be transmitted that would incline a child to stuttering.

Other findings offer evidence of the influence of environment. The incidence of stuttering appears to vary in different cultures. There is some evidence that the cultures in which there are relatively large numbers of stutterers are those characterized by outstanding competitive pressures. In addition, there is some reason to believe that in our own culture stuttering may be more common on certain socioeconomic levels, especially those marked by unusual upward mobility. In this respect, however, the evidence is decidedly less conclusive.

The consistent differences in European and American studies of the prevalence of stuttering seem to be due to more than mere coincidence and may constitute further evidence of sociocultural influences. It may be a plausible hypothesis that American children are somewhat less likely to stutter for the same reasons that they are probably somewhat more likely to be heard "talking back" to their parents. The signs that the incidence of stuttering may have declined in the past generation are also indicative of the role of environment. Perhaps the most conclusive evidence of all lies in the exceptions found in the concordance of stuttering among identical twins. Not only are such exceptions common, but the results of one recent investigation suggest that when identical twins are reared apart, discordance for stuttering may be the rule.

The probability that stuttering is related to environmental pressures for achievement and conformity of some kind appears to represent one of the fundamental pieces of information we have gained about its causation. We do not know, however, precisely what it means. Which demand is it that contributes directly to stuttering? Is it the specific demand on children to speak more fluently than they are able? Is it the more general demand that children speak more perfectly or on a more advanced or difficult level than they can from the point of view of any or all aspects of verbal communication? Or is it the still broader pressure to conform in general to standards of behavior or achievement beyond their capabilities? It is apparent that a clear choice among several different theoretical approaches to the etiology of stuttering turns on the question of which of these three possibilities is correct.

In this chapter we have been concerned with what has been learned about stuttering from studies of its prevalence and incidence in various populations. In addition to the populations we have discussed, there are a number of others with respect to which this question has been raised, consisting chiefly of persons who have specific differences—those with deafness, blindness, cerebral palsy, epilepsy, psychosis, mental deficiency, left-handedness, and bilingualism. These findings will be considered later in appropriate contexts.

Suggested Readings

Andrews, G., Epidemiology of stuttering. In Curlee, R F., and Perkins, W. H. (eds.), *Nature and Treatment of Stuttering: New Directions*. San Diego: College-Hill Press (1984).

Andrews, G., and Harris, M., *The Syndrome of Stuttering*. London: The Spastics Society Medical Education and Information Unit in association with William Heinemann Medical Books (1964), Chaps. 3, 7.

Kidd, K. K, Stuttering as a genetic disorder. In Curlee, R F., and Perkins, W. H. (eds.), *Nature and Treatment of Stuttering: New Directions*. San Diego: College-Hill Press (1984).

Kidd, K. K., Kidd, J. R, and Records, M. A., The possible causes of sex ratio in stuttering and its implications. *J. Fluency Dis.*, 3, 13–23 (1978).

Lemert, E. M., Some Indians who stutter. *J. Speech Hearing Dis.*, 1.8, 168–74 (1953).

MacFarlane,W. B., Hanson, M., Walton, W., and Mellon, C. D., Stuttering in five generations of a single family. *J. Fluency Dis.*, 16, 117–23 (1991).

Morgenstern, J. J., Socio-economic factors in stuttering. *J. Speech Hearinq Dis.*, 21, 25–33 (1956).

Sheehan, J. G., and Martyn, M. M., Spontaneous recovery from stuttering. *J. Speech Hearing Res.*, 9, 121–35 (1966).

Sheehan, J. G., and Martyn, M. M., Stuttering and its disappearance. *J. Speech Hearing Res.*, 13, 279–89 (1970).

Zimmermann, G., Lilieblad, S., Frank, A., and Cleeland, C., The Indians have many terms for it: Stuttering among the Bannock-Shoshoni. *J. Speech Hearing Res.*, 26, 315–18 (1983).

4

THE PERSON WHO STUTTERS: PHYSICAL CONSTITUTION

The next three chapters will be concerned with the question of how the person who stutters differs as an individual from others. A great many studies have addressed this basic question by comparing groups of stutterers with groups of nonstutterers with regard to an almost inexhaustible list of human traits.

Chapter 4 will be devoted to research on the stutterer's physical characteristics. This long avenue of approach to the stuttering problem began with early studies of breathing, motor capacities, and heart rate; turned to investigations of the stutterer's tissue chemistry, neuromuscular organization, handedness, and cortical potentials; and eventually led to research on more subtle aspects of auditory perception and lateral dominance for cerebral processing of speech. Some of this research was done in the hope of disposing of the question of the etiology of stuttering at one blow. There is hardly a path of scientific inquiry in the field of speech disorders more strewn with false leads, errors, conflicting replications, disappointment, confusion, and controversy. Perhaps the most important knowledge to which it has led so far is that when they are not speaking, stutterers are remarkably like other people. We shall take note of some possible exceptions to this, however.

PHYSIOLOGICAL PROCESSES

In the last chapter we saw that there is evidence of genetic influences on stuttering, and for some workers this aspect of its etiology has loomed larger than any other. For many years laboratory investigations of the stutterer's bodily processes have been conducted in pursuit of a clue to an inherited predisposing abnormality underlying the disorder. It should be noted that physiological studies may be done—for different purposes and with different implications—during stuttering, during what is judged to be the stutterer's "free" speech, or during silence. Most physiological measures are responsive to muscular effort and autonomic arousal. Consequently, if convincing evidence of an etiological factor is desired it must be obtained during silence, preferably under basal conditions and when the subjects have not been engaged in speech for several hours. In addition, it is much safer practice to compare the measures obtained in this way with those of a control group than to make use of so-called textbook norms for this purpose. The failure to adhere to these principles has sometimes resulted in disagreement and confusion in this area of research. In this discussion we will for the most part omit mention of uncontrolled studies or casual observations where better information exists.

Breathing Movements

Because of their conspicuous disturbance during stuttering, breathing movements were the first physiological phenomena to arouse the interest of research workers, and they had been studied in Europe by the end of the nineteenth century. When Travis established one of the first American laboratories for the study of speech disorders at the University of Iowa in 1927, this was among the subjects to which he immediately gave his attention. By this time any serious notion once existing that breathing abnormality was a cause of stuttering had largely fallen into disrepute, however, and the detailed pneumographic investigations of Travis and his students were undertaken primarily as studies of symptomatology (see Chapter 1).

The broad conclusions of these and other studies of the breathing movements of stutterers may be briefly stated. During stuttering there are anomalies of a number of different kinds, which were described in Chapter 1. In general, however, these anomalies are not present during silence.[1] Furthermore, many of the disturbances in the stutterer's breathing during speech are also to be found in the breathing of normal speakers during speech, although not to the same degree.

In studies of stuttering children and adolescents without controls Schilling (1960, 1962) observed abnormal diaphragmatic movements during silent breathing. Both Moore (1938) and Kurshev (1968b),

---

[1]See references in Chapter 1, footnote 8. Exceptions to this may occur during expectancy of stuttering (Van Riper, 1936) and possibly also during silent reading and reasoning (Murray, 1932).

however, found that during silence stutterers and nonstutterers did not differ in measures of breathing movement.

Cardiovascular Factors and Basal Metabolic Rate

Heart rate was another object of early laboratory investigation. In 1914 Fletcher observed an acceleration of the stutterer's pulse rate during speech, "in the period anticipatory of speaking and, in general, under those conditions that are calculated to produce stuttering." McDowell (1928) compared stutterers and nonstutterers in average heart rate and blood pressure and found no difference. Travis, Tuttle, and Cowan (1936) observed faster heart rates than normal in stuttering subjects before and during speech and, like Fletcher, attributed this chiefly to the emotional reactions and respiratory abnormalities associated with stuttering.

It seemed clear that the cardiovascular changes that had been observed during stuttering were merely symptoms of the disorder. But several years later studies by Palmer and Gillette (1938, 1939) appeared to indicate that stutterers had both faster heart rates and more sinus arrhythmia[2] than normal speakers even in silence and under basal conditions. Furthermore, unlike normal subjects, among whom there is a sex difference with respect to these factors, the male and female stutterers seemed to have cardiac rates and rhythms that were much alike. Palmer and Gillette speculated that there was a "sex-linked, neurophysiological, metabolic mechanism for stuttering."

Ritzman (1943) replicated this research with refinements in technique. He found no differences between adult male stutterers and their controls in heart rate, sinus arrhythmia, blood pressure, and basal metabolic rate (BMR). Among 4 female stutterers, however, he found less marked sinus arrhythmia and higher pulse pressure and basal metabolic rate than in their controls and a definite tendency for them to resemble the male stutterers in these measures, in general corroboration of the observations made by Palmer and Gillette. Ritzman interpreted this as a reflection of more intense sensitivity to stuttering on the part of the female stutterers. McCroskey (1957) found no differences between stutterers and nonstutterers in BMR, but did not report separately on the 3 female subjects in his group. Golub (1953), whose experimental group was made up solely of males, confirmed Ritzman's finding that their heart rates do not differ from those of nonstuttering males, as did Walker and Walker (1973). But Brunner and Frank (1976) found higher resting pulse rates in both stutterers and successfully treated stutterers than in controls. The stutterers also had greater fluctuations in pulse rate, as well as sharper increases after work.

---

[2]Sinus arrhythmia refers to normal variations in heart rate occurring regularly in the course of the respiratory cycle.

Biochemical Factors

For a brief period it appeared that clues to the etiology of stuttering might be found in the chemical make-up of the stutterer's body.

Alveolar Carbon Dioxide and Salivary pH

Biochemical research on stuttering owed its beginnings to a belief of Edwin B. Twitmyer of the University of Pennsylvania that the large majority of stutterers were shallow breathers suffering from fatigue or lethargy brought on by insufficient aeration of their blood and that the rest—a comparatively small number—were for the most part "hyperexcitable psychopaths" who tended to the opposite extreme. Twitmyer had a colleague, Henry E. Starr, who was interested in salivary pH[3] as a measure of states of emotion or excitement. Starr saw an opportunity to test both his own and Twitmyer's assumptions. He reasoned that Twitmyer's lethargic, "subbreathing" stutterers should have a low salivary pH as a consequence of their CO_2 excess, and that the "hyperexcitable psychopath" stutterers should have low alveolar CO_2 and high salivary pH. In controlled studies of both types of subjects, who were presumably selected and classified with Twitmyer's guidance, this is exactly what he found.[4]

Corroborative findings came shortly from a study of the blood cells of stutterers done by one of Twitmyer's students, Max A. Trumper.[5] Trumper based his study on the knowledge that oxygen deficit in the arterial blood results in a compensatory increase in the number and hemoglobin content of the red blood cells. Among a series of 101 cases of stuttering, he identified one-third as shallow breathers. In blood studies of this group he found that, judged by standard medical norms, there was an increased red blood cell count and relatively high hemoglobin.

With regard to salivary pH, there was some further corroboration of Starr's results in findings by Kelly (1932) of pH values that he considered "below the normal range" in a small group of stutterers. Some time later, however, Hafford (1941) obtained findings in direct conflict with those of Starr. She found no difference between stutterers and normal speakers in the distribution of salivary pH values, either under basal conditions or after a period of speech. In addition, she cited unpublished results from the doctoral dissertation of George A. Kopp, completed in 1933, which showed no difference between stutterers and controls in alveolar CO_2, a finding which was confirmed

---

[3]pH is an index of the hydrogen ion concentration; the lower the pH of a solution the higher the hydrogen ion concentration and the greater the acidity. Salivary pH is believed to be influenced by alveolar CO_2.

[4]See Starr (1922, 1928).

[5]Trumper's unpublished study, completed as a doctoral dissertation in 1928, was summarized in detail by Twitmyer (1930).

further by Johnson, Young, Sahs, and Bedell (1959). As Hill (1944a) summed it up after an exhaustive review, ". . . that stutterers as a class are in a condition of CO_2 excess is very questionable."

Chemical Composition of the Blood

A second line of biochemical inquiry concerned with blood constituents received its major impetus from the theory advanced by West and his students at the University of Wisconsin that stuttering was the symptom of a metabolic disorder whose evidences were to be found in abnormalities of tissue chemistry. The first general blood analyses of stutterers, however, were reported by Johnson, Stearns, and Warweg (1933) and had a somewhat different theoretical basis. These workers were concerned with testing the hypothesis that stuttering was due to a form of latent tetany, and their principal object was consequently to determine whether there was a deficiency of calcium in the stutterer's blood. Taking samples from fifteen adult male stutterers, they established that, judged by clinical norms, these subjects were normal in amount of serum calcium as well as such other blood constituents as inorganic phosphorus, potassium, and blood sugar.

In the same year Kopp (1934) was bringing to completion his extensive biochemical study of stutterers at the University of Wisconsin. Kopp, too, found that the blood chemistry of the stutterer was essentially normal by accepted medical standards. But when he compared his subjects with a control group of nonstutterers he discovered a variety of differences. The stutterers appeared to be not lower, but higher, in serum calcium. They were also higher in inorganic phosphorus and blood sugar and lower in potassium, total protein, albumin, and globulin, and they seemed to differ as well in the degree of relationship between some of these components. Kopp concluded that stuttering was a manifestation of a disturbed metabolism and suggested that it might one day be possible to control it by dietary means. Somewhat later, however, a study of Karlin and Sobel (1940) disclosed essentially no differences between stutterers and nonstutterers in chemical composition of the blood and failed to confirm the correlations between constituents found by Kopp.[6]

Since 1940, studies of the stutterer's tissue chemistry have been comparatively few. Anderson and Whealdon (1941) found that stut-

---

[6]Among the 22 blood constituents tested, Karlin and Sobel actually found one statistically significant difference; stutterers were lower in potassium. They attached no importance to it, however. By definition, 5 percent of the differences in a series of calculations of this sort will in the long run prove to be significant at the 5 percent level by chance. Consequently, there would be little interest in a single significant difference among twenty-two calculations, unless it represented the confirmation of a prior hypothesis with regard to that particular item.

terers did not appear to differ from the general population in distribution of blood types and therefore in the proteins controlling agglutination. Lovett Doust (1956) reported stutterers to show more marked changes than normal speakers in oxygen saturation of capillary blood in response to the stress of breath-holding and interpreted this as a sign of less stable oxidative metabolism in the stutterer. Girone and Bruno (1957) found evidence of a possible disturbance of glucose regulation. Galamon, Szulc-Kuberska, and Tronczyńliska (1969) reported an increased level of urinary histidine in some school-age children with "hereditary" stuttering. Laczkowski (1965) reported results which appear to contradict this. Finally, Podolskaya and Shklovsky (1973) obtained findings that seemed to point to a heparin deficit in the blood of stutterers and laid the blame for it on "constant and protracted emotional stress."

It is of interest that after an interval of twenty-five years Johnson, Young, Sahs, and Bedell (1959) returned to the hypothesis of latent tetany that had led to the first study of blood constituents and found a convincing refutation of it in the failure of stuttering to increase following hyperventilation. More recently, Sayles (1971) observed that overbreathing produced a decrease in stuttering in many of his subjects, possibly as a result of distraction. Lastovka (1978) found no clinical manifestations of tetany in a group of twenty-eight stutterers.

Rastatter and Harr (1988) measured neurotransmitter and amino acid blood levels in five stutterers and compared them with norms. A consistent abnormal finding was high levels of glutamine in all five subjects.

Neurophysiological Findings

Neurophysiological investigation of stuttering was pioneered by Lee E. Travis at the University of Iowa. In an intensive research program that occupied the period from about 1927 to 1937, he and his students produced a steady output of laboratory findings. The major focus for this work was provided by the theory, which Travis developed together with Samuel T. Orton, that stuttering resulted from an underlying condition in which the bilaterally paired musculatures of the organs of speech tended to work independently of each other because of the lack of a sufficient margin of cerebral dominance.

Action Potentials from the Paired Speech Musculatures

The Orton-Travis concept led to research in which the bilateral neuromuscular organization of stutterers was studied in various ways. What would seem to be the ultimate test of such a theory, however, is afforded by the electromyograph. From a recording of action potentials from the muscles on the two sides of the speech structures, it should be evident whether these muscles are starting their contractions at different times or are acting dyssynchronously in any way. Accordingly, in what was thought to be a crucial test of the cerebral dominance theory, Travis (1934) recorded electrical potentials from the left and right masseter muscles of stutterers and nonstutterers while they were speaking. He found that the recordings from the two sides were essentially identical for almost all of the nonstutterers, as well as for the stutterers when they were speaking normally. During stuttering, however, there were striking differences in the instant of appearance as well as other bilateral dissimilarities in the patterns in the majority of cases.

Events observed only during the act of stuttering, of course, always tend to raise the troublesome question of whether they are a cause or an effect. Nevertheless, these findings stood as a last support of the cerebral dominance theory long after the research on the laterality of stutterers had created serious objections to it and Travis himself had become absorbed in other etiological concepts. Finally, Williams (1955) replicated Travis's study with some additional aspects of procedure. He found many of the same action potential anomalies that Travis had observed. These anomalies, however, occurred to the same extent in the speech of the nonstutterers when they were "faking" stuttering. Furthermore, he found that they could be produced in silence in both stutterers and nonstutterers by instructing them to perform specific jaw movements.

Reflex Activities

Various autonomic reflexes have been tested in stutterers during silence. For many years Seeman and certain other European writers have commented on evidences of lability, sensitivity, or irritability of the autonomic nervous system in stutterers.[7] Confirmation from controlled studies has been essentially lacking, however. Sovak (1935) reported normal oculocardiac and positive solar plexus reflexes in the majority of a group of stuttering children and adults. Jacoby (1947) investigated the carotid sinus reflex in stutterers and found it to be normal. Walker and Walker (1973) tested stutterers' autonomic reactivity to stress by measuring the increase in their heart rates following bursts of noise. On the average their heart rates did not differ from those of nonstutterers in response to the stimulus.

Schilling (1959, 1962) reported electronystagmographic abnormalities in 47 percent of a group of stuttering children. Bruno, Carmarda, and Curi (1965) found such abnormalities in 29 of 50 stutterers. Castellini, Salami, and Ottoboni (1972) observed them in 14 of 30 cases.

---

[7]See Hogewind (1940) and Sedláčková (1963).

In none of these studies was a control group used. Široký, Langová, Morávek, and Šváb (1978), using a control group, found a considerably greater number of saddle-shaped nystagmic jerks in the records of stutterers, whether in silence or speech. In a further study, however, these researchers failed to confirm previous findings of abnormality (Langová, Široký, Šváb, and Morávek (1979).

Laštovka (1979c) recorded longer durations of the electrically evoked innervation pause[8] in stutterers than in nonstutterers, and interpreted this as indirect evidence of deviations in the central feedback function of the extrapyramidal system and the cerebellum.

Neilson, Andrews, Guitar, and Quinn (1979) found no differences between 4 stutterers and 6 normal speakers in stretch reflexes of the jaw closing muscles. Nine stutterers did not differ from controls in reflex changes in biting force in response to loud noise and tactile stimulation of the lip, tongue, and teeth in research by Smith and Luschei (1983) and McFarland, Smith, Moore, and Weber (1986). Nor were any differences found by McClean (1987) in reflexes of the orbicularis oris inferior and depressor labii inferior muscles in response to cutaneous stimulation.

McLean-Muse, Larson, and Gregory (1988) studied reflex changes in the fundamental frequency of the voice in response to auditory click stimuli (a brainstem reflex) as subjects sustained a tone at a constant pitch and intensity. There were no differences between stutterers and nonstutterers.

In general, it would appear that most studies of stutterers' reflex activities during silence have had negative results or have been imperfectly controlled and less productive of reliable knowledge than of hypotheses for investigation.

Tremors

Herren (1932) studied the occurrence of tremors in the voluntary hand movements of stutterers and normal speakers. He found that during silence as well as speech a relatively rapid tremor, at the rate of 40 to 75 per second, occurred more frequently in the records of the stutterers. Herren offered no hypothesis to account for this finding. Hill (1944b) suggested that they might be traced in part to an increased adrenalin output during stuttering.

McFarland, Smith, Moore, and Weber (1986) found no differences in amplitude of tremor of the jaw closing muscles as subjects exerted a constant force on a bite block inserted between upper and lower teeth.

---

[8]A pause that may be induced in the voluntary contraction of skeletal muscle by electrical stimulation of the nerve.

Muscular Tension

Several different methods have been used to study muscular tonus in stutterers. Travis and Fagan (1928) measured the resistance of the pendant hand to 40-ounce blows. They found that more resistance was offered by stutterers than by normal speakers during silence. This might conceivably have resulted from either situational or chronic "nervous" hypertension among the stutterers. Another inference, however, that was considered by Shackson (1936) is latent tetany. Shackson measured the time intervals between the appearance of action potentials and the beginning of muscle thickening and voluntary movement in various muscles of stutterers and controls. There was a tendency toward faster muscle contraction in the stutterers during silence, which Shackson interpreted as evidence of chronic latent tetany.

Brown and Shulman (1940) measured muscular tension by determining the pressure needed to inject a minute amount of saline solution into the body of the biceps muscle. Unlike the earlier investigators, they found no evidence that stutterers were more tense than nonstutterers.

Brain Waves

The neurophysiological investigation of stuttering begun by Travis finally culminated in a large amount of electroencephalographic research. It had been known since 1929 that the cerebral cortex was the site of a concentration of electrical activity, or "brain waves." One of these, the alpha wave, sinusoidal in form, about 10 cycles per second in frequency, and of relatively high voltage, is interesting because it is noticeably affected by varying physiological states—for example, by attention, fright, or reduced states of consciousness as in sleep, stupor, or anesthesia. The alpha rhythm has been of clinical value because it is altered by pathological conditions of the brain such as epilepsy or even, in some cases, an unsuspected proneness to epilepsy.

In view of these facts, it is not difficult to see why interest should have developed in the cortical potentials of stutterers. Since 1936, when Travis and Knott published the first of these studies, a considerable number of them have been done. The major studies—those which have employed quantitative methods and made systematic use of control groups—are summarized in Table 9 with emphasis on those findings obtained from comparisons of stutterers with normal speakers. The results of these studies are difficult to compare because of wide differences in procedure. In conducting this research there is, to begin with, a choice of various areas of the brain. Moreover, different features of the record may be chosen for study—for example, the amplitude, duration, or frequency of the waves; the percentage of the time they are present or "blocked"; their similarity to corresponding

Table 9. Cortical Potentials of Stutterers and Nonstutterers

	Electrode Placement	Brain Area	Measures	Conditions	Results*
Travis and Knott (1936)	Bipolar	Left visual and motor	Amplitude duration	Silence Speech	Found small differences that they considered difficult to interpret. The waves during the nonstuttered speech of stutterers were larger and slower than those for the speech of normal speakers.
Travis and Knott (1937)	Bipolar	Left and right visual and motor	Synchronization and similarity of the two sides	Silence Speech	During silence the stutterers were more likely than the controls to have dissimilar potentials from the two sides, and during speech (stuttered and nonstuttered) were more likely to have perfectly matched potentials.
Travis and Malamud (1937)	Bipolar	Left motor and occipital	Frequency and amplitude	Silence Fluent speech	The waves of stutterers during fluent speech were larger and slower than the waves during speech of nonstutterers.
Lindsley (1940)	Bipolar	Left and right occipital	Asynchronism and unilateral blocking	Silence Speech	During silence and speech 2 adult stutterers had more out-of-phase waves than did 48 right-handed and 8 left-handed children and the same percentage as did 9 ambidextrous children.
Freestone (1942)	Bipolar	Left and right frontal, motor, and occipital	Amount of alpha activity, amplitude, amplitude range, amount of wave similarity	Silence Speech	No clearly significant difference on any of the measures. Stutterers had more alpha similarity between areas, indicating a "lack of heightened foci of cerebral activity."
Douglass (1943)	Monopolar	Left and right occipital and motor	Bilateral and unilateral blocking	Silence Speech	The stutterers and nonstutterers did not differ in mean percent time of blocking of the alpha rhythm in silence. In speech the stutterers had greater bilateral blocking in the occipital areas. In silence the stutterers tended to show more blocking in the left occipital area; the nonstutterers, a greater amount of blocking in the right.

Study	Method	Location	Measure	Condition	Findings
Knott and Tjossem (1943)	Monopolar	Left and right occipital and motor	Percent time alpha present	Silence	Confirmed findings of Douglass that during silence there is a tendency for stutterers and nonstutterers to differ with respect to which half of the occipital areas has more alpha activity.
Rheinberger, Karlin, and Berman (1943)	Bipolar and monopolar	Left and right frontal, central, occipital, intermastoid	Dominant frequencies above 7.5 per sec., irregular mixed activity, slow waves, bilateral asymmetry, changes under hyperventilation	Silence	Comparisons disclosed an essential similarity between the two groups.
Scarbrough (1943)	Monopolar	Left frontal, motor, and occipital	Frequency, variability of frequency, qualitatively abnormal records	Silence	The stutterers did not differ significantly from their controls in frequency or variability of frequency. Three of the stutterers and one of the nonstutterers (N=20 in each group) had qualitatively abnormal records.
Jones (1949)	Bipolar and monopolar	Left and right occipital	Unilateral and bilateral blocking, amount of bilateral out-of-phaseness, clinical abnormalities	Silence	There were no significant differences for any of the measures, except that stutterers exceeded nonstutterers in amount of left unilateral blocking in bipolar recordings.
Douglass (1952)	Monopolar	Left and right occipital	Wave alterations in response to stimuli	Silence Speech	Stutterers showed greater cortical reactivity in the dominant hemisphere to emotional stimuli (e.g., words, pictures).

Table 9 (continued)

	Electrode Placement	Brain Area	Measures	Conditions	Results*
Murphy (1953)	Monopolar	Left and right occipital	Wave alterations in response to frustration	Silence	Cortical disruption during frustration was significantly greater in stutterers when like hemispheres of the two groups were compared. Following frustration, stutterers recovered cortical equilibrium to a markedly smaller degree than did nonstutterers for both like-hemisphere comparisons.
Knott, Correll, and Shepherd (1959)	Bipolar and monopolar	Left and right occipital and occipital-parietal	Amount of voltage output at various frequencies, "driving"***	Silence	On various measures presumed to indicate "anxiety-proneness," each of two stuttering groups differed from the nonstuttering group in some way, but the two stuttering groups differed from each other more than from the nonstuttering group.
Fritzell, Petersén, and Selldén (1965)	Bipolar and monopolar	Left and right frontal, central, temporal, parietal, and occipital	Incidence of atypical features	Silence	Normal EEG's were significantly more frequent among the controls. Unspecific abnormalities (increased low frequency activity) were more common among the stutterers, especially the younger ones.
Fox (1966)	Bipolar	Left and right occipital	Prominence of a dominant frequency, interhemispheric synchronization, wave quality	Silence Speech	There were no significant differences between the two groups, either in silence or in nonstuttered speech. The only intergroup differences that appeared were between the stuttered speech of the stutterers and imitation of stuttering by the controls.

Study	Type	Location	Measure	Condition	Findings
Sayles (1971)	Bipolar and monopolar	Left and right frontal, motor, parietal, occipital, anterior-temporal, mid-temporal, posterior-temporal	Incidence of atypical responses to sleep, hyperventilation, and photic stimulation	Silence Speech	Abnormal or borderline wave patterns were found in 48% of the stutterers as compared with 12% of the controls. The stutterers also showed a greater cortical sensitivity to hyperventilation. The abnormalities were unrelated to speech activity or stuttering.
Okasha, Moneim, et al (1974)	Bipolar and monopolar	Left and right frontal, central, temporal, parietal, and occipital	Incidence of atypical features	Silence	The EEG showed epileptic changes in 22% of the stutterers and none of the controls.
Zimmermann and Knott (1974)	Monopolar	Left and right inferior frontal	Amplitude of shifts in slow potentials	Anticipation of speaking	Preceding normal utterances of single words most control subjects, but only 2 of the 9 stutterers, showed a greater slow potential shift in the left hemisphere than the right.
Ponsford et al (1975)		Left and right frontal and temporal***	Averaged evoked responses	Visual presentation of the word "fire"	For nonstutterers the responses to the word "fire" in two different contexts were more different in the left hemisphere than the right. For stutterers the difference was greater in the right.
Moore and Lang (1977)	Monopolar	Left and right temporal	Percent time alpha	Between repeated oral readings	Nine of the 10 normal speakers showed greater percent time alpha over the right hemisphere, whereas 8 of the 10 stutterers showed it over the left.
Moore and Haynes (1980)	Monopolar	Left and right temporo-parietal	Integrated alpha amplitude	Stimulation by pure tones and speech	The stutterers showed less alpha in the right hemisphere than the nonstutterers for both verbal and nonverbal stimuli.
Moore and Lorendo (1980)	Monopolar	Left and right temporo-parietal	Integrated alpha amplitude	Auditory presentation of words	The nonstutterers had less alpha in the left than the right hemisphere; the stutterers, just the reverse.

Table 9 (continued)

	Electrode Placement	Brain Area	Measures	Conditions	Results*
Moore, Craven, and Faber (1982)	Monopolar	Left and right temporo-parietal	Integrated alpha amplitude	Auditory presentation, recognition and recall of words	The stutterers showed right-hemisphere alpha suppression; the nonstutterers, left-hemisphere alpha suppression.
Boberg et al (1983)	Monopolar	Left and right prefrontal, posterior frontal, temporal, parietal	Averaged alpha power	Verbal and nonverbal tasks	During verbal tasks the stutterers did not show the normal alpha relationship (right greater than left) in the posterior frontal area. After treatment they did.
Moore (1986)	Monopolar	Left and right temporo-parietal	Integrated alpha amplitude	Auditory presentation, recognition and recall of words and paragraph material	The stutterers showed right-hemisphere alpha suppression; the nonstutterers, left-hemisphere alpha suppression.

*Only those results relating to comparisons of stutterers and nonstutterers are summarized here.
**Driving occurs in response to a flashing light when the subject produces EEG rhythms at the same rate as the flashing of the light.
***The electrodes were placed over Broca's and Wernicke's areas and over the homologous points in the right hemisphere.

waves from the other hemisphere; and various other measures that may be derived from these. In addition, the subjects may be studied in silence, during speech, while stuttering, and with various alterations in the experimental conditions. Finally, some workers have used monopolar leads (one electrode over the cortex and the other at the ear), while others have preferred bipolar placement of leads (both electrodes over the cortex).

The earlier studies summarized in Table 9—most of those done through 1943—were in large part attempts to test the Orton-Travis cerebral dominance theory by determining whether stutterers differed from normal speakers in the manner in which the two hemispheres seemed to be coordinated with each other. In some cases differences were found. These tended to be unexpected and difficult to interpret, however, such as the tendency found by Travis and Knott (1937) for stutterers to have more dissimilar activity in the two halves of the brain than nonstutterers during silence, but better synchronization than nonstutterers during speech.

The investigation by Rheinberger, Karlin, and Berman (1943) appears to have been in part a straightforward attempt to analyze those aspects of the electroencephalographic (EEG) records that are significant in clinical diagnosis. The study disclosed no features distinguishing stutterers from normal speakers. In addition, they found no unusual interhemispheric relationships.

After 1950, much of the electroencephalographic research consisted of attempts, due once more chiefly to Travis and his students, to find in the EEG patterns of stutterers correlates of such behavioral tendencies as emotional reactivity, frustration, or anxiety-proneness. This is evident in the later studies summarized in Table 9, as well as in a study by Shopwin (1959) in which stutterers were judged to be higher in passive-dependency as indicated by significantly higher alpha indices.

In a different development, largely of European origin, an accumulation of EEG observations of an essentially clinical type centered on the question of pathological indications in the EEG tracings of stutterers. Quite a few workers reported abnormal records to be common among stutterers; others did not.[9] An interesting sidelight was thrown on the subject by Luchsinger and Landolt (1955), who found the EEG to be normal in the large majority of stutterers but abnormal, as a rule,

---

[9]Large proportions of stutterers with EEG abnormalities were reported by Segre (1951), Streifler and Gumpertz (1955), Bente, Schönhärl, and Krump (1956), Umeda (1962a), Schilling (1962), Hirschberg (1965), Cali, Pisana, and Tagliareni (1965), Schmoigl and Ladisch (1967), Sayles (1971), and Okasha, Moneim, et al. (1974). Essentially normal findings in the great majority of subjects were reported by Luchsinger (1954), Luchsinger and Landolt (1955), Busse and Clark (1957), Pierce and Lipcon (1959), Morávek and Langová (1962), Andrews and Harris (1964, p. 101), and Graham (1966).

in clutterers and in stutterers with a cluttering "component." Similar observations were made by Morávek and Langová (1962).

In view of the largely qualitative and uncontrolled nature of most of these clinically oriented observations, the studies of Andrews and Harris (1964, p. 101) and Graham (1966) are of special interest. Andrews and Harris randomized the EEG records of 30 stuttering children and their matched controls and gave them to an EEG consultant for blind evaluation. The records were then rearranged in matched pairs, and the consultant was asked to judge which record in each pair was "more abnormal." In neither case was there a difference between the evaluations of the stutterers and those of the nonstutterers. Graham arranged a double-blind evaluation of the EEG records of adult subjects using three neurologists as judges and found no significant differences between stutterers and controls.

On the other hand, Sayles (1971), whose EEG recordings were also evaluated by an expert without knowledge of the subjects' speech histories, found so many more abnormal wave pattems among the stutterers than the controls as to suggest that stutterers as a group "occupy a region somewhere between normal controls and epileptics." Sayles suggested that the negative findings of many previous studies were due to their failure to use such provocation techniques as hyperventilation and sleep, which are now routine in the clinical diagnosis of convulsive tendencies. Some evidence corroborating Sayles has been offered by Okasha, Moneim, et al (1974).

In the 1970s, electroencephalographic research on stuttering took still another direction, the study of cerebral processing of speech. We will consider this research shortly in connection with the subject of cerebral dominance.

Looking at the research on stutterers' cortical potentials as a whole, we might perhaps draw two conclusions. First, the weight of evidence from controlled, quantitative studies supports the view that, except for small differences that are difficult to account for, stutterers' brain potentials during silence tend to be normal. Second, there is a considerable body of additional work suggesting the presence of brain pathology in a large proportion of stutterers, but this has not received sufficient confirmation from adequately controlled studies, and conflicting findings exist.

Cerebral Blood Blow

In recent years, development of the tomograph has made possible the imaging and measurement of regional blood flow in the brain. Pool, Devous, Freeman, Watson, and Finitzo (1991) found reduced blood flow in the frontal lobes of 20 stutterers in "recognized cortical regions of speech-motor control," as well as in the left temporal lobe.

They concluded that their findings "suggest that stuttering is a neurogenic disorder."

Prevalence of Stuttering in Persons with Brain Damage

The persistent suspicion of brain abnormality among stutterers, whether or not well-founded, has received some strength from scattered reports that stuttering tends to be highly prevalent in populations with known neuropathology.

In a state hospital for persons with epilepsy Gens (1950) identified 4.5 percent who stuttered among 1,047 patients with speech. This is at least four times the usual prevalence Harrison (1947), in a more unusual report, stated that stuttering was 36 times as frequent among 60 institutionalized persons with epilepsy as in the general population.

Many who work with children who have cerebral palsy have the impression that stuttering is common in this group, but data on the subject are scarce. Rutherford (1938), in her description of 54 selected children with cerebral palsy and speech impairments, noted that 24 percent of them were stutterers, and this certainly suggests the possibility of an exceptional incidence. Heltman and Peacher (1943) found stuttering in 3.9 percent of a group of 102 individuals with cerebral palsy. Ingram (cited by Andrews and Harris, 1964, p. 7) reported a prevalence of stuttering of 15 percent in a survey of children with cerebral diplegia.

As we will see in Chapter 6, stuttering appears to have a very high incidence among persons with mental deficiency, generally, whether brain-injured or not. Schlanger and Gottsleben (1957), however, found that in an institution for individuals with mental retardation 18 percent of those with organic etiologies stuttered as compared with 10 percent who had a record of familial deficiency.

Goodall and Brobby (1982) found five stutterers among 10 West African patients with sickle cells. They speculated that stuttering in West Africa may be caused by "minimal brain damage resulting from cerebral malaria modified by sickling."

Finally, there is the report of Böhme (1968), who found a prevalence of stuttering of 19.3 percent among 802 children and adults with brain damage dating from birth or early childhood. Diagnoses of brain damage were made on the basis of electroencephalograms, observation of fine motoricity, general neuropsychiatric examination, and other tests. The majority of the group had mental deficiency. Among the 313 cases with normal intelligence 24 percent stuttered.

Summary Remarks

Numerous aspects of the stutterer's physiological processes have been subject to minute laboratory inspection in the belief that the disorder might prove to have an essentially organic etiology. The results of this research do not appear to demonstrate conclusively that the average stutterer exhibits any clinical pathology within the range of the factors that have been investigated. Whether such differences as have been reported from time to time in the areas of cardiovascular, biochemical, and neurophysiological functioning, were their existence to be confirmed, would denote the presence of an underlying constitutional basis for stuttering is also open to controversy. In his review of physiological studies of stuttering, Hill (1944a, 1944b) cited considerable evidence showing that most of the physiological and biochemical processes with respect to which stutterers had been suspected of differing from nonstutterers up to that time may be subject, in perhaps more or less pervasive and lingering as well as immediate ways, to the influence of excitement, emotion, muscular effort, or fatigue.

LATERAL DOMINANCE

Perhaps no other aspect of the person who stutters has been investigated as persistently and resourcefully as the normal tendency of certain functions to lateralize to one side of the body. Beginning with observations on the reversal of manual dexterity early in the century, this research led to investigations of handedness and other aspects of peripheral sidedness, was abandoned for a while, and is being pursued again today in studies of cerebral lateralization of language functions.

Reversal of Manual Dexterity

Although a special urgency was given to research on the laterality of stutterers by the Orton-Travis theory of cerebral dominance in the 1930s, work on the subject goes back at least as far as a systematic attempt by Ballard (1912) to verify a "frequently urged" notion that interference with handedness might cause a child to stutter. His findings added considerably to interest in the question. In a survey of schoolchildren in London Ballard found stuttering in 17 percent of the dextrosinistrals, whom he defined as congenitally left-handed children who had been forced to write with the right hand. Somewhat later Wallin (1916) reported that of the children who were found to stutter in a school survey in St. Louis, 9.5 percent had been shifted from left- to right-handed writing, as compared with only 2.0 percent of all pupils who had been shifted, but he carefully pointed out that 80 percent of the shifted stutterers had begun to stutter before receiving any instruction in writing. In 1924 Inman (cited by McAllister, 1937, p. 337) related that in an experiment at the Lingfield Colony Special Schools in England left-handed training was given to a group of children with mental deficiency and epilepsy in the hope that "additional centers in the brain might be opened up." About five months later a number of the children who were making the most rapid progress began to stutter.

Not all of the evidence pointed in the same direction. In the early decades of the century an intensive campaign was begun in the public schools of Elizabeth, N.J., to abolish left-handedness by compelling all of the pupils to write with the right hand. Some time later Parson (1924, p. 102) wrote, "Investigation showed that in the four years that the policy had been in effect in Elizabeth not a single case of defective speech could be traced to the reversal of manual habit."

In the late 1920s Travis and his students became concerned with the question of confused or ambiguous lateral dominance in stutterers. One of these students, Fagan (1931), presented a series of thirteen cases in the majority of which stuttering was said to have developed within a year after right-handed training. Travis (1931, p. 140 ff) offered various bits of anecdotal evidence, including a few contributed by Bryngelson. One of these was the case of a child who on three successive occasions between the first and sixth grades began to stutter when forced to write with his right hand and stopped stuttering when allowed to return to the use of his left. Another boy, determined to become a "southpaw" pitcher, began to stutter while zealously training himself in left-handed skills and reverted to normal speech on giving up the attempt. Still another interesting case of Bryngelson's was that of a 58-year-old man who had been a right-handed normal speaker until an injury made it necessary to amputate his right forearm. Shortly afterward he began to stutter.[10]

---

[10]To this, however, Bluemel (1933) counterposed a reference to a Professor Bestelmeyer of Munich, who described a group of 1,200 persons, each of, whom had only one arm: "Among them there is not a single case of stammering." Among 20 preferred arm amputees whom Zaner (1950) contacted through state authorities in Wisconsin, 4 told of experiencing some speech difficulty following the amputation and described it in such terms as "slight hesitancy in speaking and thinking of what to say," "stammering and failure of words," ". . . as though my mind has gone blank for a second and failed to supply me with words." Of 19 nonpreferred arm amputees none had noted any speech difficulty.

In a letter to the author, the late Dr. Bryngelson offered the following correction of the story cited above about a 58-year-old amputee: "Facts were—this patient fell in an elevator shaft and he had to have part of his fingers removed—anyway he couldn't use right hand running the elevator and other things like writing, etc. He came to me after two months of using his left hand to hold his job and had a speech defect for which he had no name—he came to me to find out what it was. It was a common kind of blocking and clonic spasm. When asked could it be eradicated I said, there is a way of trying. I sent him to a place where prongs or hooks can be used like fingers. And this he did, and it pleased him as he said he is very awkward using his left hand—although he had his job back, but didn't like to 'stutter' to his friends, etc. I could see no emotional tie-up as he was getting on well with left hand, but did not prefer it. So he went back to right and did almost as much with it as prior to accident and lo and behold (why *I* know not) he came over three months later and nary a sign of stuttering."

Handedness

The cerebral dominance theory gave a strong impetus to research on the stutterer's handedness. This research took several forms.

Surveys of Hand Usage or Preference

At first investigators simply set out to determine whether stutterers differed from nonstutterers in the proportions in each group who were right-handed, left-handed, and ambidextrous, on the assumption that people tended to belong in three more or less distinct categories with regard to handedness. The methods used to ascertain the subject's category varied. In some investigations subjects were simply asked to state their hand preference, while others made use of questionnaires or of tests in which hand usage could be observed. The results of this research proved to be rather remarkable. Before it had proceeded very far an exceedingly wide disparity began to be evident among findings reported by various workers (*see Table 10*). Estimates of left-handedness among groups of stutterers ranged from 0.9 to 21 percent. Estimates of ambidexterity varied from 0 to 61 percent. One researcher found far more ambidexterity among stutterers than among normal-speaking subjects, but comparatively little left-handedness. Another found a very large proportion of left-handed stutterers. Still a third reported little difference between stutterers and nonstutterers in the proportion of either type of handedness. Even more remarkable were the reports of percentages of stutterers whose handedness had been shifted from left to right in childhood; these ranged from 5 to 73 percent.

The reason for these differences gradually became apparent. Various definitions of ambidexterity or left-handedness were possible. How many ambidextrous stutterers one found depended in part on how one inquired about or determined ambidexterity. Furthermore, handedness was not an all-or-none property, such as maleness, but a matter of degree. It was realized that what was needed for both clinical and research purposes was a *measure* of handedness that was both objective and quantitative.

The Dextrality Quotient

Travis's students, notably Johnson, had for some time been developing a device known as a hand-usage questionnaire. This was a questionnaire instructing subjects to indicate which hand they used to perform each of a list of manual activities such as using a pencil or throwing a ball. From the subject's answers it was possible to compute a *dextrality quotient*, or D.Q., which represented essentially the proportion of right-handed responses and varied from 1.00 (perfect right-handedness) to 0.00 (complete left-handedness). The laterality

Table 10. Percentage of Stutterers and Nonstutterers Found to Be Left-Handed, Ambidextrous, and Shifted in Handedness

	Stutterers				Nonstutterers			
	N	Left-Handed	Ambidextrous	Shifted	N	Left-Handed	Ambidextrous	Shifted
Wallin (1916)	683				88,373			
Bryngelson (1935)	700	0.9	61.1	9.5				
Milisen and Johnson (1936)	23			73.1				
McAllister (1937)	139	6.5		34				
Berry (1937a)	119	21.0	17.6					
Bryngelson and Rutherford (1937)	74	4.1	34.3	71.6	74	16.7	8.3	9.5
Bryngelson (1939)	78	2.0	29.0	58.0	78	6.0	0.0	1.0
Daniels (1940)	20	5.0	20.0	5.0	1,574	10.0	1.4	4.8
Spadino (1941)	70	15.7	0.0		70			
Johnson et al (1942)	46	13.0	8.7	26.1	46	8.7	13.0	30.4
Meyer (1945)	104	11.5	7.7	16.3				
Despert (1946)	50	12.0	4.0					
Andrews and Harris (1964)	80	3.8	26.3		80	6.3	28.8	
Records, Heimbuch, and Kidd (1977)	449	12.9	4.7		356	12.1	9.3	
Accordi et al (1983)	2,802	5.1	5.1		1,602	6.4	9.7	
Adila et al (1994)	37	5.4	2.7		1,842	6.5	8.0	

questionnaire scored by means of the D.Q. appeared to offer an ideal solution to the problems that had arisen in attempts to investigate the stutterer's handedness. The results were fairly consistent in several studies in which it was used by Johnson and his co-workers *(see Table 11)*. Somewhat unexpectedly, however, the stutterers did not seem to differ from the nonstutterers at all. In most cases they turned out to be relatively right-handed, about like most other people.

Innate Lateral Dominance

The laterality questionnaire in itself did not immediately settle the handedness controversy, however. The principal reason for this was that the questionnaire was concerned almost entirely with activities highly subject to training. Proponents of the cerebral dominance theory argued that, while stutterers often seemed to be right-handed because of the influence of a right-handed society, they usually possessed an innate ambidextrous tendency that did not reveal itself on handedness inventories.

Measures of Native Laterality

Clearly, what was needed was a measure of innate, also termed *native* or *cortical*, laterality. Researchers, principally under the direction of Travis, carried on a sustained effort to devise tests of sidedness relatively uninfluenced by culture. Human structure and function were scoured for covert reflections of bilateral asymmetry, and many such evidences were found and applied in studies of stutterers. These included eyedness as measured in various ways,[11] foot preference,[12]

Table 11. Dextrality Quotients of Stutterers and Nonstutterers

	N	Stutterers	Nonstutterers
Milisen and Johnson (1936)	23, 23	.95	.78*
Morris (1938)	20	.71	
Johnson and King (1942)	98, 71	.88	.87
Johnson et al (1942)**	36, 46	.89	.94

*Normal speakers whose handedness had been changed.
**Data reported in Johnson (1955a).

---

[11]Travis (1928a).
[12]Bryngelson and Rutherford (1937).

the dominant thumb (the one uppermost when the hands are clasped),[13] simultaneous bimanual writing,[14] writing or drawing in mirror vision,[15] mirror reading ability,[16] and the relative size, strength, or skill of the two hands.[17] Several neuromuscular measures of innate laterality were tried—bilateral action potentials,[18] the relative excitability of bilaterally paired muscles on electrical stimulation,[19] and differences in motor lead of the two hands in simultaneous antitropic movements.[20] In addition, signs of deviant lateral dominance were sought in the cortical potentials of stutterers, as we have already seen, and also in certain perceptual phenomena.[21] Jasper (1932) and Morris (1938) made use of many of these measures to construct batteries of diagnostic tests of "native" sidedness.

Considerable support for the Orton-Travis theory was amassed by means of these studies. The procedure usually followed was to select control groups of right-handed, left-handed, and ambidextrous persons by means of a laterality questionnaire and to compare their performance on a given test of native dominance with that of a group of stutterers. In the main, these measures served to classify the stutterers with the ambidextrous or left-handed normal speakers. It was evident that many stutterers who were right-handed in their ordinary daily activities actually did seem to exhibit a latent ambidexterity or a mixed or confused dominance when they were given tests of this type. It would have been difficult to foresee the rather surprising conclusion to which such studies finally led.

The Critical-Angle Board Test

One of the most promising of these tests made use of simultaneous writing with both hands. It was based on the observation that in writing a word or copying a number or design simultaneously with both hands it was natural for most people to produce with one hand a mirror image of what they did with the other hand. The normal tendency was to copy the figure correctly with the dominant hand and to mirror with the other. Those who showed little tendency to mirror, or mirrored first with one hand and then with the other, could be pre-

---

[13]Johnson (1937).

[14]Jasper (1932), Fagan (1932), Van Riper (1934, 1935).

[15]Travis (1928a).

[16]Peters (1936).

[17]Cross (1936), Van Dusen (1937, 1939).

[18]Orton and Travis (1929), Travis and Lindsley (1933), Metfessel and Warren (1934).

[19]Jasper (1932).

[20]Travis and Herren (1929).

[21]Jasper (1932), Morris (1938).

sumed to be ambidextrous. Simultaneous writing, then, seemed to afford an indication of an individual's lateral dominance that was relatively uninfluenced by training.

The chief drawback of this procedure was that its success depended on the subject's cooperation in reacting quickly and spontaneously; most subjects failed to mirror if they exercised some care. This difficulty was effectively disposed of in a modification of the procedure, introduced by Van Riper (1934), which required the subjects to write simultaneously on both sides of a vertical board. It is readily seen that mirroring is difficult to avoid under these conditions. In fact, one of the problems of the vertical board test was the very difficulty that all but the most ambidextrous persons had in drawing the figure *correctly* with both hands.

Van Riper hit upon an ingenious solution to this problem. He hinged two boards together so that they could be presented to the subject open or closed at angles of varying degrees. In giving this test, which he called the "critical-angle board test," Van Riper placed the board before the subject fully opened with instructions to draw the figure correctly (i.e., without mirroring) on both surfaces at the same time. The drawing or writing was then repeated successively with the board closed at various angles until, in its fully closed position, it duplicated the conditions of the vertical board test. It is clear that at some point in this process there will be a "critical angle" at which almost every subject begins to mirror with the nondominant hand. Strongly right- or left-handed subjects could be expected to mirror with the angle board slightly closed, while highly ambidextrous ones presumably would not do so until it was almost completely closed. This proved to be precisely the case.

Van Riper (1935) gave the critical-angle board test to a number of the most highly right-handed, left-handed, and ambidextrous people he could find among several hundred college students, selecting the subjects on the basis of their dextrality quotients on hand-usage questionnaires. He found that ambidextrous subjects tended to have critical angles that were markedly larger than those of the highly unilateral subjects and that indicated that they mirrored far less readily. Now there was only one question left. How would stutterers perform on this test—essentially like right-handed, left-handed, or ambidextrous people? Van Riper gave his test to a group of stutterers. The results appeared to support the cerebral dominance hypothesis in a most convincing manner. The stutterers had critical angles that were, on the average, *almost exactly like those of the ambidextrous group*.

The matter was not to end here, however. Van Riper had compared his stutterers with three groups of nonstutterers who had been very carefully chosen as representative of three different types of handedness. In doing so he had taken for granted a premise that few people would have been inclined to dispute—that, broadly speaking, the population was divisible into three categories with respect to handedness, the great majority being both innately and outwardly right-handed to some degree. Was this assumption strictly valid? There certainly seemed little enough reason to doubt it. But several years later Daniels, who had been investigating the handedness of stuttering and nonstuttering students at Syracuse University, remarked:

> The observational procedure . . . revealed that the popular concept of kinds of handedness (right, left, and ambidextrous) is inaccurate to a degree of becoming almost meaningless. It was shown that three distinct types of handedness groups do not exist; a concept of widely varying degrees of ambidexterity among all individuals more nearly approaches the actual situation. . . . (Daniels, 1940).

That was a bold statement. Supposing it were true? In that case, any group of subjects carefully selected for their right-handedness was certainly an unusual aggregation of persons, possessing a degree of unilaterality not at all representative of the general population. There was one way to settle the question. Johnson and King (1942) gave the Van Riper critical-angle board test to a group of 98 stutterers and compared their performance with that of a group of nonstutterers who had been selected entirely *at random* with regard to handedness. Their findings bore out Daniels' contention in a manner that was arresting. Again the stutterers made responses that were similar to those of Van Riper's ambidextrous students. *And the nonstutterers performed almost exactly like the stutterers.* On a hand usage questionnaire both groups appeared essentially right-handed. The implications were clear. As Johnson and King pointed out, many stutterers did indeed have inborn ambidextrous tendencies, but that was simply because most people do.

Johnson and King were concerned specifically with the critical-angle board test. In the light of their findings, however, it becomes necessary to reevaluate the validity of a host of other indications of weak or confused innate lateral dominance among stutterers obtained in past studies in which available groups of stutterers were compared with control groups specially selected with regard to handedness. This is underscored by the results of an exhaustive study which was completed at Columbia University by Spadino (1941). Spadino studied 70 stutterers and 70 nonstutterers of elementary school age, selecting them on the same basis and without regard for handedness. On numerous tests of handedness, eyedness, footedness, simultaneous bimanual writing, and mirror reading, there were no significant differences between the two groups. In studies of simultaneous bimanual writing of more recent date, Fitzgerald, Cooke, and Greiner (1984) and Greiner,

Fitzgerald, and Cooke (1986a) found that stutterers performed as well as nonstutterers with the dominant hand, wrote more poorly with the nondominant hand, and did more mirroring with the nondominant hand. Similar results were obtained by Webster (1938). These findings conflict sharply with the Travis theory of cerebral dominance.

By the 1940s it had become apparent that stutterers as a group were not distinguished by an anomalous type of handedness. This conclusion has been confirmed by the later studies of Johnson and Associates (1959, p 84), Andrews and Harris (1964, p. 100), Records, Heimbuch, and Kidd (1977), Accordi et al. (1983), Bishop (1986), Webster and Poulos (1987), and Ardila et al. (1994). The only recent evidence of a connection between stuttering and left handedness was provided by Geschwind and Behan (1984). These workers adopted a unique approach. Whereas all other researchers has asked how many stutterers were left handed, Geschwind and Behan asked how many left-handed individuals stuttered, and focused on extreme cases. They compared 440 subjects who were very highly left handed on the Oldfield Handedness Inventory with 652 extremely right-handed persons. By self-report, 4.5 percent of the left-handed and 0.9 percent of the right-handed subjects stuttered.

Cerebral Dominance for Language and Speech

Following the early work on handedness, interest in stutterers' lateral dominance lay dormant for many years. In the 1960s, however, this interest revived, and the term cerebral dominance began to be heard again in discussions of stuttering. Ever since autopsies have been done on persons recognized to have aphasia it has been known that there is a hemispheric dominance in the cerebrum for language functions. Travis and his students did not include it in the long list of innate bilateral asymmetries which they investigated for the simple reason that there was then no useful clinical test for hemispheric language dominance aside from measures of such things as handedness itself. But we now have such tests, and in recent years researchers have administered them to stutterers.

The Wada Test

A conclusive method that has been developed for determining which half of a patient's brain is dominant for language is the intracarotid sodium amytal (Wada) test. The left and right carotid arteries, passing upward through the neck, provide the blood supply to the left and right cerebral hemispheres, respectively. If sodium amytal is injected into the left carotid artery and the patient temporarily loses the ability to speak, it is clear that the patient has a language center in the left hemisphere. By injecting each artery in turn it can be determined on which side the dominance lies, or whether, as is sometimes the case, speech is represented in both hemispheres. This, in brief, is the Wada test.

In 1966 R. K. Jones, a neurosurgeon, published an unusual report on a series of four of his cases. All of them, ranging in age from thirteen to fifty, had stuttered severely since childhood. Each one had an intracranial lesion of recent origin in the region of the presumed speech areas. In each case routine Wada testing prior to surgery showed that speech was represented in both hemispheres. Following the removal of the lesion the stuttering disappeared in each case, and the Wada test disclosed normal unilateral speech representation. On follow-up ranging from fifteen months to three years each person was still speaking normally.

Jones' report caused a stir. To former champions of the role of cerebral dominance in speech fluency it was tempting to see it as a vindication of the Orton-Travis theory, despite some puzzling aspects. Unfortunately, attempts at verification were some time in coming, in part because the Wada test is not entirely without risk. In time, however, 3 volunteers came forward from the Council of Adult Stutterers,[22] a self-help organization then affiliated with the Speech and Hearing Clinic of the Catholic University of America. Their Wada tests uniformly and unequivocally showed normal left hemispheric dominance for speech; injection of each side revealed no evidence of bilateral representation (see Luessenhop, Boggs, LaBorwit, and Walle, 1973).

Walle (1971) published a brief preliminary report of these results in order to forestall needless Wada testing of stutterers by others. In the meantime, however, a group in Sydney, Australia, had tested additional subjects who proved to have normal left-sided speech centers (Andrews and Quinn, 1972; Andrews, Quinn, and Sorby, 1972). They also tested a person who had begun to stutter at age 31 years following the onset of aphasia due to a head injury. In his case the test showed evidence of bilateral speech centers.

No doubt, anyone who looked for the meaning of these results soon made the same deduction. Stuttering did not seem to have much to do with impaired cerebral dominance for speech; brain injury possibly did.

Dichotic Listening Tests

It has been a notable and constant feature of the cerebral dominance theory of stuttering for more than 60 years that each time it is given up for dead it twitches. The question of laterality in stutterers is

---

[22]Now the National Council on Stuttering.

now being pursued in yet other forms. One of these is ear preference in dichotic listening. When normal subjects are given the task of listening to a series of words that are heard in only one ear, there is generally no appreciable difference between the number of words they hear accurately with the left and right ears. The results are quite different, however, when the task is dichotic—that is, when the subject listens simultaneously with each ear to a different series of words. In that case most subjects will tend to report accurately more words heard with the right ear than with the left. For nonspeech sounds such as environmental noises there is most often a left-ear advantage. Dichotic word tests are generally presumed to demonstrate the dominance of one-half of the brain for language, so there has been some interest in them as a safe and convenient alternative to the Wada test. They have also excited the interest of investigators of stuttering.

Curry and Gregory (1969) gave dichotic listening tests to a group of stutterers and obtained two significant findings. In the first place, only 45 percent showed the usual right-ear advantage on the dichotic word test, as compared with 75 percent of their controls. In addition, the difference between the scores for the left ear and right ear was more than twice as great, on the average, for the nonstutterers as for the stutterers. It is not difficult to interpret such results as support for a cerebral dominance theory of stuttering.

A series of further investigations of dichotic listening in stutterers have now been carried out *(see Table 12)*. Like the Curry and Gregory study, these have generally been concerned with two questions: the number of stutterers and nonstutterers who show the right-ear advantage, and the difference between the groups in amount of right-ear advantage as measured by the mean difference in score between the subjects' left and right ears. Table 12 shows conflicting positive and negative outcomes, 8 studies that found distinct differences between the groups apparently contradicted by 10 studies that did not. It has been pointed out, however (by Moore, 1976), that stutterers have generally been found to differ from nonstutterers when investigators used meaningful verbal stimuli. The table offers considerable confirmation of this. Of ten studies that used only nonsense syllables, all but two found stutterers and nonstutterers to perform essentially alike. Of the remaining eight that used words or digits only two studies—both of which, incidentally, used children as subjects—produced negative outcomes.

Although we have placed the studies of Brady and Berson (1975) and Rosenfield and Goodglass (1980) in the negative column in Table 12, in both cases a few stutterers showed a left-ear preference whereas no or fewer nonstutterers did so. Similar qualifications apply in the case of Blood, Blood, and Hood (1987), Cross (1987), and Blood and

Table 12. Studies of Stutterers' Ear Preference in Dichotic Listening: Outcome in Relatioon to Meaningfulness of Stimuli

	Outcome*		Comments
	Positive	Negative	
Curry and Gregory (1969)	Words		
Mattingly (1970)	Meaningful and meaningless stimuli		Ten nonstutterers were right-ear dominant, whereas 10 stutterers had no consistent pattern. No information given on difference between meaningful and meaningless stimuli.
Perrin and Eisenson (1970)	Words and nonsense syllables		Nonstutterers showed a right-ear preference. Stutterers showed no ear preference for nonsense syllables and a left-ear preference for words.
Slorach and Noehr (1973)		Digits	Subjects were 6- to 9-year-old children. A right-ear effect was observed equally in the stutterers and the nonstutterers.
Cerf and Prins (1974)		CV syllables	Of 19 stutterers, 17 had a right-ear preference.
Gruber and Powell (1974)		Digits	Neither stutterers nor nonstutterers showed a right-ear advantage. Subjects were mainly children.
Brady and Berson (1975)		CVC syllables	There was no difference between groups in between-ear difference scores, although 6 of 35 stutterers, and no controls, showed a left-ear preference.

Table 12 (continued)

Study	Stimulus	Results
Dorman and Porter (1975)	CV syllables	
Sommers, Brady, and Moore (1975)	Words and digits	The stutterers had fewer right-ear responses than the controls for both the words and the digits.
Sussman and MacNeilage (1975)	CV syllables	
Quinn (1976)	CVC syllables	Updates Quinn (1972) with additional subjects.
Hall and Jerger (1978)	Words	Fewer stutterers than nonstutterers showed a right-ear advantage on the staggered spondaic word test.
Davenport (1979)	Words and digits	
Pinsky and McAdam (1980)	CV syllables	The groups did not differ in dichotic indices of laterality. All 5 controls and 4 of 5 stutterers showed a right-ear advantage.
Rosenfield and Goodglass (1980)	CV syllables	The groups did not differ in degree of right-ear advantage. Five of 19 stutterers and 2 of 20 nonstutterers showed a left-ear advantage.
Liebetrau and Daly (1981)	CV syllables	The groups did not differ. The right-ear advantage was slight in both groups.
Cimorell-Strong, Gilbert, and Frick (1983)	CV syllables	Higher right-ear scores were found in 82% of controls and 55% of stutterers. The subjects were children aged 5, 7, and 9.
Blood (1985)	CV syllables	Subjects aged 7 to 12 showed fewer right-ear preferences than controls; those 13 to 15 did not.

Blood, Blood, and Hood (1987)	CV syllables	At age 7 to 9, 50% of stutterers and 80% of controls showed a right ear preference. At age 10 to 12, 60% of the same stutterers and 80% of the controls did so.
Cross (1987)	CV syllables	For accuracy of identification of syllables, 58% of stutterers and 83% of controls showed a right-ear advantage. For reaction time, 75% of stutterers and 92% of controls did so.
Blood and Blood (1989a)	Words	The groups did not differ in the percent showing a right-ear advantage, but the magnitude of the difference between ears was greater for the nonstutterers.

*Positive outcome refers to one in which a difference appeared between stutterers and controls.

Blood (1989a). Moreover, Blood and Blood (1989b) showed that the outcome of dichotic listening studies may vary with the type of data analysis used. At all events, it has long been clear that whatever anomalies of ear advantage are present among stutterers, they do not characterize all individuals. This has led to the frequent suggestion that the dichotic listening research may be revealing significant sub-types of stutterers. With this in view, Blood and Blood (1986) divided 86 stutterers into those with right-ear advantage, left-ear advantage, and no ear advantage. They found no difference among the groups in number or type of disfluencies.

Innovative variations on the dichotic listening test have been applied in the study of cerebral dominance in stutterers. Tsunoda and Moriyama (1972) devised a test in which subjects heard feedback, in the form of either a pure tone or a vowel, from their key-tapping of a simple temporal pattern. The feedback was presented to both ears, but was delayed in one ear, and the subject was told to attend to the feed-back in the other. As measured by the number of errors they made while attending to each ear, 79 percent of normal speakers had a right-ear advantage for vowels and a left-ear advantage for tones, whereas only 39 percent of the stutterers showed this pattern of dominance.

Rastatter and Dell (1987a) recorded subjects' manual reaction times as they indicated a picture that corresponded to a stimulus word. The word was introduced to one ear each time. The control subjects showed a distinct right-ear advantage with either hand, con-sistent with a concept of left hemisphere dominance for language pro-cessing. The stutterers showed no ear advantage. Their reaction time was the same for the two ears, with either hand.

Evidence from Brain Waves

Electroencephalography has proved to be still another useful means for studying cerebral asymmetry for speech-related functions in stutterers. Zimmermann and Knott (1974) measured the contingent negative variation[23] in subjects as they were about to say each of a series of words exposed in turn on a screen. In four of five normal speakers they made the expected observation of greater changes in the brain waves over the left hemisphere than the right. Before fluent utter-ances of words by stutterers, this was true in only two of nine cases. This finding was not confirmed, however, by Pinsky and McAdam (1980) or by Prescott and Andrews (1984); and Prescott (1988) found few differences between stutterers and nonstutterers in the contingent negative variation.

---

[23]The contingent negative variation is a negative wave that appears following a warning to prepare for a signal to perform a response.

Ponsford, Brown, Marsh, and Travis (1975) measured the brain potentials evoked by visual presentation of the word "fire" in the two phrases "fire is hot" and "fire the gun." For the nonstutterers the different meanings of the word produced a greater difference in potentials in the left hemisphere than in the right. For the stutterers the reverse was true.

Moore and Lang (1977) reported a suppression of alpha waves over the right hemisphere in 8 of 10 stutterers before each of several oral readings of a passage. In nonstutterers, on the other hand, they noted less alpha activity over the left hemisphere, which accords with past findings on normal speakers engaged in linguistic processing. Moore and Haynes (1980) found reduced alpha in stutterers' right hemispheres whether they listened to recorded speech or pure tones. They suggested that stutterers demonstrate, not reversed cerebral dominance for speech, but right hemisphere processing of both verbal and nonverbal stimuli. In subsequent studies Moore and his co-workers used auditory stimulation with lists of words the subjects were told they would later be asked to recall or with reading passages about which they knew they would later be questioned.[24] Again the stutterers showed more alpha suppression in the right hemisphere than in the left; the nonstutterers showed the reverse.

Few replications of Moore's research have as yet been attempted. Pinsky and McAdam (1980) found that stutterers did not differ from their controls in alpha asymmetry during verbal processing tasks. Somewhat unexpectedly, Fitch and Batson (1989) discovered little difference between the two hemispheres in alpha activity during silent verbal processing for either stutterers or nonstutterers. Results obtained by Boberg, Yeudall, Schopflocher, and Bo-Lassen (1983) agreed with those of Moore and his co-workers, but the use of expressive verbal tasks (the Wechsler vocabulary test and counting backwards by sevens) by Boberg's group makes it somewhat difficult to interpret their findings; events occurring during stuttering may be a cause, a result, or an aspect of stuttering. They reported the startling fact that, after three weeks of therapy during which stuttering was markedly reduced by training in the use of a slow speech rate and gentle onsets of phonation, the stutterers demonstrated the normal alpha relationship during performance of the verbal tasks. A similar observation was made by Moore (1984b) in a study of a single subject. Citing studies showing that stress results in greater activation of the right hemisphere, Boberg et al (1983) suggested that the finding might be due to the fact that speech tasks, even receptive ones, are threatening to stutterers as a result of past emotional conditioning.

---

[24]Moore and Lorendo (1980), Moore, Craven, and Faber (1982), Moore (1986).

In a further study of alpha asymmetry, Wells and Moore (1990) again found evidence of right hemisphere activation in stutterers during speech, using a sentence repetition task.

Auditory Tracking

In a different type of study Sussman and MacNeilage (1975) used an auditory tracking task requiring the subject to match the pitch of a tone heard in one ear to the varying pitch of a tone heard in the other. They found that when the pitch was controlled by movements of the tongue or jaw, most normal subjects did better when the varying tone was presented in the right ear. There was no lateralization effect when the hand was used to control the pitch. By contrast with the normal speakers, only 57 percent of a group of stutterers exhibited this right-ear effect on a jaw-tracking task. Sussman and MacNeilage concluded that stutterers appear to have a less distinct lateralization of a speech-related auditory sensorimotor integration.

Conflicting findings were reported by Neilson, Quinn, and Neilson (1976). They confirmed the observations of Sussman and MacNeilage for normal speakers, but found no difference between normal speakers and stutterers.

Tachistoscopic Investigations

A study by Moore (1976) reproduced the conditions of the dichotic word test in a visual mode. Pairs of words were presented simultaneously in different halves of the visual field, and the subjects were asked to say which word they saw first. Normal speakers showed a significant preference for the right half of the visual field (left hemisphere), whereas stutterers did not. A larger proportion of stutterers than nonstutterers showed a left half-field advantage. Victor and Johannsen (1984) employed nonsense syllables as visual stimuli in a study otherwise similar to Moore's. Of 42 stutterers, 11 correctly identified more syllables in the left visual field than in the right; only 4 of a like number of control subjects did so. (See also Johannsen and Victor , 1986.)

Hand and Haynes (1983) reached similar conclusions with a quite different procedure. They presented real words and nonwords (e.g., "ramy") to either the right or left visual fields of their subjects. The subject responded to real words by pressing a key (or, in a different condition, by saying /a/). The experimenters measured subjects' reaction times. As a group, the stutterers had faster reaction times when the words were presented to the left visual field (right hemisphere) than to the right. Normal speakers showed no significant difference between fields, though they tended to react faster to stimuli presented to the right visual field.

In a similar study by Wilkins, Webster, and Morgan (1984) letters and representations of faces were presented separately to subjects' left and right visual fields. Subjects were asked to respond with one button press to a target face or letter and with another button press to other stimuli. No significant difference in reaction time between visual fields for either stutterers or controls was found.

In a replication of the Hand and Haynes study with children aged 7 to 14 years, Hardin, Pindzola, and Haynes (1992) found no difference between stutterers and controls.

A series of tachistoscopic studies by Rastatter and his co-workers made use of a reaction-time format in which subjects named letters or pictures or read words presented to left and right visual fields or responded with phonation of /a/ to visual presentations of words.[25] The investigations yielded some evidence of right-hemisphere dominance in stutterers, but in somewhat inconsistent and distinctly qualified ways. Rastatter, Loren, and Colcord (1987) commented, "These processes are obviously multidimensional in nature and reach beyond current themes focusing on the relative processing superiority of one hemisphere versus the other."

Hemispheric Interference Tests

A number of studies have shown that in right-handed normal speakers verbal activity tends to reduce the rate of finger tapping with the right hand, but not with the left. This is easily seen as an interference effect resulting from the fact that the left hemisphere of the brain, which controls the right hand, is also used for speech by right-handed subjects. Such dual-task procedures presumably afford still another way of studying the cortical lateralization of speech, and they have been used in several studies of stutterers with somewhat equivocal results.

Sussman (1982) had subjects read aloud or count backwards by threes while tapping as fast as they could. During oral reading, right-handed normal speakers showed the expected reduction in tapping rate with the right hand, whereas stutterers showed the same amount of disruption in both hands, suggesting a lack of distinct cerebral dominance for speech. In counting backwards, however, the stutterers experienced much more interference with the right hand than the left.

In a study of stuttering children, Brutten and Trotter (1985, 1986) found that speaking tasks such as picture naming and storytelling reduced the rate of tapping in both hands. They found the same

---

[25]McGuire, Loren, and Rastatter (1986), Rastatter, Loren, and Colcord (1987), Rastatter and Dell (1987c, 1988), Rastatter and Loren (1988), Rastatter, McGuire, and Loren (1988).

effect, however, in a nonspeech control condition in which the children were asked to imitate the sound of a siren. Consequently, they concluded that neither their results nor Sussman's could be interpreted to support a hypothesis of bilateral representation of language in stutterers.

Replacing simple finger tapping with a task more vulnerable to interference, Greiner, Fitzgerald, and Cooke (1986b) instructed subjects to tap as rapidly as possible beginning with the index finger, tapping outward to the little finger, and beginning again with the index finger. Interference by spontaneous speech, oral reading, and singing revealed no evidence of a difference between normal speakers and stutterers in cerebral dominance for speech.

Webster (l990b) found evidence of right-hemisphere overactivation in stutterers in a different kind of study of rapid finger tapping in which subjects tapped twice with one hand for each single tap with the other. Among normal speaking right-handers, performance has been found to be better when it is the right hand that taps twice, whereas left-handers perform similarly under both conditions. Webster's control subjects performed accordingly, but the right-handed. stutterers performed like the left-handed nonstutterers.

Summary Remarks

Left-handedness and reversal of manual dexterity had been associated with stuttering by scattered observations since the early years of the twentieth century. In the late 1920s an additional emphasis on ambidexterity arose as a result of the Orton-Travis theory, and a very large amount of research was subsequently done on both the peripheral handedness of stutterers and supposed indicators of "native" laterality. By the 1940s good evidence had accumulated that stutterers did not differ from nonstutterers in their handedness. This conclusion has been confirmed by such later research as has been done, for example, by Johnson and Associates (1959, p. 84), Andrews and Harris (1964, p. 100), and Records, Heimbuch, and Kidd (1977).

As for the inference that a change of handedness may cause a child to stutter, the fact that in the end no unusual tendency toward native left-handedness seemed to characterize stutterers may indirectly cast some doubt on it. The practice of forcing left-handed children to write with the right hand has not been favored in schools for many years, and with it has gone the opportunity to study its effects on speech. In the vast majority of cases it has clearly never been an important etiological factor. That it was once thought capable of contributing significantly to the etiology of stuttering may ultimately go down as one of the curious superstitions of our time.

In late years interest in research on the lateral dominance of stutterers has been revived by the availability of tests of cerebral dominance for language and speech processing. On the intracarotid sodium amytal (Wada) test a total of six typical stutterers have shown normal unilateral representation of speech in the cerebrum. The results of a large number of dichotic listening tests have been conflicting, although there is compelling evidence that when meaningful stimuli are used in place of nonsense syllables, many stutterers show less right-ear advantage than nonstutterers. A provocative series of brain-wave studies by one researcher and his associates has yielded consistent evidence of right-hemisphere processing of speech by stutterers. As yet, relatively little unambiguous confirmation by other workers has been reported. A few tachistoscopic studies have found that at least some stutterers differ from most nonstutterers in preferring the left half of the visual field in processing visual verbal stimuli. A few studies employing hemispheric interference tasks have produced inconclusive results. In short, evidence that stutterers tend to differ from normal speakers in cerebral asymmetry for language is intriguing, but as yet somewhat fraught with inconsistencies.

MOTOR SKILLS

In the final analysis, the most valid test of the adequacy of the stutterer's neuromuscular organization is the test of what it can do. Consequently, a large amount of research has been done on various aspects of the stutterer's bodily coordination, manual skills, and control and motility of the oral structures.

General Bodily Coordination

Arps (cited by Strother and Kriegman, 1943) found stutterers to be poorer than nonstutterers in gymnastic exercises involving rhythm and coordination, and Kiehn (1935) reported slightly poorer performance in a test requiring subjects to carry a full glass of water. Bilto (1941) carried out a more detailed investigation of a group of stutterers using several standardized tests of motor ability concerned with bodily strength, agility, balance, and control. Although his stutterers tended to perform slightly below the test norms, on the average the disparities were so small that it is difficult, for the most part, to rule out the possibility that they were due to chance factors operating in the selection of subjects. Furthermore, the stutterers did as well, on the whole, as a group of children with articulatory disorders to whom the same tests were given.

In view of Bilto's observations, the findings reported by Helene Kopp (1946) were rather unexpected. Kopp administered the Oseretsky Tests of Motor Proficiency to a group of 50 stuttering children and discovered that on the basis of test norms all but 3 of the subjects were retarded in motor development by amounts ranging from 2 to 9 years, 46 percent performing more than 5 years below their age levels. The Oseretsky Tests, standardized on 5,000 Russian children in the early 1920s, is an instrument of broad scope with stress on general bodily activities requiring coordination, balance, and speed. Kopp concluded that her findings revealed a "marked disturbance of the motor function" in stutterers. Like so many other investigations of stuttering that made use of standardized tests, however, this study did not employ a control group. The omission was particularly serious in this case because the Oseretsky Tests as then formulated often allowed considerable latitude to the examiner's discretion in both the administration and scoring of items. Finkelstein and Weisberger (1954) administered the tests to 15 stuttering children and a control group of 15 nonstutterers matched for age, sex, and laterality. They found no statistically significant differences between the two groups. Comparison with the test norms showed an average retardation of three and a half months for the stutterers.

Further work using the Oseretsky-Gollnitz Tests with German children was reported by Schilling and Kruger (1960). They found that 100 stutterers performed more poorly than 100 normal controls, but better than 100 children with articulatory disorders. For example, 18 percent of the stutterers, 5 percent of the controls, and 41 percent of the children with articulatory difficulties were classified as "severely retarded" in motor development.

The findings on gross physical abilities are conflicting. While we have not had conclusive evidence that differences between stutterers and nonstutterers exist, neither has the possibility been ruled out.

Manual Skills

Investigations of the stutterers manual abilities have concerned themselves with strength, steadiness, speed and regularity of repetitive movement, hand-eye coordination, and various types of psychomotor serial discrimination tasks *(see Table 13)*.

Stutterers seem clearly normal in manual strength, regularity, and accuracy in reproducing rhythmical patterns. Several other areas of research, however, have produced conflicting results. In particular, some workers found stutterers to perform slightly more poorly in tests of manual diadochokinesis (chiefly rapid finger tapping), in tests of hand-eye coordination as in accurate aiming or tracing, and in serial discrimination tasks as in rapid sorting of cards into slots. In other studies of essentially the same abilities no differences were found.

Findings as inconclusive as these leave us with considerable freedom to speculate that stutterers tend to have a mild neuromuscular disorder, or to conclude that no deviation from the normal has been firmly established, or to infer, as did Hill (1944b) and Rotter (1955), that stutterers may exhibit some motor evidences of anxiety.

Table 13. Studies of Manual Abilities of Stutterers and Nonstutterers Classified with Regard to Whether the Stutterers Were Found to Be of Poorer (Positive Outcome) or Equal Ability (Negative Outcome)

Manual Ability	Outcome*	
	Positive	Negative
Strength		McDowell (1928) Westphal (1933)
Steadiness	Kiehn (1935) Snyder (1958)	Westphal (1933)
Speed of Repetitive Movement	West and Nusbaum (1929) Cross (1936) Snyder (1958) Borden (1983)	Strother and Kriegman (1943) Chworowsky (1952) Rotter (1955)
Regularity of Repetitive Movement	Seth (1958) Cooper and Allen (1977)	Blackburn (1931)
Accuracy of Reproduction of Temporal Patterns	Zaleski (1965)	Wulff (1935) Cross (1936) Strother and Kriegman (1943)
Hand-Eye Coordination	Bilto (1941) Carlson (1946) Snyder (1958)	Westphal (1933) Cross (1936)
Psychomotor Serial Discrimination	Bills (1934) Simon (1945) Rotter (1955) Snyder (1958)	Cross (1936) Lightfoot (1948) Ross (1955) Postma and Kolk (1991)

*Studies with more than one outcome for a given ability are classified as "positive" if any outcome was positive.

As a result of Eisenson's perseverative theory of stuttering (see Chapter 2), some interest developed in the stutterer's proficiency at making rapid shifts in motor set. This kind of ability is usually tested by first giving the subject practice in each of two motor tasks independently—for example, the writing of AAAA . . . followed by BBBB . . . then observing the number of errors the subject makes when instructed to alternate the tasks, as in writing ABAB. . . . It was in a variation of this task taken from the Mahler-Elkin Attention Test that Eisenson and Pastel (1936) first noted excessive perseverative behavior in a group of adult stutterers. Eisenson hypothesized that there was a constitutional tendency to perseverate in a substantial proportion of stutterers. King (1961) found distinct corroboration of Eisenson's earlier observations in giving a series of such alternating-activity tests to adult stutterers, but was inclined to believe that this could be adequately explained as the effect of greater anxiety-tension on the part of the stutterers. Some support may be lent to this interpretation by the fact that Martin (1962) was able to find no differences in the performance of such tasks when he administered them to stuttering and nonstuttering children. Samson and Cooper (1980) replicated King's study with adult subjects and also found no differences between stutterers and normal speakers.

More recent research on stutterers' manual skills have tended to emphasize relatively complex tasks. Williams and Bishop (1992) timed subjects as they lifted a finger from one key to press another, then touched a box and pressed another key as rapidly as possible. Stutterers proved to be slower than both normal speakers and subjects with articulatory defects. Vaughn and Webster (1989) found that more stutterers than nonstutterers showed anomalies in the way they performed tasks that required synchronous movement of the two hands, such as threading a string through a needle's eye.

On the premise that stuttering might be due to an underlying difficulty in organizing sequential motor activities in general, Webster (1985, 1986b, 1989b) had subjects tap with four fingers in various sequences. The stutterers did make more errors than their controls. Webster found the premise somewhat insufficient, however. He initiated a research program on the guiding hypothesis that stutterers' left-hemisphere mechanisms are especially subject to interference from an overactive right hemisphere. While subjects tapped out sequential patterns with the fingers of one hand, they engaged in knob turning or button pressing with the other (Webster, 1986a, 1989a). True to the hypothesis, when subjects tapped with the right hand, the concurrent activity with the left hand created more interference for the stutterers than for the controls; when they tapped with the left hand, concurrent activity with the right affected both groups equally.

Forster and Webster (1991) carried out a critical test of the theory of an interfering right hemisphere. Subjects engaged in sequential finger tapping as before, but in place of a concurrent activity with the other hand, they activated a pedal with a foot. According to the hypothesis, the stutterers should have shown more interference than the nonstutterers when using the contralateral foot, but no greater interference when using the ipsilateral foot. This did not prove to be the case. The groups did not differ, both showing more interference with the ipsilateral than the contralateral foot. Forster and Webster concluded that there may be a "generally greater susceptibility to interference of left-hemisphere mechanisms in stutterers from any ongoing neural activity regardless of hemisphere." In an earlier study Webster (1987) had obtained results which suggested that the interference might indeed be more general. The procedure of that study required subjects to transcribe sequences of letters which were presented aurally faster than they could write them down, so that subjects had to monitor and respond concurrently. Under those conditions the stutterers made more errors than the nonstutterers. The result seemed to point to an interference effect which was present regardless of whether one or both hemispheres were involved. However, Webster questioned whether there was an interference effect at all. In a further study of letter transcription (Webster, 1990a), he therefore had subjects listen to the letter sequence first and write down any that they could remember afterward. This did not result in any improvement of the stutterers' performance. The nature of the stutterers' letter transcription deficit—and of stuttering itself—remained obscure.

Motor Capacities of the Speech Musculatures

If the stutterer possesses a neuromuscular abnormality or weakness of some kind, then, regardless of its precise nature or the parts of the body whose functioning it affects, its presence must be recognizable in the defective working of the oral and other related structures if it is to be regarded as a cause of stuttering. Now it is a matter of common observation that typical stutterers, unlike so many persons who have speech impairments due to cerebral palsy, are able to use their oral structures without difficulty in such nonspeech activities as are involved in eating. There is an answer to this argument, however. The muscular adjustments involved in chewing, biting, sucking, swallowing, and the like are relatively gross ones. It may be possible to harbor a neuromuscular weakness so subtle that it reveals itself only in the rapid, fine coordinations required. for speech. This explanation is plausible enough, but a crucial test of its validity immediately suggests itself. Do stutterers tend to be less able than nonstutterers to produce rapid, fine adjustments of the articulators in nonspeech activities? So effectively does this question appear to roll up into a ball the whole issue of motor factors in the etiology of stuttering, that it has received a considerable amount of attention *(see Table 14)*.

The earliest study of the rapid repetitive movement, or diadochokinesis, of the stutterer's oral structures was reported by West and Nusbaum (1929). Using a measure consisting of the combined rate of movement of the jaw and eyebrow for each subject, they found that stutterers tended to make poorer scores than nonstutterers. Cross (1936) reported slower rates of movement of the tongue, jaw, and diaphragm among stutterers than among right-handed normal speakers. Spriestersbach (1940), however, found no differences between stutterers and nonstutterers in speed of movement of the tongue, jaw, brow, and lips. Similarly, Strother and Kriegman (1943) found no significant differences in the diadochokinesis of the tongue, jaw, and lips of stutterers and nonstutterers matched for age, sex, dextrality quotient, and rhythm discrimination. Strother and Kriegman discovered, moreover, that when comparable data of previous conflicting studies were pooled they revealed, in the aggregate, essentially no differences between stutterers and normal speakers. Finally, Chworowsky (1952) showed that stutterers performed as well as nonstutterers in the rapid repetitive articulation of isolated speech sounds and did so under both presumed emotional stress and normal conditions.

Comparable studies, with conflicting findings, have been done on stutterers' ability to move their oral structures rhythmically or to use them in reproducing temporal patterns accurately. In addition to those summarized in Table 14, a study by Zaleski (1965) found stutterers less able to reproduce rhythmic patterns with the syllables "pa," "ta," and "ka." Barrett and Stoeckel (1979) and Newman, Channell, and Palmer (1986) also reported stutterers to be less able to wink with just one eye. Mallard, Hicks, and Riggs (1982) could find no difference between stutterers and normal speakers in the ability to produce the vowel /a/ with a gentle onset of phonation.

Caruso, Gracco, and Abbs (1987) introduced a load on the lower lip of subjects as they said the /p/ in /apa/. Stutterers responded with the same compensatory adjustments as controls, but with longer latencies and smaller changes in magnitude of movement. Brown, Zimmermann, Linville, and Hegmann (1990) found stutterers slower than nonstutterers when instructed to tap with a finger, move the jaw, and say "ah" repeatedly at a comfortable rate. Riley and Riley (1991) administered their Oral Motor Assessment Scale to subjects aged 4 to 8 years. The stutterers' performance was comparable to that of children with defective articulation, but poorer than that of normal speakers.

Table 14. Studies of Motor Proficiency of the Speech Musculature of Stutterers and Nonstutterers Classified with Regard to Whether the Stutterers Were Found to Be of Poorer (Positive Outcome) or Equal Ability (Negative Outcome)*

	Tongue		Lips		Jaw		Diaphragm	
	Positive	Negative	Positive	Negative	Positive	Negative	Positive	Negative
Strength		Palmer and Osborn (1940)						
Speed of Repetitive Movement		Cross (1936), Spriestersbach (1940), Strother and Kriegman (1943)		Cross (1936), Spriestersbach (1940), Strother and Kriegman (1943)	West and Nusbaum (1929)**	Cross (1936), Spriestersbach (1940), Strother and Kriegman (1943)	Cross (1936)	Friedman (1955)
Regularity of Repetitive Movement	Blackburn (1931)		Blackburn (1931)	Seth (1934)	Blackburn (1931)	Seth (1934)	Blackburn (1931), Seth (1934)	
Accuracy of Reproduction of Temporal Patterns	Hunsley (1937)	Wulff (1935), Strother and Kriegman (1944)	Hunsley (1937)	Wulff (1935), Strother and Kriegman (1944)	Hunsley (1937)	Wulff (1935), Strother and Kriegman (1944)	Hunsley (1937)	

*Studies with more than one outcome in a given category are classified as "positive" if any outcome was positive.
**Combined jaw-brow rate. Spriestersbach (1940) found no differences for either separate or combined jaw and brow rates.

Viewed as a whole, the research on the nonspeech activities of the stutterer's speech mechanism does not lend itself to any straightforward conclusions.

Reaction Time

In our discussion of motor abilities so far, we have made no mention of a very large number of investigations of stutterers' reaction times. Following an early period of inconclusive effort, research on the motor performance of stutterers dwindled for a time. When it was resumed with enthusiasm in the 1970s, it was mainly in response to questions about stutterers' reaction time, particularly in relation to the functioning of the larynx.

Voice Initiation and Termination Time

Vocal abnormalities are a well-documented feature of stuttering behavior (see Chapter 1) and are clearly apparent to an alert observer. It is not surprising that at widely separated times in the history of thinking about stuttering, the larynx has been suspected of being the primary source of the problem.[26] A renewed flurry of interest in this hypothesis was caused in part by the electromyographic studies of Freeman and Ushijima (1975, 1978), which vividly depicted the abnormal state of the intrinsic muscles of the larynx during stuttering. One result of this interest has been an extensive series of investigations of the phonatory reaction times of stutterers (see Table 15). In this research subjects have been instructed to produce voice in various forms as quickly as possible in response to a signal. With few exceptions the results have shown stutterers to be slower on the average than nonstutterers in initiating phonation. Tests of stutterers' ability to terminate phonation have produced similar results. Stutterers have been found to differ from nonstutterers by an average order of magnitude ranging from well under one-tenth to about three-tenths of a second.

In some of these studies subjects were asked to respond with words or nonsense syllables. Only those utterances judged by the experimenters to be fluent were retained for analysis. The trouble with such observations is that they lead to the unanswerable question of whether the observed delay in phonation is a cause, a result, or a minimal form of stuttering. In search of less ambiguous data, most investigators have therefore resorted to the use of isolated vowels such as /a/ or /ʌ/. Although stutterers rarely appear to have difficulty with isolated speech sounds, it is arguable that because even saying vowels is a form of speech activity, the task is not totally free

---

[26]See Rieber and Wollock (1977) and Kenyon (1942).

Table 15. Studies of Phonatory, Oral, and Manual Reaction Times
Of Stutterers and Nonstutterers

	Subjects	Cue	Response	Results
Adams and Hayden (1976)	Adults	Tone	Initiation and termination of /a/	Stutterers were slower in both initiation and termination.
Kerr (1976)	Adults	Light	Change from one sound to another	Stutterers were slower in changing from a voiceless to a voiced sound.
Starkweather, Hirschman, and Tannenbaum (1976)	Adults	Illumination of screen	Nonsense syllables and words	Stutterers were slower.
Cross (1978)	Children aged 5 and 9; adults	Tone	Finger press	Stutterers were slower at each age level.
McFarlane and Prins (1978)	Adults	Offset of light or tone	Lip closure, /pæ/, /bæ/	Stutterers were slower (difference was significant only for tone).
Adler and Starkweather (1979)		Visual	Oral, laryngeal, linguistic, nonlinguistic	Stutterers were slower under all conditions.
Cross and Cooke (1979)	Adults	Visual or auditory	/a/ or switch press	Stutterers were slower in both vocal and manual responses, whether to visual or auditory stimulus.
Cross and Luper (1979)	Children aged 5 and 9; adults	Tone	/ʌ/	Stutterers were slower at each age level. Not all had long reaction times.

Table 15 (continued)

Cross, Shadden, and Luper (1979)	Adults	Tone	/ʌ/	Stutterers were slower, regardless of which ear received the tone.
Lewis, Ingham, and Gervens (1979)		Visual or auditory	Initiation and termination of phonation	Stutterers were slower in response to both visual and auditory cues.
Prosek, Montgomery, Walden, and Schwartz (1979)	Adults	Tone, light, or VC word	Button press or VC word	No significant differences were found.
Webster (1979b)		Visual stimulus	Syllables	Stutterers were slower.
Cullinan and Springer (1980)	Children aged 5 to 11	Tone	/a/	Stutterers with additional speech or language problems were slower. Those below age 8 did not differ from controls.
McFarlane and Shipley (1981)	Adults	Offset of light or tone	/bæ/, /pæ/	Stutterers were slower in response to auditory but not visual cues.
Murphy and Baumgartner (1981)	Children aged 4 to 6	Tone	Initiation and termination of /a/	There were no significant differences between groups in either initiation or termination.
Reich, Till, and Goldsmith (1981)	Adults	Offset of tone	Button press, throat clearing, inspiratory phonation, /ʌ/, "upper"	Stutterers were significantly slower only in the speech responses, though their reaction times were longer on all tasks. In throat clearing the difference approached significance.

	Subjects	Cue	Response	Results
Venkatagiri (1981)	Adults	Tone	Voiced and whispered /a/	Stutterers did not differ from nonstutterers in either response.
Hayden, Adams, and Jordahl (1982)	Adults	Tone	Oral reading of sentences beginning with /a/	Stutterers were slower in initiating sentences.
Venkatagiri (1982c)	Adults	Tone	/s/ and /z/	Stutterers did not differ from nonstutterers in either response.
Watson and Alfonso (1982)	Adults	Offset of tone or light	Voiced and whispered /a/, nonsense-syllable phrase	No differences between stutterers and nonstutterers were found.
Borden (1983)	Adults	Tone	Finger counting and speech counting	Stutterers were slower than nonstutterers in the execution but not in the initiation of the tasks.
Cross and Luper (1983)	Children aged 5 and 9; adults	Tone	Key press	Stutterers were slower at each age level.
Hand and Haynes (1983)	Adults	Exposure of stimulus word	Key press or /a/ if stimulus was real word	Stutterers were slower in both manual and vocal reaction time.
Till, Reich, Dickey, and Sieber (1983)	Children aged 8 to 12	Offset of tone	Button press, throat clearing, inspiratory phonation, /ʔʌ/, "upper"	Stutterers were significantly slower in throat clearing and "upper."

Table 15 (continued)

Study	Group			Results
Watson and Alfonso (1983)	Adults	Offset of /a/	/a/	Severe stutterers were slower.
Starkweather, Franklin, and Smigo (1984)	Adults	Offset of tone	Button press, /ʌ/	Stutterers were slower in both manual and vocal responses.
Wilkins, Webster, and Morgan (1984)	Adults	Exposure of letters or representations of faces	Button press on appearance of target face or letter	Stutterers were slower in reacting to faces.
Yoshiyuki (1984)	Adults	Tone	Initiation and termination of /i/	Stutterers were slower in voice initiation, but not in termination or in shadowing tone as it changed in pitch.
Hurford and Webster (1985)	Adults	Visual display of XXX	Button release	Stutterers did not differ significantly from nonstutterers and were faster after therapy.
Long and Pindzola (1985)	Children aged 4 to 8	Commands based on Token Test	Manual execution of commands	Stutterers did not differ significantly from nonstutterers.

Study	Subjects	Stimulus	Response	Findings
Bakker and Brutten (1987)	Adults	Light, tone, electric shock	/a/ or /pa/	Stutterers were slower in voice initiation, but not in lip reaction in saying /pa/.
Cross and Olson (1987b)	Adults	Tone	/ʌ/	Stutterers' voice and jaw reaction times were longer than controls' but not significantly.
McKnight and Cullinan (1987)	Children aged 6 to 12	Light, tone	/a/	Stutterers with learning disabilities had longer voice initiations times than controls and other stutterers. Stutterers without other problems had longer voice terminations times than controls.
Peters and Hulstijn (1987)	Adults	Tone	Words and Sentences	Stutterers had longer laryngeal, lip, and masseter muscle reaction times.
Stromsta (1987)	Adults	Light	/a/	Five stutterers with prolongations and tonic blocks were slower than controls. Five with repetitions were not.
Lees (1988)	Adults	Offset of tone	/a/	Stutterers were slower than controls. The difference approached statistical significance.
Bakker and Brutten (1989)	Adults	Light, tone, electric shock	/a/	Stutterers were slower than controls.
Peters, Hulstijn, and Starkweather (1989)	Adults	Tone	Words and sentences	Stutterers were slower than controls. The difference increased with increasing complexity of the response.

Table 15 (continued)

Subjects		Cue	Response	Results
Bishop, Williams, and Cooper (1991a, 1991b)	Children aged 3 to 10	Light	/a/, words, finger movements	Both stutterers and children with defective articulation were slower than controls in vocal and manual responses. The difference increased with task complexity.
Dembrowski and Watson (1991b)	Adults	Light	/a/, VCV syllables	Stutterers were slower than controls, severe stutterers more so than mild ones. Only partial support was found for the response complexity effect.
Ferrand, Gilbert, and Blood (1991)	Adults	Tone	/a/	Stutterers and controls did not differ in vocal reaction time.
Webster and Ryan (1991)	Adults	LED	Hand movement	Stutterers were slower than controls. Increasing the complexity of the task did not change the difference.
Wijnen and Boers (1994)	Adults	Visual presentation of a cue word	Words	There was no difference between stutterers and controls in reaction time.

from the possible influence of stuttering. For this reason a few studies have elicited nonlinguistic phonatory responses such as throat clearing and phonation on inspiration. In two of these studies the stutterers were found to be slower than nonstutterers; in a third the difference approached significance.[27] On the other hand, Yoshiyuki (1984) found stutterers as fast as controls in changing the pitch of the voice.

Some workers have regarded these findings as evidence that stuttering results from laryngeal dysfunction. A different interpretation was advanced by Cullinan and Springer (1980). Pointing out that many stutterers have difficulties in their early speech development (a subject we will come to in Chapter 6), they divided 20 stuttering children into a group of 11 who had mild to moderate language or articulation problems or learning disabilities and a group of 9 who did not. The stutterers with the speech or language problems proved to have significantly slower voice initiation and termination times than nonstutterers; in the case of the other stuttering children the difference was smaller and not significant. Cullinan and Springer concluded that the poorer performance of stutterers in such tasks seemed to be related to the frequency of language and articulation difficulties among them. McKnight and Cullinan (1987) found that stuttering children receiving special education services, chiefly for learning disabilities, had longer voice initiation and termination times, whereas stutterers without such problems differed from nonstutterers only in having longer voice termination times.

Cullinan and Springer also noted that the relative slowness of phonatory reactions of the stutterers was considerably more pronounced in the older subjects than in the younger ones, suggesting that it may develop as a reaction to stuttering. Their subjects ranged in age from 5 to 11 years. In a study of 4- to 6-year-old children who were free from disorders of articulation or language, Murphy and Baumgartner (1981) found no difference between stutterers and nonstutterers in vocal initiation or termination time. Cross and Luper (1979) reported slower voice reaction times in 5- and 9-year-old stutterers unselected with regard to language or articulation difficulties. Till, Reich, Dickey, and Sieber (1983) found evidence of phonatory slowness in stutterers aged 8 to 12 years who had normal language and articulation. Bishop, Williams, and Cooper (1991a, 1991b) found that both stuttering children and children with defective articulation in the age range of 3 to 10 years had longer vocal and manual reaction times than children with normal speech. The issues raised by Cullinan and Springer are as yet unresolved.

---

[27]Adler and Starkweather (1979); Reich, Till, and Goldsmith (1981); Till, Reich, Dickey, and Sieber (1983).

Initiating voice as fast as possible in response to a signal is a complex act involving, among other things, a preparatory set to respond, the perception of a stimulus, and the activation of both respiratory and laryngeal muscles. Where in this chain of events do stutterers lag? Because most studies have employed a tone as the stimulus, various workers have used both visual and auditory cues to rule out the possibility that the delay is in the auditory perception rather than in the vocal response. The effect is the same. Watson and Alfonso (1982) thought the delay might be in the stutterer's readiness to respond. Giving subjects a warning signal before presenting the cue to respond, they found no significant difference between stutterers and controls. Their subsequent replication of the study (Watson and Alfonso, 1983) did not clearly bear out this hypothesis, however; differences between the stutterers and nonstutterers appeared in severe cases despite the preparatory warning period.

A question that remains is whether the lag is in the stutterer's laryngeal or respiratory adjustments. Both Venkatagiri (1981, 1982c) and Watson and Alfonso (1982) attempted to address this question by asking subjects to respond with voiced and whispered utterances of the same sounds. Unfortunately, the results were inconclusive because in neither study did a difference between the stutterers and nonstutterers emerge for either voiced or voiceless sounds. It is noteworthy that in normal speakers laryngeal and respiratory reaction times are by no means the same. In a study of normal-speaking subjects, Shipp, Izdebski, and Morrissey (1984) timed both the occurrence of increased subglottal breath pressure and the appearance of changes in the action potentials from three intrinsic laryngeal muscles. They found respiratory response slower than laryngeal muscle response, suggesting that "it is not laryngeal adjustment time that principally determines vocal reaction time, but rather it is the temporal interval for activation of the respiratory system." Indirect support for the assumption that stutterers' slow vocal reactions may actually be slow respiratory reactions has come from some research by Prosek, Montgomery, Walden, and Schwartz (1979). They timed subjects' reactions by two measures: the start of electromyographic activity at the larynx and the actual onset of the voice. The stutterers' laryngeal responses proved to be as fast as those of the controls, but their reaction times on the acoustic measures were longer. Prosek and his co-workers suggested that "the initial gesture may occur with normal latency, but the release of the gesture or the onset of airflow may be abnormally long." In two severe stutterers, Watson and Alfonso (1987) found indications of a delay in both respiratory and laryngeal activity.

Bakker and Brutten (1989) made a similar division. They reasoned that the stutterer's increased phonatory reaction time must be due either to a lag in premotor activity (i.e., perceiving the signal and programming the response) or to slow laryngeal adjustment (posturing the larynx for phonation). Instructing subjects to say the vowel /a/ as quickly as possible in response to a signal, they measured the time interval from the onset of the signal to the point where an electroglottograph showed the first low frequency changes that marked the start of laryngeal adjustment. The beginning of vocal fold vibration gave the total laryngeal reaction time. Subtracting the premotor interval from the total reaction time then gave the laryngeal adjustment time. Analysis of the results showed that the stutterers exceeded the control subjects in both premotor and laryngeal adjustment time. In short, they took more time both in planning the response (or perceiving the signal) and in preparing the larynx for production of voice.

A few additional observations remain to be noted. Borden (1983) and Cross and Luper (1979, 1983) both pointed to a distinct overlap in voice initiation time between groups; some stutterers had faster reaction times than some nonstutterers. In three studies a severity effect was observed, the more severe stutterers tending to have slower reactions.[28] In two other investigations, however, no such relationship was found.[29] Cross and Olson (1987a) restricted subjects' jaw movement by means of a bite block on the theory that stutterers' longer vocal reaction times result from abnormal movements of the upper articulators. The effect of the bite block proved to be variable; some stutterers increased vocal reaction time, others decreased it. Finally, some provocative reports have indicated that subjects tend to initiate voice faster under conditions known to reduce stuttering markedly. Webster (1979b) noted this as an effect of masking noise. Hayden, Adams, and Jordahl (1982) and Hayden, Jordahl, and Adams (1982) were not able to confirm this, but found that stutterers' voice initiation times were faster when they spoke in time to rhythm.

Oral and Manual Reaction Time

Inevitably, the results obtained on the vocal reaction times of stutterers have led to questions about their other reaction times, specifically in oral and manual activities (*see Table 15*). With reference to oral responses, McFarlane and Prins (1978) found consistently longer reaction times for stutterers in a lip closure task regardless of whether the subject was producing a syllable such as /pæ/ or a simple movement of the lips. Likewise, Adler and Starkweather (1979) reported stutterers to be as slow in comparison with nonstutterers on an oral task as on a laryngeal one, whether the task was linguistic or nonlinguistic.

Considerably more research has been done on manual reaction times, generally by having the subject press a button with a finger. The results have been conflicting. At this writing 6 studies have

---

[28]Venkatagiri (1982c), Borden (1983), Watson and Alfonso (1983).
[29]Murphy and Baumgartner (1981), McFarlane and Lavorato (1983).

recorded slower finger reaction times in stutterers; 6 have not. The 6 failing to show any difference included a study in which stutterers were slower in the execution of finger counting tasks,[30] but not in their initiation (Borden, 1983). Another involved such complex commands as "Touch the little red circle and the big green square" (Long and Pindzola, 1985). Cross and Luper (1983) found that stutterers' voice and finger reaction times were highly correlated, but Starkweather, Franklin, and Smigo (1984) did not. Curiously, both Wilkins, Webster, and Morgan (1984) and Hurford and Webster (1985) reported that stutterers' manual reaction times were faster after speech therapy than before.

Summary Remarks

The hypothesis that laryngeal dysfunction plays a primary part in the stuttering block has lent unusual interest to the observation that stutterers tend to have longer voice reaction times than nonstutterers. That observation has now been repeatedly confirmed and even appears to extend to nonspeech activities such as throat clearing. For a number of reasons, however, the implications of this fact are far from clear.

In the first place a vocal response, even throat clearing, is obviously not a function of the larynx alone, but also of the respiratory mechanism, and when subjects are asked to produce an identifiable vowel, the oral structures are involved as well. Although the reaction times measured in these studies have sometimes been referred to as "laryngeal," there is consequently little reason to assume that these reaction times have an exclusive connection with the larynx.

Moreover, speech is so dependent on the interrelated activity of the respiratory, laryngeal, and oral musculatures that it is difficult to imagine by what observations we might determine that one part of this activity is more "important" or "necessary" for speech fluency than the others, or what meaning such words might have in this context. That the larynx participates in stuttering is certain. If we did not have other evidence of it, we would have only to note how we involuntarily constrict the glottis when we say a sound such as /b/ with extra effort. It would be futile however, to try to establish whether it was the closure of the glottis or the pressure of our lips that was the "primary" aspect of our behavior.

We are led to conclude that there is little evidence that abnormal functioning of the larynx has any sort of primacy in stuttering behavior, nor is it clear what form such evidence could take. In addition, it

---

[30]Counting by touching the thumb to the index, middle, ring, and little finger and beginning again with the index finger.

is difficult to reconcile a concept of such primacy with well-confirmed reports that some people who stutter continue to do so with esophageal speech, with a surgically constructed neoglottis, or with an electrolarynx following surgical removal of the larynx.[31] Descriptions of stutterlike reactions in the manual communication of the deaf by Silverman and Silverman (1971) and Montgomery and Fitch (1988) tend to raise the question whether it is necessary to use the speech organs at all, let alone the larynx, in order to stutter.

The delay that stutterers often manifest in their vocal reaction times is very small, but the regularity with which researchers have obtained this finding is nevertheless impressive, and we are challenged for an explanation. Some adopt the view that it reflects some type of overall neuromotor deficit in the stutterer's make-up. Investigations of manual reaction time may tell us more about this possibility, but the 12 studies that have been published to date have been so inconsistent in their outcomes that it already seems clear that if any lag in manual reaction time exists, it is not comparable to the delay in vocal reaction time. Another hypothesis that some workers find congenial at the present time is that the stutterer's slower voice initiation is due to a specific impairment of the motor speech control mechanism in the brain. Notably, Watson, Pool, Devous, Freeman, and Finitzo (1992) reported that stutterers with reduced blood flow to regions of the brain which have been implicated in conceptual models of speech motor control had longer reaction times for words and sentences.

Alternatives to organic explanations have also been considered, however. Bakker and Brutten (1989) suggested that the delay may reflect a "learned strategy . . . to slow down to reduce the risk of fluency failure." Armson and Kalinowski (1994), in a critique of the use of findings on the perceptually fluent speech of stutterers to support organic theories of stuttering, have expressed the belief that even the "fluent" phonations of isolated vowels which have generally been used in vocal reaction time studies may be contaminated by stuttering or stuttering-related events which are not evident perceptually. They point out that the question of whether such contamination has occurred in a given case may not even be answerable.

SENSORY AND PERCEPTUAL PROCESSES

Audition

The normal performance of speech activity depends in part on sensory, perceptual, and integrative skills. Is stuttering perhaps basically a receptive disorder? Some have speculated as much, inspired chiefly by

---

[31]Doms and Lissens (1973), Tuck (1979), Wingate (1981a), Rosenfield and Freeman (1983).

the theory that stuttering is analogous to the breakdown of speech under delayed auditory feedback in normal speakers *(see Chapter 2)*.

Auditory Threshold

There is an early report by Harms and Malone (1939) that each of sixty-two stutterers examined by pure-tone audiometry had an impairment of hearing, but a succession of further studies failed to disclose any significant loss.[32] Tomatis (cited by Van Riper, 1982, p. 379) stated that 90 percent of his stutterers had a hearing loss in one ear and related it to a theory involving both auditory feedback and cerebral dominance. Neither Hugo (1972) nor Aimard, Plantier, and Wittling (1966) could find any difference in sensitivity between the left and right ears of stutterers, though Hugo found that the right ears of his stutterers were poorer, on the average, than the right ears of his controls.

MacCulloch and Eaton (1971) reported a lowered auditory pain threshold for pure tones in a comparison of forty-four stutterers with a group of controls.

Phase Disparities

A literal interpretation of the analogy between stuttering and the delayed auditory feedback (DAF) effect in normal speakers would seem to imply that there is some sort of "built-in" delay in the stutterer's auditory monitoring system. Evidence suggesting that such an aberration might actually exist was obtained by Stromsta (1957). His method made use of the fact that two pure tones of equal frequency and amplitude and diametrically (i.e., 180 degrees) out of phase cancel each other out. Stutterers and normal speakers listened to an air-conducted tone and to a bone-conducted tone of the same frequency simultaneously introduced at the teeth. The subjects then varied the phase and amplitude of the air-conducted tone until a critical adjustment was achieved at which no sound was audible to them. Using this procedure at frequencies of 500, 1,000, and 2,000 Hz, Stromsta found that at 2,000 Hz there was a difference between stutterers and nonstutterers in the average relative phase angle of the air- and bone-conducted sounds as indicated by the amount of adjustment they made.

Later, by the use of a similar method, Stromsta (1972) found an unusual phase disparity between stutterers' left and right ears. His subjects adjusted the amplitude and phase of two air-conducted tones heard at either ear until they cancelled an identical bone-conducted tone. At the point of cancellation the air-conducted tones at the two

---

[32]See Bullen (1945), Sternberg (1946), Aimard, Plantier, and Wittling (1966), Asp (1968), and St. Louis and Hinzman (1988), among others.

ears had a phase disparity at several frequencies about twice as wide, on the average, for the stutterers as for the nonstutterers.

Mangan (cited by Gregory and Mangan, 1982) replicated Stromsta's earlier study and failed to find a difference between stutterers and nonstutterers in the phase and amplitude adjustments of air- and bone-conducted sound needed to obtain a null.

Effect of Auditory Feedback on Nonspeech Oral Activity

A unique approach to the investigation of the stutterer's auditory feedback mechanism was devised by Stark and Pierce (1970). It is possible to reason that if stuttering is due to the misinformation speakers get about their speech movements from a feedback system with an inherent delay, then the same delay should also create problems in their nonspeech activities if we ply them with auditory information about their performance. The rationale that Stark and Pierce gave for their study was not precisely this, but it was closely related to it. They argued that "if abnormal delays were present in the stutterer's speech feedback system, his responses to time delays artificially introduced in the auditory feedback loop would also be abnormal." The essential purpose of their study was to see if stutterers would produce deviant responses under delayed auditory feedback in a simple oral activity such as lip-closure. They trained stutterers and nonstutterers to reproduce a sequential pattern of lip-closures—silent repetitions of the syllable "muh"—with their lips positioned around an apparatus that generated an audible click with every lip-closure. The subjects then performed these temporal patterns under normal, or synchronous auditory feedback (SAF), delayed auditory feedback (DAF), and a combination of DAF by air conduction and SAF by bone conduction.

For both the stutterers and the nonstutterers the delayed feedback conditions produced disturbances in the pattern such as errors, prolonged lip-closures, and prolongations of the pattern. In general, however, the effect of DAF was about the same for both groups of subjects. It was only under SAF that any difference appeared—the stutterers tended to have longer lip-closures. In addition, a study of individual scores showed that a third of the stutterers made unusually frequent errors under SAF, both in the training period and during the experiment. This is interesting since it is under synchronous feedback—from the point of view of an outside observer—that stutterers ordinarily have difficulty with their speech. As Stark and Pierce observed, the results were inconclusive, but the method appeared to have promise.

Other Evidence of Deviant Auditory Feedback

A different kind of evidence of delay in the stutterer's auditory feedback system was sought by Dinnan, McGuiness, and Perrin (1970).

By pairing pure tones with electric shock they conditioned their subjects to emit a psychogalvanic skin response (GSR) to the auditory stimulus. They then measured the time between the pure-tone signal and the peak GSR response. On the average, it was 0.95 seconds longer for the stutterers than for the nonstutterers. This is several times longer than the most effective delay time for producing artificial stuttering in normal subjects, but the finding is interesting nonetheless.

Neilson and Neilson (1979) found that stutterers had an excessive phase lag between stimulus and response in an auditory pursuit task in which subjects had to control the pitch of one tone to match the varying pitch of another by movements of the jaw or hand. In a visual tracking task, by contrast, the performance of the stutterers and control subjects was comparable. Nudelman, Herbrich, Hoyt, and Rosenfield (1987) had 4 stutterers match the pitch of a tone that varied periodically in frequency by humming. The stutterers' tracking was more out of phase with the signal than that of 3 nonstutterers.

Fukawa, Yoshioka, Ozama, and Yoshida (1988) reported that stutterers were more susceptible than nonstutterers to delayed auditory feedback as shown by the effect on subjects' reading rates. Similarly, Jäncke (1991) found a greater lengthening of the stressed vowel of a nonsense word by stutterers under delayed auditory feedback, and also a greater shortening of the vowel when "feedback" was delivered in advance of the utterance. Jäncke suggested that there may be a greater dependence of phonation on hearing in stutterers.

Tests of Central Auditory Function

At an early date theories linking stuttering to delayed auditory feedback focused the attention of researchers on the clinical integrity of the stutterer's central auditory system. The available diagnostic tests were soon put to use. Rousey, Goetzinger, and Dirks (1959) reported that stuttering children did not perform as well as nonstutterers in making median plane sound localization responses. In a broader study of central auditory function, however, Gregory (1964) found that adult stutterers did not differ for the most part from nonstutterers on tests of sound localization, binaural loudness balance, and discrimination of speech distorted by frequency filtering. Sound localization findings by Kamiyama (1964) and Asp (1968) were in agreement with those of Gregory, although Asp observed some differences on tests of loudness balance, and Herndon (1967) found differences in the ability to discriminate between different durations of tone.

These initial efforts, then, produced largely negative results. Since the 1960s, however, a number of more sensitive clinical procedures for evaluating central auditory function have come into use through the work of Jerger and others. Hall and Jerger (1978) compared the performance of stutterers and nonstutterers on a battery of seven such tests. On most of these the stutterers' responses were normal. There were small differences between the groups, however, on three tests that are especially sensitive: the acoustic reflex amplitude function, synthetic sentence identification with ipsilateral competing message (SSI-ICM), and the staggered spondaic word (SSW) test devised by Katz (1962).[33] Although emphasizing that the overall pattern of the stutterers' test findings failed to suggest "substantial central auditory disorders," Hall and Jerger stated that the pattern was suggestive of subtle central auditory disorder at the level of the brainstem.

A study by Toscher and Rupp (1978) using identification of synthetic sentences with ipsilateral competing message (SSI-ICM) corroborated the findings of Hall and Jerger. Molt and Guilford (1979) also obtained findings essentially identical to those of Hall and Jerger on the synthetic sentence identification test: With a contralateral competing message the stutterers and nonstutterers did not differ, but with an ipsilateral competing message stutterers scored lower than nonstutterers, though within the normal range and considerably higher than subjects with known brainstem pathology. Interestingly, Wynne and Boehmler (1982) and Nuck, Blood, and Blood (1987) found that even normal speakers who exhibited some part-word repetitions in their speech had lower scores on the SSI-ICM than those who did not. Only Hannley and Dorman (1982) and Kramer, Green, and Guitar (1987) found no difference on this test.

On the staggered spondaic word (SSW) test, results conflicting with those of Hall and Jerger were reported by Karr (1977), who found no difference between stutterers and nonstutterers. On the other hand, Barrett, Keith, Agnello, and Weiler (1979), although obtaining no differences with central auditory processing tests employing frequency-filtered and time-compressed speech, found a significant difference on the SSW Test. In a study of central auditory function in eight- to eleven-year-old stutterers, G. W. Blood and Blood (1984) found no significant difference from nonstutterers on the SSW Test, the Pitch Pattern Sequencing Test, the Competing Environmental Sounds Test, or on tests involving time-compressed speech, dichotic synthetic syllables, or auditory localization. There was a subgroup of stutterers, however, who performed poorly on the SSW Test and the Competing Environmental Sounds Test.

As a result of these conflicting but provocative findings, central auditory function in stutterers has become a well worked area of re-

---

[33]The other tests were: the acoustic reflex threshold, performance-intensity functions for monosyllabic (PB) word lists (PI-PB), performance-intensity functions for synthetic sentences (PI-SSI), and synthetic sentence identification with contralateral competing message (SSI-CCM). The tests are described by Jerger (1973, 1975).

search with a variety of testing methods. On a sound fusion task, Bonin, Ramig, and Prescott (1985) found that stutterers appeared to require a longer time interval between sounds before they heard them as two sounds; the difference approached statistical significance. In a study by Cohen and Hansen (1975) stutterers performed more poorly than nonstutterers on a test of auditory-visual integration in which subjects were presented with an irregular series of taps and had to select a series of dots having the same pattern.

In a study by Kramer, Green, and Guitar (1987), stutterers performed more poorly than controls on the masking level difference task, a test of brainstem function. Liebetrau and Daly (1981) reported similar results for a subgroup of "organic" stutterers who had positive signs on the Michigan Neuropsychological Test Battery. Anderson, Hood, and Sellers (1988) obtained negative results with the Phonemic Synthesis Test, which evaluates a subject's ability to fuse separate phonemes into words, and on the Binaural Fusion Test, in which high and low frequency components of a spondaic word are presented simultaneously to different ears. In a study by Hageman and Greene (1989) there was no significant difference between groups on the Revised Token Test, but the stutterers performed more poorly on a competing message task derived from the test. Meyers, Hughes, and Schoeny (1989) found that stutterers did not differ from controls in judging which ear received the stimulus first when syllables were presented in pairs to both ears with different degrees of asynchronization between ears. Harris, Fucci, and Petrosino (1991) found that in scaling the magnitude of tones of different intensity, stutterers tended to use a restricted range of numerical values.

Finally, some research has been done on stutterers' speech discrimination and listening ability. A study by Bright (1948) appeared to show that stutterers had some difficulty on tests of listening ability involving discrimination between vowels and comprehension of paragraph material. On the other hand, Welch (1961) found stutterers to be normal in listening proficiency. Hugo (1972) likewise found no differences in speech discrimination ability except that, unlike Spielberger (1956), he found that stutterers seemed to have lower perceptual thresholds for some of their previously stuttered words.

Auditory Evoked Potentials

In a study of slow cortical auditory evoked responses, Molt and Luper (1983) found that stutterers had faster average peak latencies than normal speakers. Finitzo, Pool, Freeman, Devous, and Watson (1991) observed lower amplitudes in stutterers for all of the three major components of the auditory evoked potential. More research has been done on the early latency potentials known as the auditory brainstem response (ABR), with conflicting results. Neither Decker, Healey, and Howe (1982) nor Newman, Bunderson, and Brey (1985) observed any notable differences. I. M. Blood and Blood (1984) recorded longer Wave III and Wave V latencies for stutterers and abnormal interpeak latencies for five of eight stutterers. Stager (1990) found that stutterers as a group did not differ from controls on any of the latency and amplitude measures of brainstem auditory pathway intactness, but five of the ten stutterers were abnormal on at least one of these measures. Smith, Blood, and Blood (1990) found no differences in latencies, but greater amplitude of Wave I for stutterers.

Middle Ear Muscle Activity

Research on the stutterer's middle ear muscle function has yielded relatively little. As we have seen, Hall and Jerger (1978) found a small difference between stutterers and controls in the acoustic reflex amplitude function. They found no difference in the acoustic reflex threshold. Neither did Delaney (1979) in a study of four- to fourteen-year-old children. In Delaney's study little if any difference appeared in the latency of onset and the rise time of the reflex. The stutterers did, however, show greater amounts and rates of middle ear muscle contraction. Hannley and Dorman (1982) observed no difference in the latency or amplitude of the reflex. Mangan (cited by Gregory and Mangan, 1982) found no significant difference between stutterers and nonstutterers in the relaxation and adaptation of the acoustic reflex.

Horovitz et al. (1978) found that the threshold of reflex response of the middle ear muscles to sound was significantly lowered by induced anxiety in stutterers, but not in normal speakers. Since studies have shown that these muscles contract just prior to speech, the authors speculated that a relationship may exist between anxiety and subtle distortions of auditory feedback in stutterers.

Howell, Marchbanks, and El-Yaniv (1986) found no difference between stutterers and normal speakers in middle ear muscle activity during vocalization.

Lombard Sign

Panconcelli-Calzia (1955) found the Lombard sign in only 27 percent of a group of 80 stutterers, as compared with 78 percent of a group with normal voice and speech. This is in conflict with a considerable amount of research showing that most stutterers do increase the loudness of their voices under masking noise.[34]

---

[34]Adams and Moore (1972), Adams and Hutchinson (1974), Conture (1974), Dewar, Dewar, and Anthony (1976), Yairi (1976), Brayton and Conture (1978), Mallard and Webb (1980), Martin, Siegel, and Johnson (1984).

Prevalence of Stuttering Among Deaf Persons

In connection with the subject of audition in stutterers it is of interest that there appeared to be an unusually low prevalence of stuttering in oral schools for deaf children in two independent surveys by Harms and Malone (1939) and Backus (1938). While some stuttering was evidently to be found, it seemed particularly rare among the pupils who had little residual hearing. Varying interpretations have been offered. Shane (1955) suggested that the parent of a deaf child is relatively unlikely to become concerned about the child's fluency. Others have related this finding to the absence of auditory feedback in persons without hearing, and this has served to raise the question whether it is necessary to have some ability to monitor the sounds of one's speech in order to become a stutterer.

Montgomery and Fitch (1988) reported a prevalence of stuttering of only 0.12 percent from a questionnaire survey of schools for the deaf. Of the 12 stutterers identified, 6 were said to stutter only in signing.[35]

Vision

Stutterers as a group appear to have normal visual acuity.[36] In a comprehensive visual study, Hamilton (1940) found that they were also normal in phoria, binocular perception, and color vision.

Visual Perseveration

Eisenson and Winslow (1938) noted a tendency toward visual perseveration in stutterers. In recording colors successively exposed by means of a tachistoscope, they more often than nonstutterers erroneously named colors that had been shown earlier in the series. Goldsand (1944) also obtained evidence of visual perseveration in the adaptation stutterers made to a bright light. On the other hand, neither Sheets (1941) nor King (1961) found definite confirmation of such a tendency. While the results may appear quite inconsistent, it should be noted that essentially none of these studies was an exact replication of others, and in most cases widely differing tests were used. Research on perseveration in human behavior has cast doubt on the assumption that such a thing as sensory perseveration as a general factor exists; the various tests that have been devised for the purpose of studying it do not seem to measure the same thing.[37]

---

[35]The manual stuttering was variously described as easy, effortless repetitions; repetitions of the first syllable, perseverations, blocking, and choppy manipulations; beginning a sign, then stopping and repeating the sign.

[36]McDowell (1928), Hamilton (1940), Schindler (1955).

[37]See discussions of this question by King (1961) and Martin (1962).

One of the measures King used in evaluating sensory perseveration in stutterers was the critical flicker frequency threshold. This is
the lowest rate at which a flickering light appears steady or continuous. The lower the threshold the more lasting the after-image and the
greater the presumed perseveration. Lovett Doust and Coleman
(1955) reported that stutterers were lower than nonstutterers in critical flicker fusion threshold. No differences were found by King (1961)
or Kamiyama (1964). Subsequently, Sayles (1971) again found a lower
flicker fusion point in stutterers, which West interpreted as evidence
of muscular hypertonicity (West and Ansberry, 1968, p. 124).

Perception of Visual Symbols

Kelly (1932) found that stutterers had far greater difficulty than
their controls in a test of "visual aphasia" in which two pairs of digits
were exposed successively and the subject was required to find in the
second pair the digit that did not appear in the first pair. Spadino
(1941), however, found no differences in errors of visual perception
when subjects said or wrote words or numbers flashed on cards.
Furthermore, stutterers compared favorably with nonstutterers in
speed and comprehension of silent reading in a study by Hamilton
(1940) and have generally been found to have normal levels of reading achievement, as will be seen in Chapter 6.

Prevalence Among Blind Persons

Finally, we may note that in a survey of schools for blind and partially
sighted children, Weinberg (1964) found a prevalence of stuttering essentially within the range of expected values for the general population.

Touch and Kinesthesis

Schilling and Biener (1959) reported that in many stutterers there
seemed to be a marked difference between the thresholds of vibratory
sensation in the left and the right extremities, while this difference
appeared very rarely in their observations of nonstutterers. Fucci,
Petrosino, Gorman, and Harris (1985) had subjects adjust the magnitudes
of a vibrotactile stimulus to the hand and tongue to correspond to a scale
of six random numbers. Stutterers and nonstutterers performed the task
similarly for the hand. For the tongue, however, the stutterers used a narrower range of intensity adjustments, which the experimenters interpreted as a more "conservative" scaling behavior. Harris, Fucci, and
Petrosino (1991) again reported that stutterers used a more restricted
range of responses and lower vibrotactile magnitude values for
the tongue. In addition, Petrosino, Fucci, Gorman, and Harris (1987)

reported that stutterers showed slightly higher thresholds of sensation at three tongue sites, but gave no data.

A study of the oral sensory and perceptual abilities of stutterers and nonstutterers by Jensen, Sheehan, Williams, and LaPointe (1975) showed no differences in intra-oral two-point discrimination, weight discrimination, or interdental thickness discrimination. In subsequent studies of oral recognition of forms, Martin, Lawrence, Haroldson, and Gunderson (1981) found that stutterers made more errors; Zsilavecz (1981) reported the same, but presented no data; and Stewart, Evans, and Fitch (1985) obtained somewhat equivocal findings. Carpenter and Sommers (1987) found that stutterers discriminated forms both orally and manually as well as nonstutterers, except while hearing words to be written down.

In a study of the kinesthetic acuity of stutterers, De Nil and Abbs (1991) instructed subjects to make the smallest possible movements of the jaw, lower lip, tongue, and index finger. Without visual feedback, the stutterers made larger minimal displacements of the oral structures, but not the finger, than the nonstutterers.

CONCLUSIONS

Young (1994) has recently exposed to view the limitations of an exceedingly common type of research design in which the question is whether an average difference exists between groups of individuals. The studies we have reviewed in this chapter have been based almost exclusively on this design. No doubt, this goes far to explain why this research has been plagued from the beginning by conflicting and inconclusive findings. Yet, despite the frustrating inconsistency of the evidence concerning the stutterer's physical constitution, some of it has gathered so much weight that it urges us toward a number of broad negative and positive conclusions.

During silence, stutterers appear to be essentially similar to normal speakers with regard to various respiratory, cardiovascular, biochemical, and neurophysiological measures, despite isolated and unconfirmed reports of certain differences.

Stutterers have not been shown to differ from nonstutterers in handedness. An old contention that enforced change of handedness may cause stuttering has not been borne out by scientific research.

With regard to most types of motor ability, including bodily, manual, and oral skills, the results have been inconclusive. A notable exception is phonatory initiation time, in which stutterers, on the average, have repeatedly been observed to lag behind nonstutterers. Why they do, and whether the lag is related to an overall slowness in reaction time, is as yet undetermined.

On the average, stutterers appear to achieve poorer scores on certain sensitive tests of central auditory function, and they have tended to exhibit less right-ear advantage on dichotic listening tests employing meaningful linguistic stimuli. It is also possible that many stutterers are atypical in cerebral dominance for language as evidenced by their cortical potentials during speech processing. How such traits might be related to stutterers' slower vocal initiation, and how any of them might be related to stuttering, are questions that we have hardly begun to speculate about.

As we grope for meaning in these findings, it is important to keep in mind the overlap existing between stutterers and nonstutterers whenever physical differences between them have appeared. In other words, despite group trends to the contrary, some stutterers exhibit faster vocal reaction times, greater right-ear advantage in dichotic word tests, and the like, than some nonstutterers. This fact precludes any simple explanation of the group differences.

The overlap between stutterers and nonstutterers has been interpreted occasionally to imply the existence of subgroups of stutterers with different etiologies. On this basis, for example, investigators sometimes attempt to distinguish between "organic" and "functional" stutterers. A simpler, more parsimonious way of thinking about the overlap is to relate it to the most fundamental question we can ask regarding the etiology of a disorder: What are the conditions both necessary and sufficient to bring it about? Imagine a physical trait, say slow reaction time, in which stutterers as a group differ on the average from normal speakers as a group. Clearly, any overlap in the trait between the groups rules out the trait as a sufficient condition; if the trait, or a given amount of it, were sufficient to produce stuttering, no nonstutterers would have it in that amount. Likewise, the overlap rules out the trait as a necessary condition; if the trait were necessary to produce stuttering, no stutterer would lack it.

It follows that none of the possible or probable differences we have glimpsed between stutterers and nonstutterers represents a necessary or sufficient condition for stuttering. If the differences are not caused by stuttering, or by something else that causes stuttering as well, they may be factors that often contribute, along with others, to the etiology of the disorder in ways that will be better understood when the necessary and sufficient conditions are known. For all that the evidence has told us so far, the necessary and sufficient conditions for stuttering may yet be found in a realm far removed from those we have explored in this chapter.

At this writing much of the attention of rearchers is concentrated on what is termed the stutterer's speech motor control. By a variety of means, the possibility is being explored that stuttering results from a deficit of some type that is unique to the neuromotor mechanism for speech. The question is perfectly reasonable, but it is a curious one in that there would appear to be no technically feasible means of answering it. If the deficit is unique to speech, we obviously cannot do it by studying the nonspeech activity of the speech organs. Nor can we do it by making observations during the occurrence of stuttering; researchers recognized long ago that such observations may reflect the effort and arousal that result from stuttering, if they are not merely observations of stuttering itself. So researchers have turned in large numbers to investigations of the stutterer's "fluent" speech or speech sounds, as we saw in this chapter and in Chapter 1, usually taking precautions to ensure that the utterances are really fluent. But the precautions are increasingly being recognized to be futile because, as Armson and Kalinowski (1994) have pointed out, there is no way to be sure that unusual events recorded during these "fluent" utterances are not caused by the anticipation of stuttering or are not imperceptible stutterings themselves. How, then, are we to study the stutterer's motor speech control? It will be interesting to see if this dilemma can be resolved.

Suggested Readings

Boberg, E. (ed.), *Neuropsychology of Stuttering*. Edmonton, Alberta: Univ. Alberta Press (1993).

Moore, W. H., Jr., Central nervous system characteristics of stutterers. In Curlee, R. F., and Perkins, W. H. (eds.), *Nature and Treatment of Stuttering: New Directions*. San Diego: College-Hill Press (1984b).

Moore, W. H., Jr., and Boberg, E., Hemispheric processing and stuttering. In Rustin, L., Purser, H., and Rowley, D. (eds.), *Progress in the Treatment of Fluency Disorders*. London: Taylor and Francis; San Diego, Singular Publishing Group (1987).

Peters, H. M. F., and Hulstijn, W. (eds.), *Speech Motor Dynamics in Stuttering*. New York: Springer (1987).

Peters, H. M. F., Hulstijn, W., and Starkweather, C. W. (eds.), *Speech Motor Control and Stuttering*. Amsterdam: Elsevier (1991) .

Rosenfield, D. B., and Jerger, J., Stuttering and auditory function. In Curlee, R. F., and Perkins, W. H. (eds.) *Nature and Treatment of Stuttering: New Directions*. San Diego: College-Hill Press (1984).

Rosenfield, D. B., and Nudelman, H. B., Neuropsychological models of speech dysfluency. In Rustin, L., Purser, H., and Rowley, D. (eds.), *Progress in the Treatment of Fluency Disorders*. London: Taylor and Francis; San Diego, Singular Publishing Group (1987).

St. Louis, K. O., Linguistic and motor aspects of stuttering. In Lass, N. J. (ed.), *Speech and Language: Advances in Basic Research and Practice, Vol. 1*. New York: Academic Press (1979).

Starkweather, C. W., Stuttering and laryngeal behavior: A review. *ASHA Monographs No. 21*. Rockville, Md.: Amer. Speech-Language-Hearing Assoc. (1982).

Van Riper, C., *The Nature of Stuttering, 2nd ed*. Englewood Cliffs, N.J.: Prentice-Hall (1982), Chap. 14.

5

THE PERSON WHO STUTTERS: PERSONALITY

Some time during the 1930s a sweeping wave of interest in personality, emotional adjustment, and the psychological aspects of human illness that had been gathering momentum since the beginning of the century broke on the scientific investigation of stuttering, and from then on for a period of about twenty-five years much of the search for a common distinguishing feature of the person who stutters centered on factors of personality make-up.

ADJUSTMENT

The basic question motivating most of the research on the stutterer's personality was whether the average stutterer is to be regarded as a neurotic or severely maladjusted person on the basis of the criteria typically used to make such a determination. This might not appear to be such a difficult question, but the answer was notably elusive for more than fifty years and, even now that we can look back on enough research to make some judgments possible, they are not made with complete assurance.

In 1928 there appeared what was apparently the first published study of the emotional adjustment of stutterers.[1] This was part of an

---

[1]An earlier study by Marion McKenzie Font, done under the direction of John M. Fletcher in 1924, was published in 1955 as Chapter 34 in Johnson and Leutenegger (eds.), *Stuttering in Children and Adults*. It was an administration of the Kent-Rosanoff Word Association Test to nine stutterers and to forty-nine nonstuttering University of Iowa students. No sharp distinction appeared. Anderson (1923) made use of forty words from the Kent-Rosanoff Test in an early exploration of certain perceptual, psychomotor, and other abilities of stutterers. In a study by Travis (1928b) stutterers were given a word and asked to write word associations as fast as possible. The stutterers performed faster alone than in a group, just the opposite of Allport's findings on nonstutterers.

investigation by Elizabeth McDowell that made use of several devices for measuring emotional adjustment, including the Kent-Rosanoff Word Association Test and two early personality inventories, the Woodworth-Matthews and Woodworth-Cady questionnaires. The questionnaires contained such items as, "Does it make you uneasy to cross a bridge over water?" "Do you talk in your sleep?" "Are you bashful?" Administering these tests to stuttering and nonstuttering children in the New York City public schools, McDowell found essentially no difference in degree of adjustment between the two groups. These conclusions were substantiated by Johnson (1932) in a study of stutterers among University of Iowa students. Johnson found that on the Woodworth-House Mental Hygiene Inventory the stutterers scored as well as House's normal subjects, on the average, and tended to have distinctly more favorable scores than a group with a diagnosis of psychoneurosis whom House had tested.

In 1939, however, Bender reported results in marked disagreement. In a study of City College students with the use of the Bernreuter Personality Inventory, he found that stutterers tended to be more neurotic, more introverted, less dominant, less self-confident, and less sociable than nonstuttering students. Bender's findings were difficult to ignore. He had tested a very large number of subjects, he had employed a control group of his own in place of the risky practice of comparing subjects' scores with published test norms, and he had availed himself of what was then one of the newest and most highly regarded of adjustment inventories. Yet, despite all this, detailed inspection of his results reveals that an exceedingly important qualification must probably be attached to his conclusions. The stutterers' poorer performance on the Bernreuter Inventory was due largely to their responses to sixteen test items on which the two groups of subjects differed significantly. Of these items the great majority put a considerable premium on adequate speech or penalized subjects in some way for being stutterers. The following are some examples:

- Do you find it difficult to speak in public?
- If you are dining out do you prefer someone else to order dinner for you?
- Do you consider yourself a rather nervous person?
- Are you often in a state of excitement?
- Can you usually express yourself better in speech than in writing?

The Bernreuter, of course, did not lie about the stutterer's adjustment. In a very real sense a person whose capacity for speech is impaired is maladjusted by virtue of that problem. This was not, however, what most research workers wanted to know. When Brown and Hull (1942) tested stutterers with the Minnesota Personality Scale three years later, they confirmed the view that stutterers tend to be poor in social adjustment as opposed to most other areas of emotional health (e.g., "morale," "family relations," "emotionality"), and the same pattern has continued to show itself in greater or lesser degree in successive research studies whenever the test used has permitted distinctions of this kind to be made.

During the 1940s the scientific study of the stutterer's personality gained ground rapidly. Further research was done with adjustment inventories of improved design (see Table 16) as well as with so-called projective techniques, which will be discussed shortly. Work on the stutterer's adjustment was dominated by the Califomia Test of Personality. In three separate studies the stutterers consistently fell below the test norms. The California Test analyzed a subject's performance on the basis of twelve categories of self-adjustment and social adjustment. Although there were disparities among the findings, all three agreed in marking stutterers low in the categories of self-reliance, freedom from nervous symptoms (of which stuttering was counted as one), and social skills.

Personality research on stuttering reached a peak in the 1950s. An outstanding development was the use of the Minnesota Multiphasic Personality Inventory (MMPI). Unlike earlier personality inventories whose content was largely determined by professional judgment, the MMPI consisted of items empirically derived in research on psychoneurotic subjects, and it was standardized with careful attention to factors of reliability and validity. Furthermore, the studies in which it was administered to stutterers for the most part made use of control groups, a practice not often followed before. The results of these investigations produced a very satisfactory measure of agreement (see Table 16). By and large, stutterers showed a consistent tendency toward slightly less favorable adjustment than nonstutterers, but their scores, on the average, fell well within what is regarded as the normal range. This was demonstrated in a particularly clarifying manner by Dahlstrom and Craven (1952), who found that college stutterers were less maladjusted as a group than psychiatric patients, were not significantly more maladjusted than ordinary college freshmen, and performed most similarly to college students who had applied for counseling with personal problems.

Various other "pencil and paper" tests have been employed in the investigation of the stutterer's adjustment, as is evident in Table 16. Rarely, if ever, have these studies revealed in stutterers as a group the recognized patterns of psychoneurotic disturbance that belong to such relatively well-defined nosological categories as anxiety, depression, obsessive-compulsiveness, or the like. On the other hand, signs of mild social maladjustment have been found frequently.

Table 16.   Adjustment of Stutterers and Nonstutterers as
            Measured by Personality Inventories

	N Stutterers	Controls	Test	Results
McDowell (1928)	46	46	Woodworth-Matthews, Woodworth-Cady	No clearly significant differences were found.
Johnson (1932)	50		Woodworth-House	The stutterers did not differ from the test norms and were superior in adjustment to House's psychoneurotic group.
Fagan (1932)	33		Woodworth-House	Mild degrees of maladjustment were found in the majority.
Bender (1939)	249	303	Bernreuter Personality Inventory	The stutterers gave significant indications of maladjustment in nearly all areas tested. In particular, they had more fears, worries, and tensions, were less communicative, and were more dependent and hesitant in decision.
Brown and Hull (1942)	59		Minnesota Personality Scale	The stutterers had low scores in the area of social adjustment, but not in morale, family relations, emotionality, or economic conservatism.
Perkins (1947)	75		California Test of Personality	The stutterers revealed problems that appeared to fall consistently within the areas of self-reliance, feelings of personal worth, nervousness, social skills, and social standards.
Schultz (1947)	20		California Test of Personality	The stutterers fell below the test norms, on the average, in total adjustment. They scored poorly in self-reliance, freedom from withdrawing tendencies, nervous symptoms, and social skills.

Study			Test	Results
Cypreansen (1948)	14	14	California Test of Personality	The median of the group fell below the norm in each part of the test except one: sense of personal freedom. The greatest differences were in self-reliance, freedom from nervous symptoms, social skills, school or occupational relationships, and community relationships.
Horlick and Miller (1960)	26	30	California Test of Personality	The stutterers had slightly but not significantly lower adjustment scores than the normal speakers.
Prins (1972)	66	23	California Test of Personality	The stutterers appeared to have better adjustment, on the whole, than the control group which consisted of subjects with other disorders of speech. They tended to score low in social skills, but high in social standards. There was no relationship between adjustment and either severity of stuttering or age.
Silverman and Zimmer (1979)	10	10	California Test of Personality	Female stutterers were compared with female controls; their scores were found to be similar. Male stutterers gave evidence of lower self-esteem than female stutterers.
Richardson (1944)	30	30	Guilford Inventory of Factors STDCR	The stutterers were more socially introvertive, more depressed, and had fewer happy-go-lucky tendencies (rhathymia). There were no differences in thinking introversion and cycloid tendencies.
Shames (1951)	53		Guilford Inventory of Factors STDCR	The stutterers differed significantly from the norms only on "T" (thinking introversion).
Duncan (1949)	62	62	Bell Adjustment Inventory (Home Adjustment Items)	Of the 35 home adjustment items, 5 significantly differentiated a group of stutterers from a group of persons with articulatory impairments. The stutterers indicated the feelings, among others, that their parents did not understand them, were disappointed in them, and treated them as children.

Table 16 (continued)

	N			
	Stutterers	Controls	Test	Results
Bearss (1951)	23	23	Adams Personal Audit, Rotter Incomplete Sentences Blank	No differences were found between the stutterers and nonstutterers on either test.
Brutten (1951)	16	16	Maslow Test of Insecurity	No significant differences were found.
Thorn (1949)	21		Minnesota Multiphasic Personality Inventory (MMPI)	The scores fell within the normal range, and the composite MMPI profile revealed no evidence of neuroticism. There was no common "personality type" when the profiles were analyzed for "pattern" or any substantial difference in composite profile for the most severe and least severe stutterers.
Pizzat (1951)	53	1,400	Minnesota Multiphasic Personality Inventory (MMPI)	The stutterers had poorer scores on all clinical scales except Psychopathic Deviate, but the scores fell well within the normal range.
Dahlstrom and Craven (1952)	100	100	Minnesota Multiphasic Personality Inventory (MMPI)	The stutterers were less well adjusted than a group of 100 college freshmen, but were not as severely disturbed as a group of psychiatric patients and most closely resembled a group of college students who had sought counseling because of personal problems.
Boland (1953)	24	24	Minnesota Multiphasic Personality Inventory (MMPI)	Degree of neuroticism as measured by the Neuroticism Index failed to differentiate stutterers from nonstutterers. Stutterers were higher in measures of anxiety.
Walnut (1954)	38	52	Minnesota Multiphasic Personality Inventory (MMPI)	On all 10 clinical scales the stutterers were well within the normal range as measured by the MMPI norms. On 2 scales, Depression and Paranoia, the stutterers had significantly poorer scores than the controls.

Study	N	Test	Findings
Lanyon, Goldsworthy, and Lanyon (1978)	69	Minnesota Multiphasic Personality Inventory (MMPI)	Stutterers' scores showed no relationship to measures of overt stuttering behavior or attitudes toward stuttering of anxiety or avoidance.
Sermas and Cox (1982)	19	Minnesota Multiphasic Personality Inventory (MMPI)	Although 14 subjects had an elevated score on at least one MMPI scale, no significant elevation was found when the scores were averaged for the group.
Darley (1955)	28	Rogers Test of Personality Adjustment	More of the stuttering children had scores indicative of maladjustment, especially in the categories of social maladjustment and daydreaming. None of the differences in mean scores was statistically significant.
Sergeant (1962)*	60	Bell and Bernreuter Inventories	The stutterers had poorer social adjustment, less self-confidence, and greater emotional instability than normal speakers. This was also true in large measure of the other speech groups with speech problems studied, however.
Wingate (1962b)	70	Edwards Personal Preference Schedule	Mild to moderate maladjustment was found in the area of social relationships.
Anderson (1967)*	50	Guilford-Zimmerman Temperament Survey and Gordon Personal Profile	The stutterers did not differ from the controls in general emotional stability. The stutterers, however, tended to be more shy, less self-assured, friendlier, and more respectful toward others.
Hegde (1972)	106	Eysenck Personality Inventory	The subjects scored high on introversion, close to the anxiety group. On neuroticism they scored within normal limits, though 4 points higher than the norm, on the average.
Thomas (1976)	8	Eysenck Personality Inventory	The stutterers were higher in neuroticism and lower in extraversion, though both groups scored within normal limits.

Table 16 (continued)

Reference	N Stutterers	Controls	Test	Results
Okasha, Bishry, et al (1974)	50**	50	Junior Eysenck Personality Inventory	The stutterers, aged 8 to 12 years, were more introverted than their controls, but there was no difference in neuroticism.
Cohen, Thompson, et al (1975)	36	46	Rathus Assertiveness Schedule	The stutterers scored significantly lower in assertiveness than the controls.
Sermas and Cox (1982)	19		Revised Hopkins Symptom Checklist (SCL-90-R)	When compared with a group of nonpsychotic psychiatric patients, the stutterers had poorer scores on the Interpersonal Sensitivity Scale.
Greiner, Fitzgerald, et al (1985)	41	41	Revised Willoughby Personality Schedule	The stutterers scored higher in social anxiety and sensitivity, though there was considerable overlap between the groups.

*Cited by Bloch and Goodstein (1971).
**Values of N are approximate.

PROJECTIVE TEST FINDINGS

The study of adjustment as defined by a questionnaire yields a rather limited view of personality. For many years psychologists had been attempting to construct tests that would achieve more penetrating insights into the nature of individual character structure. Generally speaking, such attempts have proceeded on the assumption that our observable behavior must almost always contain important clues to our personality make-up, provided we are in a situation in which essentially no conventional or socially conforming responses are possible. Such "projective" tests have frequently proved to be of value to clinical workers who are skilled in their interpretation, particularly in the context of the clinical setting with the opportunities it affords for verification of test findings by means of interviews, personal observation, and other tests.

The chief disadvantage of the projective tests is that it has been difficult to develop them technically for the purpose of obtaining scientifically objective, valid, and reliable measures. In short, when subjects show a given pattern of responses on such a test, there is unfortunately not always sufficient assurance that they would show them again on future occasions, or that another clinical worker would agree on the interpretation of the responses, or that the responses actually mean what they are said to mean. As a result, projective tests in their present form have been the subject of considerable controversy, and generalizations about stutterers based on such tests must be viewed with some degree of caution.

Rorschach Research

Of all projective techniques of studying personality the most extensively developed is the well-known Rorschach Test. This consists of a series of ink blots, some in color, which are presented to the subject with the question, "What might this be?" From a variety of features of the subject's perceptions, inferences are drawn about such specific personality traits as capacity for abstract thinking, habitual concern with details, egocentricity, spontaneity, emotional stability, and so forth. This widely used test has been administered to stutterers repeatedly with findings that are conflicting and generally inconclusive.

Perhaps the earliest of these studies that could be considered a scientific investigation in any accepted sense of the term was reported by Meltzer (1934). Meltzer analyzed the Rorschach responses of 56 stuttering children and found little that was indicative of serious emotional disturbance. He wrote, "Unlike the problem children reported by Beck they are not repressed and do not lead restricted inner lives. To the small extent that neuroticism is suggested it takes what may be called an 'expressive' rather than repressive form." By contrast, Ingebregtsen (1936) found substantial evidence of neuroticism in a Rorschach study of adult stutterers.

Both of these studies were essentially clinical in nature and did not employ control groups. In 1944, however, Meltzer compared 50 stuttering children with 50 nonstutterers of like age, sex, and l.Q. on the basis of over 20 different commonly used scores or indicators of various types derived from their Rorschach records. There was essentially no distinction between the two groups with regard to the great majority of these.indicators. In three instances, however, a significant difference did appear. One of these could be interpreted to mean that the stutterers exercised somewhat poorer "control of intellectual functioning," and the other two suggested that they had somewhat greater capacity for abstract thinking. Since the two groups had been carefully matched with respect to intelligence, Meltzer concluded that the poorer intellectual control of the stutterers was of an emotional origin and that the indications of increased capacity for abstract thinking actually represented compulsive behavior to compensate for their insecurity. He pointed out that the stutterers exceeded the nonstutterers in almost every measure usually indicative of emotional instability, but these differences were for the most part very small and not significant in any statistical sense.

In the same year that Meltzer's findings appeared Richardson (1944) reported a study of adult subjects that tended to corroborate Meltzer's essential finding that there were very few differences in the Rorschach responses of stutterers and nonstutterers. Richardson, in fact, failed to find even the three differences that Meltzer had noted. She did discover, however, that in her group of 30 stutterers 7 made no use of movement or color in their responses, while this was true of only 2 of the 30 nonstutterers, and she concluded that the stutterers showed a tendency not to "recognize their inner promptings" or to "respond impulsively to their outside environment."

Two years later Krugman (1946) came to conclusions that went considerably beyond those of Meltzer and Richardson. He compared 50 stuttering children with 50 children who had behavior problems, and his basic finding was that the two groups did not differ significantly on most scores. In addition, on the basis of a qualitative evaluation of the stutterers' records, he reported that most of them were "seriously disturbed,"' that they tended to be emotionally immature and repressed, that they showed many signs of "neurotic involvement," and that one of their outstanding characteristics was their "obsessive-compulsive make-up."

Sheehan and Zussman (1951) found that stutterers exceeded nonstutterers in such tendencies as drive toward achievement, overemphasis on suppressive control, and intellectual defenses against anxiety as expressed in Rorschach responses. In related Rorschach and Thematic Apperception Test (TAT) studies at the University of Southern California, D. M. Wilson (1950) and Christensen (1952) obtained few findings that appear to lend themselves readily to the interpretation that their stuttering children were basically neurotic or markedly different from the siblings with whom they were compared. By contrast, Moller (cited by Bloch and Goodstein, 1971) found many more signs of maladjustment among stuttering boys than among predelinquent boys, including lower self-awareness and empathic ability, poorer interpersonal relationships, and higher anxiety.

It is clear from these studies and observations that a large amount of disagreement is permitted either by the Rorschach Test or by the manner in which it has been used in research with stutterers. In reviewing these studies Goodstein (1958) pointed out instances in which diametrically opposite findings were used by different workers to reach the same conclusions. In another review, Sheehan (1958b) commented that for many researchers "the Rorschach has seemed to offer an amorphous flux from which any desired interpretation could be pulled."

TAT Studies

The Thematic Apperception Test (TAT) is another well-known projective technique that consists of a series of pictures around each of which the subject is asked to make up a story indicating what is happening, the events that led up to it, the thoughts and feelings of the characters, and the outcome. The interpretation of the test is concerned essentially with the basic needs, strivings, and attitudes revealed in the subject's productions. In a TAT study of adult stutterers, Richardson (1944) found no significant differences between stutterers and controls in proportions of needs, reactions to frustrations, attitudes toward environment, adequacy of the central character, and unsatisfactory endings. In one of the few personality studies that have been done on preschool stutterers, however, Porterfield (1969) found that on the Children's Apperception Test (CAT) adaptive mechanisms of repression-denial, symbolization, and projection-introjection differentiated stutterers from normal controls, but not from a group of maladjusted children. Wyatt (1958, 1969) used pictures from the TAT and CAT, as well as a story completion test, with a group of 5- to 9-year-old stutterers and their controls; blind evaluations of the records by three judges disclosed significant distance anxiety in the stutterers—that is, fear of separation from their mothers.

In other investigations the TAT has been used chiefly for the purpose of testing hypotheses about specific character traits of stutterers. The findings of these and other projective studies will be more appropriately considered in the sections that follow.

PSYCHOSEXUAL FIXATION

After a period of broad exploration of the stutterer's personality and adjustment, the emphasis gradually shifted to studies of more specific personality dimensions. Although we will attempt to treat these dimensions individually, it will be understood that many of the findings with which we are concerned in the remaining discussion of the stutterer's personality are in various ways interrelated and overlapping, and the logic we impose on them in this way is somewhat arbitrary.

Much of this research represented efforts to verify the psychoanalytic postulates of such writers as Coriat, Fenichel, and Glauber *(see Chapter 2)*. It was therefore concerned in large part with the areas of sex and aggression and consisted in essence of attempts to identify in the stutterer's personality the classic symptoms of early psychosexual fixation (i.e., covert expressions of infantile libidinous, dependent, and aggressive needs, and their guilty repression).

Oral and Anal Eroticism

Among the most direct attempts to study repressed pregenital sexuality in stutterers have been those which made use of the Blacky Test. This test, originally designed as an aid in the objective testing of psychoanalytic hypotheses, consists of a series of cartoons depicting events of psychosexual interest in the life of a dog named Blacky. The subject is asked to tell a story about each cartoon and to answer such questions as, "What was Blacky's main reason for defecating there?" "How will Blacky feel about eating when he grows older?" In a study by Dickson (1954) stutterers significantly exceeded nonstutterers in scores indicative of anal fixation on the Blacky Test, and a tendency toward oral fixation approached significance. Merchant (cited by Blum and Hunt, 1952) found that stutterers showed evidence of disturbance in such Blacky dimensions as oral eroticism, oral sadism, castration anxiety, and penis envy and concluded that the subjects' performance was in agreement with psychoanalytic theory. In a similar investigation, Carp (1962) obtained equivocal findings.

On the TAT, Lowinger (1952) found no difference in orality between stutterers and controls. Christensen (1952), however, noted that stutterers gave more projections involving nursing at the breast.

Passive-Dependency

Shopwin (1959) found that adult male stutterers did not differ from nonstutterers in responses to the Kessler PD Scale, a questionnaire designed to reveal passive-dependency.

Katz (1966) investigated dependency and immaturity in fifty young stuttering children and fifty controls by means of the Structured

Doll Play Test. By means of mother, father, and child figures, the subjects were presented with a series of situations in which they had to make choices on behalf of an ego doll between bed and crib, glass and bottle, toilet and potty, and also between father and mother for purposes of feeding the ego doll, putting it to sleep, coming to its bed after a nightmare, and the like. Katz found no evidence of greater dependency or immaturity among the stutterers. The only difference she observed was that the stutterers made somewhat more father choices than the nonstutterers in dependency situations.

Obsessive-Compulsive Character Traits

Anal-sadistic fixation, most frequently mentioned in psychoanalytic writings as the basis of stuttering, is defined in older persons by manifestations ranging from "anal" character traits (excessive orderliness, stinginess, punctuality, acquisitiveness, moral rectitude) to the symptoms of obsessive-compulsive neurosis.

Rapaport (1946, p. 443 ff.) described a series of distinctive features of the TAT stories of persons with obsessive-compulsive character makeup. These include concern with unessential detail, expressions of doubt or uncertainty, incorrect or ostentatious use of imposing words, criticism of the picture, psychological pseudoinsights into the behavior of the characters, and various others. Using Rapaport's descriptions, Bloodstein and Schreiber (1957) drew up a checklist of obsessive-compulsive characteristics. Transcripts of the TAT stories of adult stutterers and nonstutterers were then evaluated and scored independently on the basis of the checklist by three untrained judges, two of whom had no clue to the identity of the stories as belonging to stutterers or nonstutterers. The stutterers showed no greater tendency toward obsessive-compulsive behavior than the nonstutterers.

In a study of anal fixation by Keisman (1958), adult stutterers and normal speakers rated themselves on a checklist of personality characteristics that included anal traits. In addition, Keisman used an Anal Interest Picture Test on which the criterion was the length of time the subject looked at pictures containing anal interest (e.g., a man counting bags of money) as opposed to neutral pictures. The findings were largely negative. The only qualified support for the psychoanalytic hypothesis was in the finding that the stutterers took more time to rate themselves on all traits, anal as well as others. In another study of anal fixation in stutterers, Fisher (1970) obtained somewhat equivocal results. On the semantic differential, word stimuli were rated similarly by stutterers and nonstutterers on dimensions with anal reference, such as clean-dirty. As predicted, however, the two groups assigned significantly different meanings to pictures representing anal scenes.

Hostility and Aggression

In Freudian theory a fundamental consequence of anal-sadistic fixation is the storing up of latent hostility and the distortion of hostile expressions by guilt and anxiety. From this point of view there is unusual interest in a series of investigations of stutterers employing the Rosenzweig Picture-Frustration Study. This test is made up of a series of cartoons in each of which a person is depicted making a verbal response in a frustrating situation—for example, being splashed with mud by a passing car. The response is supplied by the subject taking the test. Interpretation is concerned with the manner in which the subject appears to be in the habit of coping with his or her own hostile impulses—for example, with whether aggression is turned outward, is turned inward, or is unexpressed or denied.

Using the norms of the Rosenzweig P-F Study for purposes of comparison, Madison and Norman (1952) found that 25 stutterers performed precisely as many psychoanalysts would have predicted. As a group, their responses revealed less tendency to cope directly with frustrating obstacles, greater inclination to turn aggressive reactions against themselves, and greater tendency to be preoccupied in a compulsive way with the solution of the problem creating the frustration. Madison and Norman concluded, "These findings seem to correspond to the psychoanalytic contention that stuttering is essentially compulsive in nature, with anal-sadistic tendencies resulting in a turning inwards of aggression." On the other hand, a study by Murphy (1953) using a control group produced almost diametrically opposed findings. Murphy's stutterers seemed to show more tendency to direct aggression outward against the frustrating person or agent and to show more self-defensive responses. Finally, Lowinger (1952) and Quarrington (1953) found that groups of stutterers showed no departure at all from the test norms, while both Seaman (1956) and Emerick (cited by Bloch and Goodstein, 1971) failed to find any differences between stutterers and control subjects.

There is clearly little in the results of these studies to indicate that stutterers as a group tend to have neurotic conflicts involving aggression. Research using the TAT has also produced equivocal findings. D. M. Wilson (1950) found that stuttering children appeared to be extremely aggressive and to have more inverted hostility than their nonstuttering siblings, as judged by TAT projections. But Lowinger (1952) found no significant difference between stuttering and nonstuttering children in intensity of unconscious aggressive drives. Solomon (cited by Bloch and Goodstein, 1971) found that adult stutterers did not differ from controls on the TAT with respect to broad categories of aggression, but that they did express more themes involving subtler, less violent aggression. Porterfield (1969), on the other hand, failed to find any difference in aggression between preschool stutterers and nonstutterers on the CAT. McHale (1967) did not use the TAT pictures, but analyzed the written stories of stuttering and nonstuttering children for the needs expressed; he found no support for explanations of stuttering in terms of aggression.

On the Blacky Pictures Test, Eastman (cited by Bloch and Goodstein, 1971) obtained only partial confirmation of the hypothesis that stuttering children would show repressed hostility.

On the Rorschach Test, however, Santostefano (1960) found clear evidence of unusual degrees of hostility in adult stutterers. The instrument he used was Elizur's Rorschach Content Test (RCT), a validated method of diagnosing anxiety and hostility from the content of a subject's responses to the ink blots. Hostility is revealed by such responses as "two men fighting," "a tiger leaping on its prey," "gun," "teeth," and other explicit expressions or cultural symbolisms of aggression. Adult stutterers proved to have distinctly higher scores for hostility on the RCT than did adult nonstutterers.

Santostefano did not ascribe the difference to psychosexual fixation. Like Abbott (1947), he hypothesized that the stutterer tends to accumulate anger as a result of the frustrations of being a stutterer. The facts will support either explanation. But there is, in principle, a type of further investigation that might serve to tip the balance in favor of one or the other. The psychoanalytic hypothesis requires that the stutterer's hostility exist to a large degree in repressed form; the other does not require this as an inevitable development, even though it takes into account a normal tendency for aggression to be repressed. Criminals and delinquents tend to "act out" their aggressions; they are persons who tend to exercise too little rather than too much repressive control over their hostility. Consequently, it appears unlikely that many such persons would be stutterers if stuttering is primarily the symptom of anal-sadistic repression. The information we have on this question is meager, but suggests that there is little if any difference in the prevalence of stuttering between the criminal and noncriminal population.[2] It is true that in a study of over 2,000 case histories of children with behavior difficulties Schroeder and Ackerson (1931) found that stuttering appeared to be more characteristic of the shy, sensitive, inadequate child than of the child with aggressive conduct traits. On the other hand, fighting and overaggressive behavior ranks high in frequency among the findings of several studies of symptoms of maladjustment in stuttering children, as we will see in Chapter 6.

---

[2]Fleischman (1946), Gildston (1959).

Guilt

The presence or absence of guilt has been directly implied in most of the findings we have already discussed under the heading of psychosexual fixation. To a small extent, guilt has been investigated independently of other factors as a relatively persistent feature of the stutterer's personality. Lowinger (1952) found no significant difference between stuttering and nonstuttering children in projections of guilt on the TAT, although there appeared to be a tendency for the stutterers to be more guilt-burdened. Adams and Dietze (1965) studied stutterers' reaction times in giving written associations to words suggesting five different kinds of emotion. The stutterers reacted more slowly than the nonstutterers to all categories, including neutral words and those connoting joy. But the category that proved to be a major source of the stutterers' greater slowness were the words pertaining to guilt (i.e., "guilty," "sinner," "blamed," "misdeed").

SELF-PERCEPTIONS

Self-Concept

An important development in the study of personality is that concerned in various ways with images, perceptions, and evaluations of the self. In the numerous applications that have been made to stuttering few theories of etiology have been put to any critical test. Fiedler and Wepman (1951), who conducted the earliest self-concept research on stutterers, were in fact concerned with the hypothesis that stutterers have a characteristic view of themselves because of the social handicap of stuttering.

Most of the self-concept studies employed a unique device known as the Q-technique. The subject is presented with a set of cards on each of which is a different statement describing a personality trait—for example "I feel bored," "I am always alert," or "I believe in fate." The procedure followed is best described by quoting from Fiedler and Wepman's instructions to their subjects:

> Here are 76 statements which people have used to describe themselves. Please sort them into eight categories consisting of 1, 5, 12, 20, 12, 5 and 1 statements. Place the statement which describes you best in the first pile, the five next most descriptive statements into the second pile, and so on until you come to the one statement which is *least* applicable to you. Be sure each category contains exactly the right number of statements.

If the statements, having been forced into a normal distribution, are now given scores corresponding to their categories, the entire sort may be appropriately correlated with the sort of any other subject. Furthermore, the array of intercorrelations among a whole group of subjects, or between the subjects of two different groups, may be computed and averaged to yield measures of the congruence of their self-concepts.

By this method Fiedler and Wepman determined that the self-concepts of a group of stutterers, based on a set of seventy-six descriptions of personality traits by Murray, could not be differentiated from those of a group of nonstutterers. In addition, the stutterers' self-concepts were found to resemble those of a group of clinical psychologists, a "theoretically well-adjusted" group, more closely than they resembled those of a group of mental hygiene clinic patients.

The Q-technique has considerable versatility. The subject's sort may be correlated not only with those of others, but also to good advantage with further sorts by the same subject. In one of the most frequent applications of this procedure subjects arrange the statements once in accordance with their "actual" self-concept and again with reference to how well the statements describe how they would like to be. The amount of correlation between their "actual" and "ideal" self-concepts is then taken as a measure of their "self-acceptance" and contributes to an evaluation of their emotional adjustment. The studies of Wallen (1960) and Gildston (1967) have shown adolescent stutterers to be lower in self-acceptance than nonstutterers in this way, while Rahman (1956) found a tendency toward less self-acceptance in college stutterers that did not reach significance. It would appear that stutterers' concepts of themselves may not correspond as well with their ideals, generally speaking, as do those of nonstutterers when investigated by the Q-technique. Using conventional inventory methods of measuring self-acceptance, Berger (1952) obtained somewhat equivocal results, while Redwine (1959) found no evidence of less favorable self-concepts in stuttering children. Zelen, Sheehan, and Bugental (1954) found that stutterers undergoing group therapy expressed more positive feelings about themselves than did nonstutterers in a study employing the W-A-Y (Who are you?) technique.

Carrying applications of the Q-technique a step further, Wallen (1960) also had his subjects perform a "how I think others see me" sort and correlated this with their "actual" self-concepts. There was more disparity between the two in the case of the stutterers.

A different kind of study of the stutterer's self-concept, making use of the semantic differential and a type of repertory grid, was reported by Fransella (1968). Her essential findings were that stutterers typically see themselves differently from the way they see other stutterers. They tend to view other stutterers much as nonstutterers do, but tend to view themselves as unique individuals.

A study of 91 members of a national stutterers' self-help organization by Kalinowski, Lerman, and Watt (1987) employed a semantic differential devised by Woods and Williams (1976). The stutterers' self-perceptions did not differ significantly from those of a normal speaking control group.

Level of Aspiration and Achievement Drive

One way of studying a person's self-concept is to determine how realistic it is by comparing it with the actuality. In a sense this is done in microcosm in level of aspiration tests. These consist of a series of trials in a test of skill, after each of which subjects are asked to predict their score on the next trial. The average discrepancy between their prediction and their last performance is taken as a measure of their aspiration level. Research by Sheehan and Zelen (1951, 1955) using the Rotter Level of Aspiration Board and by Mast (1952) using the Carl Hollow Square suggested that, in general, the stutterers were less inclined than the nonstutterers to attempt what they were not sure they could do. Their attitudes, in short, tended to be somewhat overly cautious or defeatist, presumably to defend against the threat of failure. On the other hand, Emerick (cited by Bloch and Goodstein, 1971) found that they did not differ from nonstutterers in goal-setting behavior as measured by the Cassel Group Level of Aspiration Test. Moreover, Kaiser (cited by Keese and Fischer, 1976) found no difference between stutterers and controls in a level of aspiration test based on Heckhausen's labyrinth task.

These findings are inconsistent, but more than 20 years after his study using the Rotter Board, Sheehan (1979) replicated it with a group of female stutterers with the same results: The subjects showed higher levels of aspiration than female stutterers had evinced in the earlier study, but they still set lower goals than their controls. Stutterers also appeared to have lower levels of aspiration on a goal attitude inventory compiled by Trombly (1965).

If stutterers do have a tendency toward low levels of aspiration, this hardly seems consistent with the high achievement drives that are sometimes attributed to them on the basis of general observation or theory. Other data on this question are conflicting. Sheehan and Zussman (1951) found indications of a greater drive toward achievement in stutterers on the Rorschach Test. But in a study by Goodstein, Martire, and Spielberger (cited by Goodstein, 1958) stutterers did not differ from nonstutterers on two independent indices of motivation for achievement on the TAT. In another application of the TAT by Braun (1974) stuttering schoolchildren scored higher in hope for success and did not differ from control subjects in fear of failure. Luper and Chambers (1962) found adult stutterers overly sensitive to criticism and fearful of failure on a projective test in which subjects were required to identify "liked" and "disliked" photographs of people.

Stutterers also showed greater failure anxiety than nonstutterers on the Achievement Motivation Test in a study by Peters and Hulstijn (1984).

Body Image

Since its introduction for this purpose by Machover in 1949 the drawing of the human figure has been widely used as a projective personality test. Its usefulness is based in part on the assumption that when subjects respond to the request to draw a person they tend to draw a picture of themselves and that the drawing consequently contains expressions of their body needs and conflicts.

In a comparison of the figure drawings of stuttering, maladjusted, and normal adolescent boys by R. G. Wilson (1950) the stutterers' drawings, like those of the maladjusted group, contained omissions and conflict indicators and tended to be poor in movement, likeness to human beings, and detail. Putney (1955) found few differences in the self-drawings of stutterers and nonstutterers, while Fitzpatrick (1960) was concerned mainly with the distorted self-image of stutterers when asked to depict themselves in a speaking role. DePlatero (1969) found that, in comparison with normal-speaking children, stuttering children tended to produce heavy body outlines "as a defense against the menacing exterior."

Glassmann (1967) submitted the figure drawings of stuttering children and controls to three clinical psychologists for their independent, blind evaluation. The judges, each of whom employed the draw-a-person technique routinely in diagnostic work in the children's unit of a mental hospital, used a five-point scale to rate each drawing for anxiety, hostility, compulsivity, dependency, and self-concept inferiority. No significant differences were found between the two groups of drawings. The only difference approaching statistical significance was a slight tendency for the stutterers' drawings to be rated lower in compulsivity than those of the nonstutterers.

In a study of 5 stutterers aged 5 to 10 years, Devore, Nandur, and Manning (1984) employed the House-Tree-Person Technique and elicited drawings depicting both self speaking and a person of the opposite sex. The stutterers' tendency to draw smaller figures than their controls was interpreted as suggesting feelings of inadequacy. Their placement of the figures off-center toward the left of the page was said to suggest a tendency to withdraw or shun new experiences. These differences did not appear on retesting after twelve weeks of treatment for stuttering.

Body image may be studied by other means than figure drawing. Pienaar (1968) scored the Rorschach Test responses of his subjects for awareness of body boundary and awareness of body interior. The stuttering children tended to score higher on the body boundary index than either children with articulatory difficulties or those who spoke normally. Pienaar thought that either the stutterers' speech impairment tended to increase their concern about their body or more basic factors might be involved.

Role Perception

Buscaglia (1963) found that adolescent stutterers had difficulty perceiving their own life roles as well as the roles of others on the Sarbin-Hardyck Role Perception Test. However, in a study by Sheehan and Lyon (1974), there were no differences between stutterers and nonstutterers on this test. Broida (1963) made use of a number of projective techniques as well as a questionnaire administered to parents and teachers to investigate the sex role preferences of stuttering children. She reported several apparent deviations from the expected, including evidence of some ambivalence in sex role identification.

EXPRESSIVE BEHAVIOR

It is a familiar observation that people are often identifiable by their speech or handwriting or by the way they walk, laugh, or gesture. From this observation has grown an approach to psychological diagnosis that contrasts with both structured tests and projective devices, the study of so-called expressive behavior.

One of the best-known examples of this approach is the Bender Visual-Motor Gestalt Test, which approaches personality from the standpoint of the subjects' perception and organization of visual stimuli as revealed in their copying of patterns. On this test, which is sensitive to both emotional disturbance and brain damage, Burleson (1951) found no significant differences between stuttering and normal-speaking children. Likewise, Porterfield (1969) found that preschool stutterers did not differ from normal controls, but did differ significantly from a maladjusted group. R. G. Wilson (1950), however, reported that stutterers resembled maladjusted nonstutterers in "a certain motor ineptness" on the Bender-Gestalt Test, in figure drawing, and on Mira's Myokinetic Psychodiagnosis (a test of expressive movement involving the drawing of lines while blindfolded).

Handwriting Analysis

There has long been some serious interest in handwriting as an example of expressive motor behavior, although conflicting opinions have been expressed about its usefulness in the study of personality. On the basis of clinical observation, Roman (1960) suggested that stutterers' handwriting tends to be untidy, clumsy, obstructed in fluency and continuity, and marked by interruptions and repetitions. This view was not supported by a study of the quality of stutterers' handwriting by Spadino (1941), however. Eisenson (1937) found a tendency, too small for statistical significance, for stutterers to cross out more words than nonstutterers in written composition.

Painting

Laczkowska (1965) compared the watercolor paintings of stuttering and nonstuttering boys of the same elementary school grades and observed that in 80 percent of the cases the stutterers preferred cool colors such as blue, green, brown, black, or purple, while the nonstutterers tended to prefer warm colors. She interpreted this to signify a tendency on the part of the stutterers to repress their inner feelings.

Language Measures

In a broad sense, the highly personal ways in which people use language may be regarded as kinds of expressive behavior. Felstein (1950) found evidence of anxiety and poor social adjustment in the type-token ratios (number of different words in relation to total number of words) and verb-adjective ratios derived from language samples of stutterers and nonstutterers. Knabe, Nelson, and Williams (1966), however, were not able to observe any differences in similar measures of language behavior. Krause (1982) reported smaller type-token ratios for stutterers than nonstutterers in conversational speech, but suggested that their more restricted repertoires of words might have been a strategy for coping with stuttering.

Other linguistic measures applied in research on the stutterer's personality have been concerned with the meanings and affective connotations of words as perceived by the subject. Spriestersbach (1951) found indications of mild degrees of social maladjustment among stutterers whom he compared with normal and psychotic subjects with respect to the ratings they assigned to pictures as appropriate illustrations of evaluative words such as "good," "funny," "interesting," and the like. Fransella (1965) made use of the semantic differential, a technique developed by Osgood in which the subject is presented with a series of words and instructed to rate each of them on various evaluative scales, indicating, for example, the extent to which the thing referred to by the word is interesting or boring, difficult or easy, true or false, and so forth. Fransella reported that stutterers used the extreme positions of the scales more often than normal speakers, a tendency that had also been observed in persons designated as psychotic or neurotic, as well as in intelligent, anxious individuals. This is consistent with the finding of Peterson, Rieck, and

Hoff (1969) that stutterers assigned higher semantic differential ratings than did nonstutterers.

In a study of conversational behavior, Krause (1982) found stutterers reluctant to use words indicating "even a rather moderate emotional involvement."

SOME BASIC RESPONSE TENDENCIES

Anxiety

Various attempts have been made to study anxiety in stutterers as a characteristic feature of behavior, independently of its arousal in speaking situations, and various kinds of evidence of what appears to be anxiety have been found. The findings have not been conclusive, but the methods employed have differed so widely that in all probability several unrelated things have been measured.

Anxiety Questionnaires

Some workers have tried to assess the stutterer's chronic anxiety level by means of questionnaires, with generally negative results. Boland (1953) succeeded in finding evidence of a higher level of general anxiety in stutterers than in nonstutterers by making use of two indices derived from the MMPI, Welsh's Anxiety Index, and the Taylor Manifest Anxiety Scale. Negative findings were obtained by Berlinsky (1955) on the Saslow Screening Test, by Agnello (1962) and Cox, Seider, and Kidd (1984) on the Taylor Manifest Anxiety Scale, by Molt and Guilford (1979) and Miller and Watson (1992) on the State-Trait Anxiety Inventory, and by Peters and Hulstijn (1984) on the neuroticism scale and the neurotic somatic complaints scale of the Amsterdam Biographical Questionnaire.

These were all studies of adults. Andrews and Harris (1964, p. 78) found no difference between stuttering children and their controls on Sarason's General Anxiety Scale for Children, but in another study of stuttering children, Pukacova reported increased anxiety on the Taylor Manifest Anxiety Scale.

On the Likert Social Anxiety Schedule, stutterers scored higher in social anxiety than a normal speaking control group, but significantly lower than a group of "social phobics" in a study by Kraamaat, Janssen, and van Dam-Boggen (1991).

Projective Measures

Santostefano (1960) obtained indications of higher general anxiety in stutterers by means of a projective technique, the Rorschach Content

Test. Anxiety is measured on the RCT by the frequency of such responses to the blots as "a fearful monster," "a little girl running in terror," "snakes," or "blood." Moller (cited by Bloch and Goodstein, 1971) also reported greater anxiety among stutterers in a Rorschach study.

Physological Measures

In a different kind of study, Berlinsky (1955) obtained physiological measures of evoked anxiety. The subjects performed a pursuit task in which they were required to manipulate a moving spot of light within a circumscribed area under threat of electric shock, while records were made of skin conductance, pulse rate, and amplitude of respiration. Under the conditions of the experiment, the stutterers proved to have lower pulse rates, but higher respiratory rate and amplitude than the nonstutterers as well as a different pattern of relationships among the measures. For the most part, the measures were not significantly related to each other. The results clearly served to call attention to some of the problems involved in defining anxiety.

Gray and Karmen (1967), using a colorimetric index of palmar sweating, found no evidence that stutterers responded with excessive anxiety in a nonverbal situation. Their study did not attempt to introduce unusual stress. Horovitz et al (1978) induced anxiety by having subjects imagine themselves in a stressful situation such as an oral examination in which questions were being asked very rapidly. Galvanic skin response measures showed that this was effective in evoking anxiety, but stutterers and nonstutterers did not differ in mean GSR.

Peters and Hulstijn (1984) recorded subjects' heart rates, pulse volumes, and skin conductance in anticipation of and during nonverbal tasks (mirror writing and items from the Raven intelligence test). Stutterers and controls did not differ.

Behavioral Measures

Santostefano (1960) investigated anxiety evoked by laboratory stress using disruption of a previously learned response as a measure of anxiety. Subjects first learned a series of digit- symbol associations. They were then required to respond with a written word association to each of a list of words consisting in part of such "threatening" stimuli as "penis" and "intercourse." The assumption was that these would arouse anxiety and hostility. Following each word association one of the digits was presented, and a measurement was made of the amount of time the subject took to respond with the appropriate symbol. There was a general tendency in both stutterers and nonstutterers for the threat words to result in reduced efficiency of the learned responses, but this effect proved to be greater in the stutterers.

Santostefano interpreted these findings to mean that the stutterers were made more anxious and hostile by the stressful conditions. This use of both terms is important and clarifying. It would be possible to add "guilty," and perhaps others. The point to be emphasized is that physiological or behavioral measures in themselves do not permit us to make such distinctions. The distinctions can only be inferred from the experimental conditions or from subjects' reports. Such measures of "anxiety" are perhaps better referred to as measures of autonomic arousal. Brutten and Shoemaker (1967, p. 53) reviewed literature that supports a thesis of genetic differences among individuals in threshold of autonomic response to stress and discussed this in relation to stuttering from a theoretical point of view. It is within the realm of possibility that in Santostefano's work, and perhaps in some findings of Boland and Berlinsky, there is a clue to a tendency toward higher levels of autonomic reactivity in many stutterers.

Conditionability

There is evidence that anxious individuals are more readily conditioned than others and that anxiety, autonomic reactivity, and conditionability are related.[3] Moore (1938) conditioned subjects to expect an electric shock following a recorded nonsense syllable and studied the effect on their breathing movements. He noted that the stutterers were not differentiated from their controls by conditionability. On the other hand, Thomas (1976) compared the conditioning of the galvanic skin response in stutterers and nonstutterers in a nonspeech situation and found the stutterers to be more conditionable.

Defense Preference

Prins and Beaudet (1980) studied the defense mechanisms of sixteen stutterers as revealed by the Defense Preference Inquiry for the Blacky pictures. For each picture the subjects rank-ordered five statements representing alternative possible reactions of the dog Blacky to threatening psychosexual stimuli. The five statements in each class represented the defense mechanisms of regression, projection, intellectualization, reaction formation, and avoidance. Prins and Beaudet found that the stutterers' mean profile of preference for the five defensive styles was identical to the profile reported for American college students.

Rigidity

We have already touched tangentially upon certain types of rigidity in discussing motor perseveration and obsessive-compulsive char-

---

[3]See the discussion of such evidence by Brutten and Shoemaker (1967, pp. 52, 53).

acter traits. The tendency to retain habit patterns may be measured in various ways. In a study of rigidity by Solomon (1952), stutterers apparently did not differ from nonstutterers in the solution of problems requiring flexibility of attitudinal set, except in an oral test (hidden word puzzles) in which they showed more rigid behavior. Kapos and Standlee (1958) found no differences between stutterers and nonstutterers in an index of behavioral stereotypy in successive operations of a complex multiple-choice electromaze. In his study of perseveration in stutterers, King (1961) employed three tests of dispositional rigidity. Stutterers differed significantly from the nonstutterers on none. A representative example of these tasks was the working of simple addition, subtraction, multiplication, and division problems in which the mathematical symbols had assigned meanings differing from their common ones.

It is evident that rigidity is a term to which a number of different meanings may be given. Schaie (cited by Wingate, 1966a) developed a test of behavioral rigidity based on three major dimensions of the trait, which he isolated by means of factor analysis. One of these, which he termed *motor-cognitive*, is seen in adjustments to shifts in familiar patterns and continuously changing situational demands. An example is a test in which the subject writes antonyms for each of a series of words, then synonyms, and finally antonyms for words printed in lower case and synonyms for words printed in capitals. A second factor is tested by relatively simple psychomotor tasks, while a third is tested by means of a questionnaire containing such items as, "Do you feel strongly inclined to finish what you are doing in spite of being tired of it?" Schaie's Test of Behavioral Rigidity was administered to stutterers by Wingate (1966a), who found that they were distinctly more rigid than nonstutterers in the motor-cognitive area. His findings appear to be in conflict with the results of King's dispositional rigidity tests and with findings on motor perseveration in adult stutterers discussed in Chapter 4.

Suggestibility

The information we have on the suggestibility of stutterers is scanty, but interesting. It comes chiefly from an investigation by Kelly (1935), who administered the Otis Suggestibility Test and the Hull Postural Sway Test to forty-two stuttering schoolchildren and forty-two matched controls. On both tests the stutterers scored markedly higher in suggestibility. Ingebregtsen (1936), too, reported low resistance to suggestion as an experimental finding in a study of a group of stutterers, but did not describe the procedures used to measure it and did not employ controls.

Locus of Control

A trait which has acquired importance in the assessment of personality is the extent to which an individual perceives the satisfaction of needs to be under his or her personal control. Tests of this attribute measure the degree to which subjects believe that "reinforcements" depend upon their own behavior or powers as opposed to external agents such as chance or the action of others. Craig, Franklin, and Andrews (1984) found that stutterers scored slightly less favorably than control groups of nurses and university students, but distinctly more favorably than a group of diagnosed neurotic patients. McDonough and Quesal (1988) administered the Norwicki-Strickland (ANS-IE) Scale to stutterers and controls and reported no difference. Madison, Budd, and Itzkowitz (1986) also obtained negative results in a study of 6- to 16-year-old subjects with the children's form of the Norwicki-Strickland test.

Self-Monitoring Ability

Burley and Morely (1987) tested stutterers with Snyder's Self-Monitoring Scale, which evaluates subjects' concern for the appropriateness of their social behavior and their ability to modify their self-presentation appropriately for a particular social situation. The stutterers scored less favorably than the control subjects.

CONCLUSIONS

It is evident that there is considerable inconsistency in the findings resulting from research on the stutterer's personality. Yet these studies, done in such number and for so long that their account comes close to being a brief survey of personality testing itself, have made certain broad conclusions inescapable.

First, the weight of accumulated evidence does not appear to indicate that the average stutterer is a distinctly neurotic or severely maladjusted individual in the usual meanings of these terms. The evidence that most stutterers perform well within the norms on adjustment inventories is too strong to support such a view. Nor do their responses on projective tests seem to point to marked deviation from the normal or to coincide in any consistent way with the patterns of the classifiable neuroses as they are recognized on these tests.

Second, there is little conclusive evidence of any specific kind of character structure or broad-set of basic personality traits that is typical of stutterers as a group.

Third, there appears to be extreme overlapping between stuttering and nonstuttering groups with respect to adequacy of adjustment; the more adequately adjusted stutterers are in far more satisfactory emotional health than the more poorly adjusted nonstutterers.

Fourth, there would seem to be some justification for the inference that stutterers *on the average* are not quite as well adjusted as are typical normal speakers. By and large, this appears to be a matter of social adjustment to a greater degree than it affects other identifiable categories of emotional health. In addition, there appears to be evidence of tendencies on the part of many stutterers to be rather low in self-esteem and willingness to risk failure. Several explanations of the somewhat poorer average adjustment of stutterers are possible. It may be due, as has so frequently been suggested, to the eventual influence of the stuttering itself. Personality test findings on young stuttering children have not yielded conclusive evidence on this point. Or, it may be due to the fact that certain environmental influences contributing to the development of stuttering are of a type that may also sometimes contribute to insecurity and maladjustment.

The theory that stuttering reflects a deep-lying neurotic abnormality necessitating an essentially psychiatric method of treatment has been all but abandoned by professional workers who are knowledgeable about the disorder. That stutterers tend to be distinguished by specific attitudes and assumptions with regard to various features of the speech process is fairly certain. That they may often be socially maladjusted to the extent that they avoid contacts with others requiring speech is true by definition. They are also more likely than other people to be somewhat insecure generally, and it is possible that such insecurity as they have may have contributed in some manner to the development of stuttering. But that stuttering is in essence the symptom of a basic personality disorder, in the sense that a fear of crowds or a hand washing compulsion is considered to be such a symptom, is an assumption lacking adequate scientific support.

Suggested Readings

Bloch, E. L., and Goodstein, L. D., Functional speech disorders and personality: A decade of research. *J. Speech Hearing Dis., 36,* 295–314 (1971).

Goodstein, L. D., Functional speech disorders and personality: A survey of the research. *J. Speech Hearing Res., 1,* 359–76 (1958).

Sheehan, J. G., *Stuttering: Research and Therapy.* New York: Harper & Row (1970), Chap. 3.

6

THE PERSON WHO STUTTERS: DEVELOPMENTAL HISTORY AND HOME ENVIRONMENT

We will devote this chapter to the kinds of data that are to be obtained from case histories, medical and school records, routine physical examinations, clinical interviews, and diagnostic tests and to research findings relating to the early histories of stutterers.

THE IOWA AND NEWCASTLE STUDIES

Information on stutterers' early histories has been gathered in many studies, but by far the most thorough and carefully executed of these have been two extensive investigations to which we will refer throughout the remainder of this chapter as the Iowa and Newcastle studies.

The Iowa studies were conducted by Johnson and his co-workers at the University of Iowa over a period of more than twenty years on a total of 246 children and their controls and consisted of three separate investigations to which Johnson and Associates (1959) referred as Studies I, II, and III. Study I, which we have already cited as Johnson et al. (1942) and Johnson (1955a), was done between 1934 and 1940 with 46 stutterers and 46 nonstutterers. Study II was done by Darley (1955) between 1948 and 1952 with 50 stutterers and 50 controls. Study III was conducted from 1952 to 1957 with 150 subjects in each group and has been reported by Johnson and Associates (1959) together with summaries of the findings of Studies I and II.

The Newcastle study was done by Andrews and Harris (1964, Chaps. 4, 5, 6).[1] The experimental group consisted of 80 stutterers, the bulk of those found in a survey of all the children in the last two grades of primary school in Newcastle upon Tyne. For purposes of control, stutterers were paired with normal-speaking children of the same sex and closely similar age from their own class at school.

In both the Iowa and Newcastle studies, the procedure, in addition to certain tests and objective measurements, involved systematic interviewing of the parents, by means of which detailed information was collected about the birth conditions, diseases, early physical development, educational and home adjustment, family background, parental attitudes, and child training policies as well as other aspects of development and home environment. Broadly speaking and with a relatively small number of exceptions, the Iowa and Newcastle studies have shown that there is little in the case history of the typical stutterer that could be regarded as unusual, and this agrees in general with most other investigations. The outstanding exceptions, as we will see, are in the areas of speech and language development.

MEDICAL HISTORY

Birth Conditions

Attempts to determine the extent to which stutterers have births that are normal with regard to such factors as term of pregnancy, length of labor, manner of presentation of the fetus, use of instruments, injury to the infant, and the like have produced largely negative or ambiguous results. Berry (1938b) found no difference in numbers of various kinds of abnormalities in comparing the medical records of 227 stutterers and 232 controls. In the Iowa studies, mean duration of labor was significantly longer in the case of the stutterers than for the nonstutterers in Study III, but there was a marked difference in the opposite direction in Study I. The Newcastle study showed a tendency, just short of statistical significance, for the stutterers to have had more abnormal birth conditions. There were also somewhat inconclusive hints of this in studies by Milisen and Johnson (1936) and Boland (1951). No differences in conditions of birth or pregnancy were found by Accordi and his co-workers (1983), who compared the medical records of 2,802 stutterers seen over a twenty-five-year period at the Medical-Surgical Center for Phoniatrics in Padua with data obtained

---

[1]This should not be confused with the 1,000-family Newcastle upon Tyne survey cited in Chapter 3, whose findings, as they relate to speech disorders, were reported by Andrews and Harris (1964, Chap. 3) and Morley (1957).

by questionnaire on 1,602 schoolchildren. Cox, Seider, and Kidd (1984) also found no differences in birth and prenatal conditions between 37 stutterers and 54 of their nonstuttering relatives in interviews with the mothers.

Stutterers have been found not to differ essentially from nonstutterers with respect to birth weight,[2] month or season of birth,[3] and parental age at birth.[4] Allen (1948) investigated the Rh factor in mothers of stutterers with inconclusive results.

Diseases, Injuries, and Allergy

Findings with regard to the stutterer's disease history have also been largely negative. Berry (1938c), after analyzing the medical records of 430 stuttering and 462 nonstuttering children entering hospital clinics for general pediatric care or preventive medicine, reported that the stutterers were more prone to have such diseases of the respiratory system as tonsillitis, bronchitis and rheumatic fever, as well as certain disorders of the nervous system—encephalitis, epilepsy, and convulsions—which were the "accepted sequelae" of these. Berry interpreted this to mean that a genetic link existed between a constitutional predisposition to stuttering and a constitutional susceptibility to respiratory disease. Further research has failed to provide confirmation of Berry's findings, however. Both the Iowa and Newcastle studies showed a comparable incidence of diseases for stutterers and nonstutterers. In addition, the Iowa studies disclosed no difference in the incidence of injuries, surgical operations, or asthma. Cox, Seider, and Kidd (1984) reported no differences with respect to diseases and injuries in a comparison of forty adult stutterers and their nonstuttering relatives.

The Iowa finding with regard to asthma is of some importance because the observations of Kennedy and Williams (1938) and Gordon (1942) and intradermal tests by Card (1939) suggested that there may be an unusual amount of allergy among stutterers. The possibility has been of special interest because of the relationship often thought to exist between allergy and emotional factors. As a research question it is complicated considerably by difficulties in the diagnosis and ambiguities in the definition of allergy.

Mental Illness

Concerning the incidence of mental illness in stutterers we have relatively little information. Pitrelli (1948) suggested that with stutter-

---

[2]Berry (1938b), Johnson and Associates (1959, p. 50).

[3]Bryngelson and Brown (1939), Boland (1950).

[4]Everhart (1949), Morgenstern (1956), Johnson and Associates (1959, p. 75), Andrews and Harris (1964, p. 52).

ing no longer needed as a defense against a more serious disorder there should be fewer stutterers among psychotics and reported that no stutterers were to be found in a group of 311 psychotic patients in a mental hospital. Evidence that stuttering is to be found in psychotics was offered by Barbara (1946), Freund (1955), and Arnold (1958), but there are no data clearly suggesting that stutterers are either more or less likely than others to have serious mental illness.

Physical Examination

The Iowa and Newcastle studies showed stutterers to be comparable to nonstutterers in height and weight and with regard to the information about their general health that was supplied by the parents. In a series of studies that included essentially routine physical or neurological examinations stutterers have consistently been found to be in grossly normal physical health.[5] But Greene and Small (1944), Meyer (1945), and Despert (1946) all concurred in such observations as hyperactive deep tendon reflexes, perspiration and cyanosis of the hands and feet, vasomotor instability, and fine tremors of the outstretched hands, which Meyer termed the "classical manifestations of anxiety."

Finally, in a study of physical habitus by Travis, Malamud, and Thayer (1934), stutterers were found to differ markedly from nonstutterers in distribution of body types on the basis of Kretschmer's system of classification, a much larger percentage falling into the leptosome category. Bullen (1945) noted a similar distribution in a small group of stutterers and controls.

PHYSICAL AND SOCIAL DEVELOPMENT

In general, controlled studies have shown that the early development of stutterers compares favorably with that of nonstutterers with respect to the ages at which they teethe, are weaned, feed and dress themselves, acquire bowel and bladder control, sit, creep, stand, and walk, and with regard to the frequency with which difficulties are reported in connection with feeding, sleeping, or toilet training.[6] The exceptions to this have been isolated and relatively minor. On the Vineland Social Maturity Scale, McHale (1967) found that stutterers aged 7 to 15 years did not differ from nonstutterers in mean social quotient.

Berry (1938b) found that stutterers tended to have been breast-fed significantly longer, on the average, than nonstutterers, while

---

[5]McDowell (1928), Greene and Small (1944), Meyer (1945), Despert (1946), Graham (1966).

[6]See Milisen and Johnson (1936), Berry (1938b), the Iowa and Newcastle studies, Accordi et al (1983), Cox, Seider, and Kidd (1984).

in the Iowa studies the reverse proved to be true. A study by Sewell and Mussen (1952) appeared to yield little evidence that stuttering is likely to be associated in any direct way with bottle feeding, scheduled feeding as opposed to demand feeding, or abrupt weaning.

ABNORMAL BEHAVIOR SYMPTOMS

There is a relatively long list of behavior problems and symptoms of "nervousness" and maladjustment in children that are indicative of varying degrees of emotional ill health, and a few of which may in some cases be symptomatic of brain damage. These include exaggerated fears, sleep disturbances, hyperactivity, enuresis, sibling jealousy, temper tantrums, excessive thumb sucking or nail biting, lying or stealing, compulsive orderliness, difficulties in playing with other children, and a score or more of others. Stuttering and nonstuttering children have been compared with regard to these behavioral symptoms in several investigations. If we were to try to speculate about the probable outcome of such studies on the assumption that it would be consistent with the results of other research on the stutterer's personality reviewed in Chapter 5, we would be likely to predict that stuttering children as a group would not be severely affected by these problems, but might tend to have more of them, on the average, than comparable nonstutterers. This, in fact, appears to be essentially the case.

The Newcastle study found no indication of a difference between the stuttering and control groups, or even of a tendency toward a difference approaching significance. In the Iowa studies, however, as well as in an investigation by Moncur (1955), stutterers revealed somewhat more symptoms of maladjustment than did nonstutterers. In Iowa Study III both parents were asked to make ratings with regard to more than a hundred items pertaining to the emotional adjustment or social behavior of the child. In the case of 35 of these items significantly more control group children than experimental group children were rated favorably by one or both of the parents. The reverse was true on only one item. When Iowa Studies II and III and Moncur's study are compared with regard to specific behavior symptoms, there is agreement among all three only on the more frequent evaluation of the stutterers by their parents as "nervous." Two of the three studies agreed that stutterers more often exhibited fears of some kind, nightmares or sleep disturbances, compulsive orderliness, perfectionism, and fighting or overly aggressive behavior.

Fowlie and Cooper (1978) had mothers of 6- to 11-year-old stutterers and nonstutterers rate their children on a checklist of personality traits that had previously been selected by speech clinicians in characterizing stutterers. The stuttering children were perceived by their mothers as more insecure, sensitive, anxious, withdrawn, fearful, and introverted than were the nonstutterers. Fowlie and Cooper suggested that such judgments may in part reflect a general stereotype with regard to the stutterer's personality. Riley (1983) reported high self-expectations in 3- to 6-year-old stutterers compared with children with normal speech or with articulation difficultiess. Cox, Seider, and Kidd (1984), in interviews with mothers of 37 stutterers and 54 genetically related normal-speaking children, found no differences in the incidence of unusual fears or problems with feeding, sleeping, or bladder and bowel management. Accordi et al. (1983) found no difference in the occurrence of enuresis or tics in their comparison of 2,802 stuttering and 1,602 control children referred to above.

SPEECH AND LANGUAGE HISTORY

In view of all that research has revealed to date, it appears safe to say that, despite many individual exceptions, stuttering children as a group tend to be somewhat delayed in speech and language development.

Language Acquisition

Various workers have long believed that stutterers frequently tend to be slow in developing language. The support for this view, though not unqualified, has now become considerable (see Table 17). Berry (1938b) found very marked differences between stutterers and nonstutterers. The Newcastle study again produced distinct evidence of slower speech development in stutterers, corroborating Berry's findings as well as other past observations by Morley (1957, p. 411) and Milisen and Johnson (1936). Only the Iowa studies showed slight or no differences. In Study III, the last and most extensive of the Iowa studies, it was found that the stutterers had been regarded as late talkers by their parents substantially more often than had the nonstutterers, but the ages at which the parents reported the children as having said their first words and sentences proved to be much the same, suggesting that the difference was principally in the parents' evaluations of what they had observed rather than in the actualities.

We cannot be certain about the reason for the difference between the Iowa findings and those of other studies. There was, however, a difference in the nature of the populations sampled, as Andrews and Harris (1964, p. 35) pointed out. The Iowa groups tended to be representative of the higher socioeconomic levels of Midwestern society, while the Newcastle subjects were a broad sample of the population of an English industrial city. Berry's data were obtained from Chicago hospital clinics and social welfare agencies. A hypothesis to be considered is that the relatively high socioeconomic status of the Iowa sub-

Table 17. Mean or Median Number of Months of Retardation of Stutterers When Compared with Nonstutterers in the Use of First Words, Phrases, Sentences, and Speech Intelligibility Outside the Immediate Family

	N		Words	Phrases	Sentences	Intelligible Speech
	Stutterers	Nonstutterers				
Berry (1938b)	243, 140	252, 154*	7.42			12.03
Iowa Studies						
I. Johnson et al (1942)	46	46	0.0		0.0	
II. Darley (1955)	50	50	0.97	0.80	2.07	
III. Johnson and Associates (1959)	137, 136*	131	0.1		0.8	
Morley (1957)	29	111	2.7	4.9		11.2
Andrews and Harris (1964)**	78	76		4.0		

*The two values of N given are for the two items of information respectively.
**Referred to in the text as the "Newcastle study."

jects served to obscure to some extent any difference in language development that might have appeared between stutterers and nonstutterers.

More recently, in a survey of a very large number of children Accordi et al. (1983) found retarded language development in 28 percent of stutterers as opposed to 8.7 percent of a control group.

Language Ability

The apparent lateness of many stutterers in acquiring language has led to a series of comparisons of stutterers and nonstutterers on broad measures of language ability. Here the results have been equivocal. Much of this work has been done on children of school age, however. Possibly the linguistic disadvantage under which many stutterers appear to labor at the beginning tends to disappear or become more subtle in the early years. There seems to be some support for such an assumption if we review the studies with close attention to the age of the subjects.

Five investigations dealt with preschool subjects, and significant differences appeared in four of them. In a study by Murray and Reed (1977) preschool stutterers scored lower than their controls on the Peabody Picture Vocabulary Test, the Northwestern Syntax Screening Test, and the verbal abilities scale of the Zimmerman Pre-School Language Scale. Kline and Starkweather (1979) found that stutterers aged three to six years had a lower mean length of utterances than nonstutterers and lower scores on the Carrow Test for Auditory Comprehension of Language. Wall (1980) carried out a constituent syntactic analysis of the speech of four stutterers and four controls aged five to six years and found that the stutterers tended to use simpler, less mature language. Ryan (1992) found small but significant differences between 2- to 5-year-old stutterers and nonstutterers on the Peabody Picture Vocabulary Test and the Test of Language Development (TOLD). A group of 4- to 5-year-old stutterers did not differ from controls in mean length of utterance in a study by Meyers and Freeman (1985a).

We have also had two studies of kindergarten and first grade children. In a study by Westby (1979) stutterers scored lower than normal-speaking children in frequency of grammatical errors, in receptive vocabulary on the Peabody Picture Vocabulary Test, and in correct responses on semantic tasks selected from the Torrance Test of Creative Thinking. There was no significant difference on the Developmental Sentence Analysis. In an earlier study of kindergarten and first grade children E.-M. Silverman and Williams (1968) found a slight tendency for the stutterers to be poorer in such measures as mean length of response, mean of the five longest responses, and structural complexity of their utterances, but the groups differed significantly only in the number of one-word responses.

The remaining studies were carried out for the most part with elementary school children as subjects. Peters (1968), employing the same measures that had been used by E.-M. Silverman and Williams (1968) and the type-token ratio as well, found no differences between stutterers and nonstutterers of elementary school age. Perozzi and Kunze (1969) found no differences between second grade and third grade stutterers and controls on the Van Alstyne Picture Vocabulary Test and measures of verbal output and structural complexity. In a study by Pitluk (1982) 4 stutterers aged 9 to 11 years performed adequately and as well as their controls on the Reporter's Test, devised by DeRenzi and Ferrari to detect minimal expressive language impairments in persons with aphasia. Weiss and Zebrowski (1994) found 5- to 11-year-old stutterers equal to nonstutterers in narrative ability. Nippold, Schwarz, and Jescheniak (1991) found 6- to 11-year-old stutterers equal to nonstutterers in narrative ability and performance on the Clinical Evaluation of Language Fundamentals. Kadi-Hanifi and Howell (1992) reported no difference between groups in mean length of utterance among subjects who ranged in age from 2:7 to 12:6 years. By contrast, only two studies produced evidence of a language deficit in school-age stutterers. St. Louis and Hinzman (1988) reported a lower average mean length of utterance in stutterers in grades one to twelve. Byrd and Cooper (1989b) found that the performance of 5- to 9-year-old stutterers compared unfavorably with test norms on the Test of Language Development, but not on the Test of Auditory Comprehension of Language (TACL-R).

In a study of high-level linguistic production and comprehension processes in adult subjects, 11 of 19 stutterers, and no nonstutterers, were judged to be linguistically impaired by Watson, Freeman, Chapman, Miller, Finitzo, Pool, and Devous (1991).

Language-Related Abilities

Many studies have been done on more narrowly defined linguistic skills of stutterers. A few have dealt with word finding ability. Both Weuffen (1961) and Okasha, Bishry, et al (1974) reported lower scores for stuttering than for nonstuttering children in a task of finding words beginning with a given letter. Boysen and Cullinan (1971) found no group differences for 7- to 10-year-old subjects in reaction time on a picture-naming task. On the other hand, Telser (1971) obtained slower average latencies for 5- to 12-year-old stutterers on a similar task. Van Lieshout, Hulstjin, and Peters (1991) reported the same result for adults, as well as slower reaction times in uttering words displayed visually.

Stuttering children aged 9 to 12 years did not differ from normal speakers in the number of words they could write after visual presentation in a study by Knura (1970). But Bosshardt (1993) found adult stutterers inferior in the recall of consonant-vowel-consonant syllables that had been exposed visually.

Taylor, Lore, and Waldman (1970) found that stutterers did not have longer latencies of response than nonstutterers on a "cloze" test requiring them to supply words omitted from sentences.

Rastatter and Dell (1987b) studied stutterers' reaction times under two conditions. One was a simple phonation of /a/ in response to a flash of light. In the other the subject phonated /a/ if a visually presented word was a real word as opposed to a nonsense word. The difference between the two reaction times was taken to be the lexical decision time. Stutterers were slower than controls in lexical decision time.

Postma, Kolk, and Povel (1990) reported that stutterers were slower in reproducing sentences silently, forming mental auditory images of the sounds. They inferred that stutterers used more speech planning time than nonstutterers.

Crowe and Kroll (1991) administered a word association test in which subjects responded to the stimulus word with a beeper as soon as they had the response word in mind, after which they wrote the word. Measuring the time interval from presentation of the word to the beep, the experimenters determined that the stutterers had made word associations as rapidly as the controls.

Auditory Processing Ability

Conflicting findings have been reported on various auditory processing skills and other abilities thought to be related to speech and language. On the Illinois Test of Psycholinguistic Abilities (ITPA), the stuttering children investigated by Perozzi and Kunze (1969) performed more poorly than controls only on the Visual Motor Sequencing subtest, which requires the subject to reproduce in correct order a series of pictures or designs after they have been removed. On the other hand, Stocker and Parker (1977) found that stutterers, aged four to eleven years, scored lower than nonstutterers on the Sequential Memory subtest of the ITPA and on the Auditory Attention Span for Related Syllables subtest of the Detroit Tests of Learning Aptitude. Williams and Marks (1972) set out to study the ITPA profiles of stutterers rather than to compare them with others. In relation to their total performance on the test, the stutterers, aged five to nine, tended to do somewhat poorly in auditory vocal sequencing. By contrast, Manning and Riensche (1976) found no differences between 5- to 10-year-old stutterers and nonstutterers in an auditory processing task in which the subjects had to synthesize words and nonsense syllables from discrete serial presentations of their constituent sounds.

Moore, Craven, and Faber (1982) and Moore (1986) found that stutterers had poor recognition and recall of words on auditory presentation. Carpenter and Sommers (1987), on the other hand, found stutterers and normal speakers equal in auditory memory for words.

In a reaction time study by Rastatter and Dell (1985), subjects touched either of two pictures, depending on the name they heard in their headset. In one condition they knew which name they would hear; in the other they did not. The difference in the reaction times between the two conditions was considered the time required for auditory phonemic processing. The stutterers were found to be slower in auditory processing.

Postma and Kolk (1992) found that stutterers did not differ from nonstutterers in identifying phonemic errors as they recited a string of nonsense syllables, but detected fewer errors than control subjects in a tape recording of other speakers reciting the syllables.

Phonetic Ability

Tiffany (1963) devised three tests to measure a special kind of skill that he called phonetic ability or sound-mindedness. One of them, the Slurvian translations test, consists of a series of apparently meaningless "slurvianisms" such as "scene owe weevil," or "yearn ever told tool urn," which are correctly translated as "see no evil" and "you're never too old to learn." Wingate (1967a) found that adult stutterers gave significantly fewer correct translations than a group of adult nonstutterers. This was true both when the slurvianisms were received visually and by ear.

Tiffany's Backward Speech test requires the subject to reverse the sounds of a spoken word so as to produce, for example, "talk" from "caught." His Phonetic Anagrams test requires the construction of a word or words from a jumbled series of spoken sounds, for example the rearrangement of /p/, /k/, and /i/ to make "keep" and "peek." Wingate (1971) reported the performance of nonstutterers to be clearly better than that of stutterers on both tests.

All of these results were obtained from the same group of subjects. A study by Perozzi (1970) produced equivocal findings. Perozzi gave the Backward Speech test to subjects of elementary school age. The stutterers tended to do more poorly than the controls, but the difference was not statistically significant. Newman, Fawcett, and Russon (1986) found adult stutterers significantly inferior. As in essentially all studies in which differences between stutterers and nonstutterers have been reported, there was considerable overlapping between the groups.

As Wingate (1971) pointed out, these tests seem to demand an internalized manipulation of sounds to achieve a restructuring of their pattern. His results are curiously reminiscent of an all-but-forgotten report by Kelly (1932) that stutterers made far more errors than normal speakers when instructed to respond to recorded presentations of three-digit numbers by writing the number with the first two digits reversed.

Prevalence of Stuttering Among the Bilingual

Before we leave the subject of language, let us briefly note in passing that, in a group of 4,827 children about half of whom were bilingual, Travis, Johnson, and Shover (1932) found 2.8 percent of the bilinguals to be stutterers as against 1.8 percent of those who spoke only English. The difference is too great to attribute easily to chance. Moreover, Stern (1948) obtained similar findings among 1,861 children in four schools in Johannesburg. Of those who had been bilingual prior to age 6 years, 2.16 percent stuttered, while only 1.66 percent of the unilinguals stuttered. Furthermore, among the stutterers Stern judged three times as many bilinguals as unilinguals to be severe. Bilingualism, of course, may be confounded with so many other factors that we cannot be sure of the relevance of these interesting findings to the subject we have been discussing.

Articulatory Difficulties

There is hardly a finding more thoroughly confirmed in the whole range of comparative studies of stutterers and nonstutterers than the tendency of stutterers to have functional difficulties of articulation, "immature" speech, and the like (see Table 18). In addition to the findings summarized in the table, Berry (1938b) noted frequent "infantile perseveration," "very indistinct speech," and "lisping" in a survey of medical records of stutterers, and similar observations were reported by Bloodstein (1958) in a clinical study of 108 young stutterers. Kent and Williams (1963) observed that former stutterers in grade 2 were more likely to have a history of articulatory difficulties than children with no history of stuttering. McDowell (1928), whose data are not in a form permitting inclusion in Table 18, found no significant differences in the number of school-age stutterers and nonstutterers making errors on various categories of sounds in a test of articulation, though the thirty-three stutterers she tested made significantly more total errors than thirty-three nonstutterers. Ryan (1992) likewise found no difference between 20 preschool stutterers and their controls on the Arizona Articulation Proficiency Scale, but reported that 25 percent of the stutterers later required treatment for frontal lisping or difficulty with /r/.

St. Louis (1991) found severe stutterers more likely to have defective articulation than mild or moderate stutterers, but Wolk, Edwards, and Conture (1993) reported that seven preschool stutterers with disordered phonology did not differ in severity of stuttering from seven with normal phonology.

Table 18. Percentage of Stutterers and Nonstutterers Having
Other Speech Disorders, Chiefly Articulatory Difficulties,
or Having a History of Such Disorders

	N		Source of Information	% Stutterers	% Nonstutterers
	Stutterers	Nonstutterers			
Schindler (1955)	126	252	Speech Examination	49	15
Darley (1955)	50	50	Reports of Parents	26	4
Morley (1957	37	113	Speech Examination	50	31
Johnson and Associates (1959)	150	150	Reports of Parents	15.3	7.3
Andrews and Harris (1964)	77	78	Reports of Parents	29.9	10.3
Williams and Silverman (1968)	115	115	Speech Examination	23.5	8.7
Blood and Seider (1981)	1,060		Reports of Clinicians	27	
Franke (1983)	336		Speech Examination	44	
Accordi et al (1983)	2,802	1,602	Medical Records*	27.8	6.5
Louko, Edwards, and Conture (1990)	30	30	Speech Examination	40	7
St. Louis, Murray, and Ashworth (1991)	24		Speech Examination	42	

*The control data were obtained by questionnaires distributed in schools.

Interpretations

It is evident that delayed speech and language occurs with unusual frequency in stuttering children. Aside from hypothesis, we have little to go on in speculating about the meaning of this fact. One assumption, held by Bloodstein (1975) among others on the basis of clinical observation, is that children with communication disorders are more likely to acquire a sense of failure as speakers and to learn to struggle with their speech attempts. Horowitz (1965) attempted to verify this in her clinical examination of a series of children with faulty articulation. She reported that approximately 44 percent of these children "exhibited some degree of prolongations, repetitions, blockings, etc., listed by Van Riper as elements of stuttering behavior." The presence of such behavior, however, did not seem to have much to do with whether the parents had attempted to correct the child's articulation, despite the fact that the children who had been corrected were more often reluctant to speak and were more often seen to place their articulators in a deliberate way when producing certain sounds.

Comas (1974) reported on 1,050 cases of young children in whom stuttering was observed to appear while they were being treated for articulatory problems. He was also struck by the appearance of stuttering among a group of children undergoing speech therapy after cleft palate operations, though in some cases the stuttering was noted some months before speech treatment (Comas, 1975).

Another reasonable way to explain the high association between stuttering and other speech and language problems is to assume that they are caused to some extent by the same thing. This point of view was broached, for example, by West, Kennedy, and Carr (1947, p. 93), who suggested that stuttering and speech retardation often tend to appear in the same individuals because they have inherited a common predisposition to both conditions. Bloodstein (1958, p. 30) could find no indication of such a relationship in a group of 70 young stutterers. About half the group had a history of slow or abnormal speech development and half had a family background of stuttering, but there was essentially no tendency for the two to be related. This was confirmed by Seider, Gladstien, and Kidd (1982), who found no difference in the incidence of articulation and language problems between stutterers with and without a family history of stuttering. On the other hand, in both this investigation and that of Cox, Seider, and Kidd (1984), stutterers did not differ from their nonstuttering relatives in the incidence of such problems, a finding perhaps indicating that relatives of stutterers are at a higher than normal risk for speech and language retardation. Homzie, Simpson, and Hasenstab (1988) surveyed stutterers in self-help groups by questionnaire. Not only did large numbers report personal histories of delayed language and defective articulation, but 25 percent of 111 responses mentioned articulation problems in relatives.

Observations by Yoss and Darley (1974) hint that in some children articulatory problems and stuttering might both be manifestations of developmental apraxia. Among 30 children with articulation problems, 16 performed poorly on a test of oral apraxia. These children had more repetitions and prolongations in their speech than did the others. On Blakeley's Screening Test for Developmental Apraxia of Speech, Byrd and Cooper (1989a) found that the mean score of stuttering children fell between those of normal speaking and developmentally apraxic children. The performance profiles of the stutterers and apraxics appeared more similar to each other than to the profile of the normal speakers.

SCHOOL HISTORY

Grade Placement

Fairly consistent evidence has been found that stutterers, on the whole, are poorer in educational adjustment than normal speakers. The usual criterion has been amount of retardation in grade placement at school. This type of measure may be used either by comparing a child's grade placement with that of others of the same age or by comparing a child's chronological age with that of others in the same grade. Schindler (1955) found that significantly fewer stutterers were accelerated and significantly more were retarded in grade placement when compared with nonstutterers of like age. On the average, the stutterers were retarded by about one-half year, the control group by slightly less than one-quarter year. This is in general agreement with the results of previous studies. McAllister (1937, p. 11) reported that stutterers in Dunbartonshire were retarded 9.7 months, on the average. A survey of schoolchildren in 6 American cities by Conradi (1912) showed that in every grade the mean age of the stutterers was higher than that of all children in the grade, by 7 or 8 months in most grades. Comparable findings were obtained in early studies by Root, Wallin, and others (cited by Johnson, 1932). Darley (1955) found that, of 50 stuttering children and their controls, 15 stutterers and only 4 controls had repeated at least one-half grade.

It seems generally agreed that the relatively poorer educational adjustments are due directly to the difficulty of speaking in a classroom situation. The oral recitation problems of stutterers and some of their effects on academic performance were documented by Knudsen (1939).

Educational Achievement

The average retardation of stutterers in grade placement may be compared with their performance on standard tests of academic achievement. McDowell (1928) found that stutterers' overall scores on the Stanford Achievement Tests were comparable to those of nonstutterers. Schindler (1955) obtained similar findings, on the whole, using the Iowa Basic Skills Tests, but her stutterers were seven months retarded, on the average, in basic language skills[7] on the elementary level and four months retarded in basic arithmetic skills at the advanced level. Williams, Melrose, and Woods (1969) found stutterers consistently behind nonstutterers on all aspects of the Iowa Tests, although there was evidence that in the area of language skills the stutterers tended to catch up by grade 8. On a test of computational ability Schulz (1977) found no significant difference between stuttering and nonstuttering children in Germany.

In 8 studies, the silent reading ability of stutterers was found normal or not significantly below that of nonstutterers by all except those of Murray, Bosshardt, and Bosshardt and Nandyal.[8] Hamilton (1940) found also that stutterers did not differ from normal speakers in frequency of fixations and regressions or in span of fixation during silent reading. Roland (1972) observed more regressions in his group of stutterers, as did Brutten and Janssen (1979) and Brutten, Bakker, Janssen, and van der Meulen (1984).

Educational Adjustment

Somewhat unexpectedly, Cox, Seider, and Kidd (1984) reported no group difference in the school adjustment of stutterers and nonstutterers. Their experimental group was limited to families in which at least 5 members stuttered. Information was derived from interviews with stutterers and parents regarding such items as satisfaction with school achievement; attention difficulty in school; learning disability; the child's perception of teachers as unfair; adequacy in math, reading, and writing; and being difficult to control.

INTELLIGENCE

It has been asserted repeatedly that the average intelligence of stutterers does not differ from that of nonstutterers, but reports of careful investigations compel us to reexamine this assumption critically. It is true that, if comparable data from control groups are ignored, esti-

---

[7]The test of language skills is comprised of subtests on spelling, capitalization, punctuation, and usage.

[8]See McDowell (1928), Murray (1932), Hamilton (1940), Schindler (1955), Andrews and Harris (1964, p. 99), Conture and van Naerssen (1977), Janssen, Kraaimaat, and van der Meulen (1983), Bosshardt and Nandyal (1988), Bosshardt (1990). In a questionnaire survey of college students in Bogota, Columbia, by Ardila et al (1994), 27 percent of stutterers and 15.9 percent of nonstutterers indicated that they had dyslexia.

mates of the average I.Q. of stutterers in various studies fall unremarkably in the general region of 100, the theoretical average for the population at large. In the past, when small departures from this theoretical average were found they were tacitly assumed to have resulted from random sampling errors or from the manner in which subjects were obtained for study. Ultimately, however, Schindler (1955) and Andrews and Harris (1964, p. 97) drew samples of schoolchildren from large populations representing a broad range of socioeconomic backgrounds and compared their intelligence with that of similarly selected normal-speaking children, using appropriate tests of statistical inference. The results in both studies show an average I.Q. of about 95 for the stutterers as against about 100 for the nonstutterers (see Table 19). Comparable findings were reported by Okasha, Bishry, et al (1974). In each instance the difference was statistically significant.

Although an average difference of several I.Q. points is more important theoretically than practically, the striking agreement among these three studies compels us to consider seriously that there may be a small difference between stutterers and nonstutterers as groups that needs to be explained. When we examine the other findings summarized in Table 19 for a clue to the reason for which such a possibility might not have been apparent before, we see that in most cases there was no control group. In the only other controlled study, that of Johnson et al. (1942), the subjects were chosen from a relatively limited social, economic, and educational milieu. Darley's sample also represents higher socioeconomic levels, having been chosen largely from children brought to the University of Iowa Speech Clinic by their parents. Darley gives no mean or median I.Q. for his 50 stutterers, but reports that when their scores were grouped in three categories roughly representative of superior, normal, and below normal intelligence, the distribution of frequencies did not differ significantly by chi-square test from that reported by Wechsler for the general population.

By contrast with those of other studies, Schindler's subjects represented a broad cross section of the city, village, and rural population of Iowa, while those of Andrews and Harris consisted of the stutterers found in a survey of all of the children in the last two years of primary school in the city of Newcastle upon Tyne, who were matched for age and sex with control subjects from their own class at school. It is noteworthy that an average I.Q. of 96.5, only slightly higher than those obtained in the Schindler and Newcastle studies, was reported by West (1931) for a very large group of stutterers in the 1930 White House Conference survey of schoolchildren in 43 American towns and cities.

The very small amount of work that has been done on the subtest profiles and test scatter of stutterers has been sufficient to produce considerable disagreement. Scripture and Kittredge (1923) found that

Table 19. Intelligence Quotients of Stutterers and Nonstutterers

	N	Population Sampled	Stutterers		Nonstutterers	
			Mean or Median I.Q.	Range	Mean or Median I.Q.	Range
Scripture and Kittredge (1923)	62	Vanderbilt Medical Clinic	92	56-130		
McDowell (1928)	61	New York City Schools	99.1	63-156		
West (1931)	4,059	U.S. Public Schools	96.5			
Berry (1937a)	166	Chicago Hospital Clinics	99.2			
Johnson et al (1942)	46, 46	University of Iowa Outpatient Speech Clinic*	114	80-159	116	95-158
Carlson (1946)	50	Speech Improvement Classes, New York City Public Schools	109			

Table 19 (continued)

	N	Population Sampled	Stutterers		Nonstutterers	
			Mean or Median I.Q.	Range	Mean or Median I.Q.	Range
Darley (1955)	108,	University of Iowa Outpatient Speech Clinic*		54-162		50
Schlindler (1955)	23,326	Iowa Urban and Rural Schools	94.9**	55-124	99.5	50-140
Andrews and Harris (1964)	80, 80	Newcastle upon Tyne Schools	94.7**		101.8	
Hartz (1970)	126	Westphalia Schoolchildren	112			
Okasha, Bishry, et al (1974)	79, 80	Egyptian Schoolchildren	94**		101	
Pukačová (1974)	74	Czech Children	95.4			
Heinzel and Ubricht (1983)	31	West German Schoolchildren	112			

*In both the Johnson and Darley studies most of the subjects were referred by their parents. The experimental groups were representative of upper socioeconomic levels. The control groups were chosen to be comparable in socioeconomic status.

**Significantly different from the mean of the nonstuttering group.

the majority of a group of stutterers tended to have an abnormally uneven scatter of scores on the subtests of the Stanford-Binet, suggesting the possibility of brain damage or emotional instability. Furthermore, many of the stutterers tended to have particularly low scores on the vocabulary subtest, leading Scripture and Kittredge to conclude that they appeared to have a "word disability." On the other hand, an analysis by Carlson (1946) seemed to show that stutterers, as compared with children having behavior problems, performed especially poorly on the motor coordination items of the Stanford-Binet. Andrews and Harris (1964, p. 98) found essentially no differences in subtest profiles for their two groups on the Wechsler Intelligence Scale for Children. Stuttering children tested by Heinzel and Ubricht (1983) had significantly higher performance than verbal I.Q.s.

In search of evidence of brain dysfunction in stutterers, Cox (1982) employed a neurophysiological test battery consisting of the Wechsler Adult Intelligence Scale and various other tests. He found little indication of significant cerebral dysfunction.

Stuttering Among Persons with Mental Deficiency

If, as the findings we have reviewed suggest, stuttering is slightly more common in the less intelligent of the normal population, we might expect it to be especially prevalent among persons with mental deficiency. There is ample evidence that it is (see Table 20).[9] Although the prevalence figures that have been reported vary widely, almost all of them are far higher than the 1 percent that is usual in an ordinary population. Stuttering, apparently of all degrees of severity and complexity, would seem to occur more frequently in this population than in any other single identifiable group of people.

A question often raised is whether the stuttering of persons with mental retardation is the same disorder as is generally called by that name, especially since in many cases it is described as lacking much of the secondary symptomatology of ordinary stuttering. In a group of adults with mental retardation whose speech problem had been diagnosed as stuttering, Bonfanti and Culatta (1977) found few secondary features. The subjects tended to be aware of their disfluency but not concerned about it, and there was little evidence of avoidance, frustration, or anxiety. It must be kept in mind, however, that a considerable amount of "ordinary" stuttering in its early stages also exhibits few associated or reactive features (see Chapter 1). Lerman, Powers, and Rigrodsky (1965) presented evidence that much of the stuttering of school-age children with mental retardation is compar-

---

[9]See also Keane (1972) for a review that includes some unpublished studies.

Table 20. A Prevalence of Stuttering Among Persons with Mental Deficiency

	N*	Population	Percentage of Stutterers
Ballard (1912)	944	Special Schools for Mentally Defective Children	2.4
Louttit and Halls (1936)	620	Ungraded Classes for Subnormals	3.22
Wohl (1951)	145	Special Schools for Mentally and Physically Handicapped	5.5
Karlin and Strazzulla (1952)	50	Outpatient Hospital Clinic for Retarded Children	2.0
Schlanger (1953)	74	Institution for Mentally Retarded	20.3
Schlanger and Gottsleben (1957)	516	Institution for Mentally Retarded	17.0
Stark (1963)**		Educationally Subnormal Children	10.0
Schaeffer and Shearer (1968	4,307	Institution for Mentally Retarded	7.6
Sheehan, Martyn, and Kilburn (1968)	216	Institution for Mentally Retarded	0.8
Martyn, Sheehan, and Sluk (1969)	346	Institution for Mentally Retarded	1.0
Chapman and Cooper (1973)	1,467	Institution for Mentally Retarded	3.0
Brady and Hall (1976)	3,057	Educable Mentally Retarded	1.6
Brady and Hall (1976	457	Trainable Mentally Retarded in Schools	3.08
Boberg et al. (1978)	840	Classes for Educable Mentally Retarded	1.43
Boberg et al. (1978)	439	Classes for Trainable Mentally Retarded	2.51
Brindle and Dunster (1984)	351	Institution for Mentally Retarded	6.55

*Where data were obtained in institutions, N refers to the total number in the survey population who had speech.
**Cited by Andrews and Harris (1964, p. 7).

able to the early stuttering of children who have normal intelligence. They also pointed out that fears, avoidances, and secondary stuttering symptoms can and do occur in persons with mental deficiency. Schlanger and Gottsleben (1957) found such reactions in 26 percent of their stutterers with mental retardation. This should not be surprising if we recall that they may occur in mentally normal 3- or even 2-year-olds.

In an effort to find out how similar such stuttering is to that of intellectually normal subjects, Shearer and Baud (1970) investigated the adaptation effect, and Chapman and Cooper (1973) studied adaptation, consistency, and expectancy (*see Chapters 7 and 8*) in stutterers with mental deficiency. All of these phenomena were found, though not to quite the degree that is characteristic of most stutterers. Of 18 subjects tested by Chapman and Cooper only 5 indicated any expectation of stuttering, but these 5 stuttered on all words on which they had anticipated doing so.

Prevalence in Down Syndrome

Among the special classifications of mental deficiency stuttering has been reported to be unusually common in Down syndrome. A prevalence of 33 percent, based on the independent judgments of three speech pathologist, was recorded by Gottsleben (1955) for a group of 36 subjects, 45 percent by Schlanger and Gottsleben (1957) for 44 cases, and 21 percent by Lubman (1955) for 48 children with that syndrome. Rohovsky, with the help of ten other judges who listened to tape recordings, identified 48 percent as stutterers in a group of 27 (cited by Schlanger, 1973, p. 19). In two other unpublished studies cited by Van Riper (1982, p. 41), Edson found a 39 percent and Schubert a 15 percent prevalence. The only apparent exception to the general trend was the study of Martyn, Sheehan, and Slutz (1969) in which only 1 stutterer turned up among 42 subjects with Down syndrome.

In view of this remarkable prevalence, an inevitable question is whether what we are observing here is stuttering at all, in the usual sense. Cabañas (1954) noted an exceptional amount of speech interruption in a group of fifty children with Down syndrome, but regarded it as cluttering rather than as true stuttering since he found no evidence of anticipations, substitutions, or other avoidance devices or memory of past blocking. On the other hand, Rohovsky, in the study referred to above, found that of thirteen persons with Down syndrome who appeared to stutter five displayed observable reactions to their disfluency. Farmer and Brayton (1979) noted that disfluent subjects with Down syndrome achieved poorer ratings of intelligibility in conversational speech than fluent ones, and suggested that their disfluency was therefore more characteristic of cluttering than stuttering.

The most detailed examination of disfluency in Down syndrome to date was carried out by Preus (1972) on a sample of 47 individuals selected only for fairly intelligible speech. Preus studied chiefly the frequency of whole-word repetitions, part-word repetitions, and prolongations in the subjects' speech. He found a high frequency of each of these symptoms in the group as a whole. Using an arbitrary criterion of 5 instances of such disfluency per 100 words, he classified 46.8 percent of the sample as stutterers. Using the same cut-off point and excluding whole-word repetitions, he classified 34 percent as stutterers. (Institutional personnel judged 53 percent to be stutterers.) Unexpectedly, Preus found in 29.8 percent of the cases secondary symptoms consisting of associated bodily movements or of devices such as avoidance and postponement. With the aid of judges' ratings he also classified 31.9 percent of the same sample as clear or pronounced clutterers, but there was no correlation between stuttering and cluttering. Preus concluded that the disfluencies found in Down syndrome may be classified as "genuine stuttering."

Otto and Yairi (1975) analyzed the speech of subjects with Down syndrome who were judged not to be stutterers and found that it contained more part-word repetitions, word repetitions, "tensions," and other disfluencies than did the speech of control subjects of normal intelligence. Their rate of speech also tended to be more rapid.

FAMILY HISTORY

Birth Order and Sibling Relationship

There is considerable evidence that the various ordinal positions in the family are represented in about the expected proportions among stutterers.[10] Whether an only child is more likely to stutter, however, is a question that has produced conflicting findings. Among large groups of stutterers, Rotter (1939) and the Iowa studies found an unusual proportion of only children—18 or 20 percent as compared with only 10 or 12 percent among nonstutterers. Boland (1950) also found a higher percentage of only children among 262 stutterers than among a large sample of the general population, but noted that these were stutterers who had applied for treatment. In the Newcastle study, eight of the eighty stutterers and three of the control subjects were only children, not a statistically significant difference. Morgenstern (1956) observed no departure from the expected number of only children among 355 stutterers. Likewise, Accordi and his asso-

---

[10]Morgenstern (1956), Johnson and Associates (1959, p. 72), Andrews and Harris (1964, p. 54), Gladstien, Seider, and Kidd (1981).

ciates (1983) found that the same percentage of a large number of stutterers and nonstutterers were only children. Rotter and Morgenstern agreed in the finding that the average stutterer was separated from the sibling closest in age by a larger number of years than was the average nonstutterer, but this difference appeared in neither the Newcastle data nor the findings of Gladstien, Seider, and Kidd (1981).

It is difficult to reconcile such marked disparities in the outcomes of research. If there is in fact any relationship between stuttering and status as an only child, perhaps it is due to the increased parental concern to which the only child is vulnerable, as Johnson and Associates (1959, p. 225) suggested.

Familial Background

The literature contains occasional references to the incidence of such factors as left-handedness, twinning, allergies, and neurological and psychiatric disorders in the families of stutterers, but little careful investigation has been done. Bryngelson and Rutherford (1937) and Bryngelson (1939) reported findings on left-handedness that were not significant. In the Iowa and Newcastle studies there were no differences with regard to either left-handedness or twinning in the two groups of families, though there appeared to be a trend toward significantly more twins among the stutterers' relatives in the Newcastle group. The Iowa studies showed no significant difference in the incidence of either epilepsy or diabetes among the relatives of the two groups, although there were 21 cases of diabetes in the stutterers' families as against 12 in the nonstutterers'. In the families of 2,802 stutterers and a comparison group of 1,602 controls, Accordi and his co-workers (1983) found no differences in diseases, neurologic disorders, cluttering, delayed language development, or parental consanguinity.

Only with regard to the familial incidence of allergies have some findings been positive. Both Kennedy and Williams (1938) and Card (1939) found that almost all of their stuttering subjects had family histories of allergy, as compared with roughly one-third to three-fifths of their control groups. On the other hand, no indication of a difference appeared in the Iowa studies, in which about half of both groups reported some type of allergy in their families.

The family backgrounds of stutterers, of course, contain several times as many stuttering relatives as do the family backgrounds of nonstutterers (see Chapter 3).

Parents

From the point of view of any theory that regards stuttering as due chiefly or in part to environmental influences, the attitudes, child training practices, and personality make-up of the stutterer's parents are of profound interest. In the course of the development of theories of stuttering two major conceptions of the parents have emerged. In one they are viewed as basically neurotic persons whose contacts with their children are in some measure rejecting, overprotective, dominating, ambivalent, or in other ways warped by anxiety, hostility, dependence, or guilt. In the other, which is due chiefly to the work of Johnson, the parents are portrayed as largely anxious, perfectionistic, and demanding, particularly with regard to the child's speech.

Parental Adjustment

These two descriptions are clearly overlapping to some extent. One of the main differences between them lies in the degree of emotional disturbance the parents are assumed to exhibit. Johnson regarded most of them as essentially ordinary persons whose behavior simply reflects the competitive pressures of our culture to a somewhat unusual degree. On this issue the research findings are fairly clear. Although occasional observations have seemed to suggest that the stutterer's parents differ from others in typical personality make-up, the results of a series of controlled investigations in which the emotional adjustment of stutterers' parents has been systematically compared with that of parents of nonstutterers by means of personality tests have provided little support for this assumption *(see Table 21)*.

Parental Child Training Attitudes

Despite this failure to discover distinct personality deviations in most parents of stutterers, there is considerable evidence of differences in their attitudes and behavior toward their children. Some of this evidence, notably that of Kinstler (1961), is most readily interpreted as supporting a theory of stuttering as a neurotic disorder. Kinstler compared the responses of mothers of young stutterers and nonstutterers on a questionnaire designed to measure overt and covert maternal acceptance and rejection by means of ratings of agreement with such statements as, "I'd prefer not to have any more children," "A mother should sacrifice her own desires for what is best for her children," and "I do not permit my child to climb tall trees." He found that although the mothers of stutterers appeared to be superficially accepting of their children they seemed to reject their children in subtle, hidden ways to a greater extent than did the control mothers.

An appreciable body of other evidence seems to support Johnson's view of the stutterer's parents. Of more than 800 questions asked of mothers and fathers of stuttering and normal-speaking children in the Iowa studies, a large proportion dealt with the home environment, disciplinary practices, and parental attitudes and adjustments as they

Table 21. Personality and Adjustment of Parents of Stutterers and Nonstutterers

	Experimental		Control		Test	Findings
N	M	F	M	F		
Darley (1955)	48	49	43	43	Guilford Inventory of Factors STDCR	Differences between the experimental and control parents were not statistically significant for any of the five factors.
Grossman (1952)	21	21	21	21	Minnesota Multiphasic Personality Inventory (MMPI)	There was a significant difference on only one of 13 scales of the test, the parents of the stutterers having a higher average F score. (The F score is one of the four validity scales of the MMPI. A high F score is usually interpreted to mean that subjects are trying to place themselves in an unfavorable light.)
Goodstein and Dahlstrom (1956)	100	100	100	100	Minnesota Multiphasic Personality Inventory (MMPI)	The scores of the parents of stutterers closely resembled those of both their matched controls and the original standardization group of normal adults, although there were a few small differences, of which the most notable was a slight tendency, within the normal range, to be more anxious.
Goodstein (1956)	50	50	100	100*	Minnesota Multiphasic Personality Inventory (MMPI)	In a follow-up investigation the parents of 50 additional stutterers did not differ significantly from the experimental and control groups of the Goodstein and Dahlstrom study, except for a few small differences in a less abnormal direction.

Study				Test	Findings
LaFollette (1956)	85	85	50	50** California Test of Personality	There was no difference in adjustment between the experimental and control groups as a whole, mothers or fathers. The fathers of older stutterers, aged 19-30, had poorer adjustment than the fathers in the control group.
				Psycho-Somatic Inventory of McFarland and Seitz	The fathers of the stutterers exhibited poorer mental health than the fathers of the control group. There was no difference between the two groups of mothers.
				Allport Ascendance-Submission Reaction Study	The parents of the stutterers were more submissive than those of the control group, due essentially to a difference between the two groups of fathers.
Andrews and Harris (1964)	71	79		Maudsley Personality Inventory	The mothers of the stutterers did not differ from those of the nonstutterers on either of the two scales of the test (extraversion and neuroticism).
	49	62		Cattell 16 Personality Factor Inventory	No significant differences between the two groups of mothers appeared on any of the 16 factors.
Feldman (1976)	32	32	32	32 Jourard Self-Disclosure Questionnaire	Parents of stutterers and nonstutterers did not differ with respect to how much of their attitudes and concerns they confided to their spouses, friends, and children. Stutterers' parents, however, more often indicated items about which they would decline to disclose information.
Flügel (1979)	124	97		Maudsley Personality Inventory and Maudsley Medical Questionnaire	Mothers of stutterers scored higher on a combined measure of neuroticism and extraversion.
Zenner et al (1978)	7	7	14	14 State-Trait Anxiety Inventory	Parents of stutterers revealed more anxiety as a personality trait than did parents of children with articulatory difficulties and parents of normal-speaking children.

*The control group was identical with that of Goodstein and Dahlstrom (1956).
**The size of both the experimental and control groups varied somewhat from these figures from test to test.

related directly or indirectly to the children. The results showed that, while the similarities between the two groups of parents appeared to be greater than the differences, a comparatively larger number of parents of stutterers tended to impose somewhat high standards of behavior on their children or to reveal in one form or another a tendency to be critical, anxious, or perfectionistic. For example, the stutterers underwent coercive toilet training somewhat more often and were weaned somewhat sooner than the nonstutterers, and their parents expected children to walk and talk earlier and expressed more discontentment with their spouse, their children, and their socioeconomic circumstances than did the parents of the nonstutterers.

Other questionnaire data that seemed to corroborate these conclusions were obtained by Moncur (1952), who found that parents of stutterers tended to dominate, oversupervise, and be more critical of their children. This was observed also to a somewhat lesser extent by Bloom (1959).

A study by Zenner and his co-workers (1978) was concerned specifically with the factor of parental anxiety. After viewing a videotape recording of his or her own child at play with two other children, each of a group of parents of stutterers completed the A-State portion of the State-Trait Anxiety Inventory with respect to the anxiety they had experienced while watching the tape. The parents of stutterers indicated more anxiety in the situation than did parents of children with normal speech or disorders of articulation. They also revealed more anxiety as a personality trait on the A-Trait portion of the inventory.

It must be cautioned that any unqualified concept of stutterers' parents as dominating and demanding is not consistent either with clinical observation, which reveals many exceptions, or even with the results of the studies themselves. Quarrington (1974), in fact, reinterpreted the literature we have just reviewed in an attempt to show that much of it supports a view of stutterers' parents as excessively passive and permissive with respect to control of the child's behavior.

Stutterers' Perceptions of Parental Behavior

In an investigation by Gildston (1967) of adolescent stutterers by means of the Q-technique, the subjects were asked to sort the cards on the basis of how each parent "sees you and feels you really are" and on the basis of how each parent "wants you to be." The correlations between the parental actual and parental ideal sorts then yielded measures of parental acceptance as perceived by the subjects. Gildston found that perceived parental acceptance was lower in the stutterers than among the nonstutterers.

On the Children's Report of Parental Behavior Inventory, Bourdon and Silber (1970) found no differences between stuttering and nonstuttering adolescents in ratings of parental acceptance, rejection, control, possessiveness, tendency to instill anxiety, and the like. Using the same inventory in a study of eleven- to thirteen-year-old children Yairi and Williams (1971) obtained somewhat unexpected findings. The stutterers appeared to view their parents as behaving with less control and hostility and with more love and autonomy than did the nonstutterers.

Parental Level of Aspiration

A unique approach to the question of parental standards of behavior was taken by Goldman and Shames (1964a, 1964b). Employing a modified Rotter Level of Aspiration Board procedure that enabled them to control the amount of failure and success experienced by the subject, they found that parents of stutterers did not appear to set higher goals for themselves in a motor task than did parents of nonstutterers. With a similar procedure they then studied the goals that parents of stutterers set for their children. The parents were asked to predict the child's scores in operating the Rotter Board and also to predict the number of words on which the child would have difficulty in telling a story. Goldman and Shames found that the fathers of the stutterers, on the whole, appeared to exhibit unrealistic goal-setting behavior. On the speech task their estimates of the amount of difficulty their children would have was lower, despite the fact that the children were stutterers, than those of the fathers of the control group. Furthermore, on both the motor and speech tasks the fathers of the stutterers tended to persist in relatively high estimates of their children's success, in spite of failures, to a greater extent than did the fathers of the nonstutterers when confronted with their children's failures. The two groups of mothers did not differ, although the mothers of the stutterers showed a tendency to make higher initial estimates of their children's success on the Rotter Board.

Further work has failed to confirm some of these findings, however. Quarrington, Seligman, and Kosower (1969) replicated the portion of Shames' and Goldman's experiment that dealt with the goals the parents set for their children on the Rotter Board and found that the mothers of the stutterers tended to set lower goals, while the two groups of fathers did not differ.

Parents' Interactions with Children

For many years speech clinicians have advised parents of young stutterers to cultivate a warm, accepting relationship with the child, to decrease their speaking rate, and to avoid interrupting the child or bombarding the child with questions. In attempts to test the underlying assumptions of this widely accepted practice, a number of investigators have videotaped the interactions of young stuttering children and their parents in play situations. The results have been conflicting.

Kaprisin-Burrelli, Egolf, and Shames (1972) recorded the conversation between school-age children and their parents and evaluated the statements of the parents as positive or negative. Positive statements were those which encouraged verbalization, indicated understanding, gave praise, accepted feelings, demonstrated interest, and the like. Negative statements were critical, dictatorial, threatening, interrupting, lacking appropriate understanding or recognition of feeling, and so forth. The parents of stutterers were consistently found to converse with their children in a more negative manner than the parents of nonstutterers. Fifty-eight percent of their statements were classified as negative as compared with 22 percent of those made by the control group.

In a study by Meyers and Freeman (1985a) mothers of 4- to 5-year-old stutterers and nonstutterers interacted in a free play situation with their own and others' children. No differences appeared between the two groups of mothers in numbers of positive or negative statements, initiations or terminations of interactions, questions, comments, total words or utterances, or in mean length of utterances. Meyers and Freeman (1985b) found that the mothers did not differ in the frequency of interruptions of their children. Mothers of stutterers did talk faster on the average than mothers of nonstutterers, however, when speaking to both stutterers and nonstutterers (Meyers and Freeman, 1985c).

Langlois, Hanrahan, and Inouye (1986) found that mothers of stutterers made more imperative and interrogative utterances than mothers of nonstutterers. Weiss and Zebrowski (1991) found that parents of stutterers and nonstutterers did not differ in frequency of responses to children's attempts to converse as opposed to "assertive," i.e, unsolicited conversational contributions. Schulze (1991) reported no difference in parents' speaking rate, rate of turn taking, interruptions, and requests. Kelly and Conture (1992) found no difference in speaking rate, interruptions, and time taken before responding to children's utterances.

On the whole, the studies have not always found what many clinicians might have expected. This may be merely because the best experimental analogues of life situations are not the real thing. Or it may be that we are being validly admonished against the indiscriminate application of some established clinical axioms.

Parental Standards of Fluency and Attitudes Toward Stuttering

To what extent parents of stutterers are specifically perfectionistic about speech fluency is a question crucial to a diagnosogenic theory, but difficult to answer. In the Iowa studies far fewer of the stutterers' than the nonstutterers' parents agreed with the statement that "nonfluencies in speech are normal if not excessive." But the unusual concern about the fluency of their children's speech such parents expressed in response to this and other questions may just as well have been an effect of the problem as an integral part of it, as Johnson and Associates (1959, p. 85 ff.) pointed out.

Bloodstein, Jaeger, and Tureen (1952) found that parents of stutterers appeared to be somewhat unusually prone to identify tape-recorded samples of normal childhood speech as belonging to stutterers, but this was not confirmed in subsequent research by Berlin (1960). When mothers were asked to respond to individual examples of disfluency in a study by Zebrowski and Conture (1989), mothers of stutterers made more judgments of stuttering than nonstutterer's mothers in response to most disfluency types, but the difference was statistically significant only in the case of sound prolongations and broken words.

Neither Darley (1955) nor LaFollette (1956) found any difference between the two groups of parents on the Iowa Scale of Attitude Toward Stuttering. Parents of stutterers did reveal less favorable attitudes, however, on an inventory of parental attitudes toward stuttering constructed by Crowe and Cooper (1977). They also scored lower than parents of nonstutterers on a test of factual knowledge about stuttering.

Cox, Seider, and Kidd (1984) administered the revised Erickson inventory of attitudes toward speech to nonstuttering relatives, including parents, of stutterers and nonstutterers and reported no difference between the groups.

Lasalle and Conture (1991) found a significant tendency for mothers of stutterers to initiate eye contact with their children during moments of stuttering.

Parental Fluency

Knepflar (1965) found that parents of stutterers had more normal disfluencies in their speech than did parents of nonstutterers. Meyers and Freeman (1985b) failed to confirm this in their study of stutterers' mothers.

Conflicting Evidence From the Newcastle Study

On the whole, the evidence suggests that parents of stutterers often tend to impose high standards of behavior of all kinds, not speech fluency alone. Not only is this supported directly by the results of several studies, but it is particularly easy to reconcile with the sociocultural findings that suggest a relationship between stuttering and environmental pressures (see Chapter 3). Before we adopt it as a broadly valid concept of the stutterer's parental environment, however, we must take note of some sharply conflicting evidence. From the Newcastle study, which included intensive interviewing and testing of the subjects' mothers, there emerges a remarkably different picture containing little hint of perfectionism or high standards.

Like the Iowa parents, the mothers of the Newcastle stutterers were very similar to their controls with regard to most features of their personal histories, and there appeared to be about the same amount of neuroticism among them. They differed from their controls, however, in several respects. They more frequently exhibited low intelligence. They tended to have poor records of school achievement. More of them had poor work histories as indicated by frequent job changes. And finally, they more frequently failed to provide an adequate home environment, as evidenced by a greater incidence of poor housing as well as some tendency toward less unified family life and less contact with relatives outside the home. In short, the mothers of the stutterers seemed to be distinguished by a general inclination to fail—at school, at work, and in the home—and this inability to "cope" seemed to be related to low innate capacity rather than to poor emotional adjustment. Among these mothers low intelligence was significantly correlated with such factors as low intelligence and late or poor talking in the child and with abnormal personality of the husband as evidenced by psychiatric or conduct problems destructive of family functioning.[11] Clearly, the parents of the Iowa and Newcastle stutterers seem to represent two quite different groups of people.

That these two hypothetical groups may actually exist is suggested by further evidence from the Newcastle study. Andrews and Harris (1964, p. 114 ff.) carried out a factor analysis in order to determine whether they could identify subgroups of cases with respect to the array of items on which they had gathered information. Among their 80 stutterers they discovered a small delegation, as it were, from the Iowa group. Though not differentiable from the rest in any sharp or categorical way, these children tended to be marked by high social class and upward mobility, by intelligent mothers with "neurotic traits, particularly of an obsessional kind," and by good intelligence, a mild stutter, and symptoms of anxiety, aggression and disobedience, irritability, and overactivity.

The possibility that the Iowa and Newcastle findings are applicable respectively to two more or less differentiable groups of stutterers

---

[11]Fourteen of the eighty fathers of stutterers, as compared with nine in the control group, were judged to have such problems on the basis of the information obtained from the mothers. Evidently, it would have been of some interest to interview the fathers of this group. This was not possible because, as Andrews and Harris (1964, p. 39) state, "In this community, not only are children thought to be the concern of mothers alone, but the prevailing unemployment meant that few fathers were prepared to risk their jobs by taking time off to attend hospital."

may serve to raise the question of which group is more representative of stutterers "in general." The answer is not as simple as it may at first appear. The Iowa stutterers, to be sure, are from certain points of view a highly selected group. On the other hand, it is only with certain qualifications that the Newcastle subjects are to be regarded as broadly representative of whatever we mean by "the population." Andrews and Harris caution that in Newcastle upon Tyne group "geographical isolation and the harsh realities of the environment" have produced a people with a distinctive culture and that the results of their study may not be strictly comparable with those from other communities (1964, p. 36).

In their own ways both the Iowa and Newcastle groups may represent rather special cases when considered in relation to the whole range of cultural variations. It must be considered that if what we have in mind as "the population" is to be defined in terms of numbers it is very possibly best represented by people who live by the hand plow, whose likes have rarely been seen in all of England or the United States outside the pages of the *National Geographic Magazine*, and who can ill afford the luxury of being concerned about their children's stuttering.

SUMMARY

We may now restate in brief the essential facts that have been learned from research on the medical, developmental, and school histories and the home environments of stutterers.

Stutterers' medical records are for the most part similar to those of nonstutterers, despite a few vague and ambiguous suggestions of more abnormal birth conditions in the case of the stutterers in both the Iowa and Newcastle studies. The possibility of more allergy, as indicated by both personal and family histories, is also still an open one. The physical examination is apt to disclose chiefly somatic symptoms of anxiety.

Stutterers as a group appear to have normal developmental histories except with regard to speech and language. Although agreement is not complete, most research findings indicate that stutterers tend to be later than nonstutterers in saying their first words, phrases, and sentences and in acquiring intelligible speech. On tests of linguistic ability they also tend to perform more poorly at early age levels, although studies of older subjects appear to show that they soon overcome this disadvantage. Almost without exception, studies have shown that stutterers tend to have more articulatory difficulties than nonstutterers. Stutterers are often regarded by their parents as being "nervous" and as exhibiting more of such behavior as fears, nightmares, enuresis, fighting, and the like, to an extent that is probably compatible with the observation that as adults they tend to be somewhat more maladjusted, anxious, or emotionally reactive as a group than do nonstutterers. Mild degrees of educational maladjustment also appear to be more common among stutterers, probably in the main a reflection of the consequences of stuttering in a school setting.

While research findings make it quite clear that the intelligence of stutterers is generally equivalent to that of nonstutterers, close agreement among a number of studies suggests that when surveys are extended to include low as well as high socioeconomic segments of the population, the mean I.Q. of stutterers may be slightly below the general average. Moreover, stuttering appears to be unusually prevalent among those with mental deficiency.

Examination of the family environments of stutterers suggests that there may be a somewhat larger proportion of only children among them than among nonstutterers as well as a longer average separation in age from their nearest siblings, but this has not been firmly established. There is rather substantial and consistent evidence that the parents of stutterers are generally normal in adjustment, and not in any ordinary sense neurotic. But there have been conflicting findings regarding certain specific features of their personality make-up and about their behavior as parents. The studies done at the University of Iowa over a period of years, and corroborated by independent research done elsewhere, show that when compared with parents of nonstutterers from the same cultural and social background many stutterers' parents are to some extent more competitive and perfectionistic, somewhat more overconcerned about their children, and more inclined to dominate them and to set unrealistically high goals for them. On the other hand, comprehensive research on a group of children in Newcastle upon Tyne, England, offers essentially no confirmation of this view and depicts the mother instead as a person who by reason of low innate capacity tends to be poorer at creating a stable home environment than mothers of normal-speaking children.

Suggested Readings

Andrews, G., and Harris, M., *The Syndrome of Stuttering*. London: The Spastics Society Medical Education and Information Unit in association with William Heinemann Medical Books (1964), Chaps. 4, 5, 6.

Cox, N. J., Seider, R. A., and Kidd, K. K., Some environmental factors and hypotheses for stuttering in families with several stutterers. *J. Speech Hearing Res.*, 27, 543–48 (1984).

Johnson, W. and Associates, *The Onset of Stuttering*. Minneapolis: Univ. Minn. Press (1959), Chaps. 2, 3, 4.

7

STUTTERING AS
A RESPONSE

In the next two chapters we will survey a major area of research that is concerned with identifying the variables related to the precipitation of stuttering. We are shifting our attention now from stutterers to stutterings. In these chapters we will be concerned with a single basic question, What is the underlying nature of stuttering as a response?

It will be recalled that there are three general concepts about the nature of the stuttering block that have had wide influence, referred to in our discussion of them in Chapter 2 as the breakdown, the repressed need, and the anticipatory struggle hypotheses. It may be helpful to keep in mind that in large part the research on the moment of stuttering had its source in the anticipatory struggle hypothesis, particularly in a form of that hypothesis, advanced by Johnson and Knott in the 1930s which asserted that stuttering was an anticipatory avoidance reaction.[1] Much that has been discovered about stuttering as a response has resulted from attempts to verify this concept. In more recent years added impetus has been given to such studies by attempts to view stuttering in the context of learning psychology and feedback theory.

Beginning around 1935 the intensive concern with neurophysiological data that had dominated research on stuttering at the University of Iowa began to give way to an interest in the objective study of psychological variables related to stuttering. A major role in this development was played by Johnson. Johnson (1933) had suggested the notion of approaching the problem of stuttering by studying the intermittent stuttering responses or "moments" individually. This led at once to the idea of measuring the amount of stuttering by

---

[1]See Johnson and Knott (1936) and Knott and Johnson (1936).

simply counting the moments. Stuttering behavior in this way was made subject to investigation by the methods of experimental psychology, an orientation that contrasted sharply with the medical model of stuttering which up to that time had dominated its investigation as a "disorder."

The basis was thus laid for an extensive research development concerned with the frequency and distribution of stuttering, a development which was to be for many years the distinctive contribution of American workers on the stuttering problem. In the initial research reports of a series titled "Studies in the Psychology of Stuttering," Johnson and several of his students and co-workers in a single year, 1937, published so much fundamental work on stuttering as a response to stimuli that for thirty years research on the subject consisted to a considerable extent of elaboration of it.

THE DISTRIBUTION OF STUTTERINGS

If we want to learn about the nature of the stuttering response there is hardly a more fundamental question we can ask than the question of how stutterings are distributed in the speech sequence—in essence, what words are likely to be stuttered. In view of Johnson's working assumptions it was logical for him to have begun by raising the question of the extent to which stuttering occurred on words on which it was anticipated.

Anticipation in Relation to Occurrence of Stuttering

The phenomenon of anticipation may be looked at from a number of points of view. Clinically it is best known as a fearful premonition of impending blockage that most stutterers begin to experience at some time in the development of their speech problem. In the laboratory it has been studied by measurement of physiological changes occurring just prior to the block. As we will see later in this chapter, there are still other ways to examine the relationship between stuttering and anticipation. To Johnson and others at the time the question first arose, the simplest objective approach seemed to be to investigate stutterers' ability to predict the occurrence of their blocks.

In general, the procedure followed in this type of investigation was to ask stutterers to make an appropriate signal before their attempt on each word on which they thought they were going to stutter as they read aloud to the experimenter. From the resulting data for each subject one may obtain two principal findings, the percentage of signaled anticipations that were followed by stuttering and the percentage of stutterings that were anticipated. Using this method, Knott, Johnson, and Webster (1937) found that 96 percent of the signaled anticipations of their subjects were followed by stuttering (*see Table 22*). Conversely, almost 94 percent of the stutterings occurred on words on which they had been anticipated. Van Riper (1936) had reported similar findings, and Van Riper and Milisen showed that stutterers could often predict not only the occurrence, but also the length, of their blocks.

These facts are impressive. It may be argued, however, that the same facts may be interpreted as evidence against the anticipatory struggle hypothesis, since the relationship between stuttering and expectancy found in these studies, though high, is far from perfect. The observation that not all anticipations lead to stuttering is perhaps not difficult to explain since expectations of stuttering may often be held tentatively, conditionally, or with varying degrees of doubt. It is the apparently unanticipated block that poses a problem. If stutterings are caused essentially by the anticipation of stuttering, it follows that every block the stutterer has must be preceded by expectancy. This is certainly not borne out by the research findings. Not only does the average stutterer have a certain percentage of ostensibly unanticipated blocks, but Van Riper (1936) found that when such blocks occurred the stutterer frequently reported reactions of surprise. Furthermore, as Milisen (1938) demonstrated, there are stutterers who seem to be able to predict essentially none of their blockages.

Table 22. The Relationship Between Signaled Expectancy and Occurrence of Stuttering

	N	Percentage of Anticipations Followed by Stuttering	Percentage of Stutterings Anticipated
Van Riper (1936)	21	83.2	93.3
Knott, Johnson, and Webster (1937)			
Inexperienced Group	10	96.0	93.7[c]
Experienced Group[a]	12	94.0	87.3[c]
Johnson and Solomon (1937)	13	51.1[b]	62.7[b]
Milisen (1938)	26	85.0	84.6

[a]Subjects in this group had undergone considerable therapy, and several had served in another study involving prediction of stuttering.

[b]When subjects read aloud after an interval of one to seven days following the marking of words on which they expected to stutter.

[c]These percentages were not given by Knott, Johnson, and Webster, but are deducible from their data.

Anticipation as a Process Involving a Low Degree of Consciousness

As a solution to this dilemma Johnson proposed a concept of anticipation as a process that may occur on a low level of consciousness. Evidence in support of such a concept was offered by Johnson and Sinn (1937). They marked the stuttered words in the oral reading of a lengthy passage by each of a group of stutterers. The subjects were then asked to read the passage again, using a fresh unmarked copy, this time reading aloud only those words on which they did not expect to stutter. Although 98 percent of the stutterings were eliminated by this process, there remained a relatively small residue of apparently unexpected blocks. It was these blocks that formed the subject matter of the study. The outstanding fact Johnson and Sinn discovered was that to a marked extent these blocks had occurred *on words that had been stuttered in the first reading.* In addition, subjects' introspections showed that in the majority of these cases their attention had wandered, they were reading far ahead, or they had for some other reason failed to form a judgment whether they would stutter or had forgotten to indicate their anticipation by omitting the word.

The kind of interpretation Johnson placed on these findings may be elaborated by saying that it is possible for stutterers to anticipate blockages in a certain sense without being highly aware of it. Stuttering, he thought, might occur in response to a kind of anticipation that is fleeting and subliminal.

Johnson and Solomon (1937) performed a different type of experiment which they believed to be an analogue of the ordinary day-to-day situation in which stutterers seldom had time to form a deliberate, conscious judgment about the occurrence of stuttering in advance of their speech attempt. They had subjects mark the words in a reading passage on which they expected to stutter. The subjects then read the passage orally after an interval of 10 to 15 minutes and again after an interval of at least a day. In both situations stuttering occurred on about 50 percent of the words on which expectancies had been marked, as compared with about 10 percent of the words on which they had not.

Wingate (1975) found relatively little relationship between the words on which stuttering was anticipated and those that were stuttered when subjects read the words aloud in an altered sequence one and two weeks later. Both the Johnson and Solomon experiment and that of Wingate were concerned with an unusual sense of the term anticipation. The possibility that stutterings might be precipitated by expectancies that had occurred hours or days before, even in the same context, has rarely if ever been contemplated.

Anticipation in School-Age Stutterers

Whatever the merits of Johnson's concept of anticipation on a low level of consciousness, it was clearly designed to account for a relatively small number of exceptions to what seemed to be the general rule that stutterers could predict the occurrence of their stuttering. It has since developed, however, that while this may be true of adults, it is not nearly so general a rule among children.

In the first place, clinical study of the course of development of stuttering in childhood seems to show that expectancy in the usual sense of the term tends to be among the last features of the problem to develop. As a result Bloodstein (1960a) found that the question "Can you sometimes tell that you're going to stutter on a word before you say it?" got the answer yes from only 45 percent of ten- to eleven-year-old children, and only 38 percent of eight- to nine-year-olds. (The question was not asked of younger children.) Since stutterers themselves have from the beginning provided some of the strongest support for the belief that they stutter because they expect to, the fact that so many stutterers either do not have such a belief or are unable to verbalize it cannot be ignored.

In addition, we have evidence from a study by Silverman and Williams (1972b) showing that stutterers in the age range eight to sixteen vary markedly in their ability to predict the occurrence of their stuttering in reading isolated words. Although some predicted essentially all of their blocks, others predicted few or none. About half were able to predict less than 50 percent of their stutterings. Silverman and Williams questioned whether the anticipatory struggle hypothesis can apply to all stuttering children.

If it does, the evidence for it is obviously not to be found in studies of the accuracy of prediction of stuttering. As we have seen, however, prediction is not the only possible way in which we can operationalize the phenomenon of anticipation. Bakker, Brutten, Janssen, and van der Meulen (1991) attempted to do it through a study of the eye movements of school-aged stutterers. On a list of 144 words, the children first marked the words on which they thought they would stutter. Their eye movements were then recorded as they silently read a passage composed of those words. Finally they read the passage aloud. The results showed that the subjects had fixated longer on words on which they subsequently stuttered than on their fluent words. Only 10 percent of the words they had previously marked were stuttered. The experimenters believed the findings showed that school-aged children anticipate stutterings to the same extent that adult stutterers do. If so, they evidently anticipate stuttering in the sense that Johnson had in mind when he theorized that the process could occur on a low level of consciousness.

The Consistency Effect

Research on the moment of stuttering as a response had an even more fundamental beginning in the demonstration by Johnson and

Knott (1937) of the *consistency effect*. In this investigation Johnson and Knott noted the words on which stutterers had difficulty as they read a brief passage ten times in succession. They found that for most subjects the distribution of stutterings was markedly consistent from one reading to the next. In short, the places at which given subjects blocked in repeated readings of the same material were more or less the same. The words with which they had difficulty tended to be words on which they had stuttered in previous readings. If this simple observation is considered carefully it will be seen to have some significant implications. The truth might have been otherwise. It might have been found that all the words of the passage had about an equal chance of being stuttered on in any given reading. The consistency effect appears to show that there is something in the reading itself, some feature of the speech sequence—whether of form or content—that in some manner serves to elicit the stuttering block. As Johnson put it later, ". . . stuttering does not occur haphazardly or in a random or chance fashion but as a response to identifiable stimuli."

The consistency effect was confirmed by Johnson and Inness (1939) and has since been demonstrated in various other studies,[2] including two investigations of school-age stutterers by Neelley and Timmons (1967) and Williams, Silverman, and Kools (1969a). On the whole, about 65 percent of a subject's stuttering in a given reading takes place on words that were stuttered in a previous reading.[3] Zenner, Webster, and Fitzgerald (1974) showed that consistency also extends to the types of stuttering behavior that appear at the same loci.

Further work has been done in an effort to narrow down the precise meaning of the consistency effect. Johnson and Knott believed that the consistency effect showed the power of stimuli to which the stuttering had already become attached when the subject came to par-

---

[2]See, for example,Jamison (1955), Shulman (1955), Tate and Cullinan (1962), Cullinan (1963a), Martin and Haroldson (1967), Neelley and Timmons (1967), Williams, Silverman, and Kools (1969a), Rosso and Adams (1969), Adams and Brutten (1970), Prins and Lohr (1972), Seidel, Weinstein, and Bloodstein (1973), Hendel and Bloodstein (1973), Stefankiewicz and Bloodstein (1974), Wingate (1986).

[3]This percentage measure of consistency, originally employed by Johnson and Knott (1937), has been widely used because it is simple and intuitively comprehensible. A serious drawback of the measure is that it varies with the severity of a subject's stuttering merely as a computational artifact. For example, if a subject stutters on 100 percent of words in Reading 1, 100 percent of any words stuttered in Reading 2 will inevitably have been stuttered in Reading 1, and there will be a consistency score of 100 percent. Consequently, the percentage of consistency cannot be used in comparing different groups of stutterers, or stutterers under different conditions, unless the frequency of stuttering is constant. Tate and Cullinan (1962) and Wingate (1984a) suggested improved methods of measurement that overcome this disadvantage, among others, and which are especially useful in evaluating the consistency of individual stutterers. See also Cullinan (1988).

ticipate in the experiment. An alternative explanation might be that the subject remembers having stuttered on a given word in the previous reading and may respond by stuttering on it again. It is Johnson and Knott's interpretation which appears to be correct, at least in large part. Seidel, Weinstein, and Bloodstein (1973) interposed extraneous readings between subjects' first and second readings of a test passage in an attempt to interfere with their memory of the initial stutterings; this had no effect on consistency. Stefankiewicz and Bloodstein (1974) interposed a four-week interval between two readings. This resulted in somewhat lower consistency than in successive readings of a passage on a single occasion, but the bulk of it remained. After four weeks 49 percent of the subjects' stuttered words were words that had been stuttered originally.

Stuttering appears to be in large measure under the control of stimuli. When the stimulus conditions are held relatively constant, as they are in successive readings of the same passage, the distribution of stutterings tends to be relatively constant too. This seems to be the meaning of the consistency effect. To be sure, this leaves some unanswered questions. Why is the average amount of consistency not greater than it is? Is it because of our failure to control stimuli that are subtle and fleeting? Does it reflect a churning cognitive substrate of stuttering that is beyond our control? Or is there some purely random influence on stuttering? We have barely begun to think about such questions.

The Role of Cues Representative of Past Stuttering

Once the consistency effect had been established it was natural to look for more direct evidence of the role of cues in the precipitation of stuttering. Not only was such evidence found, but some interesting and basic properties of these cues also came to light in the process.

The Cues Are Learned

The special form in which Johnson and his associates developed the anticipatory struggle concept of the moment of stuttering may be written concisely,

Cue → Anticipation → Avoidance

That is, a cue representative of past difficulty leads to an anticipation of stuttering, which in turn leads to the effort to avoid stuttering, an effort which *is* stuttering. This kind of formulation clearly implies that a segment or feature of the speech sequence acquires the power to elicit stuttering through a process of learning. Johnson, Larson, and Knott (1937) succeeded in demonstrating the potentiality of neutral cues for acquiring this power. Using a passage with a colored border, they made sure that subjects would experience a large amount of stuttering on it by having them read it to an audience. Subsequently, they found that when these subjects read to a single listener the presence of a colored border resulted in increased stuttering. In a similar manner they showed that other cues, such as the content of a passage or diagonal lines drawn through words, could be made to evoke more stuttering through association with past difficulty.

Further demonstrations of this kind reported subsequently used other kinds of neutral stimuli. Goss (1956) found that once subjects had been given sufficient experience stuttering on words exposed for 12 seconds before the signal to say them was given, the 12-second interval produced more stuttering than did longer or shorter intervals. Peters and Simonson (1960) increased the frequency of stuttering on words rarely stuttered by their subjects by pairing each of these words repeatedly with a word that had often been stuttered. Fierman (1955) showed that a red border associated with *reduction* in stuttering by its presence during repeated readings of the same passage tended to cause a drop in the frequency of stuttering on a similar passage. Operant conditioning experiments later produced additional examples of reductions in stuttering through the influence of neutral discriminative stimuli (see Martin and Siegel, 1966a, 1966b, and Reed and Lingwall, 1980).

The Adjacency Effect

Johnson and his co-workers theorized that the colored border had the power that it did because it served as a reminder of previous stutterings. Strictly speaking the experiment proved only that stuttering could be influenced by learning. In the given experimental arrangement the colored border might have become a conditioned stimulus for stuttering regardless of the underlying reason for which the stuttering had occurred. This fact lends special significance to another experiment in which the role played by cues was less ambiguous.

Johnson and Millsapps (1937) had each of their subjects read the same passage nine times in succession. At intervals the words on which the subject had stuttered were blotted out by heavy pencil markings so they could not be read, and the subject was instructed to continue to read the words that were visible. In view of the consistency effect, this procedure should soon have eliminated essentially all of the stuttering. For some subjects it did, but in the majority of cases a small residue of persistent stutterings kept cropping up in new places. Examination of the words on which these residual blocks had occurred showed something unexpected. To a significant degree these words were adjacent to previously stuttered words that had been blotted out. In short, the blottings appeared to have served as cues capable of evoking new stuttering. This finding seemed to Johnson and Millsapps to epitomize stuttering as a response to cues representative of past speech failure. Moreover, it is not easily explained in terms of a simple conditioning scheme since the blot neither precedes nor coincides with the original stimulus for stuttering, but covers it up.

The inference that Johnson and Millsapps drew from their study has received some support from later research. Brutten and Gray (1961) devised an adjacency condition in which the words stuttered in repeated readings of a series of nouns could be physically removed and the remaining words respaced so as to minimize the cues representing past stuttering. They compared this with a similar condition in which the word card was merely inverted so that a colored blank remained as a visible cue to the removal of the stuttered word. Brutten and Gray found that when the visible cues were removed there was a less marked adjacency effect. The difference fell short of statistical significance, however.

Rappaport and Bloodstein (1971) put Johnson and Millsapps' inference to a different kind of test. Inferring that blots might produce stutterings for reasons other than their association with past stuttering, they compared an ordinary adjacency condition with a condition in which words were blacked out at random in a reading passage. A quite marked, unforeseen result was obtained. For half the subjects— those who had the random blots condition first—the random cues did not evoke adjacent stuttering. In the case of the remaining subjects— those for whom the random blackout cues came second—they did. In other words, blottings scattered at random do not in themselves produce adjacency. Once the subject has had the experience of having the stuttered words blotted out, however, blackout cues not only serve as stimuli for stutterings, but even have the power to do so in a new passage containing different words. It was a resounding confirmation of the conclusions to which Johnson and Millsapps had been led.

From the point of view of the anticipatory struggle hypothesis it would be difficult to overemphasize the importance of the adjacency effect. The tendency for stuttering to occur in response to the stutterer's memory of past difficulty may be said to be the essence of the assertion that it is an anticipatory struggle reaction. Furthermore, if we were to attempt to define this type of reaction in behavioral terms without the use of such words as anticipation or evaluation, we could perhaps do so only with reference to its responsiveness to cues associated with past difficulty.

This being the case, special mention should be made of the observation that the adjacency effect is apparently to be found in children as well as adults. We have discussed the inability of many school-age stutterers to predict the occurrence of their blocks and the questions this has raised. In a group of twelve stutterers of elementary school age Avari and Bloodstein (1974) were able to demonstrate the adjacency phenomenon in every case. Yet six of the twelve children were unable to predict the occurrence of any of their blocks in oral reading, and only one was able to do so with substantial accuracy. This suggests that the failure of many children to anticipate their stuttering in this type of task may not rule out the possibility that their stutterings are anticipatory struggle reactions. We will return to the complex question of anticipation and its relation to stuttering later in this chapter.

A fresh approach was taken to the investigation of adjacency by Hawkins and Brutten (1964). If the obliteration of a word by means of a heavy pencil mark may serve as a cue representative of past stuttering on a word, why should not the unobliterated word do so itself, to some extent? Hawkins and Brutten had subjects read a passage five times. For each subject they then embedded a number of stuttered words in a new passage. In the new reading the previously stuttered words produced adjacent stutterings not only horizontally, but also in other directions on the page. Horizontal adjacency was greater than vertical adjacency, and vertical greater than diagonal. In addition, more adjacency was produced by words that had been stuttered consistently and early in the previous readings than by words that had been stuttered late or only once.

Wong and Bloodstein (1977) tried to determine whether apparent departures from consistency in stuttering could be accounted for in part by an adjacency effect. It could not; they found little tendency for the new stutterings that occur in repeated readings to take place on words adjacent to those previously stuttered.

Consistency in Relation to Anticipation

One more piece of evidence was needed to close the frame of interlocking observations that Johnson and his associates marshalled in support of their conception of the moment of stuttering. If stutterings were distributed in a predictable, consistent fashion because they were responses to expectancies set off by identifiable cues, then it followed that the expectancies, too, must show a consistent distribution in repeated readings. Accordingly, Johnson and Ainsworth (1938) asked subjects to indicate in two silent inspections of the same material from two to six weeks apart the words on which they thought they would stutter if they were reading the material aloud. They found a marked tendency for anticipations to occur on the same words. Similar findings were later obtained by Peins (1961b).

A different but related question was raised by Skalbeck (1957), who found that words on which stuttering was expected were stuttered on more consistently than words on which it was not. Going a step further, Martin and Haroldson (1967) established that the stronger the subject's expectation of stutterings on a given word in a passage the more consistently the word will tend to be stuttered in successive oral readings.

The Attributes of Stuttered Words

In the stutterer's ordinary experience, colored borders or words blotted out in a reading passage do not often serve as cues for stuttering. The research we have considered so far showed clearly enough that stuttering was a response to cues, but gave little indication of the features of the speech sequence generally responsible for the consistent occurrence of stuttering in repeated oral readings or of why these and not other cues had come to be associated with past stutterings. This was the problem to which Johnson's colleague, Spencer F. Brown, turned his attention in a series of pioneering studies occupying a period of about ten years.

The question of precisely where stuttering occurs has at least two distinguishable aspects that are readily investigated—its locus within the word and the locus of the stuttered word in the larger context of speech. The first question has been of lesser concern to research workers because it is so easily answered. Over 90 percent of stutterings have been found to take place on the initial sound or syllable of the word.[4] They almost never occur on the last sound of a word. Stuttering is sometimes heard within the word, however—usually on accented syllables. Within polysyllabic words, accented syllables are more apt to be stuttered than unstressed ones.[5] That word accent exerts a distinctly secondary influence, however, was precisely demonstrated by Weiner (1984b). She compiled a list of two-syllable words, such as "contract," "address," or "permit," which can be accented on either syllable depending on meaning. Subjects pronounced each word twice with different meanings. Weiner found that 90 percent of the stutterings occurred on the first syllable, regardless of whether or not it was stressed. These results show with particular clarity the primacy of the word in stuttering. Although stutterers do at times have difficulty initiating syllables within words, stuttering in its developed form appears to be above all an incapacity to initiate words.

It was the problem of identifying the characteristics of stuttered words that presented a serious challenge. Brown approached this task with a number of hypotheses inspired by Johnson's anticipatory avoidance model of stuttering as well as by clinical observation. Some very definite predictions about the loci of stutterings are to be

---

[4]Johnson and Brown (1935), Hahn (1942b), Taylor (1966a), Sheehan (1974), Weiner (1984b).

[5]Brown (1938b), Hejna (1972), Sheehan (1974), Prins, Hubbard, and Krause (1991).

deduced from this model; namely, that the difficulty will occur whenever stutterers expect to have an interruption in their speech and are particularly anxious not to—consequently on those parts of the speech sequence that they evaluate as difficult or conspicuous. By 1945, on the basis of analysis of 10,000 words of oral reading by thirty-two adult stutterers, Brown was able to announce the confirmation of each of his hypotheses: There were four principal attributes of words that seemed to determine the loci of stuttered words in oral reading and that appeared to him to be sufficient to account for essentially all of them—the initial sound of the word, its grammatical function, its position in the sentence, and its length.

The Phonetic Factor

As early as 1935, Johnson and Brown had shown that for most stutterers the likelihood that they would block on a given word was strongly influenced by the sound with which it began. This was, however, an individual factor to a far greater degree than a group factor, the specific sounds which gave difficulty varying markedly from case to case. For stutterers as a group no one sound has as yet been established as giving appreciably more difficulty than any other. While ranks of difficulty for various sounds have sometimes been reported, there has as yet been only limited or qualified agreement on such rankings in various studies of the phonetic factor.[6] There is, however, one major group tendency on which almost all studies agree: For stutterers as a whole, initial consonants have been clearly shown to be more difficult than initial vowels.

Brown's observation that different sounds tend to occasion trouble for different stutterers lent itself readily to interpretation on the basis of the anticipatory avoidance concept since it would appear to follow from such a concept that it is the stutterer's attitude about the difficulty of a sound, rather than any inherent difficulty of the sound itself, that makes it likely that he or she will stutter on it. It is an interpretation that accords well with case history data suggesting that experiences of speech failure may instill in stutterers the conviction that they are unable to say certain specific words or sounds.[7] Further evidence of the part that attitudes and expectations play in the phonetic difficulties of stutterers comes from certain other observations. Words beginning with "ph" may be spoken fluently by some stutterers who

---

[6]See Johnson and Brown (1935), Brown (1938a), Hahn (1942b), Soderberg (1962a), Quarrington, Conway, and Siegel (1962), Taylor (1966a), Griggs and Still (1979), Jayaram (1983), Wells (1983).

[7]See Van Riper (1963) pp. 338–339. Connett (1955) attempted to increase the frequency of stuttering on the sound "t" by a discussion intended to foster the impression that it was a difficult sound, with equivocal results.

are unable to say the initial "f," while ph-words may offer difficulty to some stutterers who are able to say "f," but not words beginning with "p." One 15-year-old boy, when asked by the author if there were any sounds that gave him unusual trouble, replied, "The d-d-double-u sound. See, I couldn't say it just now." Another stutterer blocked fairly consistently on words beginning with "th," but generally not on initial "t" or "d," despite the fact that he spoke a substandard New York City dialect in which all "th" sounds were pronounced "t" or"d."

The group tendency of stutterers to have more trouble with initial consonants than initial vowels is not quite as easy to account for on an anticipatory struggle hypothesis. Brown (1938c) suggested that it was due in part to the greater importance of consonants for speech intelligibility, and hence meaning. Another possibility is that consonants are distinguished from vowels by a degree of stoppage or impedance of the airstream, involve a greater measure of articulatory tension, and consequently lend themselves more readily to the suggestion that they are difficult to say. Vowels are also fewer than consonants, and, as Taylor (1966b) has pointed out, are distributed with less "statistical uncertainty" (are easier to guess at when deleted in sentences) than consonants, and therefore carry less "information." The lesser importance of vowels for intelligibility, their lower articulatory complexity, and their smaller information value in written speech are all probably interrelated attributes; and together they probably serve to foster a folk attitude toward vowels perhaps best expressed by orthographies (e.g., Hebrew, Egyptian hieroglyphic), which either omit most vowels or represent them by means of diacritical marks.

Some findings by Uys (1970) on South African stutterers seem to show in a rather compelling way the importance of articulatory tension in producing the vowel consonant difference. Unlike English, Afrikaans is distinguished by a hard attack in the articulation of initial vowels. Uys compared Afrikaans-speaking and English-speaking stutterers in the reading of lists of words beginning with vowels and consonants. As usual, the English speakers stuttered more on initial consonants than vowels, but the Afrikaans speakers did not. The Afrikaans speakers stuttered on more initial vowels than the English speakers did. In short, when vowels were more like consonants in their manner of articulation the difference in the amounts of stuttering they produced disappeared.[8]

Whether or not this is the whole explanation, we must note that there are a certain number of stutterers who tend to have all or most of their difficulty on words beginning with vowels. Some workers take this as evidence that it is not so much the nature of consonants that usually makes them difficult as the kinds of evaluations the stutterer places on them.

---

[8]In Dutch, a language closely related to Afrikaans, Vaane and Janssen (1978) reported that vowels were among the most frequently stuttered sounds.

The Grammatical Factor

Brown discovered that most stuttering in oral reading took place on four principal parts of speech—nouns, verbs, adjectives, and adverbs—while far less difficulty was encountered on articles, prepositions, pronouns, and conjunctions. Studies by others have generally corroborated the finding that the blocks of adult stutterers occur chiefly on lexical, or content, words as opposed to function words, but have either failed to find or have failed to agree on any further ranking of difficulty of grammatical parts of speech.[9]

Brown and other proponents of the anticipatory struggle hypothesis have attributed the high frequency of stuttering on content words to the fact that these are the focal points in the stream of communication at which the meaning is most important, the speaker's emphasis is greatest, and the listener's interest is concentrated. It is here that the stutterer is therefore most likely to anticipate difficulty and to be anxious to avoid it. It may be said that the same facts would offer little difficulty to other theories of the moment of stuttering. The grammatical factor often appears to undergo a change during the course of development of stuttering, however, since many stuttering children in the earliest phase of the disorder have a considerable amount of difficulty on function words, especially pronouns and conjunctions. Whether all theories can explain this with equal readiness is a moot question. We will return to this subject in Chapter 9.

Word Position

There is more stuttering on the first word and in varying degrees on other early words of the sentence than on words in other positions.[10] Explanations that have been offered, again chiefly on the anticipatory struggle hypothesis, have stressed the conspicuousness of the beginning of the sentence. This is the point at which stutterers pass fairly noticeably from silence to speech, at which they renew their lease on the listener's attention, and at which they are therefore most likely to be conscious of themselves to some extent in their role as speakers. It is of interest that some stutterers have relatively few blocks once they

---

[9]See Brown (1937), Hahn (1942a), Eisenson and Horowitz (1945), Quarrington, Conway, and Siegel (1962), Danzger and Halpern (1973), Griggs and Still (1979), Wingate (1979). Soderberg (1967) found the grammatical factor operating within the body of the phonemic clause, but not in the initial position where many function words and pronouns were stuttered. Koopmans, Slis, and Rietveld (1991) made the same observation in a study of Dutch-speaking stutterers.

[10]Brown (1938b), Quarrington, Conway, and Siegel (1962), Quarrington (1965), Taylor (1966a), Griggs and Still (1979). Soderberg (1967) found this to be true in relation to phonemic clauses. Only Hannah and Gardner (1968), working in spontaneous speech, seem to have found conflicting results; they noted especially frequent stuttering in postverbal syntactic units.

have said the first few words of a conversation or have gotten past the first few words of a reading passage.

In apparent contradiction of past findings, Tornick and Bloodstein (1976) found essentially no tendency for the first few words of long sentences to contain proportionately more stuttering than the rest of the sentence. A plausible explanation is that each of the long sentences was constructed by adding a coordinate clause to a shorter sentence. The beginnings of constituent grammatical clauses may play a role in stuttering similar to that of the initial parts of sentences. Indeed, the position effect has been found in phrases (Taylor, 1966a), in phonemic clauses[11] (Soderberg, 1967), and even in random sequences of words (Conway and Quarrington, 1963) or in counting aloud (Borden, 1983). However, Klouda and Cooper (19878) did not find any tendency for subjects to stutter at the start of syntactic units when reading sentence pairs such as "When John leaves, Penelope will be upset," and "When John leaves Penelope, we'll be upset."

Word Length

Brown's fourth factor was word length. Longer words have been found, other things being equal, to occasion more stuttering than shorter ones.[12] Brown and Moren attributed this to the greater prominence of longer words. Long words are also, of course, inherently more difficult to articulate, are frequently evaluated as something of a challenge by stutterers and nonstutterers alike, and may be stuttered on more often because they readily evoke the threat of failure. The facts themselves unfortunately do not tell us whether it is the inherent complexity of longer words or the stutterer's evaluation of them as difficult that is primarily responsible for the increased likelihood of stuttering.

Summary Remarks and Interpretations

There is now a considerable body of evidence confirming the relationship Brown postulated to exist between the loci of stutterings and the four factors of initial sound, grammatical function, word position, and word length in oral reading. Furthermore, Hejna (1955) obtained essentially similar findings with regard to the spontaneous speech of stutterers. Trotter (1956) showed that not only the locus, but also the severity of the individual moment of stuttering, was related to the degree to which a word was characterized by these factors. Silverman

---

[11]Units of speech having only one primary stress and ending in a terminal juncture (Soderberg, 1967).

[12]Brown and Moren (1942), Soderberg (1966), Schlesinger, Melkman, and Levy (1966), Taylor (1966a), Wingate (1967b), Lanyon and Duprez (1970), Soderberg (1971), F. H. Silverman (1972), Danzger and Halpern (1973), Griggs and Still (1979). The Lanyon and Duprez study dealt with spontaneous speech.

and Williams (1967b) replicated some of Brown's basic work using alternative measures of disfluency and got the same results. Williams, Silverman, and Kools (1969b) found Brown's factors operating in the stuttering of children of elementary school age. (The early stuttering of preschool children seems to present a very different picture, however, as will become evident in Chapter 9.) Little work has been done on the subject in languages other than English, but Brown's factors were found in Norwegian by Preus and his co-workers (1970) and in Kannada by Jayaram (1981) and Venkatagiri (1982b).

As we will see shortly, there are still other attributes of words associated with the distribution of stutterings. Brown (1945), however, concluded that the likelihood of occurrence of stuttering was so highly related to the degree of presence of his four factors that any contribution made by others was small, and Taylor (1966a) found that most of the dependence of stuttering on types of words seemed to be accounted for by only three properties—the consonant-vowel difference, word position, and word length. It must be kept in mind, however, that these factors represent generalizations about groups of stutterers. Griggs and Still (1979) demonstrated that individual cases may show departures from them.

In trying to determine the meaning of Brown's four factors, a troublesome problem that has existed from the start is that of establishing to what extent these factors are independent of each other. In principle, for example, it would be possible for content words to produce more stuttering than function words largely because content words tend to be longer or because many function words begin with vowels. In the studies done since Brown's early work the kinds of controls that would permit better answers to such questions have been applied with increasing ingenuity. Taylor (1966a, 1966b) made a particularly comprehensive attack on this problem as it applies to the consonant-vowel, position, and length factors and found that all three were effective independently of each other, decreasing in influence on stuttering in the order given, with the consonant-vowel effect about twice as large as that of position and about seven times as great as that of length. As Taylor pointed out, the independent influence of the grammatical factor (content words vs. function words) has not yet been rigorously demonstrated. Evidence presented by Griggs and Still (1979) suggests, however, that it is independent of both the phonetic factor and word position.

Not only stutterings, but expectations of stuttering as well, have been found to occur in close relationship to Brown's four factors.[13]

---

[13]ee Skalbeck (1957). Also, in an early study Milisen (1937) found that stuttering was more frequently expected on longer words than on shorter ones and on the first word of the sentence, with the second, third, and fourth following in order.

This is consistent with an anticipatory struggle theory. As we have already noted, it is in this type of theory that the research on the loci of stutterings originated and in terms of which the findings have been most comprehensively interpreted. That is not to say, however, that others are not to be considered. The reader who tries to explain Brown's factors in accordance with the breakdown and the repressed need hypotheses will find that these are by no means totally lacking in the ability to account for them.

On the breakdown hypothesis one might reasonably predict the occurrence of stuttering whenever speech inherently requires more complex, precise, or difficult muscular adjustments, and also, as we must not forget, at any point in the speech sequence at which social or emotional stress is at a peak. Brown himself (1938c) undertook, for argument's sake, the most painstaking attempt to reconcile his findings with the viewpoint that stuttering is basically a physiological disorder. Perhaps the greatest difficulty such a viewpoint encounters is presented by the phonetic factor. The larger amount of stuttering on consonants than on vowels is as would be expected, and the difficulty with feared sounds could be explained fairly readily. But it might be supposed on the breakdown hypothesis that stutterers would also tend to have more difficulty as a group with certain specific consonants—those which are learned relatively late or which innately demand more complicated types of articulation. No such group tendency appears to exist.[14]

The repressed need hypothesis might lead us to expect stuttering to occur in large measure on words laden with aggressive or libidinal significance or having some relationship to the speaker's inner conflicts. Little research has been done to determine to what extent the distribution of stutterings is influenced by specific word meanings. Degree of meaningfulness of words as a whole, as measured by means of the semantic differential, does not appear to be conspicuously related to likelihood of stuttering.[15] Some of the facts we have reviewed about the loci of stutterings appear to be rather difficult to account for on the basis of the repressed need hypothesis.

Word Frequency

Since Brown completed his investigation of his four factors various others have been found or hypothesized. One of these which is well

---

[14]Fairbanks (1937), however, found some correlation between amount of stuttering on various speech sounds and certain measures of difficulty of sounds. He concluded, ". . . variations in physiological difficulty . . . may be a partial determinant of spasm distribution over the various sounds. The individual differences among stutterers are so large, however, that no single cause may be assigned."

[15]See Peterson (1969) and Peterson, Rieck, and Hoff (1969). Danzger and Halpern (1973) found no relationship between stuttering and ratings of abstractness of words.

documented is the frequency of occurrence of the word in the language. In general, the less frequently it occurs the greater the probability of stuttering on it.[16] The influence of this factor is independent of others we have mentioned, such as word length and grammatical function, and appears to occur in children as well as adults. No one to whom the other factors affecting the loci of stutterings seem comprehensible should have difficulty theorizing about possible reasons for this one. Perhaps it is worth noting that if we wanted to determine the influence of reading difficulty of words on stuttering we could hardly do it better than by studying the effect of word frequency.

Predictability of Words in Context (Information Load)

Other work on the loci of stutterings has been concerned with the factor of information value of words, in an information-theory sense. If contextual material is presented to a listener word by word, the listener will have varying degrees of success at guessing the next word from what has gone before. By using the guesses of a fairly large number of subjects, it is possible to obtain a reliable measure of the ease or difficulty with which each of the words in a given context may be predicted in sequence. Such a measure has an interesting and unique meaning. A word that is easily guessed from preceding words is relatively redundant; it adds little to what the listener already knows. A word difficult to guess, on the other hand, communicates by virtue of that fact a large amount of new information. In a highly special but useful sense, then, the predictability of words (also referred to as their statistical uncertainty or transition probability) is a measure of the information load or value they have in a given context.

In a series of independent studies it has been established that there is a degree of relationship between occurrence of stuttering and low predictability (i.e., high information value of words in oral reading).[17] This new factor may overlap considerably with those identified before. That is, there is evidence that content words, the initial position in the sentence, and perhaps the other factors associated with the loci of stutterings as well, are points of relatively high information value in language.[18] This tends to raise the question of the extent to which these factors are independent of word information in their effect on stuttering. No complete answer to this question can be given

---

[16]Hejna (1963), Schlesinger, Forte, Fried, and Melkman (1965), Schlesinger, Melkman, and Levy (1966), Soderberg (1966), Wingate (1967b), Danzger and Halpern (1973), Ronson (1976), Palen and Peterson (1982).

[17]Quarrington (1965), Schlesinger, Forte, Fried, and Melkman (1965), Soderberg (1967), Lanyon and Duprez (1970), Soderberg (1971) . Only Lanyon (1968) failed to find this in a study of three stutterers' spontaneous speech.

[18]The evidence is reviewed by Taylor (1966b).

at this writing. Quarrington (1965) showed that word position affects stuttering independently of, and more powerfully than, information value. Lanyon and Duprez (1970) found that in both spontaneous speech and oral reading stuttering was not related to information value when word length was held constant. Soderberg (1971), on the other hand, obtained evidence that both word length and information value influenced stuttering independently in oral reading.

Clearly related to information load is what Kaasin and Bjerkan (1982) were concerned with in their study of the influence of "critical words." As an example, subjects tended to stutter on "library" and "six o'clock" when conveying a message to meet there at that time.

Considerable speculation has been stirred by the relationship between information load and disfluency. This interest originally developed outside the field of speech pathology in the linguistic study of normal adult hesitation phenomena.[19] In the case of the normal phenomena the plausible inference has been drawn by linguists that hesitations occur at points of high uncertainty because the speaker is engaged in making lexical or grammatical decisions. The same reasoning may be applied to stuttering, a point of view that has been most clearly expressed by Taylor (1966b). A difficulty with the hypothesis of lexical uncertainty is that it implies a model of stuttering behavior that has not found favor among speech pathologists. It runs counter to the general clinical impression that when stutterers block on a word, they usually know very well, and often far in advance, what word they want to say and in fact tend to betray it when they stutter by repeating, prolonging, or silently mouthing the first sound of the word. Grammatical uncertainty is not a plausible explanation either, since stuttering so often occurs on the last word of a sentence or other syntactic unit.

Another interpretation is possible. When speakers come to a point of low predictability in the speech sequence, they are indeed at a point of high uncertainty as speakers. But there is an equal amount of uncertainty for the listener. It should be considered that what stutterers are reacting to when they stutter at that point may not be any type of uncertainty of their own as much as their knowledge that the listener is unable for the moment to guess what is coming next and that they, the speakers, bear alone what Eisenson has called the burden of "communicative responsibility." There are few reactions to the speech of persons who stutter more calculated to result in their stuttering than the response, "What did you say?" Conversely, it is often much easier for stutterers to tell a store clerk what they want once they have totally dispelled any possible listener uncertainty by pointing to it on the shelf.

---

[19]Lounsbury (1954), Goldman-Eisler (1958a, 1958b).

Linguistic Stress

Brown (1938b), in one of his pioneering series of studies on the loci of stutterings, noted a tendency for stuttering to occur on accented syllables of words, as we have seen. Brown did not include word accent among his four factors because it belongs to a syllable, and he was especially interested in the relationship of stuttering to properties of words (see Brown, 1945). Words differ, however, in the relative amount of stress they receive within the sentence, and Wingate (1976, 1979) speculated that this exerts an important influence on the distribution of stuttering.

From a study of the interaction of grammatical function and word position in oral reading, Wingate (1979) inferred that both owe their effect to linguistic stress. Analyzing the data of Brown (1937) on the grammatical factor, Wingate pointed out that words which received very little stress, namely, auxiliary verbs, infinitives, coordinating conjunctions, and possessive pronouns, were seldom stuttered. On the other hand, relative and personal pronouns and subordinating conjunctions, which are often stressed, were stuttered frequently, along with such other stressed words as main verbs, nouns, and adjectives. He suggested that the amount of stress that words receive may be more closely related to stuttering than is their formal designation as content or function words. In a subsequent study Wingate (1984b) found that occurrences of stuttering during oral reading of a passage corresponded closely to stress peaks recorded in a reading of the passage by a nonstutterer. Klouda and Cooper (1988) obtained similar findings in a study of stutterers' oral reading of sentences. Further confirmation came from an investigation of German-speaking stutterers by Bergmann (1986) in which subjects read the same sentence, e. g., "Mr. Vogt is cleaning the car," in response to two different questions: "Who is cleaning the car?" and "What is Mr. Vogt doing to the car?"

Explanations of the influence of linguistic stress are not far to seek. The simplest and most plausible, perhaps, is Brown's original conjecture that words that are prominent or conspicuous are most likely to be stuttered.

The Question of Phonatory Transitions

In Chapter 4 we reviewed a considerable amount of research on the voice initiation times of stutterers that stemmed from the belief that the larynx might have a critical role to play in stuttering. The same interest led Adams and Reis (1971) to raise the question whether stuttering is frequently associated with the necessity to initiate phonation during speech. They found that in five repeated readings of a passage consisting entirely of voiced sounds, subjects stuttered less than in repeated readings of an ordinary passage in which transitions from voiceless to voiced sounds were required. They also reported that more than a third of the stutterings were associated with such transitions or with the beginning of a new phrase or sentence.

In actuality the difference between the passages in frequency of stuttering was not evident on the first reading, but only appeared subsequent to it. In a later replication of their study Adams and Reis (1974) confirmed this; in their second study there was no difference until the fourth reading. They concluded that the need for rapid shifts from voiceless to voiced sounds served mainly to slow down the subjects' rate of adaptation to the passage.[20] Controversy developed when Young (1975a) applied a different method of analysis to the data of both studies and reported no significant effect on either frequency of stuttering or adaptation. Adams and Reis (1975) argued in defense of their findings, and Adams, Riemenschneider, Metz, and Conture (1975) presented additional evidence showing that there was more adaptation in an all-voiced passage. Later studies by Hutchinson and Brown (1978) and Runyan and Bonifant (1981) verified the fact that an all-voiced passage produces no change in frequency of stuttering in a single reading. In response Reis and Adams (1978) contended that the effect is not strong enough to show itself except after repeated readings. McGee, Hutchinson, and Deputy (1981), however, found no significant difference in either initial frequency or adaptation of stuttering between the all-voiced and comparison passages, though they noted a slight trend toward more adaptation on the all voiced passage.

Some other work touched more directly on the influence of phonatory transitions on the loci of stutterings. Manning and Coufal (1976) found that significantly more stuttering occurred during voiced-voiced transitions in oral reading than during voiceless-voiceless, voiceless-voiced, or voiced-voiceless. In a study of oral reading of forty-eight Dutch stutterers aged thirteen to sixteen years, Vaane and Janssen (1978) found no differences in the distribution of stuttering among the four types of phonatory transitions.

At the present writing the evidence that voice initiations in the speech sequence are especially likely to be loci of stuttering does not appear strong.

Cycles and Clustering

Finally we may note two hypotheses about the loci of stutterings that relate to temporal factors. Neither Pittenger (1940) nor Taylor and Taylor (1967) was able to find any evidence of a tendency for stuttering during oral reading to appear in periodic waves or cycles. The

---

[20]The adaptation effect is the tendency of stuttering to decrease in frequency with successive readings of the same material. We will consider it in detail later in Chapter 8.

second factor is clustering. Fein (1970) observed a tendency for stuttered words to be followed immediately by more blocks. We might expect this if the block had a stimulus value for the stutterer. Taylor and Taylor (1967), however, found no evidence of any such clustering of stuttered words. Results obtained by Still and Griggs (1979) suggest that the probability of stuttering is highest on the words immediately following a block. In 2 of their 6 subjects, however, there was first an opposite tendency, as though getting through a block conferred immunity to stuttering over the next few words.

Congruity Between Subjects—The Power of Individual Factors

We have just surveyed essentially everything we know at this writing about the reasons why stutterings occur precisely where they do in the speech sequence. What does this knowledge amount to? How well, let us say, could we predict the words on which an individual stutterer would have difficulty in reading a passage from our knowledge of the factors that we have found to influence the loci of stutterings? If we think about this something notable about these factors will soon appear. With the sole exception of the individual aspect of the phonetic factor, they are all group factors. They tell us nothing about the reasons why one person might differ from another with respect to words stuttered. To imagine that these factors would help us to predict the distribution of stutterings in an individual case, then, is to assume that this distribution is much the same from stutterer to stutterer. Is this the case?

The answer is that it is not. Hendel and Bloodstein (1973) compared the distribution of stutterings of 17 male stutterers in the reading of the same passage. On the average, 18 percent of the words stuttered by one subject were also stuttered by another. By chance alone this would have been 11 percent, so in a small measure group factors did influence the loci of their stutterings. Yet the consistency of each stutterer with himself in reading the passage again was, on the average, 48 percent. To that extent the same stimuli were operating for the average subject in both readings. To cause that much consistency these must have been largely stimuli that differed from those of the next subject. Individual factors evidently played a much larger part in the stuttering of these subjects than did group factors.

We can only infer that the various factors we have been discussing would not help us very much to predict the occurrence of stuttering in an individual case. They represent only some broad generalizations that are useful in refining our theories about stuttering. In the final analysis the loci of stutterings seem to have their main source in each stutterer's individual history of learning experiences.

We have relatively little laboratory-based information about what such individual factors might be. Clinical experience, however, suggests that a very important role is played in stuttering by specific words and sounds that vary from case to case. We have already mentioned the individual factor of phonetic difficulty, for which essentially our only source is the early study by Johnson and Brown (1935). There has been equally little study of the individual word factor. Van Riper (1972, pp. 269, 270) contributed some clinical observations suggesting that difficulties with words may arise from memories of past failure or penalty for stuttering on them. In addition, some light was shed on the potency of this factor in a study by Hamre and Wingate (1973).

Hamre and Wingate found that of the words on which subjects stuttered in a word association task 36 percent were later stuttered again when the subjects were asked to construct sentences using these words. They interpreted this as a small amount of consistency, but it must be evaluated in relation to the conditions under which it was observed. Stimuli tend to be discriminated in relation to their total contexts. It is a commonplace of clinical experience that stutterers can often avoid stuttering on some of their most difficult words simply by changing the position of the words in the same sentence. To find, then, that more than a third of the stuttered words were stuttered again in new sentences, in different tasks, on different occasions, appears to argue that the word, in and of itself, is a relatively powerful stimulus for stuttering. It may be that in the aggregate difficult words and sounds, together with all those group factors that have some influence on stuttering, go far to account for the amount of stimulus control that we see reflected in the consistency effect.

THE FREQUENCY OF STUTTERING

In considering the effect of varying conditions on the frequency of moments of stuttering we are in a sense simply extending our discussion of the basic questions with which we have been dealing. Just as stutterers do not typically block on every word in the speech sequence, they do not usually stutter in every speech situation. For very many persons there is a consistency about the conditions under which they have difficulty, suggesting that not only words and sounds, but listeners, situations, and physical environments as well may serve as cues that are capable of precipitating stuttering.

Of the observations that have been made on the subject of variations in stuttering, most by far are directly concerned with the conditions under which it diminishes or disappears. These conditions are quite numerous. Relatively speaking, it has been possible so far to submit only a small proportion of them to objective laboratory study. Consequently, we will supplement our review of laboratory findings with the results of an investigation (Bloodstein, 1950a, 1950b) that used interviews and questionnaires to study the conditions under which stuttering is reduced or absent. The observations to be reported are derived from the interviews and questionnaires used unless otherwise noted.

In that study some 115 "conditions" were described under which fairly large proportions of subjects believed that their stuttering was either absent or substantially reduced. Considerable individual variation was evident; few of these conditions produced decreases in stuttering for all subjects, by their report. Much of this variation is an artifact resulting simply from the fact that there are no definable absolute limits to what is meant by a "condition" in the context of this type of inquiry. "Speaking to your mother" is likely to represent many different conditions for different stutterers or for the same stutterer on different occasions. Even the most elaborately described conditions therefore remain abstractions that subsume innumerable others, and it is impossible either to count them or to make unqualified statements about their effects on stuttering.

The usefulness of a large number of observations of the conditions under which stuttering varies in frequency consists of the challenge they present to us to abstract their essential features and reduce them to a relatively small number of conditions of broad generality. Some of the conditions we will deal with will be more general than others. As a result they will be more abstract, hypothetical, and in some cases controversial.

Communicative Pressure

An extremely large part of what we know about the way stuttering varies in frequency can be generalized by saying that it is affected by communicative pressures. These are of many kinds, and may come from the form or content of the stutterer's message, the listener, the situation, or the nature of the social interaction.

Communicative Responsibility

The observation that frequency of stuttering seems to be related to the extent to which the stutterer is using speech to convey information to a listener has been given particular emphasis by Eisenson. Degree of communicative responsibility is itself related to a number of different kinds of variables. One of the most important of these is the meaningfulness or "propositionality" of speech. Eisenson and Horowitz (1945) found considerably more stuttering on words in a meaningful reading selection than on the same words presented in the form of a list or in a nonsense passage, and stutterers may report that they can speak words as words (i.e., when playing word games or when explaining what words "always" give them trouble). Bardrick and Sheehan found a decrease in stuttering when subjects read numbers (see

Sheehan, 1958a). Some conflicting evidence came from a study by Hegde (1970) in which ten stutterers had as much difficulty when reading a 150-word passage composed of nonsense words as in reading a meaningful paragraph.

Swearing, singing, and counting are other examples of relatively nonpropositional speech in which stuttering rarely occurs. For many stutterers there is little difficulty with the conventional verbal gestures of greeting and leave taking, commenting on the weather, or saying something "just to keep the conversation going." Stuttering may also be reduced in recitation of memorized material.

Besides reduced propositionality of speech, there are certain other variables that may serve in obvious ways to decrease communicative responsibility. Some are related to the nature of the listener. The common examples are talking to an infant or to an animal, both among the easiest of speaking situations for most stutterers. Finally, communicative responsibility may be affected by the nature of the circumstances. We have already noted that the stutterer may block severely when required to repeat something the listener has failed to "catch." Conversely, there are many conditions under which stuttering appears to be reduced essentially because the listener already knows what the stutterer is going to say; the message is redundant. Stutterers often report that they can make purchases fluently if they give the clerk their shopping list, or that they can ask for a book in the library once the person at the desk has seen the call slip, or that they can say a difficult word easily once they have spelled it aloud. It may be in part for the same reason that stutterers usually seem to be able to pronounce a word on which they are blocked if the listener supplies it. Burke (1975) noted that many stutterers could repeat sentences fluently from dictation. Stutterers can generally repeat a word without difficulty immediately after getting over a block on it.

A different type of circumstance whose effects have often been attributed to reduced communicative responsibility is chorus reading. The well-known fact that most stutterers can read fluently in unison with another person, whether a stutterer or a nonstutterer, was confirmed experimentally by Johnson and Rosen (1937). Barber (1939) found that chorus reading was decidedly more effective than reading together with others who were reading different material or in the presence of mere vocal or mechanical noise. Eisenson and Wells (1942) noted some tendency for stutterings to increase in the chorus reading situation when subjects read into a microphone by means of which they were told they would be heard individually by an audience in another room. Eisenson and Wells inferred that the reason for stutterers' fluency in chorus reading was a reduction in their responsibility for communication. On the other hand, Pattie and Knight (1944) found that in chorus reading before a small audience the accompaniment was just as effective when it was conveyed to the subject by telephone as when the accompanying reader was present in the room. They concluded that the chorus reading situation was comparable to that in which the stutterer reads in time to a metronome, the accompaniment acting as a "pacemaker."

On the whole, oral reading evokes less stuttering than self-formulated speech, as Young (1980) showed, and this too is easily imputed to a reduction of communicative responsibility. Whatever factor is at work, however, it may be outweighed by others, since some stutterers have most or all of their difficulty in oral reading.

Time Pressure

A familiar form of communicative pressure apt to have a marked effect on stuttering is time pressure. It is a common clinical observation that stutterers tend to have more trouble when they feel hurried. In a laboratory study Johnson and Rosen (1937) found that stuttering, increased when subjects were instructed to speak more rapidly.[21] There was frequently little actual increase in reading rate. Goss (1952) found that when the time interval between exposure of a word and the signal to say it was very short (less than 2 seconds) the likelihood of stuttering increased.

Difficulty of the Motor Plan

Another type of communicative pressure results when speech is made formidable by heavy demands on motor planning. Frick (1965) pointed out the relevance of motor planning to stuttering. Wingate (1967b) suggested that it helps to explain why stutterers tend to have more difficulty on long words than on short words or on unfamiliar words—that is, words of low frequency of occurrence in the language. The effect of reading difficulty of the material is no doubt a reflection of the same facts. Making use of graded reading material, Blood and Hood (1978) observed that the stuttering of school-age subjects tended to increase as the material varied in difficulty from one grade below to three grades above the readers' age levels.

Reduced demands on motor planning probably have much to do with the fact that stutterers tend to speak fluently when they use a slow rate of speech. They also generally have less difficulty in saying a series of isolated words than when speaking in phrases and sentences (Brown, 1938a), and appear to read paragraph material more fluently when they pronounce it word by word (Adams, Lewis, and

---

[21]Young (1974) failed to confirm this, but instructions to speak rapidly tended to increase the frequency of stuttering in a study by Kalinowski, Armson, Roland-Mieszkowski, Stuart, and Gracco (1993).

Besozzi, 1973). There is rarely any difficulty at all in saying speech sounds or isolated syllables of words. Furthermore, it may be of interest from this point of view that when a difficult word is pronounced "for" stutterers—that is, when they are presumably making use of auditory assistance in their motor planning of the word, they can often say it fluently. As we have seen, they also tend to be able to say a stuttered word fluently after one or more successive pronunciations of it on their own. Silverman and Williams (1972a) had stutterers repeat a stuttered word 180 times. Most of them quickly became fluent, though they then tended to have alternating periods of stuttering and fluency.

Stuttering also appears to be influenced by the length and complexity of sentences. Tornick and Bloodstein (1976) found that less stuttering occurred in the reading of a short sentence (e.g., "She learned to swim") when it stood alone than when it was made the initial part of a longer sentence (e.g., "She learned to swim in the clear water of the lake"). Jayaram (1984) confirmed this effect in both English and Kannada speakers and found in addition that when the short sentence was made the end of a longer sentence rather than the beginning, it occasioned not more but less stuttering than when it stood alone. It is evidently not length or complexity per se that is the potent factor, but the anticipation of and planning for it.

Postma and Kolk (1990) found that "tongue twisters" produced more stuttering, but instructions stressing accuracy in the repetition of sentences had no effect.

Wells (1979) examined six sentences containing only one relative clause and six sentences with two relative clauses from the recorded spontaneous speech of each of a group of stutterers. A higher percentage of stuttered syllables was found on the more complex sentences. Ronson (1975), however, found no differences in stuttering in the reading of simple, active, affirmative, declarative sentences, negative sentences, and passive sentences by adult subjects. In a similar study with 8- to 12-year-old children, on the other hand, Palen and Peterson (1982) reported a trend for severe stutterers to have more difficulty in the oral reading of sentences as the level of transformational processing increased. In studies of types of sentences in relation to stuttering it is difficult to separate syntactic complexity from motor planning difficulty, since sentences that contain more complex language are inevitably longer. The use of oral reading, however, would seem to minimize complexity on the level of purely linguistic formulation.

In sum, essentially any kind of speech whose automatic serial ordering is easier is likely to occasion less stuttering. Healey, Mallard, and Adams (1976) found more fluency in the oral reading of song lyrics with which stutterers were highly familiar than in the reading of unfamiliar lyrics. As we will see later, the simplification of motor planning may also have something to do with the much-discussed adaptation and metronome effects.

Listener Reactions to Stuttering

Stuttering often appears to vary with social pressures in the form of unfavorable listener reactions, or what the stutterer perceives as social penalties for stuttering. Porter (1939) showed that the amount of difficulty subjects experienced in reading to various listeners was consistent with their previous evaluations of the listeners as "hard" or "easy" to talk to, and Berwick (1955) found that this extended even to a situation in which the stutterer read to photographs of such listeners. It is evident that listeners or cues representative of them may become capable of consistently evoking stuttering. This raises the question of whether there are any definable features of the listeners that tend to make them "hard" or "easy" for stutterers as a group. Comments of adult subjects appear to indicate that one important feature of this kind is the listener's reactions to the stutterer's speech difficulty. Generally speaking, the stutterer in an advanced phase of the disorder has more difficulty when noting or expecting reactions of impatience, embarrassment, pity, shock, or the like in the behavior of the listener. In contrast, a close friend who no longer appears to notice the stuttering may be quite easy to talk to; so, in some cases, may a stranger who is not expecting the person to block.

Stutterers' comments about the amount of difficulty experienced in speaking to their parents are often revealing. Parents characterized as easy to speak to are often described as easygoing, understanding, or the like. On the other hand, those with whom there is a great deal of stuttering tend to be described as distressed, critical, or impatient. One stutterer who found it difficult to talk to his mother said, "When I go into a block she goes into it with me." Another said about his father, "I seem to feel that when I talk to him I must choose my words carefully." In general, it may be said that stutterers typically have less difficulty to the extent that their listeners appear to be accepting them as individuals rather than reacting to them as stutterers.

An experimental study of the effect of listener reactions on stuttering in an audience situation was reported by Hansen (1956). By actuating appropriate lights and counters of the Wisconsin Sequential Sampling Analyzer, Hansen presented stutterers with what they believed to be a quantitative measure of the reactions of their audience from moment to moment as they spoke or read. When unfavorable audience reactions were presented during intervals of speech difficulty, the stuttering seemed to increase. To a lesser extent, favorable reactions during fluent periods appeared to result in a decrease in stuttering.

Concern About Social Approval

Communication is a social act. Communicative pressure is increased when the speaker is ill at ease, feels inferior, or expects social disapproval or rejection. Under such conditions stuttering is liable to be intensified.

One of the outstanding examples is speaking to a person whom the stutterer perceives as important, superior, or in a position of authority. Sheehan, Hadley, and Gould (1967) showed that college stutterers had more speech difficulty when speaking to faculty members dressed in suit or sport jacket and tie and addressed by the title of "Doctor" than they did in speaking to students dressed in sports shirts without jacket or tie and introduced only as "Tom Brown" or the like. They concluded that the lower the speaker's self-esteem, or the more authority-laden the listener's status, the greater the amount of stuttering.

Conversely, there is likely to be less speech difficulty when stutterers have reason to be confident about their status. They usually report that they tend to speak more fluently with people who are younger or who are in some measure subservient to them. Ramig, Krieger, and Adams (1982) verified the observation that stutterers generally have less difficulty with children than adults. Officers who stutter are often able to give orders fluently to soldiers they command, and in varying degrees this may apply to a foreman in a factory, an overseer of hired help on a farm, or even a monitor at school. One stutterer when interviewed was experiencing a marked reduction of stuttering that he attributed to the wearing of a pair of hunting boots. His explanation was that they had virtually "the same feel" as the paratroop boots he had worn for four months in an airborne unit in the Army two years earlier during World War II. During those four months he had had very little difficulty with his speech "partially, I suppose, because other people didn't do things such as jumping out of an airplane." Soon after his return to civilian life his stuttering became more severe, but about a month or two later he noticed that whenever he wore his hunting boots he spoke more fluently.

Speaking to members of the opposite sex represents a different type of circumstance in which concern about the listener's approval often appears to result in considerable stuttering. On the other hand, stutterers are sometimes encountered who almost never block or have any tendency to do so when on dates, and it is interesting to note in such cases that the person frequently has a history of success in social situations of this type, is confident of his or her ability to impress the opposite sex, and seems, in general, to be gifted with ease and assurance in such situations. An attractive young female subject accounted for her fluency when speaking to members of the opposite sex by explaining that she felt "more free to speak" with men than with women.

There are still other conditions that illustrate the manner in which stuttering may be related to desire for approval. The difficulty of the audience situation for most stutterers is an example about which we will say more shortly. For some stutterers speaking to a stranger appears to be an easy speech situation; they become relatively unconcerned about the listener's approval, feeling that they are unlikely to meet the person again. Stutterers also frequently explain the favorable effect of alcoholic intoxication on their speech in this way. One subject commented, "You don't care if you stutter or what you do."

Audience Size

Stuttering tends to increase when there is more than one listener and apparently becomes radically reduced when no listener is present. There can hardly be any better example of the effect of communicative pressure. As audience size increases so does communicative responsibility, the threat of unfavorable listener reactions to stuttering, and concern about social approval.

Increases in stuttering in audience situations have been observed in a series of studies.[22] Porter (1939) found that frequency of stuttering increased progressively with audience sizes of 1, 2, 4, and 8 listeners, although the difference between 4 and 8 listeners was small and not significant (see Figure 9). Only Young (1965) obtained findings to the contrary. He arranged a series of oral reading conditions in such a way that the subjects had no way of anticipating beforehand how many listeners there would be, with the startling result that variations in audience size had essentially no effect on stuttering.

Reports by stutterers that their difficulty is very markedly reduced when they are alone have also been confirmed repeatedly.[23] The usual procedure in these studies has been to monitor stuttering by means of a concealed listener or microphone, after instructing subjects to check their own stuttered words in order to preserve the impression that hey were not being observed. Bergmann (1987) observed a marked reduction in stuttering when subjects' reading was recorded in a sound-isolated booth without direct contact with the experimenter. Martin and Haroldson (1988) even found some reduction in stuttering when they had subjects engage in monologue, apparently with no effort to convince them that they were alone. In an experiment by Hood (1975) stutterers were found to speak more fluently in the presence of a person whose hearing was masked and whose eyes were

---

[22]Steer and Johnson (1936), Porter (1939), Hahn (1940), Dixon (1955), Shulman (1955), Van Riper and Hull (1955), Siegel and Haugen (1964), Commodore (1980).

[23]Steer and Johnson (1936), Porter (1939), Hahn (1940), Razdolsky (1965), Quinn (1971), Sváb, Gross, and Langová (1972), Langová and Sváb (1973).

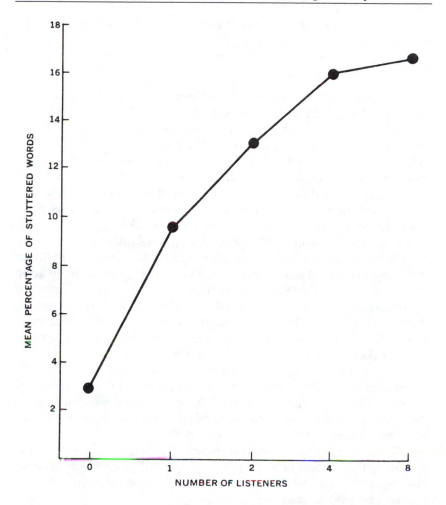

Figure 9. Mean percentage of Stuttering of thirteen stuttnerers in oral reading to vary-ing numbers of listeners. Plotted from data of Porter. Copyright 1939 by the American Speech-Language-Hearing Association. Reprinted by permission.

blindfolded than in the presence of someone who could see and hear them. Being heard alone evoked more stuttering than did just being seen. That there is any stuttering at all when stutterers are alone is perhaps due in part to the fact that they may serve to some extent as their own critical listeners. Some stutterers say that they have no blocks whatever if they are absolutely sure they are alone, but that they may stutter if they hear a footstep down the hall, or if they talk "as though" to a listener, or even if they think, "If somebody were listening to me I would be stuttering."[24]

The Factor of Attention

Another statement of very broad generality that we can make about the frequency of stuttering is that it tends to vary with the amount of attention stutterers give to their speech, the cues that evoke stuttering, their role as speakers, or their self-concept as stutterers. When they forget that they are stutterers—for example, when acting in a play or in some cases when talking to total strangers—they may have little or no difficulty with speech. One stutterer commented that if a teacher called on him unexpectedly for a response it was often possible for him to say three or four sentences fluently until it suddenly "dawned" on him and he would begin to stutter.

On the other hand, if the total stranger with whom the stutterer is talking fluently should turn out at some point in the conversation to be a speech pathologist, there is liable to be an abrupt recurrence of stuttering. As we have seen, there is likely to be a sharp increase in difficulty if we fail to hear the initial message and ask the stutterer to repeat it. We have made the person more conscious of his or her role as a speaker. Similarly, stutterers are apt to have exceptional trouble on the telephone, which reduces a person to a voice. Maddox (1938) found that blocks increased in oral reading when stutterers observed themselves in a mirror. Van Riper (1937c) reported more stuttering on words dictated to subjects by stutterers than on words dictated by nonstutterers.

There is an almost endless number of examples of reduction in stuttering that appear to be due to displacement of attention, or what has generally been called "distraction." It is possible to group them into several well-defined categories.

Novel Modes of Speaking

Virtually any change that can be made in the way a person normally talks is apt to result in much improved or essentially fluent speech for the majority of stutterers, provided the change does not lose its novelty.[25] Such changes include singing, speaking in a sing-song or with other unusual inflectional patterns, speaking in a monotone, whispering,

---

[24]See Bluemel (1935, p. 86) and Blanton and Blamon (1936, p. 79).

[25]Novel speech patterns may fail to work if they are used repeatedly. One stutterer, newly arrived in New York City from a small town in the Midwest and anticipating an exceptional amount of difficulty speaking, adopted the habit of talking in a Texas "drawl" and spoke quite fluently for about a month in this way. He began to stutter again, however, as soon as the drawl became an accustomed manner of speaking.

shouting, using an abnormally high pitch or an abnormally low pitch, adopting an unusual voice quality, speaking with exaggerated articulatory movements or with "slurred" articulation, with objects in the mouth, at a slow rate, on inspiration of air, with altered breathing, or in time to rhythmical movements such as those of a metronome. Perhaps the only important exception is rapid speech which, as we have seen, may be a source of speech pressure for many stutterers as they try to "get their words out" hastily before impatient listeners. Garber and Martin (1977) found no reduction in stuttering when subjects increased their vocal intensity. Shouting, however, has often been observed to result in more fluency.

There are many other examples of the immediate effectiveness of a change in speech pattern. Stutterers can often speak fluently when they imitate a foreign dialect, impersonate someone else, speak in a declamatory manner on the stage, or adopt an unaccustomed manner of behavior—for example, clowning, assertiveness, or the like. Cherry and Sayers (1956) found that many stutterers spoke fluently while "shadowing" or concurrently repeating another person's speech, and this was confirmed by Kondas (1971), Healey and Howe (1987), and others. Dixon (1957) obtained a reduction in stuttering in oral reading by having subjects shout "Hey!" at the beginning of each sentence. In studies by Ingham, Montgomery, and Ulliana (1983) and Gow and Ingham (1992), stuttering was reduced by instructions, aided by visual and auditory feedback, to vary the frequency of intervals of phonation of prescribed durations. Stutterers who underwent laryngectomies and did not stutter when they learned to use esophageal speech have been mentioned by various writers, along with some counterexamples of stuttering that persisted after laryngectomy.[26]

A number of the effects we have mentioned have been the subjects of experimental investigations. Johnson and Rosen (1937) demonstrated the effects of singing, whispering, choral speaking, and changes in rate, pitch, loudness, and inflection. Other studies have been done on whispering,[27] singing,[28] high and low pitch,[29] reduction of speaking rate,[30] and the use of a monotone.[31] Speaking in time to a

---

[26]Irving and Webb (1961), Doms and Lissens (1973), Wingate (1981a), Rosenfield and Freeman (1983).

[27]Witt (1925), May and Hackwood (1968), Perkins, Rudas, Johnson, and Bell (1976), Commodore and Cooper (1978), Commodore (1980).

[28]Witt (1925), Wiechmann and Richter (1966), Healey, Mallard, and Adams (1976), Colcord and Adams (1979), Wingate (1981b).

[29]Ramig and Adams (1980, 1981).

[30]Ingham, Martin, and Kuhl (1974), Perkins, Bell, Johnson, and Stocks (1979).

[31]Adams, Sears, and Ramig (1982).

metronome has also been repeatedly investigated, as will be seen in Chapter 8. Perkins, Bell, Johnson, and Stocks (1979) found that reducing reading rate by pausing between words reduced stuttering, but doing so by prolonging the sounds in each syllable reduced stuttering far more. Healey, Mallard, and Adams (1976) showed that fluency in singing was not due merely to familiarity with the lyrics. Several studies have attempted to pursue a suggestion by Wingate (1969, 1981b) that the chorus reading effect in stuttering results from changes in the vocal pattern. Ingham and Carroll (1977) and Ingham and Packman (1979) reported that the nonstuttered speech of stutterers in solo and chorus reading could not always be differentiated by listeners. Adams and Ramig (1980) found decreased vowel durations in the chorus reading of stutterers. By controlling subjects' reading rates, Ingham and Packman (1979) showed that the chorus reading effect could not be attributed simply to reduced rate.

The assumption that the novelty of the speech patterns we have been discussing is the chief reason for their effectiveness is based in part on the fact that practically any alteration in speech seems capable of producing fluency. Although the best evidence that the effect of a mode of speech is due to its novelty is probably its failure to be of help after prolonged use, there is little reliable evidence of this kind outside of clinical experience, since it is essentially impossible to devise a satisfactory laboratory analogue of prolonged use. As is true of so many other reductions of stuttering, moreover, some of these are attributable and may indeed be due to more than one factor. Some speech patterns, such as speaking slowly, make reduced demands on motor planning, as we have already seen. Others are probably incompatible with stuttering behavior on the level of sheer execution of speech movements; examples are legato speech, speaking with gentle phonatory onsets, using soft articulatory contacts, or initiating airflow before speech attempts.

In addition, Wingate (1969, 1970) offered the view that many such reductions in stuttering result specifically from altered vocalization and prosody. In a study of the speech patterns of three stutterers under a large number of fluency-inducing conditions, Andrews, Howie, Dozsa, and Guitar (1982) searched for temporal characteristics (e.g., speech rate, articulation rate, duration of phonation) common to all of them, but could find none. Wingate (1981b) studied the speech of four subjects in shadowing, singing, speaking in time to rhythm, and unison speaking. Qualitative analysis of spectrograms seemed to show some common features, chiefly reduced vocal inflection and concentration of energy in the lower harmonics.

Although other factors besides novelty may thus account for a part of the fluency produced by certain altered speech patterns, these factors can play a part in only a relatively small number of them. The best explanation is one that will help us understand why almost any and all unaccustomed ways of speaking, even imitation of the normal speech of another person, will cause an abrupt decrease in stuttering in most cases. The only explanation of this kind that has ever been offered is the novelty of the pattern.

That such novelty in itself can be the cause of fluent speech implies that some type of distraction of attention is operating. Generally, the stutterer's attention has been thought to be distracted from speech or stuttering. It is well to consider that if novel speech mannerisms owe their effect to distraction it can hardly be because of the very small amount of attention it takes to talk in a high pitch, in a foreign accent, or in time to rhythm, or the like. It seems far more likely that the interference with stuttering comes mainly from the impression stutterers receive from hearing themselves talk in a strange way and from awareness of the strange impression they are making on others. The same effect is to be seen in the adolescent boy who distracts himself from a feeling of social inadequacy by clowning. To change one's voice or speech is to assume a masquerade so extravagant that for most people it serves to hide for a moment the person they feel themselves to be. In short, it is perhaps not so much the difference in their speech that makes stutterers fluent as much as the perception that they are speaking differently.[32] This masquerade effect may be glimpsed with particular clarity in a report of Scripture (1931, p. 60) about a stutterer who was unable to dictate to his stenographer. Finding that his client was almost totally lacking in musical ability or a singing voice, Scripture advised him to sing what he wanted to dictate. This he was able to do without the slightest stuttering, in what he supposed was a singing voice. As long as he thought he was singing he spoke fluently, in a voice that did not differ from his ordinary one except that it was slightly easier and more natural. The treatment did not succeed because he refused to make a fool of himself by singing to his stenographer.

Associated Activity

A second category of reductions in stuttering which seem to be attributable to distraction includes associated physical activities of various kinds. For example, there may be little stuttering when speech is accompanied by dancing, piano playing, or swimming or when the stutterer is demonstrating how to play a musical instrument or operate a machine. Geniesse (1935) reported a laboratory investiga-

---

[32]In Chapter 8 we will encounter further evidence of this effect in the observation that essentially any change in auditory speech feedback that causes stutterers to hear themselves in a strange way appears to reduce stuttering.

tion showing that stutterers tended to be able to speak fluently while walking on all fours. In a study by Arends, Povel, and Kolk (1988), stuttering was significantly reduced when subjects spoke while engaged in a manual tracking task that consisted of keeping a dot on a screen within a moving square.

The effectiveness of some of these conditions appears to stem from the fact that stutterers are able to time their word attempts with part of the action. For example, a stutterer reported that while playing the piano he avoided stuttering by striking the keys when he was about to block. When every syllable of speech is timed with a rhythmical activity—for example, with walking or periodic movements of the arm, hand, or foot—there is particularly little probability that stuttering will occur, as Barber (1940) demonstrated experimentally. The only stutterer ever seen by the author who had blocks when talking in time to a rhythmic swing of the arm was a person who had been trained to do this at a "stammering school."

Emotional Arousal

Stuttering is likely to be reduced or absent under conditions that generate motivation, excitement, or emotion so strong as to make stutterers "forget themselves." Stutterers may be able to express themselves fluently when angry or when carried away by enthusiasm. It is particularly instructive that they often tend to speak well under conditions of fear. One stutterer said that during World War II his speech had been good enough for him to do mortar communications work, but only in the heat of combat. Another said that as a navigator on a heavy bomber he had never stuttered when there was doubt about whether they would get back to their base. Even stage fright is occasionally mentioned by stutterers as a condition that eliminates stuttering. A commonplace example of distraction through emotional arousal may be glimpsed in the following dialogue between a rehabilitation counselor and a young woman with a stuttering problem.

Counselor: How do you feel about drugs?

Client: (stuttering) I wouldn't have anything to do with them.

Counselor: Why not?

Client: (stuttering) Well, just because everybody else takes drugs doesn't mean I have to.

Counselor: Is that the only reason?

Client: (stuttering) They're no good. They can kill you.

Counselor: You know that, because your sister died of an overdose.

Client: (fluent for the first time in the interview) *How did you know that?*

Intense or Unusual Stimuli

A variety of sensory stimuli appear to be capable of reducing stuttering. Among examples reported by stutterers are severe pain and extreme fatigue.[33] The use of drugs producing narcosis, anesthesia, sedation, vasoconstriction, and other effects have all been observed clinically to remove stuttering in certain instances.[34] Hyperventilation caused a drop in stuttering in a study by Sayles (1971). Many other examples of reductions in stuttering associated with extraneous stimulation are to be found in literature on stuttering going back many years. Gutzmann (1898, p. 433) found that some stutterers were able to speak fluently under the influence of a small but steady electric current from electrodes at the larynx and on the nape of the neck. In a few cases he was astonished to find that mere application of the electrodes without the electrical current had almost the same effect.

Loud noise and many other kinds of alteration of the stutterer's auditory feedback are also capable of reducing stuttering. As we will see later in this chapter, however, the reasons for this are a matter of debate. Webster and Gould (1975) reported a marked reduction in the blocks of a severe stutterer following anesthetization of his larynx. On the other hand, Hutchinson and Ringel (1975) found an increase in the stuttering of six subjects as a result of anesthesia of the oral structures.

Can Someone Be Distracted from Stuttering?

Throughout this discussion we have been assuming that there is an important factor of attention in stuttering and that fluency is often achieved by distraction of this attention. This assumption has been widely held and until recently little questioned. In recent years, however, a tendency has been evident on the part of some workers to regard such explanations of fluency with suspicion. Three different and mutually incompatible objections to distraction have been raised—that it plays no part in stuttering, that it is meaningless, and that it is inadequate to explain all of the phenomena that have been attributed to it. We will consider each of these criticisms in turn.

Doubts about the existence of distraction as a factor in stuttering were based initially on some experimentation by Beech and Fransella, who were primarily concerned with the reason for the metronome effect. After demonstrating that stutterers could speak fluently in time

---

[33]See Bloodstein (1950a, 1950b). In an experimental study Curtis (1942) found a tendency, short of statistical significance, for stuttering to decrease following muscular exercise.

[34]See Bloodstein (1949). In a laboratory study by Love (1955), however, neither Nembutal (a depressant) nor Benzedrine (a stimulant) was found to have any significant effect on stuttering.

to a rhythmic metronome, Fransella and Beech (1965) attempted to rule out distraction as a cause of their findings by showing that fluency did not result when the subjects were instructed to listen attentively to an arrhythmic metronome beat. Recognizing that listening to an arrhythmic beat might simply not be as distracting as talking in time to rhythm, Fransella (1967) had stutterers write down a series of tape-recorded numbers while reading aloud. Again there was no effect on stuttering. Fransella concluded that the metronome effect had not been caused by distraction.

The same argument can be used equally well to reject distraction as a cause of any other effect in stuttering, of course. It therefore raises a very broad issue. If a certain degree of attention is required in order for stuttering to take place this is a fundamental and revealing fact, though one that we have long taken for granted. If it were true that a person could not be distracted from stuttering this would be bound to influence our perspective on it profoundly. It would make stuttering unique among behaviors that are as responsive to environmental stimuli as stuttering has been found to be.

In the opinion of this writer the task of writing numbers while reading does not put distraction to any such critical test. There are several reasons for this. Not only must we consider the factor of the strength or magnitude of a distractor, but we must also take into account that if activities are capable of interfering with stuttering the reverse must also be true. Unfortunately, we cannot judge from Fransella's study to what extent her subjects' stuttering interfered with the response of writing numbers—that is, to what extent such responses were delayed while blocks were occurring.

There is, however, an even more urgent question that arises in relation to this experiment. It is quite possible that the writing of numbers was distracting enough to interfere with the act of oral reading itself. If the subject had a tendency to stop reading momentarily when it was time to write down a number, the writing activity could not conceivably have reduced the stuttering. It is self-evident that a condition so distracting that it compels the stutterer to take time out from speaking or reading cannot interfere with stuttering. In fact, the reason why unusual patterns of speaking give the appearance of being such powerful distractors is in all probability that they are among the few competing responses which by definition do not distract from talking.

Two more recent attempts have been made to determine whether subjects can be distracted from stuttering. Kamhi and McOsker (1982) had stutterers step on and off a 10-inch platform while reading aloud, and Thompson (1985) had them manually track an irregular line on a rotating drum while speaking. In neither case was there any effect on stuttering. These experiments, like those of Beech and Fransella, demonstrate the peculiar difficulty of doing research regarding distraction. It is clear that the conditions employed did not interfere with stuttering; yet neither these nor an endless number of similar demonstrations could prove that there are not other conditions capable of distracting from stuttering. On the other hand, it would be easy to point to a great many conditions that do interfere with stuttering, but these are the very conditions about which controversy exists regarding whether they are examples of distraction. We are forced to conclude that this type of research is incapable of determining whether stuttering requires attention and can be reduced by diverting the stutterer's attention. Until a better approach to the problem can be devised, our only alternative may be to evaluate the concept of distraction by considering what it helps us to explain. We may now place in the balance a compelling amount of evidence in its favor.

In brief, distraction helps us to account for a very wide range of observations. We may sum these up by saying that stutterers are likely to talk more fluently when they adopt virtually any novel speech pattern or mannerism, when they are in vigorous action, when they are carried away by emotion or excitement, or when they are reacting to novel or powerful stimuli. It enables us to understand why some of these factors have a tendency to "wear out" when they are overused. In addition, it meshes with another set of observations which seem to be merely the obverse of the distraction effect. As we saw in Chapter 1, stuttering is capable of interfering with voluntary manual activities such as the alternate squeezing and releasing of a rubber ball. It may interfere with the perception of the passage of time. In some cases it may reduce the perception of visual and auditory stimuli. Finally, the concept of distraction is consistent with the many indications that stuttering tends to increase in real life circumstances that draw stutterers' attention to their speech.

We have been discussing the most sweeping objection to the concept of distraction; namely, that stutterers cannot be distracted from stuttering. A second and more valid objection to the concept is its vagueness of definition. Writers who have used the term through the years have variously held that stutterers were being distracted from their speech, their stuttering, or their anticipation of stuttering. As the work of Fransella and Beech has served to show, there is little agreement on any precise operational meaning of distraction.

The problem of describing what we mean by distraction in adequately scientific terms does not seem insurmountable, however. It reduces essentially to a description of interference between competing stimuli or competing responses. This has been a matter of concern in other areas of research also. For example, Norman and Waugh (1968)

identified both a stimulus-produced and a response-produced interference with recognition memory. Keele (1972), also concerned with
the subject of memory, wrote, "When the processing of one stimulus
interferes with processing another, the processing is said to take attention," and also, "When performing one task interferes with performing another, the tasks are said to require attention."

This may be applied directly to stuttering. What we have called distraction appears to consist of two broad observations. One is that competing stimuli of sufficient strength or novelty may interfere with attention to
the stimuli that evoke stuttering. The other is that competing responses
requiring sufficient attention may interfere with the response of stuttering.

Finally, an objection to the concept of distraction that may be
raised with some justification is that it has tended to be overused. Its
capability to cover a multitude of circumstances makes it all too easy
to invoke it as a reason for observations of fluency having no other
readily apparent explanation. Alternative explanations may prove to
be better in some instances. In many cases several influences probably
contribute equally to a reduction in stuttering, and distraction may
serve merely as one factor. For this reason we need to be skeptical of
the uncritical use of explanations based on distraction.

Suggestion

Hypnotic suggestion was used widely in attempts to treat stuttering as early as the beginning of the nineteenth century. Its effects are
often striking, though usually temporary. Moore (1946) reported a clinical investigation of hypnotic suggestion with 40 stutterers; each was
worked with repeatedly for a period of at least seven weeks. Of the 40,
9 were not adequately responsive to hypnosis. Twelve spoke fluently
when the suggestion was given that "hesitances would not bother," but
failed to respond to posthypnotic suggestions. Eleven not only spoke to
audiences without stuttering, but usually carried out posthypnotic suggestions fluently. Eight remaining subjects with "apparently little limit"
to hypnotic behavior carried out posthypnotic suggestions fluently
before audiences and reported that their speech continued to be "easy
and relaxed" for two or three days following hypnotic sessions.

Various forms of nonhypnotic suggestion have been observed to
be equally potent in removing stuttering for brief periods. Emile
Coué, a Frenchman famous for his feats of suggestion, once persuaded a severe stutterer to speak before an audience by leading him
to the stage and assuring him that he did not stutter. The stutterer
spoke without difficulty, but within a week he appeared at a speech
clinic for help, blocking more severely than before.[35] The effects of

---

[35]See Heltman (1943, p. 78).

suggestion on stuttering are perhaps best known in the form of the observation that literally any form of therapy appears to be capable of producing sudden and largely temporary "cures" in certain instances.

Tension, Stress, and Generalized Anxiety

Stutterers often report that their speech improves when they are calm and relaxed. Some are benefitted by training in voluntary relaxation of their muscles. Six stutterers who were engaged in the regular practice of transcendental meditation all reported to McIntyre, Silverman, and Trotter (1974) that the stuttering had been reduced as a result. This finding was confirmed by Allen and Daly (1978). Treon and Tamayo (1975) reported that two subjects reduced their stuttering moderately by self-regulation of their galvanic skin response.

Conversely, clinical observation suggests that an increase in general tension may result in more frequent blocks. For example, stutterers who tell of speaking fluently under conditions of acute fear or emotional stress sometimes report more stuttering "after it was all over." One subject who had no stuttering immediately after an automobile accident said, "And then when I got home I was shot. I could hardly say one word without having a bad block." In some cases stuttering appears to increase on almost every occasion on which the stutterer is generally tense, anxious, or upset; stuttering may become virtually a daily barometer of the person's frame of mind.

Research findings that bear on the effect of stress tend to be equivocal, but this is perhaps to be expected in view of the variety of ways in which it can be defined and the difficulty of creating stress in the laboratory. Random electric shock seems to have limited effect on stuttering.[36] Toomey and Sidman (1970) studied the frequency of stuttering during the sounding of a buzzer warning the subjects of impending shock. Of four subjects only one showed an increase in stuttering; two stuttered less. Stressful conditions such as fatigue, pain, or hyperventilation appear to be more likely to decrease stuttering than to increase it, as we have seen. Laboratory experiences of failure seem to have little effect.[37] Confronting the stutterer with discomforting silence does seem to produce more stuttering, according to a report by Gould and Sheehan (1967), though somewhat conflicting findings were obtained by Adams and Brutten (1970). On the basis of the well-documented premise that women tend to have higher anxiety levels at premenstruation than at ovulation, Silverman, Zimmer, and Silverman (1974) recorded the speech of four female stutterers at these two points in their menstrual cycles and found more stuttering at premenstruation in each case.

---

[36]Frick (1951), Bearss (1952).
[37]Lerea (1955), Trombly (1959).

The Presence or Absence of Cues

Among the conditions under which stuttering may be markedly reduced are a number that differ considerably from each other, yet seem to owe their effect on stuttering to a common underlying factor; in all of them, many of the cues to which the person habitually responds by stuttering have been removed. For example, some stutterers are able to avoid stuttering effectively at times by using word substitutions. Some stutterers have difficulty at home but not at school, while in other cases the reverse may be true. Stutterers are to be found who have essentially all of their difficulty in oral reading, none in spontaneous speech. Cases have been reported in which the person stuttered only on the telephone, or only when ordering a meal, or only when riding in elevator;[38] such stutterers appear to speak normally in most situations for the same reason that most of us are non-stutterers in all of them—there are no cue-stimuli for speech difficulty. Presumably under all of these conditions the stutterer has learned to respond discriminatively to cues associated with them as a result of specific past experiences.

A stutterer may have difficulty speaking one language but not another. Sometimes it is the first-learned language in which stuttering occurs and sometimes the second. Dale (1977) described the cases of four Cuban-American adolescent boys who stuttered in Spanish but not English. All had been born in the United States, but spoke only Spanish in the home. Dale related their stuttering to home pressures, reported by both the boys and their parents, to retain proficiency in the Spanish language. Nwokah (1988) noted that among 16 stutterers in Anambra State, Nigeria, who were equally proficient in English and Igbo, some stuttered more in one language and some in the other.

Finally, some stutterers speak better in new surroundings—for example, on vacation trips, when enrolling in a new school, or on entering the armed services. One stutterer interviewed by the author had virtually lived a nomadic life for this reason. Whenever he stayed in one place for more than a few months his stuttering became so severe that he could hardly talk. He would then quit his job, pack his belongings, and move away to begin all over again in a new town.

Anticipation of Stuttering

It is an old observation, long antedating current anticipatory struggle theories of stuttering, that stutterers' expectations of difficulty with their speech may be a powerful force in bringing it about. This is an assumption of rather broad reach since it can be viewed as

---

[38]Blanton (1931), Bender and Kleinfeld (1938, p. 243).

encompassing many of the generalizations we have already made. If blocks can be evoked by the anticipation of stuttering it is only reasonable to assume that they may come and go with fluctuations in stutterers' attention to their speech, with suggestions that instill the conviction that they will or will not stutter, with the cues to which their anticipations have become attached, and even with generalized states of tension or anxiety that are conducive to expectancy.

Ironically, it is the very prominence of this factor in stuttering that has given it its controversial aspects, since it has led to the theory that it is the essence of the difficulty. This has tended to carry with it the implication that every block the stutterer has must be preceded by anticipation. This is a far more debatable point than the assumption that anticipation is an influential factor, and research findings have not produced conclusive evidence with regard to it. Earlier in this chapter we saw that while many stutterers can predict the occurrence of their stuttering there are many exceptions to this, particularly in children and even in adults. There are, however, other ways besides the stutterer's predictions by which anticipation of stuttering can be studied.

The Effect of Varying the Duration of Expectancy

Within certain limits, the longer the time interval elapsing between the moment stutterers intend to plan their speech response and the moment they attempt it, the greater appears to be the probability of stuttering. Stutterers who wait a long time for their turn to recite in the classroom because their name begins with "W" are apt to have a great deal of difficulty when finally called on. An observation of this sort serves both to define anticipation operationally and to suggest a systematic way to study its effect on stuttering.

Goss (1952) studied this effect experimentally by varying the time interval between the exposure of a stimulus word and a signal to the subject to say the word. For intervals from 2 to 10 seconds, he found that the amount of stuttering progressively increased with the length of time the stutterer waited to say the word. For intervals shorter than 2 seconds there was another increase in stuttering as the interval was decreased to 1 and then 0 seconds, a finding that suggests that with the demand for an immediate or rapid response a new source of speech pressure makes itself felt *(see Figure 10)*.

In a further study Goss (1956) varied the time interval between a warning signal and the exposure of the word, the word being spoken as soon as it was seen. Again there was more stuttering with longer intervals. It appears that not only waiting to say a specific word, but merely waiting to speak, tends to increase the probability of stuttering.

These findings appear to show not only that a relationship between stuttering and anticipation exists, but also that the relation-

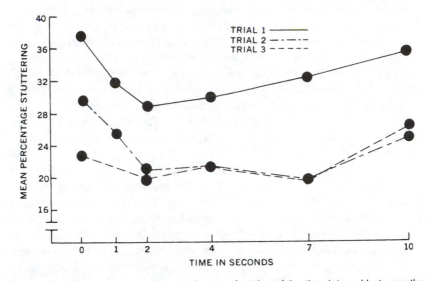

Figure 10. Mean percentage ot stuttering as a function of the time interval between the exposure of stimulus words and the signal to say them, during three successive trials. Reproduced from Goss (1952). Copyright 1952 by the American Psychological Association. By permission.

ship is dependent. Consequently, they are of considerable importance. In a somewhat similar study, however, Fransella (1971) obtained negative results. Time intervals ranging from 5 to 13 seconds between word presentation and signal to speak did not differ in their effects on stuttering, either when subjects could predict the moment of occurrence of the signal or when they could not.[39]

On the other hand, Forte and Schlesinger (1972) found the effect again. Furthermore, they found it in children. Their subjects were twenty school-aged stutterers. Each subject took turns reading aloud with five normal-speaking classmates on a series of occasions. The order in which the children read was determined by their seating arrangement, and this was systematically varied from one time to the next. The results were similar to those of Goss. The first position produced more stuttering than the second, but from the second to the sixth the stuttering increased progressively again *(see Figure 11)*.

Autonomic Arousal as a Measure of Anticipation

The objectivity of measures of autonomic arousal has long been appealing to workers who have been interested in the subject of antici-

---

[39]Fransella's experiment was chiefly concerned with the effect of ability to predict the occurrence of the signal to speak, and it differed from Goss's in certain features of procedure. For example, the subjects were allowed 10 seconds to say the word on receiving the signal.

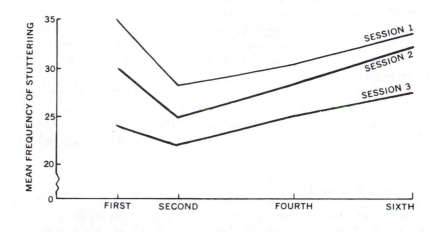

Figure 11. Mean frequency of stuttering of twenty school-aged stutterers in relation to the order in which they took their turn in oral reading with five classmates, during three reading sessions. Reproduced by permission of the publisher from "Stuttering as a function of time of expectation" by Forte and Schlesinger. *J. Communic. Dis.*, 5, 347-58. Copyright 1972 by Elsevier Science Publishing Co., Inc.

pation of stuttering. In general, laboratory investigations have produced a great deal of evidence of physiological arousal just prior to the block. At an early date Van Riper and Milisen (1939) were able to review a considerable amount of research showing that stuttering was often preceded by accelerations in pulse rate, vasoconstriction, unusual eye-movements, electrodermal responses, and disturbances of breathing. Later Tanberg (1955) reported manual motor disturbances prior to stuttering. Kurshev (1968a) and Ickes and Pierce (1973) found additional evidence of vasoconstriction. Kurshev (1969) studied GSR measures accompanying expectation of stuttering, and Brutten (1963) traced the decline in palmar sweating as subjects' predictions of stuttering decreased in repeated silent readings of a passage. Gray and Williams (1969), however, could find no evidence of pupil dilation preceding the block. Myers (1978) studied the relationship of the severity of stutterings to various measures of respiration, blood volume, skin conductance, and heart rate just prior to stuttering.

As useful as these studies have been, they have not provided any critical tests of the hypothesis that stutterings are precipitated by anticipation. To find changes in the GSR preceding the block is interesting, and it would be even more so if we found them when the subject did not consciously anticipate stuttering. But finding such changes frequently is not the same as finding them in every case. Furthermore, the absence of such signs might merely mean that anticipation may occur without a detectable degree of emotional arousal. In a study of three subjects who reported that they consistently anticipated their stutterings, Baumgartner and Brutten (1983) found that in two cases there was no relationship between cognitive expectancy and changes in heart rate prior to stuttering. They concluded that "for some stutterers, expectancy may reflect an objective rather than an emotional belief that speech will be difficult." The theory that stuttering blocks are caused by speakers' convictions that the words they are attempting will be difficult, and that they must therefore use some effort, care, or special strategy for saying them, does not necessitate the assumption that stutterers are emotionally aroused, but only that they want to talk and mistakenly believe there are obstacles in the way.

Preparatory Muscular Activity

Perhaps more crucial than autonomic arousal to an anticipatory concept of stuttering is some kind of inappropriate muscular preparation for speech. In an electromyographic study of a single stutterer, Bar, Singer, and Feldman (1969) found evidence of unusual laryngeal muscle activity during anticipation of stuttering. A study of nineteen subjects by McLean and Cooper (1978) failed to confirm this. On the other hand, Shrum (cited by Guitar, 1975) obtained action potentials from subjects' facial, neck, and chest muscles and found a rise in their amplitude preceding stuttering in almost all the muscles studied. More recently an electromyographic study of forty-two subjects by Thurmer, Thumfart, and Kittel (1983) showed muscular hyperactivity at the larynx, tongue, and lip prior to stuttering. Murray, Empson, and Weaver (1987), too, found evidence in action potentials at the larynx that muscular preparedness for speech may play an important role in stuttering.

A series of studies has also demonstrated that subjects can generally reduce their stuttering by using auditory or visual feedback to lower the electromyographic signal from their laryngeal, masseter muscle, lip, or chin areas prior to utterances.[40] The precise reasons for all such reductions in stuttering are in some doubt however, due to a number of further observations. For example, Guitar (1975) noted that the sites at which reduced preparatory muscle activity resulted in decreased stuttering were not necessarily the sites where speech was blocked. Pachman, Oelschlaeger, Hughes, and Hughes (1978) reported on two subjects for whom training of the frontalis muscle was effective in reducing stuttering and for whom such training worked whether the subject raised or lowered the activity of the muscle. Both Craig and Cleary (1982) and Moore (1984) noted instances in which there appeared to be fluency even though muscle tension was high.

---

[40]Guitar (1975) Hanna, Wilfling, and McNeil (1975), Lanyon, Barrington, and Newman (1976), Cross (1977), Lanyon (1977), Moore (1978), Craig and Cleary (1982), Moore (1984).

Shearer and Simmons (1965) obtained negative findings in a study of the stapedius muscle of the middle ear, which has been found to be activated concurrently with the speech musculature. Acoustic impedance measurements showed that middle ear muscle activity did not precede speech output in stutterers by a longer interval than it did in nonstutterers. Their results were confirmed by Quinn and Andrews (1976).

Other Evidence of Anticipation

Peters et al. (1976) found changes in stutterers' brain potentials prior to attempts on words the subjects had rated as frequently stuttered. These changes appeared even when the word was not actually stuttered.

Brutten and Janssen (1979) showed that in silent reading adult stutterers tended to have longer eye fixations on words on which they had indicated expectancy of stuttering than on words on which they had not. The subjects also showed longer fixations on words on which they subsequently stuttered than on nonstuttered words when they read the passage aloud. Janssen and Brutten (1981) reported similar results for stuttering children aged 6 to 12 years, as did Bakker, Brutten, Janssen, and van der Meulen (1991).

On spectrograms of syllables spoken just prior to stutterings, Knox (1976) found increases in fundamental frequency, decreased rate, and eccentric transitions. Falck, Lawler, and Yonovitz (1985) found, for the most part, decreases in fundamental frequency and decreased voicing prior to blocks. The pattern of change varied, however, depending on whether the block that followed involved prolongation, repetition, or absence of phonation, suggesting that the moment of stuttering begins its characteristic pattern "considerably before it is easily identifiable." In summary, the anticipation of stuttering manifests itself in a wide variety of ways. There is little doubt that, in older subjects at least, stutterings tend to be closely associated with anticipatory events. Unfortunately, relatively little research has yet been done with specific reference to such questions as whether such events occur preceding ostensibly unexpected blocks, how frequently they are to be observed in young children, and whether stutterings ever appear in the absence of any such events.

Anxiety About Stuttering

Since the precise role of anticipation in stuttering has not been established, it stands to reason that this is also true of that special kind of anticipation called anxiety about stuttering. In at least a loose sense, stuttering in its developed form often appears to be a kind of speech anxiety reaction. To many who have worked with stutterers clinically this impression seems very strong. Furthermore, a difficulty which varies with communicative pressures, with attention to speech, and to a large extent with anticipation of stuttering might perhaps hardly be thought at a glance to be anything else. Bloodstein (1950b) made an elaborate attempt to show that the broadest possible generalization about the multitude of conditions under which stuttering is reduced or absent is that it declines with reduction in anxiety about stuttering. So close has such a relationship appeared to be that the anticipatory struggle hypothesis has often been expressed as the inference that stuttering is a reaction of anxiety about speech or stuttering.

It is, in fact, the very closeness of the relationship that makes counterexamples so striking. And counterexamples are to be found in ample number, even on the level of clinical observation. They are especially common in our experience with children. Although stuttering children are capable of intense speech anxiety reactions, many show little outward sign of anxiety on most occasions. The tendency of stutterers to have more severe difficulty as a result of obvious fear of stuttering is characteristic of its most advanced forms. Moreover, even adult stutterers are to be found who have some of their most severe difficulty in such situations as the speech clinic, in which their attention is strongly focused on their speech, but in which they seem to experience little if any anxiety as that term is commonly understood.

We also find counterexamples when we define anxiety in terms of objective signs of autonomic arousal. In general, such measures do tend to give abundant evidence of anxiety accompanying stuttering. We reviewed this evidence in our description of the visceral concomitants of stuttering blocks in Chapter 1 and in our discussion of the physiological studies of anticipation in the preceding section. Furthermore, certain studies have shown in a rather pointed way a tendency for GSR measures to vary concomitantly with the stutterer's speech or stuttering.[41] In other research, however, such a tendency has been missing or equivocal. For example, Gray and Brutten (1965) did not find a consistent reduction in palmar sweat measures of anxiety as the frequency of stuttering decreased with repeated readings of a passage. Neither did Ritterman and Reidenbach (1975). Nor was there any reduction in palmar sweating under white noise in a study by Adams and Moore (1972), although the noise reduced the stuttering markedly. Reed and Lingwall (1976, 1980) found no consistent tendency for GSR measures to decrease with reduction in stuttering in "punishment" experiments. Similarly, palmar sweat measures of anxiety have failed to decline concomitantly with improvement in speech during treatment.[42] In an experiment by Ickes (1975) the administration of Nembutal lowered subjects' palmar sweat indices even though

---

[41]Berlinsky (1955), Kline (1959), Valyo (1964), Treon and Tamayo (1975).

[42]See Gray and England (1972) and Gregory (cited by Ingham and Andrews, 1971a).

it increased stuttering in some cases. Janssen and Kraaimaat (1980) found that, although the self-rated anxiety of stutterers exceeded that of nonstutterers during oral reading, their skin conductance and heart rates increased no more than did their controls'. Similar results were obtained by Peters and Hulstijn (1984). During and just before speech tasks stutterers and nonstutterers differed only in self-ratings of anxiety. Heart rate, pulse volume, and skin conductance increased to the same extent in both groups. Murray, Empson, and Weaver (1987) found that stutterers did not have elevated heart rates when anticipating speaking. Weber and Smith (1990) recorded palmar skin conductance, peripheral blood volume, and heart rate before, during, and after reading and speaking. They found correlations between these arousal measures and stuttering that were significant but quite low. The relationship varied considerably among individuals.

We can add to this the observation that tranquilizing drugs appear to be quite variable in their influence on stuttering. Some stutterers appear to be benefitted by them, while some do not. Clinical reports of successful use of tranquilizers are common, but some studies have shown little effect (see Chapter 11).

It is evident that anxiety is a term with many meanings. As a result the question of how stuttering varies with anxiety about stuttering is far from simple. All we can say is that by the definitions of anxiety that are usual in clinical and experimental work, anxiety about stuttering has a distinct but inconsistent, limited, and qualified relationship to stuttering.

CONCLUSIONS

Summary

In this chapter we have dealt with the basic question of the nature of stuttering as a response. The facts that have been discovered may be summarized as follows:

The Distribution of Stuttering

In general, there is a strong tendency for stutterings to occur on words on which the stutterer predicts they will occur. Stutterings that are not predicted occur often, however, particularly in the case of children. Some older and many younger stutterers are able to predict the occurrence of few of their blocks. Nevertheless there is evidence that many of these individuals may respond to subliminal anticipations of stuttering.

In both children and adults, stutterings tend to occur as relatively consistent responses to cues in the speech context. The same cues have been found to evoke stuttering over periods of weeks, though some change appears to take place in them with the passage of time. In the laboratory new cues may be given the power to elicit stuttering by association with conditions under which frequent stuttering occurs. There is evidence that in both children and adults stuttering may take place in response to cues for no other reason than that they are evocative of past stuttering.

Studies of the loci of stuttering in the speech sequence show that the blocks are likely to occur on the first syllable of the word, although they may sometimes be found on accented syllables in other positions within polysyllabic words. Various attributes of words have been found to influence the distribution of stuttering in adults and children of school age. Stuttering tends to occur more often on words beginning with consonants than on words beginning with vowels (at least in English), on content words than on function words, on long words than on short ones, on words at the beginning of the sentence than elsewhere, on words of lower frequency of occurrence in the language, on words carrying more information load as defined by their predictability in context, and probably on words that receive more stress. It is not entirely clear to what extent these factors are overlapping and interdependent. In any case, since the distribution of stutterings in the same reading material varies widely among different individuals, it is evident that these general features of words do not wield as strong an influence as do individual factors. Although relatively little research has been done on factors that vary from case to case, it is known that there is a marked tendency for stutterers as individuals to have special difficulty with certain words or sounds, apparently because of personal histories of past failure on them, and there is some evidence that this has a fairly strong effect on the distribution of stutterings.

The fact that the distribution of stuttering is influenced by so many attributes of words may perhaps be interpreted to mean that, whatever its origin, stuttering is above all a difficulty in the initiation of words, rather than the execution of sounds, syllables, or other units of speech. This is corroborated by the observation that stuttering usually occurs at the beginning of a word and virtually never at the end. There is some evidence, however, that stuttering may be influenced by certain features of sentences, particularly their length or complexity, and in Chapter 9 we will see that the early stuttering of young children may consist to a large degree of difficulty with whole syntactic structures.

The Frequency of Stuttering

The frequency of stuttering tends to vary markedly in response to a very large number of identifiable situational factors. All or most of these appear to be subsumed under a number of general conditions:

The frequency of stuttering tends to vary with the amount of communicative pressure imposed on the stutterer by such factors as audience size, listener reactions, concern about social approval, time pressures, the degree to which the stutterer is responsible for conveying a meaningful message to a listener, and the demands which the encoding of the message makes on motor planning.

The frequency of stuttering is also affected markedly by a factor of attention, most clearly exemplified by conditions which tend to interfere with stuttering. This interference, generally known as distraction, may come from competing stimuli or competing responses. It may take the, form of novel speech patterns or mannerisms of almost any kind, associated activities, emotional arousal, or strange or intense sensory stimuli.

The frequency of stuttering may be influenced by suggestion, by the presence or absence of the cues to which it has become attached, and probably also to some degree by generalized tension and anxiety.

Finally, the frequency of developed stuttering often seems to vary, at least to a considerable degree, with anticipation of stuttering, and that appears to be the most general statement we are at present able to make about it.

Alternative Models of the Stuttering Response

In Chapter 2 we described three basic conceptual models which have been advanced to account for the moment of stuttering. The information outlined in Chapter 7 represents almost all the data in our possession by which these models may be tested. We may now ask how good an explanation of the data each of them provides.

The Anticipatory Struggle Hypothesis

It was largely out of efforts to substantiate a form of the anticipatory struggle hypothesis that research on stuttering as a response originated. How well has this model succeeded? On the credit side it takes little effort of interpretation to make it fit most of the facts in an illuminating way. Stuttering appears to be a response to cues representative of past difficulty, a property that uniquely defines anticipatory struggle reactions among learned responses. The blocks appear to occur chiefly on those segments of the speech sequence that stutterers tend to evaluate as difficult or important, which evoke the threat of failure, or on which stuttering is likely to be conspicuous or embarrassing. The frequency of stuttering seems to vary largely with communicative pressures and with the attention stutterers give to their stuttering, their speech, or their role as speakers. In many individuals stuttering seems to vary with fear or expectancy of stuttering. On the whole, the anticipatory struggle model appears to achieve a parsimonious integration of a very broad range of observations.

The model also meets with some notable difficulties, however. One of them is that stuttering can and evidently often does occur in the absence of anxiety as that term is ordinarily defined. Some might argue that essentially any awareness of the threat of something even slightly annoying or frustrating must be considered mild amiety, regardless of what the GSR reading or the subject says. At all events, this problem does not appear to be critical. Johnson's concept of stuttering as an anxiety-motivated avoidance reaction received wide currency, but it is not the only way to state the anticipatory struggle hypothesis. It can be expressed adequately by saying that the stuttering block results from speakers' convictions, preconceptions, or expectations about the difficulty of the utterance they are about to attempt or from their doubts about their ability to succeed at it. Stated in terms of anxiety, the model will fit many cases. It is not without any foundation in fact. It is simply not general enough.

Perhaps a more serious difficulty is that stutterings can occur in the absence of expectancy of stuttering as defined by stutterers' reports or by their ability to predict the occurrence of their blocks. It can be argued that conscious expectancy of stuttering is not necessarily implied by the theory that stuttering is due to a belief in the difficulty of speech or by the hypothesis that it is a response to cues representative of past speech failure. Nevertheless, some form of anticipation would seem to be implied. As we have seen, there are numerous ways in which anticipation may be defined operationally for the purpose of verifying its relationship to stuttering. One can, for example, vary the amount of time the stutterer waits to say a word and see how that affects the probability of stuttering. Researchers have also investigated stutterers' brain waves, muscle potentials, visceral reactions, and eye movements just prior to stuttering and have made spectrographic analyses of their phonations preceding blocks. All of these studies have resulted in demonstrations of the anticipatory activity for which the investigators were searching. As yet, however, conclusive evidence in support of the anticipatory struggle hypothesis is lacking.

Another problem encountered by this model has to do with the role of punishment in stuttering. According to the anticipatory struggle hypothesis stuttering should increase as a result of punishment for stuttering. There is considerable clinical impression and some experimental evidence that it does. Yet research has shown that electric shock, verbal punishers, and other aversive stimuli tend to reduce stuttering very markedly when administered contingently, as we will see in Chapter 8. The issue is clouded by the observation that such presumably reinforcing stimuli as cessation of loud tone and the word "right" have been found to do the same thing. It is possible that what has been called punishment is in fact stimulus-based distraction. In any case, laboratory conditions of punishment may represent poor analogues of social penalty in the world outside.

The Breakdown Hypothesis

The breakdown model of stuttering implies that the block is primarily a response to stress. Perhaps all of the observations that appear to support the anticipatory struggle hypothesis can be explained without difficulty by this theory too. It is possible to assume that anticipations of difficulty or memories of past failure in speech are factors that may powerfully affect stuttering but are not the essence of it. The essence of it may be a predisposition to motor disintegration of speech. Speech anxieties may serve, with other stresses, to trigger such disintegration.

One issue which this point of view raises concerns the relative influence on stuttering of speech-related stress and stress from other sources. In our review of the variables related to stuttering speech-related pressures appeared to predominate by far. This may only be, however, because the stutterer encounters speech-related stress far more often than other kinds.

The same ambiguities with regard to punishment, expectancy, and anxiety which are an embarrassment to the anticipatory struggle hypothesis create problems for the breakdown model. Perhaps particular difficulty is offered by the inconsistent relationship between stuttering and signs of autonomic arousal.

The Repressed Need Hypothesis

Psychoanalytic theories of stuttering have been concerned with few of the phenomena that have been discussed in this chapter and do not appear to afford a satisfactory integration of many of them. There are frequent allusions in psychoanalytic writings to fluency under conditions of anger and to the ability of some stutterers to act a role in a play. In addition there is the general implication that the difficulty varies with the ideational or emotional content of the stutterer's speech. Compared with other factors, only a small amount of research has been done on the influence of speech content on stuttering. Bernhardt (1954) reported that in response to the Blacky Test certain areas of psychosexual conflict evoked more stuttering than others. In a word association study using words related to speech, security seeking, obstacle surmounting, and sex, Kline (1959) found significant differences in the amount of stuttering in verbal associations to the various word groups. On the other hand, Weisberger (1967) did not find increased stuttering in Thematic Apperception Test responses involving themes of sexuality, aggression, and parental authority. Other studies of the effect of speech content have not been directly relevant to the repressed need hypothesis.[43]

Perkins and Hagen (1965) permitted subjects to overhear a derogatory impression of their personal adequacy. Immediately afterward, subjects who were allowed to vent aggression directly by giving their frustrator an electric shock stuttered less in oral reading than those who were not. L. H. Silverman et al (1972) found increased stuttering in spontaneous speech immediately after subliminal exposures of anal and oral aggressive pictures.

Suggested Readlngs

Bloodstein, O., Conditions under which stuttering is reduced or absent: A review of literature. *J. Speech Hearing Dis., 14*, 295–302 (1949).

Bloodstein, O., Hypothetical conditions under which stuttering is reduced or absent. *J. Speech Hearing Dis., 15*, 142–53 (1950).

Van Riper, C., *The Nature of Stuttering, 2nd ed.* Englewood Cliffs, N.J.: Prentice-Hall (1982), Chaps. 7, 8.

Young, M. A., Increasing the frequency of stuttering. *J. Speech Hearing Res., 28*, 282–293 (1985).

---

[43]Moore, Soderberg, and Powell (1952), Moore (1954, 1959), Bar (1969), MacKay (1969).

8

STUTTERING AS A RESPONSE: SOME CONTROVERSIAL PHENOMENA

In the general review of variations in the frequency of stuttering just concluded we have purposely put off any systematic discussion of four specific conditions under which stuttering tends to diminish. Although they represent only a few of scores of such conditions they are especially important because they have lent themselves to a great deal of research and speculation concerning their meaning. Knowing what causes them would give us deeper insight into the causes of other changes in the frequency of stuttering.

THE ADAPTATION EFFECT

In 1937 Johnson and Knott issued the first published report of the bservation that a reduction in stuttering usually takes place in successive oral readings of the same material.[1] Further research on the effect was done byJohnson and Inness (1939). In these and other studies that soon followed, several basic facts about adaptation became clear. It tends to be very marked during the first few readings and becomes progressively less so, generally reaching a limit beyond which repeated readings have little or no further effect. Most of the reduc-

---

[1]According to an editorial note by Johnson, the study by Van Riper and Hull (1955) was probably the first investigation of the adaptation effect, though it remained unreported for many years.

tion that is to take place will be evident in most cases by the fifth reading. On the average, this decrease in stuttering is roughly 50 percent of the frequency of stuttering in the initial reading.

Johnson's curiosity was aroused by the adaptation effect, and it occupied his attention for a considerable time. But it was principally due to the important role that adaptation played in the learning-based formulations of Wischner (1950, 1952b) somewhat later that extraordinary interest developed in studies of this effect. As a result of more than three decades of research we now probably know more about adaptation than about almost any other comparable aspect of stuttering.

Among the basic facts that have been learned are that the rate of adaptation decreases with an increase in the time interval between successive readings.[2] The length of the passage does not seem to be an important factor.[3] There is relatively little transfer of the adaptation effect to readings of different material.[4] Adaptation is only temporary; if the passage is read again after an interval, the frequency of stuttering will have increased again in amounts varying with the length of the interval and will be fully restored to its original level with a few hours.[5] This "spontaneous recovery" of stuttering has been of exceptional interest to those to whom it has appeared analogous to the spontaneous recovery of a conditioned response following experimental extinction trials.

The adaptation effect is to be found in the stuttering of children as well as adults.[6] Although it has been studied chiefly in oral reading, it has also been demonstrated in spontaneous speech by various means.[7] In general, during adaptation there is a reduction in essentially all of the various types of disfluency (part-word repetitions, word repetitions, phrase repetitions, etc.),[8] although some differential effects have been shown to occur in individual cases.[9]

Stutterers differ widely in the extent to which they adapt; many do not appear to show any adaptation at all, and some may show increased stuttering with repeated readings.[10] There has been a good

---

[2]Shulman (1955).

[3]Shulman (1955) demonstrated this with passages varying from 200 to 1,000 words in length. Brutten and Dancer (1980) showed, however, that repeating each of a series of words individually results in a greater reduction of stuttering than repeating the same words the same number of times as a list.

[4]Harris (1942).

[5]Newman (1954), Jones (1955), Jamison (1955), Frick (1955), Leutenegger (1957), Peins (1961a), Gray and Brutten (1965).

[6]Neeley and Timmons (1967), Williams, Silverman, and Kools (1968).

[7]Moore (1954), Newman (1954), Schaef (1955), Bloom and Silverman (1973), Coppa and Bar (1974), Kroll and Hood (1974).

[8]Timmons (1967), Silverman and Williams (1971), Kroll and Hood (1974).

[9]Sakata and Adams (1972), Webster and Brutten (1972).

[10]Newman (1963), Bloom and Silverman (1973), Moore, Flowers, and Cunko (1981).

deal of curiosity about the reasons for this individual variation. Attention has been given to the possibility that adaptation scores might be useful in measuring or predicting response to therapy, on the assumption that adaptation represents a "miniature model" of improvement. Findings so far have not provided much support for such an assumption.[11] Some attempt has been made to relate amount of adaptation to certain personality measures and behavioral characteristics.[12] The only relationship on which there is as yet consistent evidence is that less severe stuttering is associated with a more marked tendency to adapt.[13] Work has also been done on problems relating to the measurement of adaptation, and various ways of measuring it have been proposed.[14]

Theories of Adaptation

A variety of theories have been offered to account for the adaptation effect. The theory advanced by Wischner (1950) was that it represents the experimental extinction of a learned anxiety-motivated response. This point of view asserts that adaptation is an actual on-the-spot unlearning of stuttering behavior and implies that whatever reinforcement serves to maintain this behavior is diminished during successive readings of the same material.

A second theory, suggested byJohnson,[15] is that stutterers' anxieties about stuttering are reduced through deconfirmation of their expectancies. That is, their stuttering or its consequences may fail to live up to their expectations in the sense that we tend to exaggerate what we dread, and so they tend to be less fearful of stuttering and less concerned with avoiding it.

A third proposal, by Sheehan (1958a, p. 132), was that the occurrence of stuttering in itself is fear reducing. The stuttering during the first reading thus reduces fear enough to permit less stuttering on the second, and so on.

A fourth theory is that adaptation is due to reactive inhibition. In his theory of learning, Hull postulated that massed repetitions of a response produced an inhibitory potential, related to fatigue, which temporarily reduced the strength of a response in the absence of any

---

[11]Van Riper and Hull (1955), Quarrington (1956), Johnson, Darley, and Spriesterbach (1963, p. 268), Prins and McQuiston (1964), Lanyon (1965), Prins (1968).

[12]Falck (1956), Quarrington (1956,1962), Agnello (1962), Gray and Karmen (1967), Sayles (1971).

[13]Van Riper and Hull (1955), Shulman (1955), Oxtoby (1955), Quarrington (1959), Siegel and Haugen (1964).Gray (1965a, 1965b) showed that it is possible to predict the course of adaptation from a subject's initial frequency of stuttering.

[14]Trotter (1955), Quarrington (1959), Tate, Cullinan, and Ahlstrand (1961), Cullinan (1963a), Silverman and, Williams (1968), Bloom and Silverman (1979).

[15]See Johnson et al. (1967, p. 276) and Johnson, Darley, and Spriestersbach (1963, p. 268).

change in learning or motivational states. This explanation of stuttering adaptation, originally weighed by Wischner (1947), was particularly developed and extended by Brutten and his co-workers.[16]

A fifth theory is that adaptation is due to rehearsal of the reading material. Various reasons why this might reduce the frequency of stuttering have been suggested. Perhaps the earliest proponent of such a theory was Eisenson (1958, p. 240 ff.), who stated that repeated readings of a passage reduce its propositional value and tend to "establish an articulatory and vocal set that approaches the automatic." Eisenson suggested that adaptation was related to the effect on stuttering of memorization of reading material.

The Effect of Varying the Reading Material

Precisely what is it that the stutterer adapts to? The most direct approach to an understanding of adaptation has been made in studies that have attempted to answer this question by varying one feature or another of the adaptation condition. One way to do this is by varying the reading material. Experiments in which stutterers have read continuously changing material have established that far less adaptation— only 10 to 20 percent, on the average—takes place under these conditions.[17]

These findings show clearly that while some adaptation takes place to the speech situation, most of it is to the speech context. We are left, however, with the question of precisely what features of the speech context are adapted to. It is interesting from this point of view that adaptation takes place even in the repeated reading of word lists.[18] On the other hand, there is evidence that some of the adaptation to be observed in connected reading is adaptation to its prosodic features. Wingate (1966b) conducted an adaptation experiment with a series of reading passages that contained the identical sequence of words, but each of which was punctuated differently to produce a different pattern of meanings. Less adaptation occurred under this condition than in the reading of a passage that was not successively altered in this way. It would seem that the stutterer adapts to any or all features of the reading material.

The Effect of Varying the Situation

A different type of experimental attack on the problem of adaptation is one in which the speech content is held constant and some fea-

---

[16]See Gray and Brutten (1965) and Brutten and Shoemaker (1967, p. 67 ff.).

[17]Johnson and Innes (1939), Cohen (1953), Donohue (1955), Golub (1955), Hegde (1971c). There is even less adaptation in continuously changing spontaneous speech (Cohen, 1953; Rousey, 1958)

[18]Wischner (1947), Golub (1955), Peterson, Rieck, and Hoff (1969), Brutten and Dancer (1980).

ture of the situation is systematically varied from reading to reading. Shulman (1955) took this approach in a study in which the stutterer's audience was increased by one person with each of five successive readings of a passage to a maximum of five listeners in the last reading. The stutterings decreased from reading to reading despite the progressive increase in the size of the audience, but the amount and rate of adaptation were decidedly less than in an ordinary adaptation sequence. This finding was confirmed by Siegel and Haugen (1964). Wischner (1952b) interpreted Shulman's results as reflecting the interaction between specific word anxiety, which was decreased by the successive readings, and general situational anxiety, which was increased by the audience factor.

Wischner (1947) found that a sudden loud noise during the course of the readings tended to arrest the course of adaptation temporarily, and inferred that this was analogous to the phenomenon of disinhibition in classical conditioning experiments—the arrest of experimental extinction of a response by distracting stimuli. Wingate (1972) reported a similar finding, but attributed it to interference with "general psychophysiological adaptation" to the situation during the initial reading.

Daly and Cooper (1967) administered electric shock to subjects during and following stuttering blocks in the course of successive readings. They were attempting to test Wischner's nonreinforcement theory of adaptation and hypothesized that the contingent shock would prevent reinforcement and lead to an increase in the adaptation rate. It did not do so.

Kroll and Hood (1976) reported that when subjects were not told beforehand that they would be required to read the passage repeatedly, adaptation was preceded by an increase of stuttering on the second reading.

The Role of Anxiety and Expectancy in Adaptation

The adaptation theories of Wischner, Sheehan, and Johnson implied that adaptation is associated with a progressive decrease in anxiety. Brutten and his co-workers attempted to check this assumption directly by means of measures of palmar sweating taken during adaptation and obtained inconsistent results. Sometimes adaptation was accompanied by a decline in the palmar sweat measures and sometimes not.[19] They drew the conclusion that reduction in anxiety is not a necessary condition for adaptation.

---

[19]Brutten (1963), Gray and Brutten (1965), Brutten and Shoemaker (1967, pp. 75, 76). See also Ritterman and Reidenbach (1975).

Somewhat related to this is the question of whether there is an "expectancy adaptation effect." Wischner (1952b), who related expectancy to anxiety about stuttering, found that there was. He reported that when stutterers were asked to pick out the words on which they would expect to stutter, they tended to mark progressively fewer words in repeated silent inspections of the same reading material. While this effect was not found by Peins (1961a), Brutten (1963) found a tendency toward expectancy adaptation which approached significance.

Is the Stutterer Adapting to Stuttering?

Let us come back to the question of what stutterers are adapting to. So far we have seen that they are adapting for the most part to the reading material and to some extent also to the situation. Yet if we examine the theories of adaptation enumerated earlier it will be clear that almost all of them view stutterers as adapting primarily to neither, but to their stuttering. With the exception of the point of view that the adaptation effect is due to rehearsal of the reading material, they all impute the effect for different reasons to the fact that in the course of successive readings the subject repeatedly experiences stuttering. Whether it is the fact that the stuttering fails to receive reinforcement, or that the consequences of stuttering are not as fearful as expected, or that the stuttering serves to reduce anxiety, or that the stuttering creates reactive inhibition, in all these cases it is the experience of stuttering itself that is viewed as bringing about its reduction. There is a simple way to tell whether adaptation is due to repeated stuttering, and that is to see what happens if the stutterer reads a passage repeatedly with little or no stuttering.

Frank and Bloodstein (1971) attempted to do this by having the stutterer read in unison with an experimenter. After five unison readings during which there was little stuttering the subjects read the passage once more independently. Their stuttering was compared with their performance in an ordinary adaptation condition. The results were instructive. In the sixth reading of the unison condition, when the subjects read independently, the average frequency of stuttering was almost exactly equal to the average amount of stuttering in the sixth reading of the ordinary adaptation condition (see Figure 12). In brief, their stuttering had been reduced to the same extent by repeated reading regardless of how much stuttering they had done along the way. They had adapted to the reading, not the stuttering.

Rehearsal Theories of Adaptation

Identical results were obtained in a replication of the Frank and Bloodstein study by Gold (1994). If it is not too rash to accept the

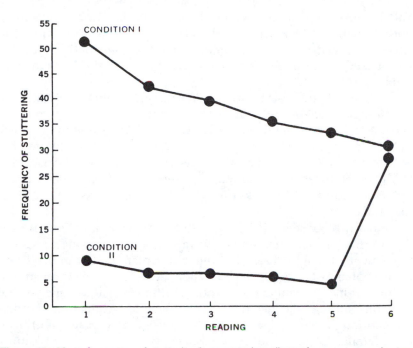

Figure 12. Mean frequency of stuttering in repeated readings of a passage under two conditions. Condition I was an ordinary adaptation series. In Condition II the subjects read in unison with an experimenter in all readings but the last. The two curves end at approximately the same point even though there has been a difference in the amount of stuttering along the way. Reproduced from Frank and Bloodstein (1971). Copyright 1971 by the American Speech-Language-Hearing Association. Reprinted by permission.

sweeping implications of these findings without further verification by others, it would appear that the rehearsal theory of adaptation is the only one that has merit. If so, this raises the question of exactly how rehearsal might lead to a reduction in stuttering. Again we have plunged into the depths of speculation since it is possible to identify some five theories about the answer to this question.

One is Eisenson's theory, already alluded to, that rehearsal minimizes the propositional value of the reading material.

A related theory, proposed by Jakobovits (1966), is that the individual words tend to lose much of their meaning through "semantic satiation." The theory is based on the observation that through repetition words tend to decrease in meaningfulness as measured by the semantic differential. Like Eisenson's hypothesis, it assumes that stuttering is influenced by the propositionality of speech.

A third theory with some connection to the first two is that in repeated reading of a passage the words become more predictable and lower in information value. It was advanced by Schlesinger, Forte, Fried, and Melkman (1965). Soderberg (1969a) showed that in successive readings of the same passage the information value of words tends to decrease according to a curve that is similar to the typical curve of adaptation.

A fourth hypothesis is that of Webster and Lubker (1968a), who speculated that through successive rehearsals stutterers tend to become less dependent on auditory cues for guidance of their speech output. It is based on the premise that stuttering is due to interference with speech by defective auditory feedback. Webster and Dorman (1971) demonstrated that normal speakers make fewer errors under delayed auditory feedback after they have rehearsed the reading material orally.

Finally, Bloodstein (1972) suggested that the adaptation effect is due to greater ease and conviction in the serial ordering of speech movements through rehearsal of the motor plan. Earlier in this chapter we noted instances in which fluency seemed to come from simplification of motor planning due to the stutterer's manner of speaking or to the nature of the material. Another way to facilitate serial ordering is through rehearsal, as anyone who has ever repeated a difficult or unfamiliar word aloud in order to master its motor plan knows. This explanation is related to one that was offered by Wingate (1966b), and it was clearly anticipated by Eisenson's view that the repeated readings "establish an articulatory and vocal set that approaches the automatic."

What Is the Stutterer Rehearsing?

All the evidence we have reviewed hints that adaptation is basically a matter of familiarization. But with precisely what? Is it necessary, for example, for subjects to read the passage orally, or is it enough for them to read it silently or mark the words on which they think they would stutter? We can give a conclusive answer to this question. Peins (1961a) found that successive silent markings of anticipation had no influence on frequency of stuttering when the subjects began to read the passage aloud, and a series of further studies has confirmed the ineffectiveness of passive silent rehearsal.[20]

The rehearsal must be oral. Must it also be vocal, or will repetition of silent speech movements do? Wischner (1947) found that after two rehearsals of a passage with silent "lip" movements there was a reduction of stuttering which did not quite attain statistical signifi-

---

[20]Besozzi and Adams (1969), Robbins (1971), Brenner, Perkins, and Soderberg (1972). Moss (1976), Murray, Empson, and Weaver (1987).

cance. With four lipped rehearsals Robbins (1971) found distinct evidence of such an effect. Brenner, Perkins, and Soderberg (1972) found that neither lipped nor whispered rehearsal reduced stuttering. Analysis of the data presented by Moss (1976) showed that lipped and whispered rehearsal had significant effects, but Moss found that vocal rehearsal reduced stuttering even more. In a study by Bruce and Adams (1978) whispered rehearsal had no effect. The issue is in doubt. All we can say for sure is that adaptation requires some type of active rehearsal. The more closely such rehearsal approaches the stutterer's ordinary speech the more unequivocal appears to be its benefit.

While the fact that active rehearsal is necessary may seem to give more support to some of the rehearsal theories of adaptation than to others, it will not, perhaps, serve to rule out any of them conclusively. Other kinds of information tend to weigh against several of these theories, however. The well-established fact that adaptation occurs in the repeated reading of word lists appears to make it unlikely that reduced contextual propositionality is a factor of major importance. In addition, the theory of increased predictability (reduced information load) is difficult to apply meaningfully in the case of a list of words.

This does not rule out reduced propositionality through semantic satiation of words, but Peterson, Rieck, and Hoff (1969) have cast some doubt on such a theory. They had stutterers rate selected words of a passage on the semantic differential both before and after repeated readings. In some cases the adaptation trials produced some semantic satiation of the words; in an equal number of cases it did not, though the stuttering declined.

On the assumption that the critical factor in the rehearsal effect is improved control of phonation, Ciambrone, Adams, and Berkowitz (1983) correlated thirteen subjects' adaptation scores with their improvement with practice in voice initiation time (see Chapter 4). The correlation coefficient (+0.445) was too small to demonstrate that improvement in vocal initiation time is a good predictor of amount of adaptation.

Zimmermann and Hanley (1983) theorized that the adaptation effect would be accompanied by changes in the velocities, displacements, and durations of movement of the tongue, jaw, and lip. In a study of three subjects the hypothesis was not borne out.

Horii and Ramig (1987) found that in the course of repeated readings, both stutterers and nonstutterers increased the duration of utterances between pauses. No change occurred in the fundamental frequency of the voice.

Prins and Hubbard (1990, 1992) reported that the duration of various speech segments did not change during adaptation, that adapting and non-adapting stutterers did not differ in the duration of speech segments, and that speech did not become more rhythmic during adaptation.

RESPONSE-CONTINGENT STIMULATION

In all of the attention we have given to the conditions under which stuttering varies in frequency we have not yet considered whether it is amenable to punishment and reinforcement. Yet, as we saw in Chapter 2, the broad issue of whether stuttering is an operant response, subject to prediction and control within the framework of B. F. Skinner's operant analysis of behavior, hinges on this question. The first answer came in a report by Flanagan, Goldiamond, and Azrin (1958) that they had produced temporary fluency in three stutterers by contingent presentations of a 105 dB tone and had increased the frequency of stuttering by contingent cessation of the tone. Following this announcement and the publication of a theoretical paper on stuttering and normal disfluency as operant behavior by Shames and Sherrick (1963) unusual interest developed in verifying the observations of Flanagan, Goldiamond, and Azrin.

The first to do so were Martin and Siegel (1966a, 1966b). Their subjects were five adult stutterers, each of whom spoke continuously in 40-minute to 1-hour sessions at intervals of a day to more than a week. With their first two subjects they made electric shock contingent upon specific stuttering behaviors such as nose wrinkling, tongue protrusion, or prolongation of the sound "s." In each case, within the first several minutes of shock the behavior rapidly decreased in frequency until it had virtually disappeared. In each case the behavior continued to be essentially absent in subsequent sessions, whether or not shocks were given, as long as the electrodes remained in place on the subject's wrist (*see Figure 13*). Each time the electrodes were removed the behavior rapidly increased in frequency to its original level. The only exception to this occurred after a plain nylon strap had been attached to one subject's wrist during a single 22-minute contingent shock session. In subsequent sessions there was a marked reduction of his behaviors even when the electrodes were removed, as long as the nylon strap remained in place.

With a third subject, shock was given during continuous spontaneous speech for any stuttering in any observable form, and virtually all stuttering was soon eliminated. In a later session during which the subject stuttered and was shocked on five occasions, a blue light was turned on during the procedure. On a subsequent occasion the presentation of the blue light alone produced a reduction in stuttering almost to zero for a time, despite the fact that the electrodes were not in place and the subject knew that he could not possibly be shocked. Whenever the electrodes and the blue light were both removed the stuttering returned to its usual level.

With the two remaining subjects (Martin and Siegel, 1966b) a more complex contingency using verbal punishment and reinforcement was

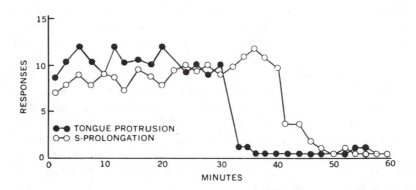

Figure 13. Number of tongue protrusion and s-prolongation responses per 2 minutes made by one subject during a 60-minute session of contingent electric shock. He had already been shocked for tongue protrusion in previous sessions. During the first 30 minutes the electrodes were off. For the next 10 minutes the electrodes were attached and shock was delivered contingent on tongue protrusion, which immediately decreased essentially to zero. During the last 20 minutes the shock was made contingent on s-prolongation for the first time, resulting in a rapid decline in the frequency of that response. Reproduced from Martin and Siegel (1966a). Copyright 1966 by the American Speech-Language-Hearing Association. Reprinted by permission.

arranged. The shock was replaced by the words "not good," and the word "good" was spoken at the end of every 30-second interval of oral reading during which no stuttering had occurred. In addition, at the start of experimental sessions the subjects received instructions to read carefully and fluently, and in some of the sessions a nylon strap was fastened to their wrists with the explanation that it was a "reminder to say each word as fluently as possible." The stuttering of both subjects fell off rapidly to a very low level under these conditions.

In three later sessions the nylon strap alone, without initial instructions or contingent verbal reward and punishment, produced a marked reduction in stuttering even when the subjects read to new listeners in a different room or into a telephone. Whenever the strap, instructions, and contingent verbal stimuli were removed the stuttering returned to its former level. When the instructions to "read fluently" were presented alone the stuttering dropped rather sharply to about a third of its original frequency, but the reduction was not as marked as under the other experimental conditions, and the stuttering steadily rose to its base level over the next 15 minutes.

These findings of Martin and Siegel had weighty theoretical implications concerning the nature of the moment of stuttering. They served in a most compelling way to raise the question whether stuttering is to be regarded, in behavioral terms, as an operant response, subject to positive or negative reinforcement and to punishment like the instrumental lever-pressing activity of a hungry rat. Such a model appears to suggest what in everyday terms is called a "simple" habit—that is, a habit simple enough to eliminate by paying attention to it and trying hard not to do it again. To all appearances it is in direct conflict with a considerable amount of clinical experience suggesting that stutterers are often likely to have their most severe difficulty when fearful of stuttering, aware of the probability of severe penalties for it, and strongly motivated to avoid it. Moreover, it runs counter to the experimental data of Van Riper (1937b) and Frick (1951), which showed that, when stutterers were told that at the end of their reading they were to receive as many electric shocks as they had blocks, their stuttering tended to increase.

There have been other experimental findings, however, which are in apparent conflict with those of Van Riper. Oxtoby (1955) reported that instructions to "try to avoid stuttering" had no effect on the frequency of blocks. Steer and Johnson (1936) found that in a series of 15 situations of varying difficulty there was a correlation of only 0.36 between subjects' severity of stuttering and reported desire to talk without stuttering. Wingate (1959) found a decrease in stuttering when the subjects were penalized after each block by an interruption in an electronic communication link with a listener or when each block was simply called to their attention by a recording counter. Furthermore, the results of Van Riper's experiment on the effect of penalty on stuttering were not confirmed either by Gross and Holland (1965) or by Williams and Martin (1974).

Additional Evidence in Support of the Operant View

A large amount of further research has been done on the question of whether stuttering may be modified by its contingent consequences, and almost invariably the answer has been that it can. Most of these studies have dealt with punishment for stuttering. This has taken the form of electric shock,[21] reprimands such as "wrong,"[22] loud noise,[23] intervals of delayed auditory feedback,[24] response-cost (money taken away),[25] time-out (an interval of several seconds during which the subject is not permitted to speak),[26] and recorded laugh-

---

[21]Gross and Holland (1965), Daly and Cooper (1967), Daly and Frick (1970), Moore and Ritterman (1973).

[22]Quist and Martin (1967), Reed and Lingwall (1976), Mowrer (1978), Martin and Haroldson (1979), Christensen and Lingwall (1982, 1983).

[23]Murray (1969), Hegde (1971b), Reed and Lingwall (1976), Stephen and Haggard (1980).

[24]Goldiamond (1965).

[25]Gross (1969), Halvorson (1971).

[26]Haroldson, Martin, and Starr (1968), Adams and Popelka (1971), Martin and Haroldson (1971), James and Ingham (1974), James (1976), Martin and Haroldson (1979), Costello and Hurst (1981), James (1981a, 1983).

ter.[27] It should be added that as soon as the punishment is discontinued the stuttering generally tends to return to its original level. Hegde (1971b) found no lasting effect on stuttering in oral reading after three months of daily application of contingent noise with five subjects.

Christensen and Lingwall (1983) found that contingent presentations of the word "wrong" produced its maximum effect in 20 minutes of conditioning; no further reduction in stuttering occurred after that. Christensen and Lingwall (1982) also reported that the conditioning was more effective in a laboratory than in a homelike setting, particularly when the verbal punisher was presented remotely by headset.

Gross and Holland (1965) found not only that contingent electroshock reduced stuttering, but also that it did so even when the listener was the one who received the shock. LaCroix (1973) observed that stutterers can reduce their own stuttering by activating a hand counter each time they stutter. Similar results have been described by Mowrer (1978) with the self-administered verbal punisher "stop," by Hanson (1978) and James (1981b) using self-recording of stuttering, and by Martin and Haroldson (1982) and James (1983) using self-administered time-out.

Stuttering has been reduced in laboratory investigations not only by punishment, but also by reinforcing fluency. The reinforcement has generally consisted of the word "good" or a small amount of money, and the reinforced response has been a predetermined period of fluency or number of consecutive fluent words. Reinforcement of fluency has either been given alone or combined with punishment for stuttering.[28] Self-reinforcement for fluency with tokens produced reductions in stuttering in a study by Cross and Cooper (1976).

Other demonstrations of the effect of contingent stimuli on stuttering have taken a considerable variety of forms. Hutchinson and Mackay (1973) brought about increased stuttering on subjects' fluent words in repeated readings by shocking them for saying the words fluently. Hasbrouck, Graham, and Brooks (1976) reduced the stuttering of three subjects by punishing them only for their normal disfluencies. In a study by Martin and Haroldson (1977) a group of subjects stuttered less after watching a video tape recording of a severe stutterer who experienced a marked reduction in stuttering under a contingent time-out procedure.

A unique application of punishment was made by Curlee and Perkins (1968). After being instructed to signal expectancies of stuttering prior to speech attempts, subjects were intermittently shocked for

---

[27]Reed and Lingwall (1980).

[28]Russell, Clark, and van Sommers (1968), Gross (1969), Halvorson (1971), Moore and Ritterman (1973), Lanyon and Barocas (1975), Hegde and Brutten (1977), Bastijens, Brutten, and Stés (1978), Mowrer (1978). See also Chapter 11.

doing so. Both the frequency of signaled anticipations and the frequency of stuttering decreased as a result. Daly and Frick (1970), however, obtained only a moderate reduction in expectancies and no reduction in stuttering in such a study, while Harris, Martin, and Haroldson (1971), using time-out from speaking as a punisher of expectancy, obtained variable results with three subjects. Earlier, Williams (1962) had found a marked decrease in stuttering when electric shock was made contingent on any anticipatory behavior such as tensing the jaw muscles, holding the breath, or changing the speaking rate prior to stuttering.

Dissenting Views and Counterexamples

Not all workers are agreed that the operant control of stuttering has been adequately demonstrated by the research we have just reviewed. The mildest demurrers have been on purely methodological grounds. For example, Starkweather (1971) argued that for several reasons the usual practice of making base-rate comparisons in operant conditioning studies may be of questionable validity in research on stuttering. Adams and Popelka (1971) showed that there is some difficulty involved in making a stimulus contingent on stuttering and that attempts to do so are frequently unsuccessful. James and Ingham (1974) questioned whether stutterers' expectations of fluency might account for some of the results attributed to punishment. They found, however, that manipulating their subjects' expectations did not influence the results of a time-out study.

Is Operant Stuttering Limited to the Secondary Features?

A different kind of qualification was urged by Brutten and Shoemaker (1969), who argued that only the associated symptoms of stuttering are subject to modification by response-contingent stimuli and that the repetitions and prolongations are not. This is consistent with their theory that the integral symptoms of stuttering are classically conditioned, while the secondary features are acquired through instrumental (operant) conditioning (*see Chapter 2*). In support of this view Janssen and Brutten (1973) reported a study of four stutterers in which shocks made selectively contingent on prolongations of sound had no systematic effect on the prolongations themselves; there was an increase in the case of two subjects and no change in the other two. For three of the subjects there was a decrease in the total number of moments of stuttering. Janssen and Brutten also cited an unpublished study of a single subject by Webster in which part-word repetitions failed to decrease under contingent aversive stimulation. Also consistent with this point of view is the finding by Oelschlaeger and Brutten (1976) that instructions to two stutterers to try to avoid repetitions of sounds were of no avail, whereas instructions to avoid interjections such as "uh" and "um" significantly reduced these reactions. Finally, Brutten (1980) presented data on a subject whose prolongations increased in frequency under contingent presentation of the word "wrong."

Costello and Hurst (1981) obtained somewhat contrary results in a study of three subjects. In two cases, target behaviors such as jaw tremors and repetitions of sounds, syllables, and words were reduced by contingent time-out, along with other symptoms that were not targeted for punishment. Subject 3 was given time-out for prolongations. There was no consistent effect on the prolongations, and her hard contacts increased. The experimenters then tried to punish the prolongations with a 90-decibel burst of tone. Prolongations, repetitions, and hard contacts decreased as a result, but only moderately. Finally, the experimenters had a talk with Subject 3 "to encourage harder work at fluency," following which all types of disfluency decreased further. Eventually the experimenters were able to demonstrate a distinct reduction in all disfluencies in response to the tone.

Punishment or Distraction?

A more sweeping skepticism was expressed by Biggs and Sheehan (1969), who contended that the reason for the punishment effect in stuttering is not the relationship of response and aversive stimulus at all. In a modified replication of the original study of Flanagan, Goldiamond, and Azrin (1958) they placed 6 adult stutterers under three conditions of 4000 Hz, 108 dB tone: presentation of the tone contingent on stuttering, cessation of the tone contingent on stuttering, and random presentation of the tone. The three conditions resulted in approximately the same amount of suppression of stuttering. Biggs and Sheehan concluded that the decrease in stuttering as a result of response-contingent stimulation is not the effect of punishment, but of distraction.

Effect of Neutral and Rewarding Stimuli

There is another reason why questions have been raised about the meaning of the research findings on punishment. In many studies the stimuli responsible for producing fluency have apparently had little aversive quality. Biggs and Sheehan's subjects generally rated the loud tone as only mildly aversive. In a study by Reed and Lingwall (1976) the punishment, consisting, of 95 dB noise or the word "wrong," failed to elevate GSR measures in 6 of 10 subjects. In 4 cases the GSR was actually lowered. In a later study Reed and Lingwall (1980) again found that punishment, in the form of recorded female laughter, had inconsistent, variable effects on the GSR although stuttering was consistently reduced. Adams and Popelka (1971) questioned 8 subjects who had served in a study of the effect of time-out from speaking and found that 6 had failed to perceive the time-out as punishment, evaluating it instead as a chance to, relax. In a similar study by James and Ingham (1974) only 6 of 14 subjects evaluated the time-out in terms suggesting unpleasantness. Martin and Gaviser (1971) showed that time-out was aversive enough so that normal speakers engaged in a free-choice button-pressing activity during spontaneous speech learned to avoid the button that signaled time-out from speaking and to press the one that did not. Nonstutterers questioned by Yonovitz and Shepherd (1977) also tended to regard time-out as annoying, but stutterers did not have definite reactions, and measures of their GSR and heart rate showed little evidence that the time-out was aversive.

If the mild aversiveness of some punishing stimuli tends to raise some questions, what is the meaning of the "punishers" that are on their face neutral or even rewarding? The outstanding case in point was supplied by Cooper, Cady, and Robbins (1970). They tested the effect of the words "wrong," "right," and "tree" and found that they all reduced stuttering equally. Siegel and Martin (1966) encountered a similar phenomenon in normal speakers when a "neutral" buzzer reduced the frequency of disfluencies. They offered the explanation that a neutral stimulus may have an alerting or "highlighting" value in the case of responses that are socially disapproved and which therefore "carry their own punishment."[29] Cooper, Cady, and Robbins suggested that a similar explanation might possibly do for their findings. This cannot be denied, and if it is true it is important, the more so since it seems to run counter to long-standing expectations about stuttering that have stemmed from ordinary clinical observation. We cannot overlook the fact, however, that this type of explanation has little place in the operant analysis of behavior which is concerned only with the effects of observable consequences. To resort to such an explanation is therefore to abandon the hope of prediction and control within a Skinnerian system that has been the ultimate goal of efforts to demonstrate the operant nature of stuttering.

Within the operant framework a punisher is defined only as a contingent stimulus which reduces the rate of responding. To remain within this frame we must forego any "explanation" of the Cooper, Cady, and Robbins findings and simply define them as punishment. It is irrelevant that the words "right" and "tree" do not strike us as punishing or may not be evaluated negatively by the subjects. At first

---

[29]See also Siegel (1970).

glance this may seem to be a simple way to dispose of a troublesome problem, but the impression proves to be illusory. The difficulty is not merely the artificiality of this use of the term punishment, but the conclusions to which it leads. It is paradoxical within the operant frame to find that a stimulus that decreases the rate of occurrence of one response increases the rate of another. Judged by its consequences the word "right" is as effective a generalized reinforcer as can be found. To observe it acting as a punisher is anomalous and contradictory.

Daly and Kimbarow (1978) replicated the Cooper, Cady, and Robbins experiment with school-age subjects and obtained the same results. Several additional attempts have been made to test the effect of contingent presentation of stimuli that are presumably neutral or reinforcing.[30] The reinforcers have usually been money or a signal in lieu of money. The results have been somewhat inconsistent and confusing, but there is a distinct tendency for the stuttering of most subjects to decrease just as it does when presumably aversive stimuli are used. Lanyon and Barocas (1975) found that an audible signal contingent on stuttering reduced stuttering about equally whether it meant monetary gain or loss, but that random presentation of the signal had no effect.

No satisfactory explanation has yet been advanced for the fact that virtually any contingent stimulus seems capable of reducing the stuttering of most subjects. Hanson (1978) attempted to test the hypothesis, already mentioned, that by drawing the speaker's attention to the stutterings, the stimulus somehow makes it possible for the stutterer to speak more fluently. Hanson reasoned that if this were the case, stutterers' heightened awareness of their stuttering would be reflected in a tendency to identify more blocks in their own speech. In an experiment, 2 subjects were instructed to first depress a handswitch to note each stuttering block they detected in their own speech. In a subsequent session Hanson administered a neutral stimulus in the form of a brief flash of a small jewel light. The subjects' attentiveness to stuttering was then measured once again by having them detect the blocks in their speech. In the case of one subject the light flash reduced the stuttering, but had no effect on her subsequent count of her own blocks. In the other case the light flash had no effect on the stuttering, but the subject's count of her blocks increased. As Hanson concluded, each subject failed in a different way to confirm the hypothesis that contingent stimuli reduce stuttering by calling the subjects' attention to their blocks.

In a study by James, Ricciardelli, Rogers, and Hunter (1989), a group of stutterers who were not highly responsive to time-out from speaking

---

[30]Patty and Quarrington (1974), Lanyon and Barocas (1975), Oelschlaeger and Brutten (1975), Starkweather and Lucker (1978), Corcoran (1980), James (1981a).

became more so after completing a program of training in syllable prolongation. It was concluded that the contingent stimulus became more effective because it encouraged the subjects to use "fluency skills."

Summary Remarks

The results of a number of studies have caused some workers to be skeptical about the interpretation placed on the effects of contingent stimuli in so much past research on stuttering and to question whether the operant model of behavior is an adequate representation of the stuttering response. Such doubts have been strengthened by other apparent discrepancies between predictions from the model and observation. It would be reasonable to predict, for example, that punishment for operant behavior would be more effective if delivered immediately contingent on the response than if it were delayed. Williams and Martin (1974) compared the effect of electric shock immediately after each block with a condition in which the subjects received the appropriate number of shocks following every sentence. Stuttering was reduced by the same amount under both conditions.

We would also expect a large amount of punishment to have a greater effect than a small one. Yet, in a study of the effect of time-out from speaking, James (1976) found that enforced interruptions of speech of 1, 5, 10, and 30 seconds reduced stuttering to about the same extent. James suggested that the punishment in this procedure might be the initial interruption rather than the time-out from speaking.

Finally, it has been difficult for researchers to account for anomalous and idiosyncratic responses of individual stutterers to the operant conditioning paradigm. One example was a study of punishment and negative reinforcement of stuttering with 5 subjects by Martin, St. Louis, Haroldson, and Hasbrouck (1975). Punishment consisted of electric shock. Negative reinforcement, under which stuttering should have increased, took the form of brief periods of cessation, contingent on stuttering, of a steady electric shock. Under negative reinforcement there was an increase in stuttering in 2 subjects, a decrease in 1, and no change in 2. In the punishment condition 2 subjects stuttered less, 2 stuttered more, and 1 was not affected. The authors concluded, "Results of the present experiment yield only very equivocal support to the notion that stuttering is an operant response class." Equally contradictory or inconsistent results of response-contingent stimulation were reported by Hegde (1971a), Cross and Cooper (1976), and others.

Conclusions

Almost all research findings point to the conclusion that response-contingent stimuli have a broad potential for reducing the frequency of stuttering. The reason for this reduction, however, is far from clear.

What was at first widely thought to be a punishment effect that contradicted long-standing clinical assumptions about the effect of aversive reactions to stuttering now seems more and more to represent another kind of process, as yet poorly understood, in which the aversiveness of the contingent stimulus is irrelevant and which has little in common with the social penalty that often appears to increase the severity of stuttering. Three alternative hypotheses have been advanced to account for the effect of contingent stimuli. One is that it represents a form of operant conditioning. A second is that contingent stimuli help the speaker to avoid stuttering by calling attention to it. A third is that some type of distraction is at work.[31] As yet there is little evidence to support any of these explanations. Stuttering is an ephemeral, elusive phenomenon that is responsive to subtle psychological states. The application of contingent stimuli, whether aversive or not, generally appears to create a psychological state in which stuttering tends to diminish. The nature of that state remains to be clarified.

The outstanding triumph of the operant model of stuttering was the unexpected demonstration that stuttering appeared to be subject to punishment within B. F. Skinner's operant conditioning paradigm. The model would now seem to have produced research findings that are anomalous within this paradigm, and not everyone is agreed that what is taking place in so-called operant conditioning experiments is learning or conditioning.

There is a further problem with which the operant model must deal. Operants represent an extremely broad category of behavior. The statement that stuttering is operant behavior is therefore relatively empty in itself. It acquires significant content only to the extent that we can specify at least in general terms the contingencies by which the behavior is governed. At this writing we do not seem to be closer to being able to do so than we were in 1958 when it was first reported that stuttering had been brought under "operant control." That is, we lack elementary knowledge of the reinforcements by which stuttering is maintained. We could not take any steps to extinguish it by withholding reinforcement. We do not know what satiations would serve to decrease it or what deprivations would tend to make it more frequent.

THE WHITE NOISE EFFECT

For many years it had occasionally been noted that stutterers are likely to have less speech difficulty in the presence of loud noise—for

---

[31]The distraction hypothesis should not be dismissed lightly. Subjects receiving an unusual or inappropriate stimulus immediately after every stuttering block are soon conditioned to expect the stimulus at each instant they expect to stutter. The distraction, if distraction it is, may thus come at a critical moment.

example, near ocean surf, a waterfall, or a passing train. Kern (1932) demonstrated this effect experimentally by means of a Barany drum. Then in 1955 Shane in the United States and Cherry, Sayers, and Marland in England reported that binaural masking with white noise at high intensity brought about the virtual elimination of stuttering in most subjects. In both cases the inference was drawn that it was the subjects' inability to hear their own speech that produced the effect, rather than mere distraction. Since then the white noise effect has been verified repeatedly.[32] The reductions in stuttering achieved tend to vary from subject to subject and often fall considerably short of complete fluency. Conture and Brayton (1975) observed the chief effect of the noise to be on part-word repetitions, but in a study by Hutchinson and Norris (1977) most disfluency types were found to be reduced.

The great majority of studies have been concerned with oral reading. In spontaneous speech both Hutchinson and Norris (1977) and Mallard and Webb (1980) found no significant reduction in stuttering for stutterers as a group. That the white noise effect can be demonstrated in the spontaneous speech of stutterers is evident, however, from a series of studies.[33]

Theories of the White Noise Effect

Several points of view have developed about the reason for reductions in stuttering under masking noise. The conclusion to which Cherry and Sayers came from their study in 1956 was that stuttering is a perceptual rather than a motor abnormality. At about that time interest had begun to develop in Lee's discovery that delayed auditory feedback could produce "artificial stutter" in many normal speakers, and an analogy with clinical stuttering had already been drawn (see Chapter 2). To some workers the white noise effect seemed an illuminating confirmation of the hypothesis that the stutterer's basic trouble was a disturbance of auditory feedback, since it was easy to imagine that the noise served to mask the interfering feedback. Maraist and Hutton (1957) put this in servo-theory terms when they said that in stuttering a person "misevaluates his own speech

---

[32]Maraist and Hutton (1957), Sutton and Chase (1961), Shrum (1962), May and Hackwood (1968), Burke (1969), Murray (1969), Webster and Dorman (1970), Adams and Moore (1972), Adams and Hutchinson (1974), Conture (1974), Garber and Martin (1974), Conture and Brayton (1975), Dewar, Dewar, and Anthony (1976), Dewar, Dewar, and Barnes (1976), Yairi (1976), Altrows and Bryden (1977), Garber and Martin (1977), Hutchinson and Norris (1977), Brayton and Conture (1978), Lechner (1979), Martin and Haroldson (1979), Ingham, Southwood, and Horsburgh (1981), Zsilavecz (1981), Martin, Siegel, Johnson, and Haroldson (1984), Martin, Johnson, Siegel, and Haroldson (1985).

[33]Garber and Martin (1974, 1977), Dewar, Dewar, and Barnes (1976), Martin and Haroldson (1979), Ingham, Southwood, and Horsburgh (1981), Martin, Siegel, Johnson, and Haroldson (1984), Martin, Johnson, Siegel, and Haroldson (1985).

output at some point in the control system and finds error where, in reality, no error exists." When their auditory feedback is interrupted stutterers cease their efforts to correct their nonexistent error and so temporarily stop stuttering. It is this general point of view, expressed in various ways by Yates (1963), Webster and Lubker (1968a), and others, that has perhaps been chiefly responsible for the continued interest in the white noise effect.

A second interpretation was advanced by Shane (1955). She suggested that when stutterers were unable to hear their own speech they were "relatively free from the anxiety-producing cues involved" in hearing themselves stutter. Others would have said hearing themselves "speak." In either case the explanation is based on the anticipatory struggle concept of stuttering, particularly as expressed by Johnson.

A third possibility, suggested by Wingate (1970), is that fluency under white noise results from an increase in the intensity of the subject's voice or from other vocal changes of the Lombard effect.

A fourth theory is that the noise acts as a distraction. This simple viewpoint has not often been advocated, but it has been recognized from the beginning as a possibility.

Must Subjects Fail to Hear Their Own Speech?

In trying to narrow down the possible reasons for the white noise effect we would obviously find it helpful to know if the critical factor is the subjects' inability to hear their own speech. Shane (1955) believed it was and offered as evidence the finding that white noise which had a marked effect on stuttering at 95 dB had essentially no effect at 25 dB. Cherry and Sayers (1956) found that high-frequency masking noise was considerably less effective than low-frequency noise (below 500 Hz) They concluded that the reduction in stuttering was due to the stutterers' failure to hear the low-frequency components of their speech.

On the other hand, the research findings as a whole have tended to weigh against the assumption that subjects must fail to hear their own speech. In the first place, both Shane (1955) and Adams and Moore (1972) found that the great majority of their subjects reported hearing their own speech above the noise. In addition ample evidence exists that white noise will reduce stuttering in forms allowing the subjects considerable ability to hear their speech. Maraist and Hutton (1957) studied the effect at masking levels of 30, 50, 70, and 90 dB above normal threshold and observed a progressive decrease in the amount of stuttering, with a particularly marked decline beginning at 50 dB, where the subjects' speech must have been clearly audible to them. Murray (1969) found that random bursts of noise produced a decided reduction of stuttering, though not as much as continuous noise. Both May and Hackwood (1968) and Conture (1974) found that high-frequency masking (above 500 Hz) resulted in as much fluency as low-frequency masking. This conflicts with Cherry and Sayers' results referred to above, but even Cherry and Sayers observed distinctly reduced stuttering under high-frequency noise. Moreover, Barr and Carmel (1969) reported a decrease in stuttering with only 50 dB of high-frequency narrow-band masking noise delivered to only one ear. Yairi (1976) also found that stuttering decreased under monaural noise, though not to the same extent as under binaural masking.

These conditions did not all reduce stuttering equally, and it might be argued that there are various possible degrees of interference with the ability to hear one's own speech. For this reason exceptional interest was stirred by the study of Sutton and Chase (1961), in which reduced stuttering was apparently achieved by white noise without any masking of speech at all. Using a voice-actuated relay to turn the noise either on or off while the subjects read aloud, Sutton and Chase tested the effect of three experimental conditions: continuous noise, noise present only during the phonation of sounds, and noise present only during the silent periods. They found that all three conditions were equally effective.

This prompted a rejoinder by Yates (1963) that we normally hear the feedback from our speech with a slight delay; moments of feedback do not coincide exactly with moments of phonation. For this reason Yates believed that at least part of this feedback was masked in both of Sutton and Chase's discontinuous noise conditions. Later a somewhat similar objection was raised by Webster and Lubker (1968b). They pointed out that it takes time for a voice-actuated relay to respond to phonation since the intensity of the voice must reach a required level. Consequently, they reasoned, in the condition in which the noise was turned off by phonation, the subjects' auditory feedback must have been masked during the critical fraction of a second when phonation was being initiated. In reply, Chase and Sutton (1968) agreed that such a delay existed and that it was added to by mechanical lag in the relay itself. With reason, however, they pointed out that the same delay that was present when voice turned the masking off must also have been present in the condition in which voice turned it on. Using the argument that the initial part of the phonation is critical for stuttering, it thus becomes difficult to explain why stuttering was reduced when noise was present only during phonations, the initial portions of these phonations not having been masked.

Subsequently Webster and Dorman (1970) performed the same experiment using a list of single words in place of connected reading material and obtained the same results: Stuttering was reduced equally whether the noise was started by onset of phonation, stopped by phonation, or continuous. Altrows and Bryden (1977) repeated this experiment using sentences in place of words. Controlling the noise manually, they found that noise presented only before initiation of a sentence and terminated following the first audible speech sound had no effect on stuttering in the sentence as a whole. This is perhaps no more than would be expected considering that there was no noise during almost the entire reading of the sentence, but they also found no effect on stuttering on the first word, despite the masking of its initial sound. When they presented the noise continuously or concurrently with the reading of each sentence, stuttering was reduced.

What results of these three studies suggest is that the noise works grossly and not by virtue of any selective effect on the initial portion of a word, that the noise must be present for a substantial part of the time during which the subject is speaking, but that it need not be concurrent with intervals of phonation. If this is so, our best judgment at present would probably have to be that the white noise effect does not depend on masking of speech. This means that neither Cherry and Sayers' theory that the noise masks a perceptual defect nor Shane's inference that it obliterates anxiety-producing cues would seem to have sufficient support. With respect to anxiety reduction, it may be pertinent that Adams and Moore (1972) found that the white noise had little effect on stutterers' levels of autonomic arousal as measured by palmar sweating.

The Influence of Vocal Changes

If stutterers' fluency under white noise has little to do with difficulty in hearing their own speech, it is perhaps unlikely that it is due to the Lombard effect. Nevertheless, the increase in vocal intensity that usually occurs with exposure to loud noise had frequently been considered as a possible cause of the reduction in stuttering. There is ample evidence that, at least as a group, stutterers do increase their vocal loudness under masking (*see Chapter 4, footnote 34*). The question is whether this is the factor responsible for the gain in fluency. One way to test such an assumption is to instruct or train subjects to maintain a normal level of vocal intensity while exposed to the noise. This was done in three separate studies with the same result: The stuttering decreased in noise despite the absence of increased vocal intensity.[34] An exception was an unpublished study of Anthony cited by Adams and Moore (1972). A second strategy is to study the effect of raising vocal intensity without masking noise. Again the results conflict with the vocal intensity hypothesis. Shrum (1962) found significantly greater reduction of stuttering in subjects under masking than when they read at the same high intensity level without masking.

---

[34]Cherry and Sayers (1956), Dewar, Dewar, and Anthony (1976), Garber and Martin (1977).

Garber and Martin (1977) found no decrease in stuttering with increased vocal intensity and no masking. Further difficulties for the hypothesis are presented by reports of individual cases in which the subject's vocal intensity in noise failed to vary concomitantly with stuttering frequency. For example, Yairi (1976) noted that in 2 of his 6 subjects decreases in stuttering in noise were not always accompanied by increases in vocal level, and in a study by Martin, Siegel, Johnson, and Haroldson (1984) the amount of reduction in stuttering was unrelated to the change in intensity of the subjects' voices.[35]

There seems, then, to be little evidence to support the hypothesis that increased vocal loudness alone can account for the white noise effect. Wingate (1970) pointed out that we must also consider the effects of noise on the stutterer's vocal pitch and duration, but relevant research findings as yet have been sparse and ambiguous. Brayton and Conture (1978) found (as did Lechner, 1979) that the fundamental frequency of stutterers' voices did tend to rise in noise, but the subjects with greater increases in fundamental frequency tended to show smaller decreases in stuttering. For seven subjects decreases in stuttering showed a modest correlation with increases in vowel duration ($r = 0.41$), but in the remaining two cases there was apparently little relationship between the two measures. Increased vowel duration may possibly be part of the reason stutterers tend to speak more fluently in noise, but, as is true of increased vocal intensity, it is evidently not the whole reason.

Finally, Hayden, Jordahl, and Adams (1982) explored the possibility that stutterers' fluency in masking noise is due to a favorable effect of noise on voice initiation time (see Chapter 4). Contrary to their hypothesis, however, subjects' vocal initiation time proved to be slower rather than faster under noise.

White Noise as a Novel Form of Auditory Feedback

We are left with one remaining explanation—that the white noise is distracting. This is a prosaic hypothesis, but it has at least one strong source of support. Evidence suggests that almost any novel form of auditory feedback is capable of reducing stuttering. Harris (1955) found that merely amplifying the stutterer's voice had this effect. Ham and Steer (1967) observed less stuttering in some subjects with amplification, delay, or frequency filtering of their auditory feed-

---

[34]Cherry and Sayers (1956), Dewar, Dewar, and Anthony (1976), Garber and Martin (1977)

[35]See also Conture (1974) and Mallard and Webb (1980). Moore and Adarns (1985), however, found that instructions and practice did not completely reduce subjects' vocal intensities to prenoise levels, although the difference was not apparent to the ear.

back. The effect of distorting the stutterer's auditory feedback by frequency filtering was confirmed by Howell, El-Yaniv, and Powell (1987) and by Kalinowski, Armson, Roland-Mieszkowski, Stuart, and Gracco (1993). Unison reading reduces stuttering even when the second person reads different material.[36] Adamczyk and his colleagues found that reverberation had a marked effect on stuttering.[37] Stephen and Haggard (1980) obtained reductions in stuttering with delayed auditory feedback; with a four-speaker babble of voices played backwards, delayed or synchronous, contingent on speech or continuous; with a speech-contingent low-frequency tone that was either synchronous or delayed; and with a continuous low-frequency tone. Stuttering has also been reduced by frequency filtered delayed auditory feedback (Adamczyk and Kuniszyk-Jóźkowiak, 1987); by phase shifted feedback of the vocal tone (Webster, 1991); and by a click at the onset of each syllable activated by the intensity of the sound (Howell and El-Yaniv, 1987). Not all of these conditions reduced stuttering to the same degree, but the observations suggest that just as it is difficult to find a novel method of speaking that does not alleviate stuttering, it may be difficult to find an unusual kind of auditory speech feedback or auditory perceptual field that does not do the same thing.[38]

Martin, Siegel, Johnson, and Haroldson (1984) found that amplification of stutterers' feedback of their own voices resulted in greater fluency only when following a condition in which their stuttering had been reduced by masking noise. Curious about whether it was the noise or the fluency that had caused this effect, they repeated the study with the addition of a rhythmic speech condition. Again the amplified side-tone reduced the subjects' stuttering when preceded by the noise condition, but not when preceded by rhythmic speech (Martin, Johnson, Siegel, and Haroldson, 1985).

Howell (1990) investigated the effect of altered feedback of several kinds on the intensity of the voice. He found that stutterers and normal speakers increased their voice levels under delayed feedback and white noise and reduced them slightly under frequency shifted and amplified speech feedback.

One of the most thoroughly investigated of these altered feedback effects, because of the applications it has found in the treatment of stut-

---

[36]Barber (1939), Cherry and Sayers (1956), May and Hackwood (1968). The effect is greater when the material is the same, however.

[37]Adamczyk, Sadowska, and Kuniszyk-Jóźkowiak (1975), Adamczyk, Kuniszyk-Jóźkowiak, and Smolka (1979), Admczyk and Kuniszyk-Jóźkowiak (1987).

[38]The author was acquainted with a stutterer who was in the habit of drawing his record player up to the telephone when he had a call to make.

tering, is delayed auditory feedback (DAF).[39] Its effect on the stutterer is often just the reverse of its effect on the nonstutterer, despite some inconsistency. A frequent report is that some stutterers, especially in milder cases, tend to expence increased difficulty, much as do nornal speakers. Most stutterers appear to improve under DAF, however. There is reason to believe that more than just novel auditory feedback is involved in this improvement. In the effort to overcome the disruptive effect of the DAF most speakers tend to slow their rate of speech, concentrate on proprioceptive and tactile monitoring, or overarticulate.[40] Stutterers who do these things in order to "beat" the DAF effect are incidentally doing things that are likely to decrease their stuttering as well. This may be the reason stutterers who speak fluently under DAF appear to be miraculously avoiding both their stuttering and the disfluencies that are a usual consequence of DAF. Nevertheless, DAF may also derive a large share of its power over stuttering simply as a novel change in the stutterer's auditory perceptual field, since Langová, Morávek, Novák, and Petřík (1970) found that DAF that had been made almost unintelligible by frequency filtering had as beneficial an effect on the speech of stutterers as did unfiltered DAF.

In view of all these findings, it is perhaps not to soon to conclude that virtually any change in stutterers' accustomed way of hearing themselves speak is likely to alleviate their speech difficulty. This calls to mind a similar observation we made in Chapter 7—namely, that any change in the stutterer's accustomed way of speaking is likely to result in immediate fluency. Is the parallelism merely a matter of chance? In Chapter 7 we ventured to suggest that it is not the negligible effort it takes to adopt an artificial speech pattern that diverts the stutterer's attention from stuttering, but the bizarre way in which he hears himself talking. It may not be far fetched to suggest that in reviewing the effects of altered speech and altered speech feedback on stuttering, we are dealing with one and the same observation.

Returning to the white noise effect and the supposition that it acts as a novel form of feedback, there is one final question that is crucial for essentially all explanations based on distraction but rarely easy to answer. Does the effect wear off with loss of novelty? The evidence

---

[39]Nessel (1958), Soderberg (1960), Chase, Sutton, and Rapin (1961), Lotzmann (1961), Neelley (1961), Goldiamond (1965), Ham and Steer (1967), Webster and Lubker (1968a), Curlee and Perkins (1969), Soderberg (1969b), Langová, Morávek, Novák, and Petřík (1970), Webster, Schumacher, and Lubker (1970), Gibney (1973), Hutchinson and Burk (1973), Macioszek (1973), Burke (1975), Treon and Tamayo (1975), Hayden, Scott, and Addicott (1977) Hutchinson and Norris (1977), Novák (1978), Timmons and Boudreau (1978a, 1978b), Lechner (1979), Martin and Haroldson (1979), Stephen and Haggard (1980), Zsilavecz (1981) Howell, El-Yaniv, and Powell (1987), Kalinowski, Armson, Roland-Mieszkowski, Stuart, and Gracco (1993).

[40]See discussions by Soderberg (1969b), Van Riper (1970), and Wingate (1970).

we have is too meager to permit a confident answer. We know that of the subjects tested by Cherry, Sayers, and Marland (1955) the only one who failed to improve under white noise worked in surroundings with a high ambient noise level. We also have a report by Guttman (1960) that in Leningrad portable hearing-aid-like masking devices for stutterers were abandoned after a few years "because stutterers did not experience lasting improvement and found it cumbersome." On the other hand, Trotter and Lesch (1967) reported the successful use of such a device by a college teacher for two and a half years. He normally used it during lectures, committee meetings, and telephone conversations, turning it on whenever he blocked or thought he was about to stutter. Garber and, Martin (1974) had three subjects talk spontaneously during a series of 6 to 11 50-minute sessions in which white noise was on continuously for alternate 5-minute periods. In 2 of the the 3 cases there was no substantial "long-term" effect on stuttering, although their stuttering had been reduced by 82, 15, and 38 percent, respectively, during the first 5 minutes in which noise had been presented. By contrast, a stutterer tested by Dewar, Dewar, and Bames (1976) showed no habituation to the noise in twenty-two biweekly sessions. The difficulty with all such observations is that we know too little about the effect of novel conditions on stuttering to say whether an adequate test of this effect requires days, weeks, or many months.

The Auditory Feedback Theory of Stuttering

In stuttering theory, the white noise effect has been important chiefly in relation to speculations about defective auditory feedback mechanisms as the underlying cause of stuttering (see Chapter 2). A theory has several possible relationships to the facts. It may be in conflict with them, it may be irrelevant to them, it may manage to account for them, and it may illuminate them with meaning. The auditory feedback model is the kind of theory that brightly illuminates a few facts, but stands in weak or ambiguous relationship to most of them. It has given a simple meaning both to the white noise effect and to what would otherwise have been merely a chance resemblance between stuttering and the speech breakdown of normal speakers under delayed auditory feedback. It has also been made to account for several other facts about stuttering, but appears irrelevant to most of them. Since it is questionable whether the white noise effect depends on masking of speech, the explanation provided for it by the theory seems to be of doubtful validity. It remains to be seen whether the resemblance of DAF speech disruptions to stuttering fares better with careful investigation.

Hutchinson and Ringel (1975) reported that complete deprivation of oral sensation in six stutterers caused an increase in the frequency and severity of stuttering. Although the significance of this finding is obscure, some workers may be inclined to speculate that the loss of oral sensation increased the subjects' dependence on their auditory feedback.[41] If the finding is confirrned, the theory of defective auditory feedback may therefore have scored another enlightening explanation. On the debit side, no satisfactory answer has yet been made to the objection of Moravek and Langova (1967) that stuttering tends to occur at the moment of initiation of speech units before auditory feedback has begun to arrive.

THE METRONOME EFFECT

Most stutterers can talk with exceptional fluency when they time their speech to a rhythmic beat such as the ticking of a metronome. This played a part in both early and more recent attempts to treat stuttering. In modern times laboratory studies have repeatedly confirmed the metronome effect.[42] Both syllables and words have been timed with the metronome with striking results. Auditory, visual, or tactile rhythmic stimuli have all been found equally effective. The effect has been demonstrated in both oral reading and spontaneous speech. Trotter and Silverman (1974) reported that a portable metronome device continued to reduce stuttering after sixteen months of continuous use by one of the authors (Silverman), but the effect was greatest during the first three months. Later, Silverman (1976b) related that over a three-year period the benefit he received from the device steadily decreased, and in the final six months it had very little effect on the frequency or severity of his stuttering. Barber (1940) and others have regarded the metronome effect as an example of distraction. Fransella and Beech (1965) questioned whether this is an adequate explanation, however, and so have others since. In discussions of distraction as a possible cause there has sometimes been some confusion between the distraction, if any, that might come from the sound of the rhythmic beat and the distraction that might be involved in the use of the rhythmical pattern of speech. Experimental work attempting to rule out distraction has been inconclusive, as we saw in our discussion of distraction in Chapter 7. Perhaps the only undisputed fact that has been learned from explorations of the basis for the metronome

---

[41]The interpretation suggested by Hutchinson and Ringel was that the loss of sensory feedback may have impaired the subjects' ability to minimize stutterings by appropriate oral movements.

[42]Barber (1940), Fransella and Beech (1965), Azrin, Jones, and Flye (1968), Brady (1969), Jones and Azrin (1969), Greenberg (1970), Silverman and Umberger (1974), Trotter and Siiverman (1974), Silverman (1976b), Hanna and Morris (1977), Hutchinson and Navarre (1977), Hutchinson and Norris (1977), Brayton and Conture (1978), Martin and Haroldson (1979), Wingate (1981b), Hayden, Adams, and Jordahl (1982), Martin, Johnson, Siegel, and Haroldson (1985).

effect is that it is not due primarily to reduced rate of speech. Brady (1969) set the metronome at a rate corresponding to that of the subjects' unaided oral reading. Fransella and Beech (1965) used their subjects' rates of nonstuttered reading as predicted from their silent reading rates. Hanna and Morris (1977) used their reading rates in free speech. Both Barber (1940) and Hanna and Morris (1977) tested the effect of a metronome rate that made subjects speak even faster than usual. In all cases the metronome remained highly effective, though slower rates tended to result in still less stuttering.

There are two other identifiable effects of the metronome condition besides the effect it may have on rate. One, of course, is the unusual regularity or rhythm it imparts to speech. The other is the effect it has of breaking speech up into very small units for isolated articulation, particularly when subjects time their speech to the metronome syllable by syllable. It is a good guess that something might be learned by separating the effects of these two factors.

The Factor of Syllabification

The separation of syllabification from rhythmicity was accomplished by two studies, one of which was done by Brady (1969). He had subjects speak one syllable per beat in time to both a rhythmic metronome and a metronome that produced beats in accordance with no regular pattern. In both cases there was little stuttering. Significantly fewer blocks occurred in the rhythmic condition, but the difference was slight.

It might have appeared from Brady's study that rhythm had little to do with the metronome effect. He suggested that the beat had a "cue" function, signaling to the subject when the next sound was to be said. Fransella (1971), however, found that such a signal has little effect on stuttering, even when it is predictable. Brady's findings are not difficult to account for on the basis of the observation that under both of his metronome conditions speech was reduced to a string of isolated syllables. Syllables tend to be extremely easy for most stutterers to say in isolation. In part, it appears to illustrate a general factor that we discussed earlier in this chapter, the tendency for stuttering to diminish as the motor plan of speech becomes easier.

The Factor of Rhythmicity

As we have seen, Brady studied the effect of syllabification removed from rhythmicity. Azrin, Jones, and Flye (1968) did the opposite; they studied the effect of rhythmicity independently of syllabification. Like Brady, they had subjects speak in time to a rhythmic and arrhythmic metronome—in actuality a vibrotactile pulse. Unlike

Brady, however, they instructed subjects to speak one whole word to each beat, except that words that were too long were to be syllabically divided between beats.[43] This was an important difference in procedure. Isolated words tend to be stuttered far more often than isolated syllables, probably because many of them are polysyllabic and require more complex serial ordering and because they have more meaning. The results were instructive. The rhythmic condition reduced stuttering sharply. In the arrhythmic condition, however, with neither syllabification nor rhythmicity to help them, the subjects stuttered as much as they did without any metronome.

It is evident that rhythmicity has a very strong effect of its own on stuttering, apart from the powerful effect of syllabification. Why this is so may be open to debate. When virtually every unusual pattern of articulation, voice, stress, inflection, or phrasing that can be invented for that purpose seems to reduce stuttering markedly, however, it would be gratuitous to assume that speaking rhythmically is an exception. On the other hand, Brady (1969) argued that the metronome effect is greater in magnitude than that of most other speech patterns. This gains support from the study of Johnson and Rosen (1937) in which a metronome condition produced more fluency than high or low pitch, high or low intensity, slow rate, or whispering. It was on a par with singing, speaking in time to an arm-swing, and speaking in a sing-song, all of which have a rhythmic element.

Considered solely as an unusual speech pattern, however, rhythmic speech is obviously a compelling one. Perhaps the reason for this can be glimpsed in the finding of Azrin, Jones, and Flye (1968) that a rhythmic beat produces a synchronization effect; vocal and motor responses of normal subjects tend to become timed with it. In contrast, speaking in time to an arrhythmic beat, though it is difficult and confusing as Brady remarked, is hardly a speech pattern at all, in the usual sense. Since the beat is unpredictable, subjects are forced to wait for it and then say their word or syllable. In the rhythmic condition, on the other hand, they do not literally time each word or syllable to the beat. They extract from the beat the information they need to program their speech so that its rhythm coincides with that of the metronome. It is this programmed aspect that gives it the character of a speech pattern. As unusual patterns go, it can hardly be denied that rhythmic speech is a bizarre one.

The evidence we have considered suggests, then, that at least two factors underlie the metronome effect. One is that stutterers tend to

---

[43]The subjects were reported to have followed these instructions with no apparent difficulty. When a word was long either one or two syllables were usually spoken during a beat.

become fluent when they find themselves speaking in almost any way strange to them. In this respect the metronome effect is allied to the fluency stutterers experience when they assume a dialect or imitate another person's speech. The other factor, especially strong when the stutterer times each syllable to the beat, is a drastically reduced demand on motor planning.

Throughout this discussion we have tacitly discounted the effect of any distraction that might come merely from hearing a rhythmic metronome. Although such an effect seems improbable, studies by Greenberg (1970) and Brayton and Conture (1978) force us to think about it since they found that a rhythmic metronome reduced stuttering even when the subjects were not instructed to pace their speech with it. We must recall that Azrin, Jones, and Flye (1968) found a rhythmic beat to have a synchronization effect on vocal responses. Greenberg's comments, furthermore, suggest that the subjects often spontaneously "fell into rhythm" with the metronome. Presumably, this was the cause of their fluency.

Suggested Readings

Beech, H. R, and Fransella, F., *Research and Experiment in Stuttering*. Oxford: Pergamon (1969), Chap. 7.

Costello, J. M., and Ingham, R J., Stuttering as an operant disorder. In Curlee R. F., and Perkins, W. H. (eds.), *Nature and Treatment of Stuttering: New Directions*. San Diego: College-Hill Press (1984).

Prins, D., and Hubbard, C. P., Response contingent stimuli and stuttering: Issues and implications. *J. Speech Hearing Res., 31*, 696–709 (1988) .

Siegel, G. M., Punishment, stuttering, and disfluency. *J. Speech Hearing Res., 13*, 677-714 (1970).

Van Riper, C., *The Nature of Stuttering, 2nd ed*. Englewood Cliffs, NJ.: Prentice-Hall (1982), Chaps. 13, 15.

9

EARLY STUTTERING AND NORMAL DISFLUENCY

Stuttering usually develops in the early years of childhood, as we have seen. It tends to undergo many changes in the course of time. To try to glimpse something of its etiology in the mass of information we have accumulated on adults and school-aged children is a little like viewing it through a dense screen. In this chapter we will be concerned with the relatively small but increasing amount of knowledge we have about the moment of stuttering in its earliest forms.

Most of the work that has been done on early stuttering has been inspired by theories about its relationship to the disfluency that is so common in the speech of young children. We will therefore need to be concerned with this as well. It is possible to take essentially three points of view about normal disfluency in relation to early stuttering: l) that it has nothing to do with stuttering, 2) that stuttering begins as an effort to avoid it, and 3) that stuttering develops as certain forms of normal disfluency become more frequent and severe. We might narrow the search for the cause of stuttering considerably if we could choose among these points of view.

THE AVOIDANCE HYPOTHESIS

Johnson was not the first to take notice of the fact that most young children are exceptionally disfluent at the same age at which a certain number of them begin to stutter, but it was the central role that this fact played in his diagnosogenic theory that was primarily responsible for the important place that normal disfluency assumed in thinking and research on stuttering. His theory stated that certain parents or other adults are unusually anxious or perfectionistic about the child's speech fluency. Such adults tend to react to the child's essentially normal disfluencies as a speech impairment. The child may then develop anticipatory avoidance reactions through anxiety about the speech hesitancy. Before its diagnosis as stuttering, this hesitancy may be of greater or lesser degree depending upon factors of environment, personality, or heredity, but in most cases, according to this theory, it does not differ markedly in amount or quality from that of other children who do not come to be regarded by their parents as stutterers.

Johnson's theory challenged an older viewpoint about the origin of anticipatory struggle behavior, one which assumed that it came about as a reaction of fear and avoidance to a stage of *abnormal* repetitions or prolongations in a child's speech. In short, one of the most basic issues that his theory raised was whether a so-called primary stage of stuttering existed. Johnson said it did not; the disfluencies others had described as primary stuttering Johnson regarded as normal. This theoretical issue had a clinical counterpart. How did one tell the difference between a normally disfluent child and an incipient stutterer? Prior to Johnson it was widely assumed that if the parents said the child was a stutterer their word could be taken for it. Johnson's theory made it plain that the question was not so simple. True enough, a great many youngsters brought for treatment as stutterers could have raised few doubts in anyone's mind about the difference in their speech. Furthermore, when speech interruptions did appear to leave room for some uncertainty, the parent was apt to state flatly that the child was not stuttering that day. Nevertheless, there were instances in which many speech clinicians believed they had genuine reason to be perplexed, and it was soon evident that little agreement existed on any reliable objective criteria for making a distinction between a stutterer and a nonstutterer in early childhood.

Other questions, more easily answered by investigation, were raised by the diagnosogenic theory. The theory implied that a relatively large amount of disfluency was to be found in the speech of normally developing children. This was amply confirmed in a series of studies.[1] It had also been suggested by the early research of Adams (1932) and Fisher (1932) showing that speech repetitions in children tended to decrease with age. Other students of early childhood development described what they called "stuttering" as a common occurrence in preschool children.[2] They seemed to be referring to identifiable episodes of speech difficulty contrasting with the subject matter

---

[1]Davis (1939, 1940), Branscom, Hughes, and Oxtoby (1955), Egland (1955), Mann (1955), Johnson and Associates (1959, Chap. 8), Winita (1961).

[2]Ilg, Learned, Lockwood, and Ames (1949), Métraux (1950).

of the other studies, but it was difficult to know to exactly what extent this was so.

The diagnosogenic theory also implied that adult listeners were apt to differ appreciably with regard to their concepts of the kind of speech behavior that warranted the label of stuttering. Tuthill (1940, 1946) found evidence that this was true not only of ordinary listeners, but also of so-called experts. Various efforts to determine whether parents of stutterers had higher standards of fluency than parents of nonstutterers produced results that were inconsistent or difficult to interpret.[3] Some indirect support for this assumption came from the large amount of research that we have examined in different forms indicating that stutterers are often subject to pressures from their environment to live up to high standards of behavior.

When all of these pieces of evidence are carefully weighed, however, it is apparent that they fall short of furnishing conclusive proof of Johnson's theory. Furthermore, not one of them is, strictly speaking, necessary to the proposition that stuttering is caused by a misdiagnosis of normal disfluency. There is perhaps only one underlying assumption crucially important to the theory; namely, that *at the moment of initial diagnosis the speech of children who come to be regarded as stutterers does not differ in essential respects from that of children who do not come to be so regarded*. This is the essence of the diagnosogenic concept, upon which it stands or falls.

Unfortunately, it is extremely difficult to submit such an assumption to an objective scientific test since the investigator is almost never present in the role of a detached observer at the moment of original diagnosis. We cannot do it in a speech clinic since, as Johnson emphasized, children's speech a month, a week, or even a day following the diagnosis may differ from their speech prior to the diagnosis as a result of the negative evaluations placed upon it. The only method found practicable to date, that used by Johnson and his co-workers, has been based upon parents' descriptions, supplemented by imitations, of the earliest stutterings of their children obtained some time after the onset of the problem. The disadvantage of such a procedure is partly in its reliance on subjects' memories, which are notorious for distortion of past events. A further weakness of such a procedure results from the fact that language, which in large part intervenes between the observer and the observed, is a great leveler of distinctions. Nevertheless, the issue involved has been of such importance to

---

[3]Bloodstein, Jaeger, and Tureen (1952), Berlin (1960), Johnson and Associates (1959, p. 85 ff).

many workers that the findings have been of outstanding interest despite these limitations.[4]

In Chapter 6 we cited the greater part of the findings of a series of investigations referred to as the Iowa studies, in which parents of stutterers and nonstutterers were interviewed intensively by Johnson and his co-workers. If our interest were solely in the validity of the diagnosogenic theory, essentially all of these findings could probably be ignored except for one particular portion of the results obtained in Study III (Johnson and Associates, 1959, Chap. 6). In this portion of the study, mothers and fathers of stutterers, interviewed, on the average, about eighteen months after the reported onset of stuttering, were asked to "imitate and describe what the child was doing in his speech when he first stuttered." A control group of mothers and fathers of nonstutterers were asked to report similarly on the first nonfluencies that they recalled having observed in their children's speech.

The results are summarized in Table 23. It takes hardly more than a glance at the table to see that there were distinct differences in the descriptions offered by the two groups of parents. The earliest normal disfluencies were characterized by phrase repetitions, pauses, and interjections far more often than were the earliest remembered stutterings. The earliest stutterings, on the other hand, were more often described as syllable repetitions and sound prolongations. Word repetitions were identified as stutterings with great frequency and with about equal frequency as normal disfluencies. In addition to the differences shown in Table 23, the parents' responses indicated that the earliest stutterings were more frequently accompanied by unusual force, effort, or muscular tension in "getting words out" than were the earliest normal nonfluencies. This was reported by 36 percent of the mothers and 34 percent of the fathers of the stutterers, as compared with 17 percent of the mothers and 13 percent of the fathers in the control group (Johnson and Associates, 1959, Table 47, p. 145).

In short, the central premise of the diagnosogenic theory would not appear to have been borne out by the group data. Did this mean that the theory had been proved wrong? Johnson argued staunchly that it did not. He reasoned that there was not a single type of nonfluency that separated the two groups of subjects without very considerable overlapping between them. The very same things most parents had described as initial stutterings had been classified by some others

---

[4]Johnson himself was well aware of these limitations; his defense of the method was, in essence: If you don't study it this way, how do you study it? Since Johnson, there has been little attempt to study the "onset" of stuttering through interviews with parents. See Yairi (1983) and Yairi and Ambrose (1992b), however.

Table 23. Percentages of Control and Experimental Group Parents Who Reported That the Child Was Performing Each of the Indicated Speech Reactions When They First Thought the Child Was Nonfluent or Stuttering, Respectively

| | Repetition | | | Sound Prolongations | Other Nonfluency | | |
					Silent Intervals, Pauses	Interjections	"Complete Blocks"
	Syllable	Word	Phrase				
Control							
Fathers (N = 69)	4	59	23	3	36	30	0
Mothers (N = 80)	10	41	24	4	41	21	0
Experimental							
Fathers (N = 143)	57	48	8	15	7	8	3
Mothers (N = 146)	59	50	8	12	3	9	3

From: Wendell Johnson and Associates, *The Onset of Stuttering*, University of Minnesota Press, Minneapolis. Copyright © 1959 by the University of Minnesota. By permission.

as normal disfluencies, and the same things most parents had described as normal disfluencies had been identified by some as stutterings; consequently, stuttering was, at least in part, a perceptual problem.

The same overlapping extended to reports of "unusual effort or tension." Not only did most parents of stutterers report that the earliest stutterings they remembered were devoid of any signs of tension, but, curiously, a few of the *nonstutterers* were reported to have shown signs of tension, awareness of speaking differently or incorrectly, surprise, irritation, or displeasure in connection with their earliest nonfluencies, despite the fact that any child who had ever even briefly been regarded by anyone as a stutterer had been systematically excluded from the control group (Johnson and Associates, 1959, Appendix, pp. 79, 80). Clearly, the overlapping required as much explanation as did the differences. Johnson's point was, in essence, that if the parents' evaluation of a child as a stutterer were influenced solely by the child's excessive or unusual disfluencies, there should have been little or no overlapping between the two groups with respect to the phenomena they had respectively labeled stuttering and normal disfluency.

Accordingly, Johnson did not abandon his theory. He did revise it, however. In place of the simple statement that stuttering was caused chiefly by its own diagnosis, he substituted an "interaction hypothesis." This said that stuttering was most appropriately defined, not as a feature of a child's speech, but as a perceptual and evaluative problem that arises for a listener as the result of an interaction involving three major variables—the listener's sensitivity to the speaker's nonfluency, the degree of nonfluency of the speaker, and the speaker's sensitivity to his or her own nonfluency and to the listener's evaluative reactions to the nonfluency (Johnson and Associates, 1959, Chap. 10).

THE CONTINUITY HYPOTHESIS

Johnson might have drawn a different conclusion from the overlapping he observed. If parents of stutterers and nonstutterers tended to a notable extent to describe the same disfluencies in their children's speech this might have been because stuttering and certain kinds of normal disfluency in young children are not categorically different things. Johnson did not draw this conclusion. His basic philosophy about stuttering was that it was something to be sharply differentiated from the normal. This dichotomous view had been inherent from the start in his theory that stuttering was the child's effort to avoid normal disfluency. When the overlapping he found between stutterers and nonstutterers seemed to show that no feature of speech would serve to differentiate them categorically, he defined stuttering as a problem that arose for a listener. It was the only way to maintain a clear-cut distinction between them.

Consequently it remained for others to propose the continuity hypothesis on the basis of the work Johnson had done to make such a theory virtually inevitable. The suggestion has been made in more than one form. It was discussed by Bloodstein (1961a, 1970, 1975) as the view that mild tensions and fragmentations are an ordinary feature of the speech of young children as a result of commonplace communicative pressures and difficulties. When the tensions and fragmentations become magnified by communicative pressures or failures that are severe and chronic they tend to be identified as episodes of stuttering, according to this viewpoint.

Shames and Sherrick (1963) advanced a continuity hypothesis in the context of their analysis of stuttering and normal disfluency as operant behavior (see Chapter 2). They suggested that what comes to be called stuttering may be normal disfluency that has increased in frequency due to inadvertent reinforcement by individuals in the child's environment.

LISTENER IDENTIFICATION OF STUTTERING

The moment it was recognized that there was such a thing as normal disfluency in the speech of young children, the words *stutterer* and *stuttering* acquired a degree of ambiguity that they have never lost. The fact that this ambiguity played a special part in Johnson's theory, furthermore, insured that it would become an important subject for research. The usual procedure in such studies has been to present recorded samples of speech to listeners for identification. Both the identification of disfluencies as stutterings and the identification of speakers as stutterers have been investigated. The speakers have been adults more often than children, but in either case the ultimate focus of the research has been the diagnosis of stuttering in young children.

Listener Agreement

The initial study of listener identification, done by Tuthill (1940, 1946) under Johnson's direction, was concerned almost solely with determining how well listeners tend to agree on the occurrence of stuttering blocks. For this purpose Tuthill performed three experiments. In the first one he made a phonograph recording of the speech of adult stutterers and normal speakers. He played this recording to three groups of listeners: speech clinicians, normal speakers with no training in speech pathology, and stutterers. As the subjects listened they marked the stuttered words on a transcript of the recording. The results showed marked disagreement among listeners in all three groups on the places at which stuttering had occurred. A considerable number of "stutterings" were identified in the speech of nonstutterers. The clinicians showed no more agreement than the untrained normal speakers.

In the second experiment Tuthill played a recording of a stutterer's speech to eleven experts on stuttering, to 7 janitors, and to 6 mothers of preschool children. Each of the experts had a Ph.D. in speech pathology, seven were directors of university speech clinics, and four were fellows of what was then called the American Speech Correction Association. Despite this, the experts ranged from 34 to 89 in the number of blocks heard and did not agree better among themselves on the occurrence of stuttering than did the untrained listeners.

Tuthill's third experiment was essentially a replication of the first —with sound film replacing a phonograph recording. The addition of visual cues did not increase observer agreement materially. Of 219 words marked as stuttered half were marked by less than 25 percent of the subjects, only 39 were agreed on by 75 percent of subjects, and 45 were identified in "normal" speech.

Further evidence of listener disagreement on the occurrence of stuttering has been obtained in successive studies.[5] In an investigation by MacDonald and Martin (1973) a group of college students observed videotaped samples of the speech of adult stutterers and identified both the "speech disfluency" and the "stuttering." No more than 13 percent of all the events judged as stuttering were agreed on by the majority of observers. Curlee (1981) reported that giving observers a definition of stuttering had no effect on extent of agreement; Martin and Haroldson (1981) found that it actually resulted in significantly lower agreement.

It should be noted that the evidence of observer disagreement relates mainly to the identification of individual moments of stuttering. In contrast, Wingate (1977) found relatively high agreement and accuracy among judges asked to identify samples of the speech of adolescent and adult individuals as belonging to stutterers or nonstutterers. Curlee (1981) obtained high agreement among observers on frequency counts of stuttering despite low observer agreement on individual occurrences of stuttering. Ingham and Cordes (1992) reported marked differences in frequency counts of stuttering by different judges, however.

Variables Related to the Identification of Stuttering

In other work the disagreement among listeners has generally been taken for granted, and interest has centered around the question of what factors tend to influence the identification of stuttering.

---

[5]Emerick (1960), MacDonald and Martin (1973), Young (1975b), Coyle and Mallard 979), Curlee (1981), Martin and Haroldson (1981), Martin, Haroldson, and Woessner (1988).

Speech Variables

As might be expected, the identification of speakers as stutterers from recorded samples of their speech increases with the frequency, extent, or rated severity of their disfluency.[6] The type of disfluency is also a factor. In general, sound or syllable repetitions and sound prolongations tend to incline listeners to identify stuttering more than do revisions and interjections, which are more likely to be evaluated as normal disfluencies.[7] With respect to syllable repetition, however Sander (1963) found that it made a considerable difference whether the speaker used single-unit repetitions like th-this or double-unit repetitions like th-th-this. Sound prolongations, in research by Lingwall and Bergstrand (1979), were judged to be stutterings if they exceeded 912 milliseconds in duration.

In some of the studies we have cited, word repetitions occupied a somewhat anomalous position with respect to listener judgments, since they were readily evaluated as either stutterings or normal disfluencies. In more recent research the frequency and extent of such repetitions have proved to be critical factors. Curran and Hood (1977b) found that double-unit word repetitions (like like like this) tended to be identified as stutterings, whereas single-unit word repetitions did not. In a study by Hegde and Hartman (1979b), however, even single-unit word repetitions were judged to be stutterings when they were frequent enough; a majority of listeners judged speech samples as stuttered when 15 percent of the words were repeated. Hegde and Hartman (1979a) and DeJoy and Jordan (1988) found that even interjections of "uh" evoked a judgment of stuttering by large numbers of listeners.

Listener Variables: The Set to Observe Stuttering

From the point of view of Johnson's avoidance or interaction hypothesis the effect of listener variables on the identification of stuttering is of particular interest. Several listener variables have been studied. One of these is the set that may be given to listeners by instructing them to listen for stuttering. In a study by Williams and Kent (1958) college students listened to a recording of an adult speaker imitating various types of disfluency. On one occasion they were instructed to mark all "stuttered" interruptions on a transcript of the recording. On another presentation of the same recording they were told to mark all "normal" interruptions. The results showed that

---

[6]Boehmler (1958), Berlin (1960), Sander (1963), Hoops and Wilkinson (1973), Huffman and Perkins (1974).

[7]Boehmler (1958), Williams and Kent (1958), Huffman and Perkins (1974).

to a considerable degree they tended to hear what they were instructed to listen for. Many of the interruptions marked as stuttered under one set of instructions were marked as normal interruptions under the other.

The tendency of observers to identify the same interruptions as both stuttering and normal disfluency on different occasions was referred to as "confusion" by Williams and Kent (1958) and as "ambiguity" by MacDonald and Martin (1973). In the study of MacDonald and Martin, college students observed videotaped samples of the speech of adult stutterers and evaluated them once for the occurrence of "speech disfluency" as differentiated from stuttering, and again for the occurrence of "stuttering." They found that of all the events identified as stutterings 29 percent were also judged to be disfluencies by one or more of the observers. A similar investigation by Curlee (1981) with some improvements in procedure produced considerably higher measures of ambiguity.

In a different type of study by Berlin (1960) several groups of mothers evaluated recorded samples of children's speech. Berlin found that mothers of children who stuttered or had other speech impairments were more likely to evaluate a child as a stutterer if the word stuttering were used in the instructions than if it were not.

Findings of Curran and Hood (1977a) conflicted with those of previous studies. College students listened to samples of the speech of three young children who had been trained to imitate various disfluency types. Attempts to influence the listeners' judgments by telling them that the children were stutterers or nonstutterers had little effect on the evaluation of the speech as stuttered or normal. In a study by Bar (1967) listeners who were instructed to attend to the manner of a stutterer's speech and listeners who were instructed to attend to the content did not differ significantly in their estimates of the percentage of stuttering.

Other Listener Variables

It has generally been found that speech clinicians, students of speech pathology, or others who have some professional knowledge about stuttering tend to make more identifications of stuttering or stutterers than do laypersons.[8] Tuthill (1940) also found this to be true of stutterers. Similar findings with regard to parents of stutterers were obtained by Bloodstein, Jaeger, and Tureen (1952), but not by Berlin (1960) or by Curran and Hood (1977b).

Sander (1968) had mothers of normal-speaking children listen to a recording of a child with mild and ambiguous disfluencies and then

---

[8]Tuthill (1940), Boehmler (1958), Emerick (1960), Ward (1967), Hoops and Wilkinson (1973). Conflicting findings were obtained by Schiavetti (1975) and Curran and Hood (1977b).

questioned them about some of their attitudes and reactions. He found two assumptions significantly related to a judgment that the child was stuttering—that the child not only looked upon speaking as something difficult to do, but also showed an emotional disturbance. Sander discovered, in addition, that mothers who did not believe that the child was stuttering were just as likely to say that they would try to correct the child's speech as were mothers who did feel that the child was stuttering. In short, the failure to apply the label stuttering did not necessarily mean the absence of concern.

Gately (1967) found that the recorded speech of a stutterer more often evoked a judgment of stuttering from listeners who had high scores on the Taylor Anxiety Scale than from those with low scores, but this tendency did not reach statistical significance. Responses to questions about the speaker and his manner of speaking suggested that the anxious listeners were more sensitive to and critical of the disfluencies.

Giolas and Williams (1958) investigated the reactions of kindergarten and grade 2 children to adult disfluencies. They reasoned that if children tend to label the disfluencies of others as "different" they may react similarly to disfluencies in their own speech. The children listened to tape-recorded stories told by fluent and disfluent speakers and were then asked which stories they liked best and which person they would prefer as a teacher. The disfluencies markedly affected the subjects' choice of a teacher, and their comments showed that they were aware of the disfluencies and reacted to them. Several of the second graders were already using the term stuttering. Culatta and Sloan (1977) obtained similar findings in a study of children from grades 1 to 4, and Norbut (1976) reported that children from kindergarten to sixth grade readily differentiated fluency from disfluency. Langer (1969) even found expressions of negative attitudes in preschool children when he questioned them about their reactions to filmed examples of stuttering.

THE FEATURES OF EARLY DISFLUENCY

The findings we have just reviewed show that listeners may experience a certain amount of confusion about what to call stuttering and normal disfluency, even in the speech of adults. This suggests that even adults, and so presumably young children as well, are not divided into two totally distinct categories with respect to the amount or kind of disfluency they exhibit in their speech. Such an assumption was basic to Johnson's hypothesis that stuttering is largely a disorder in the evaluations placed upon a child's fluency. It is also basic to the outlook that what are called stuttering and normal disfluency in young children are largely different degrees of the same thing. We will now take stock of the information we have about the early disfluencies of children from this point of view.

The Iowa Study

Normative data on the types of disfluency observable in the speech of young stutterers and nonstutterers are not abundant. Most of the data—and in the case of stutterers virtually all of the data—come from the study by Johnson and Associates (1959, Chap. 8). That study consisted in part of an analysis of recorded samples of the speech of sixty-eight boys and twenty-one girls "alleged" to have been stuttering for periods ranging from a month to over three years and a like number of nonstuttering children matched for age, sex, and socioeconomic status of the family. The children's speech samples, about 500 words in length on the average, were analyzed for the occurrence of the eight kinds of disfluency listed in Table 24 and described in Chapter 1.

Two cautions should be observed in accepting the data of this analysis as a valid description of early disfluency. One is that it omitted both silent intervals and such symptoms of effort or tension as hard attacks on sound, gasping, or audible glottal straining. All of these are to be heard in examples of early stuttering and possibly also, in varying degrees, in normal childhood disfluency. The other caution is that the subjects,

Table 24. Mean Number of Disfluencies Per 100 Words of 68 Male Stuttering and 68 Male Nonstuttering Children

From: Wendell Johnson and Associates, *The Onset of Stuttering*, University of Minnesota Press, Minneapolis. Copyright © 1959 by the University of Minnesota. By permission.

	Stutterers	Nonstutterers	P*
Interjections	3.62	3.13	NS
Sound and syllable repetitions	5.44	.61	.01
Word repetitions	4.28	1.07	.01
Phrase repetitions	1.14	.61	.01
Revisions	1.30	1.43	NS
Incomplete phrases	.34	.23	NS
Broken words	.12	.04	.05
Prolonged sounds	1.67	.16	.01
All categories	17.91	7.28	.01

*Level of significance of the difference between stutterers and nonstutterers.

though five years old on the average, ranged from about two and a half to slightly more than eight. As we will see, there is evidence that well before the age of eight changes occurring in early stuttering may affect the relative frequency of certain disfluency types.

Differences Between Stutterers and Nonstutterers

With these qualifications in mind, we may review the results of the Iowa study. A significant portion is summarized in Table 24. The table shows the mean number of disfluencies of each type per 100 words for the male stutterers and nonstutterers.[9] The stutterers exceeded the nonstutterers in the frequency of most types of disfluency. There was no significant difference, however, in the case of interjections (such as "uh"), revisions, and incomplete phrases. The data provide an empirical basis for excluding these types from a definition of stuttering. Significant differences between the two groups appeared in the case of sound and syllable repetitions, word repetitions, phrase repetitions, broken words, and prolonged sounds. If we take into consideration the fact that certain disfluency types were far more frequent than others in general, the groups differed mainly in the number of sound, syllable, and word repetitions. Not only did the stutterers tend to have more of these repetitions, as shown in Table 24, but they also significantly exceeded the nonstutterers in the mean number of units per repetition. This was also true of interjections and, in the case of female subjects, phrase repetition. The average stutterer tended to have one- to three-unit repetitions, while the average nonstutterer tended to have repetitions of one or two units (Johnson and Associates, 1959, pp. 212–14).

So much for the differences. Johnson considered them to be the result of an "undeliberated experiment" in which two groups of children whose speech was "presumably more or less similar" to begin with were subject to different evaluative reactions to their speech by parents for varying periods of time.

Stutterers Have More of the Same Disfluencies That Nonstutterers Do

In addition to statements about differences, two general statements can be made regarding similarities between the two groups of children. One is that, as Table 24 shows, no types of disfluency exhibited by the stutterers were absent from the speech of the nonstutterers, not even those most clearly differentiating the two groups. As far

---

[9]The data for the female subjects were essentially the same, except that the groups were smaller and that two differences significant in the case of the boys (phrase repetitions and broken words) were not significant for the girls.

as it goes, this observation makes it possible to entertain a continuity hypothesis about the relationship between stuttering and normal disfluency. Stutterers appear to do the same things nonstutterers do, only—in the case of some of these things—more so. It does not lend particular support to Johnson's interaction or avoidance hypothesis, since it is possible to assume that whether children come to be perceived as stutterers is essentially a matter of how much of certain kinds of disfluency they exhibit in their speech and has little to do with any eccentricity of the perceiver.

The Overlapping of the Distributions

There is, however, a second statement that can be made about the relationship between the two groups of children that supports the interaction theory, and Johnson gave it great emphasis. It was the observation that even where the stutterers showed more of a given type of disfluency than the nonstutterers there was a marked overlap of the two distributions. In the case of sound or syllable repetitions, for example, about 20 percent of the male nonstutterers had more of them in their speech than did 20 percent of the male stutterers. In the case of word repetitions again 20 percent of the male nonstutterers exhibited more than did 20 percent of the male stutterers. With respect to total number of disfluencies of all kinds 20 percent of the male nonstutterers exceeded 30 percent of the male stutterers. The fact that certain children bore the label "stutterer" though they were more fluent than certain children who were called "normal speakers" seemed to Johnson to be evidence of perceptual and evaluative factors at work. He argued that there were no "natural lines of demarcation" between "normal" and "abnormal" fluency. Consequently there was no way to define stuttering as a feature of a child's speech that would serve to differentiate it operationally from normal disfluency. Stuttering therefore could only be defined, he said, as an evaluative reaction of a listener (Johnson and Associates, 1959, pp. 205, 218–20). As we have seen, for Johnson the distinction between stuttering and normal disfluency was by definition a sharp and categorical one.

Further Work on the Features of Early Disfluency

All subsequent work has left little doubt that young stutterers tend to have more disfluencies in their speech than young nonstutterers. The questions that have arisen have been concerned mainly with the form of the disfluencies. Yairi (1972) and F. H. Silverman (1974) gathered data on subjects of elementary school age which appear to be in general agreement with Johnson's with respect to the disfluency types that tend to differentiate groups of stutterers and nonstutterers.

Unfortunately, we still lack the kind of normative data needed most urgently—that relating to the disfluencies of preschool children. In lieu of it we must continue to form our conception of early stuttering from the data gathered by Johnson and Associates (1959) on a group of subjects ranging upward to as much as eight years in age. At least with respect to the frequency of word repetitions, the information may be misleading. Although Johnson's data showed word repetitions to be very prominent in the speech of stutterers and indicated that they are more than four times as frequent as in the speech of non-stutterers, the data showed them to be less common than sound and syllable repetitions. Clinical experience suggests that in the very earliest phase of stuttering, between ages 2 and 5 years, the reverse may be true in many if not most cases. In an analysis of the disfluencies of five preschool stutterers by Bloodstein and Grossman (1981) word repetition proved to be the most frequent aspect of the disfluency in three cases, part-word repetition in only one. Word repetition was the only feature forming a conspicuous element of the pattern for all five subjects. Part-word repetition was a prominent element in two cases. This is in agreement with the observations of Westby (1979), but conflicts with those of Culp (1984) and Meyers (1986), who reported part-word repetition the most common type of disfluency in preschool stutterers. Part-word repetitions were also the most frequent type in the speech of ten 2- and 3-year-old stutterers studied by Yairi and Lewis (1984), but these unusual cases, collected over a ten-year period, involved children brought for examination only two months or less after the reported "onset" of stuttering. Few parents seek help quite so soon if the child's difficulty is largely confined to whole word repetitions. These observations underscore the need for an adequate normative study of early stuttering.

Much of the relevant research has served mainly to emphasize that the kinds of disfluency most typical of stuttering are also found abundantly in the speech of nonstuttering children. E.-M. Silverman (1972a) found that so-called stuttering-type disfluencies occurred frequently in the speech of ten 4-year-old normal-speaking children. She observed marked variation from child to child and from one speech situation to another in the most frequently occurring types of disfluency and found that almost all of the children exhibited "stuttering-type" interruptions—chiefly part-word repetitions and prolongations—as their most frequently occurring disfluency types on at least one of three days on which their speech was sampled.

Westby (1979) examined the disfluencies of three groups of kindergarten and first grade children: 10 stutterers; 10 children who were not regarded as stutterers, but who were judged by their teachers to be highly disfluent; and 10 typically disfluent children. She found that both the stutterers and the highly disfluent normal speakers had more disfluencies of all types than the typically disfluent normal speakers, but were quite similar to each other in both amount and type of disfluency. Word repetitions and interjections were the most frequent types of disfluency for both stutterers and highly disfluent normal speakers, and interjections were the most common type for the typical normal speakers. The stutterers and highly disfluent normal speakers differed most from the typical normal speakers in frequency of word and part-word repetitions. The suggestion clearly emerging from Westby's study is that it is not difficult to find children in whom stuttering lies latent during their early years, although they are by any ordinary definition normal speakers.

Similarly, Yairi (1982), in following the development of fluency in 33 2-year-old children for the space of a year, observed disfluencies that "may be regarded by parents or other observers as stuttering." Large increases and decreases in disfluency occurred in the speech of many of the children, although part-word repetitions decreased progressively with age. Yairi (1981) noted the possible existence of two sub-populations of children, a large number of fluent children and a much smaller number of highly disfluent ones.

In a study of 50 normal speaking 2- to 6-year-olds, Ito (1986) found that disfluency increased with age until it reached a peak at age 4 years, then decreased in the 5- and 6-year-old children. At the early age levels those using more complex sentences exhibited the largest amounts of disfluency. Of one particularly disfluent child who was studied over time, Ito reported, "The highest observed frequency of dysfluency corresponded with the period when she began to use longer and more complicated sentences. Furthermore, her dysfluency began to improve at approximately the same time that she began to use those sentences constantly."

Additional studies of the disfluencies of normal-speaking preschool children have been reported. Like those already mentioned, they have shown that young nonstutterers exhibit all of the types of disfluency found in the speech of children who stutter.[10]

Not everyone has accepted the assertion that early stuttering cannot be categorically distinguished from normal disfluency on the basis of features of a child's speech. To some, for example Wingate (1962a), McDearmon (1968), and Kools and Berryman (1971), the evidence that certain types of interruption are more typical of children called stutterers while others are equally characteristic of stutterers and nonstutterers seems to justify the outlook that there is a differ-

---

[10]Haynes and Hood (1977), Colburn and Mysak (1982a), Wexler (1982), Wexler and Mysak (1982), Yairi (1982), Culp (1984).

ence in kind between stuttering and normal disfluency as forms of speech behavior. Floyd and Perkins (1974) found no evidence suggesting overlap or even continuity between the disfluencies of four preschool stutterers and twenty preschool nonstutterers. The lowest percentage of disfluent syllables of a stutterer was 7.28, whereas the highest among the nonstutterers was 2.58. Although recognizing that their sample was too small for generalization, they pointed out, "The fact that within each group the scores are closely spaced, whereas between the two groups a large gap in the scores exists, suggests that the preschool stutterers and nonstutterers of this study were discretely different."

Bjerkan (1980) identified virtually no part-word repetitions, sound prolongations, or blockings in the speech of 108 normal-speaking nursery school children, although the speech samples were, on the average, over 300 words in length. At the same time, he found that two children who were regarded as stutterers exhibited no more "word repetitions" (by which Bjerkan meant repetitions of words, phrases, or sentences) than did the nonstutterers. Bjerkan concluded that early stuttering is qualitatively distinguishable from normal disfluency as fragmentation of words.

It is evident that the question of how to draw a line between cases of early stuttering and normal disfluency has continued to challenge workers who are skeptical about both the avoidance and continuity hypotheses. Stromsta (1965, 1986) suggested that such a distinction might be made by spectrographic study of children's disfluencies. Of 38 children who were examined because their parents were concerned about their disfluencies, 27 yielded spectrograms characterized by experienced judges as having "a lack of formant transitions and abrupt phonatory stoppages in association with prolongation and clonic-type disfluencies." Ten years later Stromsta determined the status of these children by questionnaire. Of the 27 children with abnormal spectrograms 24 were still stuttering, while of the remaining 4 cases 10 were not. Yaruss and Conture (1993) found the same spectrographic features that Stromsta had observed, but the abnormalities failed to distinguish a group of children thought to be at high risk from a group thought to be at low risk for continuing to stutter.

Researchers have continued to look for evidence of specific features of early disfluency that differentiate the normal from the abnormal in a categorical way, but with little success. Caruso, Conture, and Colton (1988) compared the respiratory, laryngeal, and labial activity of 3-year-old stutterers during stuttering with that of nonstutterers' fluent speech. They observed essential similarity of functioning between the two and concluded that the speech coordinations of the stutterers and nonstutterers differed in degree rather than kind.

Hubbard and Yairi (1988) found that disfluencies occurred in clusters in both stutterers' and nonstutterers' speech, although this tendency was greater in the case of the stutterers. Healey and Bernstein (1991) reported no differences between the repetitions of preschool stutterers and controls in variability of the fundamental frequency of the voice. Zebrowski (1991) found that young stutterers and normal speakers did not differ in the length of their sound prolongations or the number of repeated units of sound or word repetitions. Yairi and Hall (1993) found no difference in durational features of children's word repetitions, except for a possible tendency for stutterers to have faster repetitions.

THE DISTRIBUTION OF EARLY DISFLUENCIES

The question we have been discussing is whether stuttering and stuttering-like normal disfluencies are merely different degrees of the same thing, or whether they are two quite different kinds of speech behavior, with entirely different sources, which by accident resemble each other. Can there be "stuttering" and "nonstuttering" repetitions? This serves to raise the question whether the disfluencies of stuttering and normal-speaking young children tend to vary under the same conditions and in general respond to the same stimuli. The question can be raised separately for different types of disfluency. There are large gaps in our knowledge of this broad subject. Such information as we have is chiefly about the distribution of the disfluencies in the speech sequence.

Consistency and Congruity

Stutterers

The evidence about the consistency effect, though meager, suggests that it is present in the disfluencies of young stutterers. Bloodstein (1960a) tested 14 stutterers between the ages of 3 and 6 years by having them repeat a list of simple sentences from dictation twice in succession, and found percentages of consistency ranging from 50 to 100 with a mean of 71. Neelley and Timmons (1967) found a mean consistency of about 40 percent in 30 3- to 8-year-old stutterers, using a similar method. None of the individual consistency scores of their subjects was statistically significant, but the test was very brief. It appears likely, as Neelley and Timmons stated, that the consistency effect as it is found in young stutterers is an early form of the adult phenomenon. The findings therefore suggest that stuttering is a response to stimuli even in its incipient stages.

Is it heavily influenced by individual factors, as is fully developed stuttering? To answer this question the author reanalyzed the data of the Bloodstein (1960a) study of the consistency effect in young stutterers to compute the amount of congruity among subjects. By eliminating some subjects and some sentences it was possible to isolate a series of 5 consecutive sentences that had been said in identical form by 7 subjects. The average congruity was 42 percent. That is, on the average each child had stuttered on 42 percent of the words that were stuttered by any of the other six children. This was significantly higher than chance. The average consistency of these children, however, was signiflcantly higher still, amounting to 75 percent in their two utterances of these sentences. Just as in the case of older stutterers (*see Chapter 7*), the responsiveness to cues that was evident in their consistency scores appeared to reflect their unique learning experiences as individuals to a greater extent than it reflected the influence of factors operating for the subjects as a group.

Nonstutterers

The consistency effect has also been found repeatedly in the disfluencies of normal-speaking children. It was reported in children of elementary school age by Williams, Silverman, and Kools (1969a), in 5- to 8-year-olds by Neelley and Timmons (1967), in 4- to 6-year-olds by Bloodstein, Alper, and Zisk (1965), and in 3- to 4-year-olds by Wynia (1964). Neelley and Timmons observed that it tended to be lower in magnitude than the consistency of stutterers of comparable age. None of the subjects had consistency scores which passed individual tests of statistical significance, but it is difficult to tell to what extent this was due merely to inadequate sampling of their performance.

The Loci of Disfluencies in the Speech Sequence

There appears to be a broad similarity between the factors affecting the loci of disfluencies of stutterers and nonstutterers at various age levels, as well as a few differences. In normal-speaking adults and schoolchildren the factors seem to be essentially the same as those discussed in Chapter 7 in connection with stuttering. In this age range normal disfluencies are more likely to occur on content words, longer words, words beginning with consonants, and words of lower predictability in context.[11] One exception is position of the word in the sentence, which seems to be an important factor only in the youngest nonstutterers.[12] Another unexpected observation made by Lanyon (1968) was that in the spontaneous

---

[11]Lounsbury (1954), Mann (1955). Goldman-Eisler (1958a, 1958b, 1961), Maclay and Osgood (1959), Blankenship (1964), Blankenship and Kay (1964), Silverman and Williams (1968), Chaney (1969), Williams, Silverman, and Kools (1969b), F. H. Silverman (1972).

[12]Silverman and Williams (1968), Chaney (1969), Williams, Silverman, and Kools (1969b) .

speech of adult nonstutterers disfluency was not related to the predictability of words in context, as it was in oral reading.

The outstanding difference in the loci of disfluency, however, is not between stutterers and nonstutterers. It is between children of preschool age and older subjects, whether stutterers or not.

The Loci of Disfluencies in Preschool Children Are Anomalous

It was in stutterers that the anomalous pattern of distribution of early disfluencies first showed itself. In a clinical study of developmental forms of stuttering by Bloodstein (1960b) several distinctive aspects of the earliest phase of the disorder appeared to emerge. Among these was a tendency for almost all of the stutterings to take place at the beginning of the sentence in many cases. A second feature was a tendency for many stutterings to occur on function words, especially pronouns, conjunctions, and prepositions. Still another was a tendency toward a great deal of repetition of whole words. This all added up simply to the frequent occurrence of stutterings such as "And-and-and-and Ira's cousin came too," or "Her-her-her-her name is Leslie. I-I-I-I-I told you already." These were by no means wholly new observations. Bluemel (1932), in his original description of what he termed "primary" stuttering, said ". . . it commonly assumes the form of repetition of the first word of the sentence. . . . Often we hear repetition of initial consonants or initial syllables of words, and especially of introductory words to sentences."

Furthermore, the statement that referred to prepositions in the same breath as pronouns and conjunctions eventually needed to be qualified. Several years later Bloodstein and Gantwerk (1967) did a quantitative study of the grammatical factor in the disfluencies of 13 stutterers from about 3 to 6.5 years of age. Two main findings appeared. In the first place the grammatical factor as it exists in developed stuttering was absent. The stutterings tended to occur on all parts of speech, for the most part in proportion to how frequently the various parts of speech were represented in the child's verbal output. Second, there was a distinct tendency for pronouns and conjunctions (but not prepositions) to be stuttered on more often than would have been expected by chance.

This was an unusual departure from previous findings on older stutterers, and it seemed even more remarkable when a study of elementary school children by Williams, Silverman, and Kools (1969b) showed that with just a few years of development the grammatical factor seemed to change abruptly to conform to the adult pattern. What did it mean? The interpretation that Bloodstein and Gantwerk (1967) offered of their findings on preschool stutterers was based on the premise that when stutterers repeat a sound or syllable they are repeating the initial fragment of a word because they feel helpless to say the word in its entirety. They speculated that young children often tend to fragment sentences rather than words. This would explain the unusually frequent repetition of the first words of sentences. Since the first words of sentences are often pronouns or conjunctions this seemed to them to account for the high frequency of repetition of these parts of speech. Inspection of the transcripts confirmed that stuttered words at the beginnings of sentences were indeed often pronouns and conjunctions. Bloodstein and Gantwerk suggested that the grammatical functions of words acquire their influence on stuttering only as the child begins to find individual words forbidding and to fragment words rather than sentences. It was an explanation that seemed to catch a number of elusive facts in one net, but it ultimately proved to be in need of refinement. Bloodstein and Gantwerk did not suspect that in obtaining their findings they had touched the edge of something that probably involves much more than just the grammatical factor alone.

Anyone interested in the relationship between stuttering and normal disfluency would have been concerned to find out whether these curious features of early stuttering were present in the disfluencies of preschool nonstutterers as well. In time it became clear that they were. In the first place, E.-M. Silverman (1972b) reported that word repetition was exceedingly common in a group of 4-year-old nonstutterers. Then Helmreich and Bloodstein (1973) and E.-M. Silverman (1974) independently investigated the grammatical factor in the disfluencies of 4-year-old normal speakers, and both found an unusually large amount of disfluency in only two categories—pronouns and conjunctions.[13]

Word Repetitions Occur at the Beginnings of Syntactic Units

E.-M. Silverman (1974) reported two other notable findings. One was that there was a significant tendency for the normal disfluencies of 4-year-olds to occur on the first words of sentences. This was as expected. In addition, however, she reported that her subjects' disfluent pronouns and conjunctions very frequently occurred within the sentence as well as at the beginning. This observation, if it were to prove true of stutterers as well, would of course give little support to Bloodstein and Gantwerk's attempt to explain the high frequency of stuttering on pronouns and conjunctions as a consequence of the occurrence of these parts of speech at the beginnings of sentences.

---

[13]There were also some respects in which the findings differed from those that had been obtained on stutterers. In the Bloodstein and Gantwerk study the increase in disfluency on pronouns and conjunctions was at the expense of nouns and interjections. In the Helmreich and Bloodstein study it was largely at the expense of nouns, verbs, and prepositions.

Why would a child repeat a pronoun or conjunction in the middle of a sentence? At one time the author had thought that fragmentations of prepositional phrases such as "in-in-in the morning" or "by-by-by-by myself" played an important part in early stuttering, but had discarded the notion when investigation failed to show an unusual amount of stuttering on prepositions. Silverman's findings, however, thrust the question to the fore again. Perhaps other phrases were fragmented as well. To answer this question the author examined six available samples of the recorded speech of preschool stutterers. These were transcribed and notations were made of the stutterings. It took hardly more than a glance at the transcripts to show that all of the word repetitions, and even the majority of the part-word repetitions, had occurred at the beginnings of syntactic units—that is, at the beginnings of sentences, clauses, verb phrases, noun phrases, or prepositional phrases. As an illustration we may examine one of the samples.[14] In the following transcript an arrow following a sound means a prolongation of the sound. The horizontal line indicates a silent interval.

> Once upon a time there w . . . th-there-there-there was a _____ a sailor, and he . . . and his name was Ira, and-and then a-a big whale and . . . came along, and-and-and no one could catch that whale e-except-except Ira, and it was Mo→by Dick. N-no sai→lors could catch him. And so once upon a time all the sailors came out to see Ira catch that whale, and (swallow, gasp) and-and-and-and Ira's cousin came too. So they . . . I-Ira (unintelligible fragment) with the harpoons, and Ira got a harpoon, a-and-and they . . . But Moby Dick has-has-has harpoons in-in himself, Moby Dick.

This sample abounds in word repetitions. Note that each one occurs at the beginning of a clause such as "and no one could catch that whale," a verb phrase such as "has harpoons in himself," a noun phrase such as "a big whale," or a prepositional phrase such as "in himself." In no case is a word repeated at the end of a sentence or at the end of a constituent syntactic unit within a sentence. That is, there are no utterances such as "Once upon a time-time all the sailors . . . ," or "No sailors could catch him-him," or "Moby Dick-Dick has harpoons in himself." As examples of stuttering these are as eccentric as "look-k-k" or "Bob-b-b."

In the other samples the same rules were observed. Four were fairly good illustrations of the tendency of word and part-word repetitions to occur very frequently on the first words of sentences There were many examples such as "He-he-he-he . . . h→is fathers' _____

---

[14]For a more detailed report of this study see Bloodstein (1974).

name _____ is Stevie too," "'Cause-'cause-'cause-'cause I'll get sick," and "Weh-weh-weh well I think you forgot wuh-one other thing."

The remaining case was in marked contrast to the others. There were no word repetitions. The stutterings consisted chiefly of sound repetitions, prolongations, and hard attacks on sound. An example was "I → have t→wo s→s-sisters." The stutterings were not confined to the first words of syntactic units, but were distributed as they typically are in developed stuttering. If the child's repetitions were fragmentations of anything they were clearly fragmentations of words. It was an example of stuttering in a more advanced form. In the author's experience such early cases of more advanced stuttering are not rare, but they are not typical of children brought for treatment as stutterers in the earliest years.

In brief, these observations suggested that there are certain regularities that govern the distribution of early stuttering in its typical form. To verify them Bloodstein and Grossman (1981) subsequently examined longer samples of the speech of five additional preschool stutterers. Of the 135 words which these children were heard to repeat, all except one were the first word of a syntactic unit.[15] To be sure, the other features of their disfluency, such as part-word repetitions and prolongations, also showed a strong tendency to occur at the beginnings of syntactic units, but 18 percent of such features appeared at other loci. In the case of word repetitions we seem to be dealing, not with a tendency, but essentially with a rule. Word repetitions appear to occur at the beginnings of syntactic structures as often as sound or syllable repetitions occur at the beginnings of words.

Further Inferences and Questions

What does this regularity mean? In the first place it would seem that the features of early stuttering that appear anomalous—its frequent occurrence on function words, its strong affinity for the beginnings of sentences, and the numerous repetitions of whole words—can all be accounted for by supposing that stuttering has its origin in an early stage of fragmentation of syntactic units. The essence of this assumption is that children repeat the initial word of the unit because for the moment they feel that to attempt the unit as a whole is too difficult.

Sometimes children may repeat whole phrases for the same apparent reason; phrase repetitions occur regularly at the beginnings of syntactic units too. It also seems probable that many if not most of

---

[15]One child repeated the word "school" at the end of a noun phrase: "My school school my my my my my → school's gonna have a big cake . . ."

the sound and syllable repetitions of young children have the same meaning. The great majority of them occur at the beginnings of syntactic units, often in conjunction with word repetitions (as in "a-and-and-a-a-a-and"). Wall, Starkweather, and Cairns (1981) found them in nine young stutterers mainly at the beginnings of clauses, especially "and" clauses. Bernstein (1981) found them chiefly at the beginnings of sentences in nonstutterers and at the beginnings of sentences and verb phrases in stutterers. Bloodstein and Grossman (1981) found them in five stutterers primarily at the beginnings of sentences or clauses and also at the beginnings of verb phrases, noun phrases within sentences, prepositional phrases, and infinitive constructions beginning with "to." There was essential consistency among all three studies.

The difference in the case of part-word repetitions is that they can also be viewed as fragmentations of words. When a part-word repetition occurs on the last word of a syntactic unit (as in "I painted a h-house") it must, in fact, be viewed as such if it is a fragmentation at all. Sound and syllable repetitions in places other than the beginnings of syntactic units are far more frequent, however, in the stuttering of older children and adults.

While the hypothesis that early stuttering represents the fragmentation of syntactic units may give us an inkling of what the child is doing, we are left with the question of the ultimate reasons for the behavior. Since syntactic units are likely to be natural units of motor planning, one possibility is that the child's fragmentations may reflect a sense of inadequacy in the skillful execution of speech as a motor task. The results of a study by DeJoy and Gregory (1973) on normal-speaking four-year-old children seem to support this view. They found that the amount of disfluency in the initial segments of the children's sentences increased with the length of the sentences, but had no relationship to their syntactic complexity. On the other hand, the basic problem might be more closely related to grammatical uncertainty, since this would seem to accord well with the fact that many stutterers experience some early difficulty with language acquisition *(see Chapter 6)* No confident answer to this question can be given.

There is another pressing question. What is the reason for the early transition that stutterers seem to make from fragmentation of syntactic units to fragmentation of words? Again we are without an answer, but not totally without some basis for speculation. Few persons are aware of syntactic units as such, but essentially all speakers of a language develop an awareness of individual words. Speech consciousness means, above all, word consciousness. As Kahmi, Lee, and Nelson (1985) have shown, however, preschool children tend to have an incompletely developed awareness of words. Perhaps as this awareness grows, whatever generalized sense of difficulty in speaking they have acquired therefore begins more and more to develop into a sense of the formidability of words. This feeling may be exaggerated in the case of stutterers, but it may also have much to do with the part-word repetitions of children who are regarded as normal speakers.

Do Word-Bound Factors Influence the Loci of Early Disfluencies?

In Chapter 7 we saw that the stuttering of older children and adults tends to be influenced by certain attributes of words. For example, they are more likely to stutter on content words, words beginning with consonants, and longer words. If early stuttering consists for the most part of fragmentation of syntactic units rather than words, this would appear to imply an easily verifiable prediction. The loci of early stutterings should not be strongly influenced by word-bound factors, except to the extent that such factors may happen to characterize the first words of syntactic units. It would also be of interest to learn to what extent this is true of the early disfluency of normal speakers, since we would like to know whether normal disfluency is related to stuttering.

The evidence so far indicates that this prediction will probably be confirmed for both stutterers and nonstutterers. In the case of stuttering, an analysis by Bloodstein and Grossman (1981) of five subjects' repetitions, prolongations, and hard attacks on sound showed little influence of word-bound factors. As in the study by Bloodstein and Gantwerk (1967), there was no grammatical factor as such; not content words but pronouns and conjunctions were stuttered on to an unusual degree, evidently because they were so often the first words of syntactic units. Only one child showed any significant preponderance of stuttering on consonants over vowels. None of the subjects stuttered more on polysyllabic than monosyllabic words; there was, in fact, a distinct tendency in the opposite direction, apparently because so many of these children's sentences and clauses began with such words as "he," "and," "but," and "so." As expected, stuttering occurred with great frequency on the first words of sentences. The failure of initial consonants to elicit more stuttering than initial vowels was also reported by Wall, Starkweather, and Harris (1981) in their study of nine preschool stutterers.

In the case of normal disfluency, independent investigations by E.-M. Silverman (1974) and Helmreich and Bloodstein (1973) showed, as we have already seen, that the grammatical factor is absent. In addition, Sichel (1973) investigated the phonetic (consonant versus vowel) factor in a group of normal-speaking preschool children. This too was absent. The subjects tended to have a somewhat unexpected amount of disfluency on words beginning with vowels, in large part because of the frequency with which they repeated the word "and" at the beginnings of sentences and clauses. Finally, E.-M. Silverman (1975) studied both the phonetic factor and the influence of word length in normal-speaking four-year-olds in a preschool classroom situation and in a structured interview situation. There was no phonetic factor in either situation. Word length had no influence on disfluency in the classroom situation. In the interview situation there was slightly more than expected disfluency on monosyllabic words, an effect not likely to have resulted directly from the fact that the words were monosyllabic.

So far in our research, neither early stuttering nor the disfluencies of normal-speaking young children seem to be notably influenced by the word-bound factors that operate in the case of older subjects. The assumption that early disfluency represents the fragmentation of syntactic units appears likely to be confirmed. More investigation with larger groups of subjects is needed.

Other Factors

A number of attempts have been made to test additional hypotheses about the loci of early disfluencies. In a study of nine preschool stutterers Wall, Starkweather, and Harris (1981) were concerned with the influence of voicing transitions. Their main finding was that stuttering most often occurred following a pause, regardless of the type of voicing transition.

The remaining investigations were concerned with normal speakers. In a study of four children aged two to three years, Colburn and Mysak (1982b) found little support for the hypothesis that normal disfluencies would be associated with semantic structures just emerging in the children's grammar (e.g., action, intention, negation, etc.). Disfluency occurred more often on well-leamed and practiced structures. Both E.-M. Silverman (1973a) and Colburn (1985) found a significant tendency for early normal disfluencies to cluster on the same or consecutive words.

VARIATIONS IN FREQUENCY

A great deal is yet to be learned about early stuttering and its relationship to normal disfluency through research on the conditions under which the disfluencies of stuttering and nonstuttering children vary in frequency. The promise of this approach is underscored by the very considerable amount of data showing that among adults and older children normal disfluencies tend to vary under some of the same conditions as does stuttering. For example, there is a large amount of evidence that normal speakers exhibit something highly similar if not identical to the adaptation effect in stutterers.[16] Normal disfluencies of adults are also influenced by response-contingent stimuli in essentially the same way as are stutterings.[17] F. H. Silverman (1971) showed that the normal disfluencies of adults diminish when speech is timed to a rhythmic stimulus, and both Silverman and Goodban (1972) and Sherrard (1975) found that normal disfluency in oral reading was reduced under masking noise. The relationship of normal speech interruptions to anxiety has been extensively studied, chiefly in adults, by Mahl (1956, 1961) and his co-workers, and others.

Despite the many similarities found in these and other studies between the variables affecting the frequency of stuttering and normal disfluency in adults, research has also disclosed occasional differences. It is impossible to know whether such differences are basic or merely reflect divergent processes of development. It is only in the study of the relationship between stuttering and normal disfluency in their earliest phases that some possibility exists for obtaining answers to questions about the origin of stuttering.

In the case of young children far less work has yet been done, and most of it has been concerned only with normal disfluency.

Nonstutterers

Davis (1940) observed the situations in which each of 62 normal 2- to 5-year-old children exhibited speech repetitions of all types during an hour of free play in a preschool situation. She found that repetitions tended to occur with outstanding frequency under certain conditions—for example, when the child was excited over his or her own activity, wanted to direct the activity of another child, was attempting to attract the attention of another child or of the teacher, was forced by the teacher to change an activity, or wanted an object in the possession of another child. In a study of children's interactions with their own and other children's mothers, Meyers and Freeman (1985b) observed that normal-speaking 4 to 5 year-olds tended to be more disfluent when interrupting a mother.

Other studies have attempted to vary the frequency of normal childhood disfluency experimentally by varying the listeners or situa-

---

[16]Starbuck and Steer (1953, 1954) Brutten (1963), Gray (1965a), Gray and Karmen (1967), Williams, Silverman, and Kools (1968), Soderberg (1969a), F. H. Silverman (1970b, 1970c,1970d), Silverman and Williams (1971), Silverman and Bloom (1973), Kroll and Hood (1976), Miller and Miller (1977), Moore, Cunko, and Flowers (1979).

[17]Siegel and Martin (1965a, 1965b, 1966, 1967,1968), Brookshire and Martin (1967), Brookshire (1969), Brookshire and Eveslage (1969), Siegel, Lenske, and Broen (1969), Siegel and Hanson (1972), Hutchinson and Mackay (1973), Kazdin (1973), Hasbrouck and Martin (1974).

tions.[18] In this way more disfluency has been found in a structured interview than in a preschool classroom situation, in socialized than in egocentric speech, and in solitary play than in conversation with an adult. Newman and Smit (1989) found increases in the disfluency of normal speaking 4-year-olds when the experimenter decreased her response time from 3 seconds to 1 second in conversational interaction with the subjects. Neelley and Timmons (1967) found evidence of the adaptation effect in nonstutterers who were 5 to 8 years of age.

Among the more interesting findings have been those dealing with the influence of language complexity on normal disfluency. Haynes and Hood (1978) studied the effect of adult modeling of simple and complex language on the fluency of normal-speaking 5-year-old children. The instructions to each child were, in part: "I'm going to look at these pictures and say something about each one. Listen very carefully to my sentences so you will know what kinds they are. Later, we will take turns making sentences and I want you to try to make your sentences like mine." After listening to the experimenter model a series of sentences, the children were asked to make up their own sentences for each of a new series of pictures. In the simple condition the experimenter used sentences that contained no major transformations and few pronouns or auxiliary verbs. In the complex condition sentences were of comparable length and involved pronouns, negatives, and more difficult transformational rules. Analysis showed that the two conditions did, in fact, produce a difference in the syntactic complexity of the children's language, their mean length of response, and their disfluency. The disfluencies that increased in frequency in the complex condition were chiefly word repetitions, revisions, incomplete phrases, and "disrhythmic phonations" (prolongations, hard attacks, or broken words).

In a study by Pearl and Bernthal (1980) normal-speaking 3- and 4-year-old children repeated after the examiner sentences representing several transformational types. The passive sentences, reported to be among the last to be acquired by children, occasioned more disfluency than the others. Simple, affirmative, active sentences were the most fluently produced. The 5-year-olds studied by Gordon, Luper, and Peterson (1986) did not reveal this effect when simply repeating sentences after an experimenter, but did so in a sentence modeling procedure similar to that used by Haynes and Hood. The passive construction also elicited more stuttering in a study by Gordon and Luper (1989), although Gordon (1991) failed to confirm this. Ratner and Sih (1987), using a sentence imitation procedure, and McLaughlin

---

[18]Egland (1955), E.-M. Silverman (1971,1972a, 1973b), Martin, Haroldson, and Kuhl (1972a, 1972b), Martin and Haroldson (1975), Wexler (1982).

and Cullinan (1989), using a sentence modeling procedure, found that the disfluencies of preschool nonstutterers increased with sentence complexity.

Modeling of sentences produces more stuttering than simple sentence imitation, as Gordon, Luper, and Peterson (1986), Gordon and Luper (1989), and Gordon (1991) all showed.

With children of reading age (grades 3 to 6) Cecconi, Hood, and Tucker (1977) found that the amount of disfluency in oral reading varied with the reading difficulty of the material. The disfluencies affected were word and part-word repetitions, "disrhythmic phonations," and "tense pauses." In a single-subject investigation of the oral reading of a five-year old boy, Hegde (1982) analyzed the antecedents of disfluencies of various types. By far the most frequent antecedent was poor lexical control (unacceptable pronunciations of unfamiliar words), which resulted in disfluencies of all types.

Stutterers

With respect to the conditions under which the frequency of stuttering varies in young children there is a growing but still quite meager amount to report. A tendency of 5- to 8-year-old stutterers to show adaptation was reported by Neelley and Timmons (1967). In 2 preschool stutterers Martin, Kuhl, and Haroldson (1972) found a decrease in stuttering as a result of contingent time-out procedures. Razdolsky (1965) reported the interesting observation that of a group of 32 stutterers between 2 and 6 years of age the majority stuttered as much or almost as much when they were alone as when they were speaking to a listener. By contrast, most of a group of school-age stutterers spoke appreciably more easily when they were alone. The only preschool stutterers who did so to a marked degree were said to be three bright 6-year-olds who were embarrassed by their stuttering.

In a study of 9 stutterers aged 4 to 7 years, Stocker and Usprich (1976) employed a series of questions with increasing levels of communicative demand[19]—for example, about a toy car: 1) Is it hard or soft? 2) What is it? 3) Where would you keep one? 4) Tell me everything you know about it. 5) Make up your own story about it. The frequency of stuttering increased with levels of demand, a particularly marked increase occurring between levels 3 and 5. There was much less stuttering in a similar test requesting responses identical to those given previously (e.g., "This is what you told me about the car last time . . . Now tell it to me again").

---

[19]The Stocker Probe technique. See Stocker and Gerstman (1983).

A replication of the Stocker and Usprich study by Martin, Parlour, and Haroldson (1990) did not unequivocally confirm the inference that early stuttering varies with level of linguistic demand, but the question of a link to language difficulty was pursued in other forms. Ratner and Sih (1987) had 3- to 6-year-old children imitate utterances varying in syntactic complexity from simple active affirmative declarative sentences to those involving embedded clauses. In stutterers and nonstutterers alike, the amount of disfluency was generally correlated with order of development of the sentence types. Gaines, Runyan, and Meyers (1991) found that young children's stuttered sentences in spontaneous speech tended to be longer and more complex than their fluent sentences. Weiss and Zebrowski (1992) also observed more stuttering on longer and more complex utterances of subjects aged 4 to 10 years. Gordon (1991) reported that preschool subjects stuttered more on a sentence modeling than a sentence imitation task but failed to find that syntactic complexity of sentences had any effect. Kadi-Hanifi and Howell (1992) found that 2- to 6-year-old stutterers and nonstutterers were more disfluent on simple sentences in spontaneous speech than on complex ones. Older subjects were more disfluent on complex sentences.

Meyers (1989, 1990) studied the disfluencies of 12 2- to 6-year-old stutterers in dyadic interactions with mother, father, and a familiar playmate. Frequency of stuttering did not vary with conversational partner, nor was there any evidence that stuttering was affected by the positive or negative intent of the partner's verbal interactions or by whether the partner's interactions consisted of comments, questions, interruptions, or imperatives.

ATTRIBUTES OF DISFLUENT CHILDREN

If stuttering and normal disfluency in early childhood are related kinds of behavior we might reasonably expect the more disfluent of a representative sample of normal speakers to have some of the same personal attributes that distinguish stuttering children as a group. As yet, research in this area is in its incipient stages, and there is a relatively small amount of information to review.

One basic personal attribute is age. Since there is a decline in the frequency with which cases of onset of stuttering are reported from year to year during childhood (see Chapter 3) it may be of some significance that with few exceptions studies have found that the disfluency of normal speaking children also tends to decrease with age. For a brief period at about age 2 years children may show considerable variation in amount of disfluency with age, as both Colburn and Mysak (1982a) and Yairi (1982) observed in longitudinal studies.

Evidently some children become more disfluent as language emerges. However, across the early childhood period as a whole the decrease has been clearly apparent in most investigations.[20] DeJoy and Gregory (1985) found the decrease to be in word, part-word, and phrase repetitions, incomplete phrases, and "disrhythmic phonations" (prolongations, broken words, or hard attacks).

Another attribute is sex. In view of the sex ratio in the incidence of stuttering it would be interesting to know whether there is a difference in the amount of disfluency in the speech of normal-speaking boys and girls. Unfortunately, we are faced with two sources of uncertainty in dealing with this question. There is evidence that the sex ratio in stuttering tends to decrease as we go back into childhood from age level to age level, as we saw in Chapter 3, and we do not know for sure whether it is present in any substantial degree among preschool cases. Glasner and Rosenthal (1957) found that among 153 children who were reported by their parents to have stuttered at some time before entering the first grade, the sex ratio was only 1.4 to 1 when corrected for a sex difference in the total sample surveyed.[21] The other uncertainty is about the extent to which boys and girls differ in degree of normal disfluency. Fisher (1932) and Davis (1939) found somewhat more repetition, chiefly of syllables, among boys than girls. Essentially no sex differences were found, however, in later studies of young children by Johnson and Associates (1959, p. 208), Kools and Berryman (1971), Haynes and Hood (1977), or Ratusnik, Kiriluk, and Ratusnik (1979).

Still a third characteristic about which we have some information is language and speech development. Young stutterers often tend to be somewhat slow in the development of linguistic and articulatory skills, as we saw in Chapter 6. With respect to normal disfluency there have been somewhat inconsistent findings. In 62 2- to 5-year-old children, Davis (1940) found essentially no relationship between amount of speech repetition and such measures of language maturity as mean length of response, amount of verbal output, vocabulary, number of correct speech sounds, intelligibility, and percentage of functionally complete responses. Likewise, Berryman and Kools (1975) found that among 92 first graders disfluency was unrelated to reading ability, intelligence, or judges" ratings of language level, while among children aged 4, 6, and 8 years examined by Haynes and

---

[20]Adams (1932), Fisher (1932), Davis (1939), Branscom, Hughes, and Oxtoby (1955), Yairi and Clifton (1972), Haynes and Hood (1977), Wexler (1982), DeJoy and Gregory (1985).

[21]Andrews and Harris (1964, p. 31) found, however, that sex ratios based on incidence figures such as these tend to be lower than ratios based on the prevalence of stuttering at a given time, possibly because episodes of stuttering tend to be briefer in girls than in boys. They reported that for small numbers of children who were stuttering in a given year during the first five years of the Newcastle survey the sex ratio averaged 2.6 to 1.

Hood (1977) there was no relationship between disfluency and syntactic proficiency as measured by Lee's Developmental Sentence Score. Enger, Hood, and Shulman (1988) reported no significant difference in language measures between highly fluent and highly disfluent young subjects in a school program with a preponderance of gifted children with advanced language development.

On the other hand, Borack (1969) found that elementary school children with articulatory problems were significantly more disfluent than a comparable group with normal articulation. Muma (1971) carried out a transformational analysis of the language performance of carefully selected highly fluent and disfluent normal-speaking 4-year-olds. The two groups did not differ in their use of various sentence types, but the highly fluent group tended to use more double-base transformations. Similarly, DeJoy and Gregory (1976) selected from a group of 60 samples of the speech of 3-year-old and 5-year-old children the 10 with the highest number and the ten with the lowest number of disfluencies of various types and compared the 2 groups of samples with respect to the Developmental Sentence Score. The disfluent children scored lower in syntactic maturity than the fluent ones in the case of word repetitions, pauses, incomplete phrases, and, for the 5-year-olds, in the case of part-word repetitions. Stocker and Usprich (1976) found more disfluencies in preschool children who had articulatory problems and delayed language development than in children who did not. Similar findings were obtained by Ragsdale and Sisterhen (1984) for 5- and 6-year-olds with articulatory difficulties and by Lybolt (1986) for 8 children with expressive language deficits. Merits-Patterson and Reed (1981) reported the interesting finding that young children receiving language therapy had more disfluencies, in the form of word and part-word repetitions, than children with normal language development, whereas comparably language-delayed children not getting treatment did not.

The findings of these studies suggest that a relationship does exist between normal childhood disfluency and speech and language skill, but that it can be demonstrated only in subjects with wide disparities either in fluency or in speech and language skill. This was given a special kind of emphasis in a study by Westby (1979) in which stutterers, highly disfluent normal speakers, and typically disfluent normal speakers in kindergarten and first grade were compared on several measures of grammar, vocabulary, and semantic aspects of language. The highly disfluent normals scored significantly lower than the typical normals on most of the measures. There was no difference between the highly disfluent normal speakers and the stutterers.

Finally, the familial tendency in the incidence of stuttering suggests the possibility that more disfluent children in general tend to have more disfluent parents. Yairi and Jennings (1974) correlated the number of disfluencies of various types to be found in the speech of a group of normal-speaking preschool boys with the amount in the speech of their mothers and fathers, but could find essentially no evidence of a relationship.

CONCLUDING REMARKS

The main purpose of this chapter has been to consider what relationship, if any, there is between stuttering and normal disfluency in young children. The basic empirical question is whether any "natural lines of demarcation" exist between the disfluency of those who are called stutterers and those who are called normal speakers. If, as Johnson asserted, there were not, we could draw either of two conclusions. These would depend on how we define what we mean by "abnormal" in relation to fluent speech. If, like Johnson, we viewed the abnormal as something that is by definition qualitatively distinct from the normal, we would have to conclude that stuttering could not be defined in terms of any feature of a child's speech and consequently had to be defined at least in part on the basis of the evaluative judgments of listeners. If, on the other hand, we were willing to accept a relative, quantitative, or dimensional concept of abnormality, we could if we wished define stuttering in young children as a relatively severe degree of normal disfluency or of those specific types of normal disfluency from which it could not be readily demarcated.

The first alternative is embodied in Johnson's avoidance or interaction hypothesis. The second is what we have called the continuity hypothesis. In effect, the avoidance theory says that if one child's speech repetitions are normal there is little justification for calling another child's speech repetitions anything else just because there are more of them. By contrast, the continuity hypothesis says that if one child's speech repetitions are stuttering there is little reason to call another child's repetitions anything else merely because there is a relatively normal amount of them. While these two statements appear to represent only differences in definition of stuttering there is a vast distinction between them in their ultimate implications for theory and therapy. In the first instance we must look for the source of the child's problem largely in the perceptual distortions of a listener by reason of which the child comes to regard disfluencies as a matter for concern and to struggle to avoid them. In the second case we must look for the causes of the problem largely in the nature of the stutterings that are latent in almost all children's speech and in the variety of possible factors that might tend to increase them.

Some workers would reject both of these approaches to the etiology of stuttering because they do not accept the assumption that stutterers' and nonstutterers' disfluencies cannot be sharply differentiated empirically in early childhood. Increasing efforts have been made to find out whether any natural lines of demarcation between the two exist, either in the nature of the disfluencies themselves or in the stimulus variables which determine their distribution and frequency. Considerable evidence has accumulated that the essential features of what is generally called stuttering in young children are similar in kind to some of the features of disfluency that appear in the speech of many children who are not called stutterers. There also appears to be a striking similarity in the manner in which these features are distributed in stutterers' and nonstutterers' speech. Nevertheless, no broad consensus exists on the question of whether early stuttering and certain types of normal disfluency are united by a single continuum. The question has many aspects still open to further investigation.

It may not have been lost on the reader that in pursuing the main purpose of this chapter we have been led repeatedly by different paths to another subject, the relationship between stuttering and language development in young children. The pieces of evidence suggesting that early stutterings may be fragmentations of syntactic structures, that the more disfluent normal-speaking children are poorer in language skill, that normal disfluency varies in frequency with changes in language complexity, that stutterers are more often delayed in language development than nonstutterers—all these observations are obviously capable of being related to each other. As to whether and how they are connected, however, all that anyone can as yet offer are inferences and speculations.

Suggested Readings

Bloodstein, O., The rules of early stuttering. *J. Speech Hearing Dis., 39,* 379–94 (1974).

Bloodstein, O., and Grossman, M., Early stutterings: Some aspects of their form and distribution. *J. Speech Hearing Res., 24,* 298–302 (1981).

Haynes, W.O., and Hood, S. B., Disfluency changes in children as a function of the systematic modification of linguistic complexity. *J. Commun. Dis., 11,* 79–93 (1978).

Johnson, W. and Associates, *The Onset of Stuttering.* Minneapolis: Univ. Minn. Press (1959), Chaps. 6, 8, 9, 10.

Westby, C. E., Language performance of stuttering and nonstuttering children. *J. Commun. Dis., 12,* 133–45 (1979).

Young, M. A., Identification of stuttering and stutterers. In Curlee, R. F., and Perkins, W. H. (eds.), *Nature and Treatment of Stuttering. New Directions.* San Diego: College-Hill Press (1984).

10

INFERENCES AND CONCLUSIONS

From the standpoint of those whose chief interest is in the significant thinking and research that have been done on the nature and etiology of stuttering, this book has now been finished and may be put down. It may be appropriate, however, to try to draw some inferences about the ultimate meaning of the information we have reviewed. That is the purpose of this chapter. It hardly needs to be said that no final conclusions about the nature and etiology of stuttering are yet possible and that much of what is contained here must necessarily consist of viewpoints with which perhaps few other workers would agree. Students who have been conditioned by their years of schooling to react with an attitude of submission to expressions of opinion that are set in 10-point roman are strongly advised to skip this chapter.

SUMMARY OF CURRENT KNOWLEDGE ABOUT STUTTERING

We may begin by taking stock of what we know. If we summarize the general conclusions of the last seven chapters, most of the significant information we have gained in our review of research may be contained in the following statements:

Stuttering is predominantly a disorder of childhood, more common in males than females.

There is evidence that both genetic and environmental factors play a part in its etiology.

No major personality differences between stutterers and nonstutterers have been discovered, although mild degrees of maladjustment seem to be fairly common among stutterers.

There may be subtle constitutional differences between stutterers and nonstutterers as groups, but research has not yet revealed any organic abnormality that is a necessary and sufficient condition for stuttering (i.e., a condition possessed by all stutterers and no nonstutterers).

Stutterers are often somewhat delayed in speech and language development and often tend to have early difficulties of articulation.

In its developed form, stuttering is distributed in the speech sequence largely in response to features of words that tend to make them difficult, conspicuous, or evocative of past speech failure. It varies in frequency from situation to situation chiefly in response to such factors as communicative pressure and awareness of oneself as a speaker or stutterer. In the absence of such factors it may be absent altogether.

In early childhood it is possible to identify certain types of disfluency—especially part-word repetition, repetition of whole words, and prolongation of sounds—which tend to occur more often in the speech of children regarded as stutterers than in the speech of children who are not. No reliable way has yet been found, however, for distinguishing these "stutter-type" disfluencies qualitatively from similar ones in normal speakers.

Evidence suggests that the speech repetitions of young children are related to some type of difficulty with whole syntactic units to a greater extent than to difficulty with words.

While some of these conclusions may be perplexing, many of them seem to fit together fairly well. They appear to lend themselves to the inference that stuttering usually develops at least in part because of environmental pressures imposed in some manner on the child's speech. It is this general interpretation of the facts, which obviously leaves many questions unanswered, that we will develop in this chapter.

THE PROVOCATIONS MAY NOT BE LIMITED TO DISFLUENCY

To try to make sense of what we know, we must have a working hypothesis about the nature of stuttering. It is the author's working hypothesis that, whatever else is involved in stuttering, it is in large part a type of anticipatory struggle reaction. Although this model has some difficulties to overcome, it seems to him to have fewer problems than any of the others and to account most simply and satisfactorily for the facts known about stuttering.

On this premise, the question of the etiology of stuttering in its most general form is the question of how a child acquires a disabling belief in the difficulty of speech. In the preceding chapter we gave detailed consideration to one answer to this question that is embodied in Johnson's interaction hypothesis. This hypothesis states in essence that the onset of stuttering may be a joint product of the parents' high standards of fluency, the child's unusual kind or degree of disfluency, and the child's proneness to react to either or both of these. Taking this hypothesis as a point of departure for thinking further, it is difficult to avoid the question of which of these factors contributes most significantly to the etiology of reactive struggle behavior in the child's speech—the parental evaluations as Johnson believed, the abnormal disfluencies, perhaps even the third of these factors.

If we continue to think about this question, however, we are liable to be struck by the realization that it takes for granted an assumption gratuitous and contrary to a good deal of clinical experience. It seems to assume that fluency is the only aspect of a child's speech about which a parent may become concerned or that only penalties for disfluency may result in anticipatory struggle reactions. Yet it is possible to think of a good many other factors besides "normal" or "abnormal" disfluency that might in certain instances serve as provocations to such behavior.

One of these is delayed development of speech. In the course of remedial work with children who have developmental problems related to language or articulation, it is not exceptionally rare for stuttering to seem to begin virtually before the clinician's eyes as the child begins to make progress in overcoming these difficulties. Such instances have been described by Van Riper (1963, p. 318), Curtis (1967), and Hall (1977), among others, and have been observed by the author and various of his colleagues. A report by Merits-Patterson and Reed (1981) is provocative in this regard. They studied the disfluencies in the speech of children with delayed language who were receiving language therapy, a group with equally delayed language who were not, and a control group of children with normal language development. Only the group receiving therapy had more disfluencies than the control group. Van Riper also gave some emphasis to another clinical observation that cannot be sharply separated from this one; namely, that stuttering frequently follows in the wake of parental efforts to hasten the normal process of language development in children who by ordinary standards have quite adequate speech (1963, p. 319). In either case it is not difficult to understand why the child might come to regard speech as a formidable undertaking and to respond with the tense and fragmented reactions of stuttering.

Of all provocations to stuttering, faulty articulation is the one detected most frequently in parents' accounts of the onset of the disorder. Two examples will serve to illustrate the nature of some of these observations. The mother of a 3 year-old boy was sufficiently overwrought by his inability to say the "l" and "g" sounds to undertake her own program of remedial speech training. Not only did she persistently correct the child's pronunciation of words beginning with "l" and "g," but she attempted to do so by showing him how she "put her mouth" when she said them. The boy had barely learned how to produce these sounds when he was observed to have begun to stutter. The earliest symptoms recalled by the mother were repetitions on words beginning with "l" and "g." Another case was that of a six-year-old girl who was brought to the speech clinic because of her immature articulation. During the examination she appeared to exhibit, in addition, frequent struggle reactions including gasping and exaggerated pausing. The mother, however, emphatically denied that the child ever "stuttered or stammered." She was a dominating parent and a compulsive talker who continually interrupted the child to correct her articulation or to exclaim, "Now, you can say it better than that!"

A third type of speech failure that may be a frequent instigator of stuttering reactions is cluttering. These two symptoms are not infrequently observed together in both children and adults, and the author has seen cases appearing to lend support to Deso Weiss' contention that stuttering often begins as the child's effort to avoid cluttering (see Chapter 2). One of the most convincing examples was the case of a boy who began to stutter when he was 16 years of age. Since early childhood he had been known as a rapid speaker. As he grew older his jerky, staccato utterances began to attract more attention, and finally a concerted effort to slow him down was made by his parents, sister, aunt, and even a few of his friends. For a time he could scarcely speak without being accused of "swallowing" his words or trying to say one word before finishing the last. It was during this time that he began to stutter.

Still a fourth precipitating agent of some importance appears to be oral reading difficulty in the classroom, particularly when the constant threat of failure present in such a situation is intensified by a teacher's impatience or the child's emotional insecurity. Cases of this kind assume particular significance in the light of the familiar observation that stuttering sometimes appears to start at school rather than at home. It is also significant that some stutterers have all or most of their blocks in oral reading. Finally, we must take note of the occasional instances in which a child exhibits stuttering and a reading disability as well. That this may frequently be more than mere coincidence is suggested by the case of a fifteen-year-old stutterer with a reading disability who was seen by the author. He stuttered mostly in oral reading and blocked most severely on words for which he had no sight recognition. After several months of therapy consisting in part of an attempt to increase his reading vocabulary, his clinician reported that fear of reading and stuttering were much reduced.

Up to this point we have considered four conditions under which stuttering appears to be provoked by the threat of speech failure. A plausible implication appears to be that stuttering may stem from almost any situation that forces children to labor over their utterances or in some way establishes the invidious suggestion that speech requires effort and care. This is borne out by a variety of further observations. The author recalls one case in which stuttering was said to have stopped when the mother persuaded her husband to stop correcting the child's pronunciation of difficult polysyllabic words. In another case a child of 4 years was brought for examination with the unusual complaint that he spoke too slowly. The mother said that she had recently tried to "help him to talk faster," but had found that he began to stutter when she did so. The child spoke noticeably slowly, in a manner typical of some young children.

In a third case a 3-year-old girl began to stutter during a period of severe throat infections. Just prior to the reported onset of stuttering she had been exceedingly hoarse, had been unable to phonate at times, and had had to struggle in order to be heard. The earliest symptoms of stuttering were said to have been complete stoppages of speech. In still another case a 4-year-old girl was taken to visit relatives in Norway during a summer vacation. After some initial lack of success in making the other children understand English, she learned to speak fluent Norwegian. On her return that fall, however, she found it difficult to speak English. While relearning English she was first noticed to stutter.

In addition, clinical experience suggests that stuttering may sometimes develop as a reaction to cleft palate speech, the labored articulation of cerebral palsy, or the speechlessness of intense shock or fright. Instances such as these are not common, of course, but they are instructive because they suggest that a very broad range of provocations may be capable of precipitating stuttering reactions. Freeman and Rosenfield (1982) and Rosenfield and Freeman (1983) called attention to cases in which persons who had undergone laryngectomies developed apparent symptoms of stuttering while attempting to learn alaryngeal forms of speech. Even the speech failures resulting from delayed auditory feedback may apparently have this potentiality, as Tiffany and Hanley inadvertently discovered through their experience with one subject in a study of the DAF effect in normal speakers:

> This subject had experienced increasing difficulty with the side-tone readings, particularly on one word—pony. Following the delayed sidetone readings, he continued to experience great difficulty with this word even though no sidetone delay was present. He exhibited stuttering-like symptoms, as though the experimental readings had produced a kind of specific anxiety for this word. He not only appeared to be more non-fluent than before the sidetone experience but also appeared to show tension and avoidance behavior consistent with accepted descriptions of stuttering patterns (Tiffany and Hanley, 1956).

THE ROLE OF SPEECH PRESSURES

Despite all this, it is by no means true that provocations comparable to the ones cited may be readily identified in all cases of stuttering in children. Furthermore, we must not forget that many children have slow speech development, articulatory problems, reading difficulties, or the like, but never become stutterers. Evidently, there are other factors that play a significant part in the etiology of stuttering. In view of all that we have previously learned about stuttering it is not a far-fetched assumption that another factor of major importance is some source of pressure, whether from within children or directly from their environment, that fosters in them a somewhat more-than-average need for approval of their speech and a predisposition to evaluate any real, imagined, alleged, or anticipated speech deviations as failures.

There is by now ample evidence to indicate what some of these sources might be. Like Johnson, we may infer that in many cases children's exaggerated concern about their speech stems chiefly from their parents' tendency to be dominating, overanxious, or striving and to impose rather high standards of behavior. In other instances the most important cause of pressure may be the child's own basic anxiety, sensitivity, perfectionism, or excessive need for approval. This is sometimes brought out with particular clarity when stutterers have an identical twin with normal speech. The following are two brief examples:

Boyd and Floyd were identical twins in their twenties. Boyd had stuttered since about the age of 2.5 years, according to his mother. He had been a breech delivery. From the parents' earliest observation he had been an anxious child. His toilet training was made difficult by his fear of falling into the toilet. He was afraid of his barber. For a few weeks after he entered kindergarten his mother had to stay with him in the classroom. Floyd, on the other hand, had had an uneventful birth, had not had any of the anxieties that troubled his brother, was a confident young man, and had never stuttered. The other case was that of a 6-year-old stutterer with a normal-speaking brother who was said to be an identical twin and who looked so much like him that they were often mistaken for each other by their teacher and classmates. Asked whether there was anything else that differentiated the two children besides the stuttering, the mother unhesitatingly declared that the twin who stuttered was much more "sensitive," while the other was more "aggressive."'

Clinical observation reveals that speech pressures may come from any number of other sources besides parental perfectionism or the personality of the child. One of these is chronic recitation fright stemming from an unfavorable classroom atmosphere. Another is the need to keep up with a twin sibling who is more advanced in speech. Still another is the presence in the home of an adult model whose speech is a matter of family pride. Some stutterers appear to have attached excessive importance to perfection in speech mainly because the excellence of their own speech made it an object of unusual accolades. A parent may become overly concerned about the child's speech because there have been memorable instances of stuttering in the family, as Johnson has suggested. In other cases it may be merely ignorance of the normal process of speech development that leads a parent to expect too much of a child.

In one case a severe stutterer, aged 12 years, was in a special class for children with mental retardation. His mother, a schoolteacher, and his father, an intelligent and articulate person, had apparently subjected the boy to severe pressures to live up to standards of language use that were unrealistic in view of his problem. He was said to have spoken "beautifully" until he began to stutter at age 7 years, although he had been a late talker. The father said, "He would never say a two-syllable word if he could use a four-syllable word."

STUTTERING AS TENSION AND FRAGMENTATION

In summary, we are suggesting that neither excessive disfluency nor its evaluation as stuttering is necessary in order for anticipatory struggle reactions to develop; all that may be needed is a set of circumstances in which a child is chronically vulnerable to the threat of speech failure in essentially any form. In developing this hypothesis, however, we have tacitly made some assumptions about the moment of stuttering. We have, in effect, denied that stuttering at its inception is necessarily a reaction of avoidance—whether of simple repetitions or anything else.

It will be recalled from Chapter 2 that there are many ways of expressing what we have referred to in this book as the anticipatory struggle hypothesis. One of the most widely used has been Johnson's description of the moment of stuttering as an anticipatory avoidance reaction, a description whose antecedent is to be found in the older concept that "secondary" stuttering is the effort to avoid "primary" stuttering. The idea of avoidance seems to work well enough as long as we are talking about stuttering in a relatively developed form. That is, if we assume that stuttering behavior is occasioned chiefly by stuttering itself or by cues representative of it, the block is conveniently regarded as an attempt to avoid stuttering. When we try to apply the concept of avoidance to the problem of the etiology of the disorder, however, it tends to distort our perception by making it difficult to view incipient stuttering as a reaction to anything but simpler speech disfluencies.

Avoidance is an ambiguous term. When we say that a motorist avoids an obstacle or a rat avoids an electrified grid, we are using the term avoid in a manner fairly descriptive of behavior. But the statement that we "avoided" falling into debt or getting sunburned gives little specific information about what we did; it tells chiefly about our motivations, fears, or anticipations. Similarly, the statement that stuttering begins as the avoidance of repetitions, or disfluencies, does not describe the stuttering behavior. It merely represents an inference about the motive lying behind it. When we ask precisely how children thought to be so motivated actually behave, we find that they stop, repeat, strain, and so forth. But these are precisely the same things they might do if they were motivated by a fear that they were going to have difficulty articulating a word or phrase or that they were going to encounter any other kind of speech failure. In short, there is essentially nothing in stutterers' observable speech behavior that necessitates the assumption that they are avoiding something, except in the rather indirect sense that a person struggling to open a pickle jar may be said to be trying to avoid the consequences of failing to open it.

It is evident that we need a term more descriptive than avoidance if we are to be free to consider the theory that pressures and provocations other than those that relate to disfluency may contribute to the etiology of stuttering. On the assumptions we have adopted in this chapter, it might be appropriate to describe stuttering as behavior consisting in some measure of *tension* and *fragmentation* in speech. The most important value of the term "fragmentation" is that it expresses the particular sense in which repetitions may be regarded as reactions to a belief in the difficulty of speech. To some extent virtually every type of stuttered response is both tense and fragmented. But repetitions exhibit most conspicuously that fragmented, discontinuous type of articulation which we may speculate to result from the stutterer's conviction that a word (or phrase, or sentence) is too difficult to attempt in its entirety. This view of repetitions is supported by the observation of Sheehan (1974) that some repetitions involve successively larger samples of the word, as in "th-thir-thirty-five."

We may sum it up most succinctly by saying that the repetitions of stuttering are not so much repeated utterances as repeated stoppages. This concept is useful for both theory and therapy. It makes it possible to regard even the "simple" repetitions of early stuttering as anticipatory struggle behavior. It serves to explain why the final syllables or sounds of words are almost never repeated. It also helps to account for the fact that stutterers continue to produce utterances of sounds that they have already said perfectly several times.[1] Moreover, as we saw in the preceding chapter, by extending the concept of fragmentation of words to fragmentation of syntactic units we appear to gain insight into some of the most curious features of stuttering in its earliest phase of development.

In formulating a general model of stuttering behavior as tension and fragmentation in speech we may, like Chomsky, borrow from structuralist philosophy the idea of deep and surface structure. Tension and fragmentation relate to the underlying structure of stuttering. As we are using these terms, they do not refer to anything directly visible or audible. We might conceivably feel tension in the stutterer's oral musculatures if we palpated them, but we cannot see or hear it in the stuttering; we can only see or hear its effects. Nor can we identify by direct observation the speech elements that the stutterer is fragmenting; we can only infer them from the fragments that the stutterer repeats. The observable features of stuttering, if we exclude the extraneous secondary aspects, consist of repetition of speech units, prolongation of sounds, hard attack on sounds, and silent interval or stoppage. These four include substantially all of the surface features of stuttering. They appear when normal speech segments are transformed by tension and fragmentation.

Tension in the articulation of continuant sounds results in their prolongation. In the case of stop-plosive consonants the same tension generates a hard attack—essentially a lengthened stop phase followed by an overaspirated plosive phase. Fragmentation of syntactic units generates repetition of their initial syllables, words, or phrases. Fragmentation of words results in repetition of their initial sounds or syllables. Sometimes fragmentation of syllables within words results in repetition of initial sounds of syllables, as in "inv-v-vite." Silent intervals are rather obvious surface realizations of tension and fragmentation, but even more than most features of stuttering are difficult to characterize in a simple way as either one or the other. In many cases they seem chiefly to express a type of fragmentation, as in "a a _____ sailor," or "I'm ———— I'm a big girl." But complete stoppage may also reflect tension, as when a hard attack on a stop-plosive con-

---

[1]Another explanation sometimes offered is that stutterers do not have difficulty with a sound as such, but with the transition to the next sound. This seems to us not so much an explanation as a description, however. Why are stutterers unable to make this transition? We believe it is a failure of conviction about their ability to say the word as a whole, rather than any difficulty with transitions as such. Otherwise transitions would give difficulty at all places in the word rather than at the beginning.

sonant results in an exceptionally prolonged stop phase or when the stutterer attempts speech with a tightly closed glottis.

This conceptual model is at best an oversimplification taking little account of various complex interactions that might be involved in the genesis of stuttering blocks. Prins (1983) has shown how the model might be extended to include the frustration that results from stuttering and how frustration might directly and indirectly exacerbate the tensions and fragmentations.

THE POWER OF THE CONTINUITY HYPOTHESIS

By giving up the assumption that anticipatory struggle behavior is the avoidance of normal disfluency, then, and talking instead of tensions and fragmentations in speech, we open the way for consideration of the wide range of provocations to stuttering that seem to be suggested by clinical experience. In the author's view another significant advantage is that it permits us to adopt the continuity hypothesis. The avoidance theory implied that a clearly defined difference existed between stuttering and normal disfluency. There is hardly any sharper distinction than that drawn between the avoidance of something and the thing being avoided. Once the notion of avoidance is removed we are free to consider the point of view that what is usually called stuttering in young children is essentially a somewhat extreme degree of certain types of disfluency to be found in the speech of most young children. There appear to be a number of compelling reasons for assuming that this is true.

In the first place, we have seen *(Chapter 3)* that parents of preschool children tend to report numerous episodes of stuttering of such brief duration that the incidence of the disorder in the earliest years is a matter of considerable vagueness and appears to depend in part on what we are willing to call stuttering. We are perhaps justified in wondering how much more often young children experience intervals of difficulty so inconsequential that they escape even the parents' notice or are shortly forgotten. It appears to be a reasonable inference that we are dealing here with something essentially equatable with the "stuttering" which Metraux (1950) and others have studied as a characteristic phenomenon in the speech of preschool children and which may in turn be identical or continuous with what others have termed normal disfluency.

In the second place, we may recall the overlapping Johnson and his associates found to exist between the early disfluencies of stutterers and those of nonstutterers as described by the parents. A considerable portion of the nonstutterers were reported to have had more prolongations and sound and syllable repetitions in their speech than did many of the stutterers. It is an exceedingly interesting feature of this overlap that not only some of the stutterers, but some of the nonstutterers as well, were said to have shown signs of effort, tension, awareness, bewilderment, irritation, or the like in connection with their earliest disfluencies, despite the fact that all children who had ever been regarded as stutterers had been excluded from the control group. How is this to be explained? A plausible interpretation would seem to be that a very large number of ordinary young children frequently "stutter" somewhat (i.e., that a sharp distinction between the "normal" and the "abnormal" is simply not to be made).

Third, while certain "stutter-type" disfluencies—chiefly repetitions of all types and prolongations of sound—have been found to distinguish groups of stutterers clearly from groups of nonstutterers, this appears to be entirely a difference in degree. There are no stutter-type disfluencies that are not to be found in the speech of many nonstutterers.

Fourth, there are growing indications of marked congruity between the patterns of distribution of early stutterings and normal disfluencies in the speech sequence. So far the evidence seems to show that in both cases speech repetitions observe the same distributional regularities. In stutterers and nonstutterers alike, early disfluency appears to be dominated by the fragmentation of syntactic units.

Finally, the continuity hypothesis is consistent with a theory that stuttering is largely due to speech pressures and provocations of the kind we have discussed in this chapter. Most of these factors are essentially commonplace. It stands to reason that whatever speech difficulty they caused would be commonplace too, in some measure.

> . . . it seems an extremely plausible assumption that the reason the symptoms of some children referred to the speech clinic do not contrast sharply with the hesitations of many normal youngsters is that anticipatory struggle behavior is characteristic to some degree of the speech of almost all young children. It would be rather curious if this were not so. One may be fairly sure that the influences which produce stuttering are present to a small extent in almost every child's environment. Consequently, almost every child can be expected to exhibit mildly and fleetingly the tensions and fragmentations which develop into identifiable episodes of stuttering in a few. It would hardly be profitable to discuss whether or not these reactions of the normal child are stuttering, although stuttering may be a convenient enough name for behavior which differs only in degree from that for which parents usually seek clinical help.
>
> Ever since such a thing as normal nonfluency was recognized, it appears to have been assumed that it was something to be distinguished categorically from "stuttering." This has given rise to one of the most taxing problems with which speech clinicians have been beset in recent years—the problem of determining what, precisely, is the difference between the two, and of making a judgment in the speech clinic as to

whether a given pattern of speech interruptions in a young child is or is not "stuttering." Actually, it appears to be far more natural to assume that there exists only a difference of degree between the normal and abnormal. In all probability, the question of how to differentiate between stuttering and normal nonfluency can never have an absolute answer. The only distinction which one can validly make appears to be a purely relative one between struggle reactions which are mild and occasional and those which are more severe and persistent (Bloodstein, 1961a).

The question, quite simply, is whether we are dealing with a problem like a broken collarbone or a case of pneumonia, in which the diagnosis is either yes or no, or whether stuttering is more like hearing loss, high blood pressure, emotional maladjustment, mental retardation, or innumerable other ills that merge by fine degrees with the normal. The continuity hypothesis holds that stuttering belongs to the second group. From a clinical point of view this implies that the techniques appropriate to the differentiation of abnormal from normal disfluency must be similar to those used in the diagnosis of hearing loss. That is to say, the differentiation must be quantitative. It can only be based on the number of disfluencies of specified kinds that are counted in the child's speech under definable conditions.[2] In such a process, of course, the numbers that signify abnormality are selected on the basis of norms and with the aid of information about the social consequences of disfluency of different amounts and kinds under different conditions; but ultimately, like the decibel level that separates normal hearing from mild hearing loss, such numbers are somewhat arbitrary.

CONCLUSIONS

We began this chapter by summarizing the most important facts about stuttering that have emerged in the course of our review of the research findings. Trying to be consistent with these facts, we have attempted to outline a general hypothesis about the etiology of stuttering that may be stated briefly as follows:

> *Stuttering is an anticipatory struggle reaction. In its clinical form it represents a relatively severe degree of tensions and fragmentations that are a common occurrence in the speech of young children. It develops readily in circumstances in which speech pressures are unusually heavy, the child's vulnerability to them unusually high, or the provocations in the form of communicative difficulties or failures unusually frequent, severe, or chronic.*

---

[2]In the case of stuttering, unfortunately, such a process is likely to be vastly more difficult in practice than in principle because of the way the disfluencies of young children tend to fluctuate from day to day and week to week. Even sampling a child's speech on successive occasions may provide only a partial solution to this problem.

We may check back now to see how well this hypothesis accords with our factual information. That stuttering is predominantly a disorder of childhood is readily understood as a consequence of the fact that the younger the child the less secure is the mastery of speech and language, the more fraught with difficulties is the communicative process, and the more malleable are the child's speech attitudes and behavior in response to environmental demands. The sex ratio in stuttering may be related to the slower speech and language development of the male and his greater proneness to speech and language failures, as well as to the heavier speech pressures that he encounters or is led to impose upon himself. The findings that appear to show that stutterers as a group exhibit an unusual amount of delayed speech or articulatory difficulty are obviously consistent with our hypothesis. So is the general observation that the incidence of the disorder is related to environmental pressures. If some stuttering children tend to be somewhat insecure, anxious, or sensitive, it is not difficult to account for this on the assumption that such children may be more vulnerable to threats or suggestions of speech failure.

On the whole, our hypothesis does not as readily account for the familial incidence of stuttering or other evidence of possible genetic influences. While the theory can be reconciled with such facts by various means, it does not afford any special insight into them, and we are left in doubt as to their precise meaning. Evidence from two independent studies shows that the presence of a family history of stuttering in a given case is not related to either of the other two major factors that appear to be conducive to the development of stuttering—parental pressures and late-developing or faulty speech.[3]

Finally, we must remember that our hypothesis rests upon the premise that the moment of stuttering is an anticipatory struggle reaction. This premise is based upon a multitude of observations about stuttering behavior that were considered in Chapter 7. While it appears to this author to be the most satisfactory choice among alternative concepts of the moment of stuttering, it remains an inference of a high order of abstraction to which there adheres a measure of doubt. Above all, whatever appeal the anticipatory struggle hypothesis or any other concept may have for us as a means of accounting for the facts, we must not allow it to dull the sharpness of our perception that the stuttering block remains a baffling and mysterious phenomenon and that there are as yet no conclusive answers to such seemingly basic questions as whether it is essentially "voluntary" or "involuntary" in nature, autonomically or centrally controlled, respondent or operant, learned in itself or an unlearned resultant of learned behaviors.

---

[3]Bloodstein (1958, p. 30), Andrews and Harris (1964, p. 115).

The same may be said about the etiology of stuttering. Although we have developed a number of inferences about it, we must conclude that there are few grounds for zeal in support of any theory. It is hoped, however, that this book has at least helped to clarify some of the questions that are central to a solution of the problem.

Suggested Readings

Bloodstein, O., Stuttering as tension and fragmentation. In Eisenson, J. (ed.), *Stuttering: A Second Symposium*. New York: Harper Row (1975).

Bloodstein, O., Stuttering as an anticipatory struggle disorder. In Curlee, R. F., and Perkins, W. H. (eds.), *Nature and Treatment of Stuttering: New Directions*. San Diego: College-Hill Press (1984).

Bloodstein, O., Stuttering: *The Search for a Cause and Cure*. Boston: Allyn & Bacon (1993), Chap. 15.

11

TREATMENT

The treatment of stuttering, like its etiology, is a matter of considerable controversy. The methods that have been attempted with some degree of success are extremely varied, and the recorded history of their use goes back in some cases to classical antiquity. In this chapter we will briefly survey some of the principal remedial approaches, with emphasis on current practices.

METHODS IN EARLY USE

Modiflcatlons of the Speech Pattern

In Chapter 7 we saw that stutterers are likely to speak fluently as soon as they adopt almost any novel manner of speaking. From ancient times to the present this has been persistently discovered and rediscovered as a remedy for stuttering in a variety of ingenious forms. Demosthenes's famous pebbles, if the old story is true, were an expedient of this type. Two thousand years later they appeared in more refined form as an ivory "support" for the tongue. In the past two hundred years this general approach to therapy has been represented chiefly by methods that teach the stutterer to talk in time to rhythmic movements of the arm, hand, or finger or to adopt other unusual speech patterns. Stutterers have been advised to speak slowly, in a sing-song, or in a monotone; to slur the consonants and prolong the vowels; to shorten the vowels and stress the consonants; to hold the tongue this way or that way; or to pay attention in one manner or another to their rate, phrasing, or breathing.

Almost nothing appears to remove stuttering as quickly and completely as do devices of this kind. Unfortunately, in many cases the benefit proves to be merely temporary. Furthermore, when stutterers relapse after having been "cured" in this way there is often a tendency for the arm-swing, drawl, or other mannerism that they have habituated to become part of their stuttering pattern and to increase the abnormality of their speech. For these reasons a strong suspicion of such methods for many years characterized the attitudes of clinical workers, particularly in the United States where this kind of therapy was largely confined to commercial "stammering schools" until the 1960s.

The invention of new ways of altering stutterers' speech patterns was never completely abandoned, however. Froeschels's chewing method was a well-known example of comparatively modern date. Stutterers learned to speak fluently by performing chewing movements together with speech. They then gradually attenuated the chewing activity and finally merely imagined themselves to be chewing (Froeschels, 1943). Ventriloquism, another technique suggested by Froeschels (1950), made use of the art of speaking with a minimum of lip movement. Cherry and Sayers (1956) introduced a therapy they called "shadowing," based on their observation that stutterers tend to speak fluently when producing a running copy of another person's speech. Eventually the advent of "behavior therapy" for stuttering brought various modifications of the speech pattern into frequent use again, as we will see.

Suggestion

Another powerful method of eliminating stuttering temporarily is suggestion. This has been used consciously and deliberately with stutterers ever since the phenomenon of hypnotism became widely known in the early nineteenth century. It was probably employed long before that, however, unwittingly and in nonhypnotic forms. The older literature on stuttering contains references to a large variety of therapeutic techniques that apparently owed whatever effectiveness they had to the stutterer's belief that they would help. Among these were "hunger cures" and other forms of punishment, regulation of diet, periods of enforced. silence, bloodletting, tongue surgery, articulatory drills, and breathing exercises. In modern times there have been many attempts to treat stuttering by posthypnotic suggestions of fluency, hypnotic suggestions repeated regularly over long periods, and autosuggestion.

Those who can be hypnotized tend to gain marked relief from their difficulty, but the majority relapse fairly soon. At least part of the reason for the temporary nature of the recovery appears to be that this type of therapy makes little fundamental change in the fear of stuttering that adult stutterers are likely to have. They may tell themselves with conviction that they will not stutter and talk fluently while the conviction remains strong; however, as long as they still regard stuttering as an intolerable stigma the most trifling countersuggestions of imminent failure in the form of certain sounds, words, situations, or listeners to which they had learned to react with expectancy may be enough to undermine their synthetic "confidence" and precipitate a new onset of the disorder. Furthermore, when recovery has been based for the most part on hope and faith, relapse may be accompanied by severe demoralization.

The fact that stutterers may be helped for some time by practically any type of therapy in which they believe strongly has some important implications. It means that they may be especially likely to obtain short-term benefit from a therapist who is deeply convinced of the effectiveness of the methods used, who happens to be charismatic, or who has a prestigious role (e.g., physician, psychiatrist, or the like). A corollary hypothesis for which there is considerable evidence in the history of treatment of stuttering is that almost every new movement in therapy is likely to enjoy a kind of honeymoon during which successes occur in part as a result of the hope and enthusiasm of clinicians. To the extent that this is true, evaluating the results of any new departure in therapy is obviously no simple matter.

Relaxation

An old method still in fairly wide use in the day-to-day practice of speech pathologists is relaxation. This would seem to have a certain basic appropriateness in the case of a disorder consisting essentially of struggle behavior. It is almost impossible to be relaxed and to stutter in the usual sense at the same time. As a result of long experience, however, considerable dissatisfaction with this approach has arisen among clinical workers. A few stutterers seem to learn the trick of relaxing their muscles so effectively that they have little further difficulty with their speech. But such persons appear to be rare. Usually, stutterers tend to speak better in a treatment environment while practicing relaxation. Outside that environment, however, they may find it impossible to relax precisely in those situations where it is most important for them to do so. Anxiety and tension are difficult to separate. Consequently, most workers employ relaxation only in certain special forms or in conjunction with other types of therapy. As we will see later in this chapter, relaxation has been used in recent years as a feature of a conditioning therapy known as systematic desensitization, and it has also been employed with specific speech muscles through electromyographic feedback.

PSYCHOTHERAPY

Early in the twentieth century a radically new method of treating stutterers was tried for the first time. Freud wrote comparatively little about stuttering, but what he did write left little doubt that he considered it a neurotic symptom rooted in unconscious conflicts. By 1920 various followers of Freud, among them Brill and Coriat, had treated a considerable number of stutterers by psychoanalytic therapy, and thereafter this gained recognition rapidly as a method of treatment for the disorder. The psychoanalysts from the beginning directed their efforts against what they regarded as the cause of stuttering through the resolution of inner personality conflicts. The older methods of distraction, suggestion, and relaxation were for the most part rejected as superficial attempts to deal with symptoms alone, and some psychoanalysts warned that the elimination of stuttering by such techniques represented a premature and dangerous removal of the stutterer's neurotic defenses.

Perhaps the best way to sum up the results of psychoanalytic treatment of stutterers to date is by saying that they appear to have been too good to warrant outright rejection and too poor to warrant any substantial amount of satisfaction. If hope ever existed that psychoanalysis would immediately provide an essential solution to the stutterer's problem, this hope was soon dispelled by Brill (1923).

Brill, who clearly understood that the difficulty of stutterers was not so much their lack of amenability to improvement as their great tendency to relapse, was one of the few workers of his day employing any type of stuttering therapy to make careful follow-up studies. He reported that of sixty-nine adult stutterers whom he had treated regularly "for a few months to a year or even longer" the great majority at first appeared to have regained essentially normal speech, but that after eleven years only five of the sixty-nine patients whom he had discharged as recovered were "really well." He commented, "Most of the others seem to be satisfied that they have been improved, although they have their ups and downs."

Other workers—for example, Travis (1957) and Glauber (1958)—have been more optimistic about the results of psychoanalysis, and it might reasonably be argued that clinical techniques of psychoanalysis are now much advanced over those available to Brill, but further follow-up studies of any importance have not been reported. Many psychoanalysts appear to have come to the conclusion from their experience with stutterers that the majority of them are unusually resistant to therapy.

Classical Freudian psychoanalysis is not, of course, the only existing form of psychotherapy. By now stutterers have been treated by various neo-Freudian forms of psychoanalysis, by group psychotherapy, by nondirective therapy, psychodrama, gestalt therapy, rational-emotive therapy, and most other varieties of psychotherapy. There is as yet little evidence that any of these has proved outstandingly successful or has more of the usual potential for reducing stuttering temporarily that is inherent in virtually any remedial measure. Furthermore, the absence of conclusive research evidence that stuttering is an attempt to satisfy unconscious needs or that it is wholly or necessarily a symptom of personality conflict does not make for confidence that future efforts to treat it through psychotherapy will be more successful.

THE IOWA DEVELOPMENT

In the 1930s there arose another challenge to the older methods of treating stuttering. Although this was primarily the work of three persons, Bryng Bryngelson, Wendell Johnson, and Charles Van Riper, it may be best understood in the context of certain broader historical events to which it was related. In the early decades of this century speech and language pathology as a profession did not exist. Although a number of phoneticians, psychiatrists, and other professional workers were making significant early contributions to this area of knowledge, whatever correction of speech disorders took place was largely in the hands of classroom teachers with more good intentions than training and commercial speech "specialists" who frequently had neither. During the 1920s the first active stirrings that were to develop into the scientific study and treatment of speech, language, and hearing problems as a nonmedical field of professional specialization made themselves felt.

One of the more significant of these beginnings took place at the University of Iowa as a clearly deliberated step undertaken by the noted psychologist Carl Emil Seashore as dean of the Graduate College. Johnson (1955b) told the absorbing story of the manner in which Seashore's special kind of imagination contributed to the establishment of a new academic and professional study at the University of Iowa. Recognizing that the initial need was for a research program to provide a better scientific understanding of speech and hearing disorders and that no single academic department then existing could offer all of the basic knowledge and skills for such a program, Seashore proceeded to break down departmental barriers. He selected a promising student to direct the development of the program and, with the cooperation of the departments of psychology, speech, physics, psychiatry, neurology, otolaryngology, and other university departments, he prepared him for a career as a new kind of specialist.

That student, Lee Edward Travis, was, in Johnson's words, probably "the first individual in the world to be trained by clearly conscious design at the doctoral level for the definite and specific professional objective of working experimentally and clinically with speech and hearing disorders." In 1927 Travis became the first director of the University of Iowa Speech Clinic. Under his supervision a group of researchers and clinicians was soon engaged in work on a variety of problems of speech and voice. Chief among Travis's own personal interests was stuttering, and the decade that he remained at the University of Iowa was a period of unparalleled ferment in research, theoretical speculation, and clinical experimentation in this area. In all of this intense activity the remarkable scope of the training Travis had received by Seashore's careful design was clearly visible, but the new concepts of therapy that emanated from this activity, and which were so profoundly to influence the treatment of stuttering in the United States, have come to be associated with the names of three of Travis's early students who were directly responsible for the development and elaboration of these concepts.

In brief, the new therapeutic approach for which Bryngelson, Johnson, and Van Riper opened the way was aimed at a reduction in the fear and avoidance of stuttering while at the same time attempting to reduce the stuttering itself directly through gradual modification based on study and understanding of the behavior of which stuttering consisted. This approach represented a sharp departure from the philosophy on which the older methods were based. Bryngelson, Johnson, and Van Riper were severely critical of those methods. They argued that they merely gave the stutterer a temporary crutch on which to lean and that quick recovery almost inevitably portended sudden relapse. Above all, such methods served in the long run to intensify rather than decrease fear because in effect they said to the stutterer, "Don't stutter. Swing your arms or talk in some odd and unnatural way, but whatever you do, don't stutter." And the implication was that hardly anything was more unusual or grotesque or more to be feared and avoided than stuttering. By contrast, the new approach was to say to the stutterer, "Go ahead and stutter. But learn to do so without fear and embarrassment and with a minimum of abnormality."

In precisely what manner and for what reasons this particular point of view arose in the atmosphere of the University of Iowa Speech Clinic of the 1930s is a difficult question to answer simply. Unquestionably, an influence of the utmost significance was Travis's interest in "mental hygiene" and the psychology of adjustment. Another factor of probable importance was that two of the three chief promulgators of this point of view began their professional careers as severe stutterers who had had personal experiences of short-lived success and intense discouragement with older methods of therapy and who, moreover, had intimate knowledge of the manner in which fear and stuttering were related. At any rate, this was the general clinical outlook that they more or less jointly formulated. It was an outlook that lent itself with great vitality to modification and development in highly individual ways, and anything further that is to be said about it must concern itself with the distinctive contributions of the three men who shared it.

Bryngelson: Voluntary Stuttering and the Objective Attitude

The phrase "objective attitude" in connection with stuttering therapy appears to have been first used, at least with the precise systematic implications that it came to have for most speech pathologists, by Bryngelson. Oddly enough, this basic goal of stuttering therapy initially took on significance in conjunction with the attempts to treat stutterers by means of laterality training that were made at the University of Iowa during the 1930s. Shortly after the Iowa clinical and research program was established, Travis, together with Samuel T. Orton, head of the department of psychiatry at the University of Iowa, formulated a concept of stuttering as a symptom of conflict between the two cerebral hemispheres (*see Chapter 2*). It is a curious feature of an essentially neurophysiological breakdown theory that it permits considerable emphasis in therapy on the stutterer's attitudes and adjustments. One reason for this is that if stutterers can avoid some of the strong emotional reactions that ordinarily accompany stuttering, they may thereby eliminate a major source of the external pressures presumed to precipitate breakdowns of their vulnerable neuromuscular organization.

Bryngelson, as Travis's student, followed his lead in attempting to develop the "native dominance" of stutterers as a major concern of therapy, but he also put very great stress on the cultivation of attitudes of acceptance and objectivity in relation to their speech difficulty. To Bryngelson an objective attitude on the part of stutterers meant the ability to discuss their stuttering freely and casually with others. It meant the willingness to enter difficult speech situations and the refusal to make use of word substitutions or other tricks for avoiding stuttering. In general, the goal was to bring the problem out into the open and to be willing to stutter. This lent itself to the use of group therapy in which stutterers were encouraged to ventilate their feelings about their speech problem before an audience of other stutterers and in which they could be helped to gain objectivity by the examples set by others. It also led to a great emphasis on "situational" work in which stutterers were taken outside the speech clinic and challenged to demonstrate their ability to maintain an objective attitude in feared situations. The elements of Bryngelson's remedial program that were concerned with laterality have passed into disuse, but the teaching of an objective attitude through situational work is today still used by many speech pathologists as a major aspect of therapy with stutterers in the most advanced phase of the disorder.

A particularly distinctive contribution Bryngelson made to this type of therapy was a technique he termed "voluntary stuttering." Practically as soon as it became evident to the Iowa group that the stutterer's fear of speaking could often be very markedly reduced, it was apparently recognized that this approach when used alone had its limitations. Not only was it useless to try to eliminate all fear of stuttering in most cases, but very frequently a considerable amount of stuttering remained after the fear had been substantially reduced. From the very beginning, therefore, the work on attitudes toward speech was combined with efforts to modify the stuttering behavior directly. This was the primary purpose of voluntary stuttering as it was first suggested by Bryngelson. In 1932 there had appeared a book by Knight Dunlap entitled *Habits: Their Making and Unmaking* proposing a technique termed "negative practice" for the elimination of an undesirable habit. Dunlap's principle was that by practicing the error deliberately it could be brought from the realm of the habitual and automatic and dealt with appropriately in a conscious, purposeful way. Bryngelson took this device and applied it to stuttering with a somewhat modified rationale. He suggested that stutterers learn to stutter voluntarily as a means of fighting for conscious control of their "spasms." This exercise of control was for Bryngelson the principal objective.

Stutterers were to practice the technique before a mirror until they had thoroughly mastered it. They were then to use it in speech situations outside the clinic. If attempts to stutter voluntarily on a difficult word resulted in an involuntary reaction, they were to repeat the attempt until the block was completely under their control. In principle, Bryngelson advocated that stutterers learn to imitate the basic components of their own characteristic stuttering behavior, but he found that it was usually easier for stutterers to block on purpose when they produced a simple, effortless repetition of initial sounds. Bryngelson was not oblivious to other benefits that voluntary stuttering had in addition to the element of control. He saw it as a means of learning to stutter without the avoidances, starters, and other tricks and devices with which stutterers frequently complicated their difficulty. He also recognized in it the psychological benefit of deliberately facing what one was ordinarily inclined to avoid or hide.

Voluntary stuttering has been employed widely in stuttering therapy, particularly by clinicians who are able to develop a high level of morale in the stutterer. It is not, as may be imagined, an easy discipline for the typical stutterer to learn or for parents to understand when the need for this arises. In more recent years a tendency toward less use of voluntary stuttering in its original form has been discernible, perhaps as part of a trend on the part of some speech pathologists toward greater concern about the clinician-stutterer relationship.[1] As will be seen, however, the technique exerted considerable influence on Johnson and Van Riper as they developed their therapeutic approaches, and in direct and indirect ways it has played an important part in the history of stuttering therapy.

Johnson: Perceptual and Evaluative Reorientation

A product of substantially the same influences that motivated Bryngelson to advocate voluntary stuttering and the objective attitude, Wendell Johnson formulated a therapeutic program based on similar goals, but with certain differences that were eventually to lead to his own distinctive form of treatment. Johnson's outlook on therapy was markedly affected by his growing conviction that there was little physical or organic basis for stuttering and by his development in the late 1930s of a "diagnosogenic" theory of its origin *(see Chapter 2)*. Like Bryngelson, he believed that it was necessary to reduce the fear of stuttering as much as possible and that among stutterers' chief objectives in therapy was to learn to handle speech situations adequately as stutterers without apologizing for their blocks or allowing themselves to be handicapped by their speech difficulty. For Johnson, however, fear was at the heart of the problem. He believed that stuttering was an avoidance reaction motivated by anxious anticipation of speech interruption and that the way to start talking normally was to stop trying to avoid stuttering.

This premise also lay behind the particular kind of use that Johnson made of Bryngelson's voluntary stuttering. For Johnson, the value of voluntary stuttering had little to do with the aim of gaining control over the stuttering reactions. The very notion of control was one to which he was unsympathetic. He felt that stutterers tended to be overly cautious and perfectionistic in the manner in which they went about speaking to begin with and that what they needed was to be not less but more spontaneous about it. Voluntary stuttering, as Johnson applied it, was an exercise in throwing caution to the winds. In being disfluent on purpose stutterers were weakening their tendency to avoid disfluency and consequently their tendency to stutter. From this point of view it was desirable for stutterers to perform the voluntary pattern simply and easily, without the hurry and tension that characterized avoidance behavior. Gradually, Johnson believed, it would be possible for stutterers by this means to slow down, delay, and simplify their stuttering reactions until they became essentially like normal disfluencies.

----

[1]See, for example, Cooper and Cooper (1969), Cooper (1966, 1968, 1971), and Manning and Cooper (1969) for work on this relationship.

In this connection he pointed out that most normal speech contained hesitancies. The difference between stutterers and normal speakers was that stutterers reacted emotionally to their hesitations. By the same token, leaming to speak normally was ultimately in large measure a matter of stutterers' evaluations; it was something that occurred when they began to perform their interruptions without reacting to them as a speech difficulty.

Perhaps the most potent factor that contributed to the development of Johnson's thinking about stuttering was the general semantics of Alfred Korzybski (1941), and it is with an essentially semantic approach to therapy that he is generally identified. As Johnson saw it, the things that prevented stutterers from talking normally were simply the things they did to keep themselves from stuttering; if they were to go ahead on the assumption that there was nothing to prevent them from talking adequately they would speak without any trouble. Consequently, stuttering was caused by a peculiar set of perceptions and evaluations that stutterers entertained about their speech. As such, it was a kind of behavior influenced by the language they used in talking and thinking about their speech and subtly and pervasively conditioned by primitive, animistic, and naive conceptions inherent in that language.

For example, Johnson pointed out, stutterers often tended to talk about their speech difficulty very much as though it were caused by demons inside of them that played hob with their oral apparatus; they were likely to say, not "I press my lips together too hard when I talk sometimes," but "My lips come together too hard," or "My tongue pushes against my teeth," or "My throat shuts tight." If stuttering were chiefly a matter of erroneous assumptions or inferences, then its chief antidote was the checking of these inferences by means of scientific observations, or what as a general semanticist he called "extensionalization," and in time this became an important feature of Johnson's therapy. Stutterers carefully observed their stuttering behavior before a mirror and by means of tape recording to determine just what they did to prevent themselves from speaking. They systematically observed what happened when they spoke in time to rhythms or when they were alone in order to verify the fact that there was nothing wrong "inside" to keep them from talking normally. They observed the disfluencies of normal speakers in order to discover that normal speech was not perfect speech. They made scientific observations of the reactions of their listeners to find out that, by and large, listeners were more tolerant of their stuttering than they had assumed.

This type of treatment involved the bringing about of certain important changes in the stutterer's perceptual and evaluative reactions. Ultimately, perceptual and evaluative reorientation based upon general semantics became Johnson's chief method of attack on the problem. In this he was influenced considerably by the work of Dean E. Williams (1957) who extended and developed this approach to therapy. Johnson finally discarded much of his earlier therapy, including the technique of voluntary stuttering. His basic clinical procedure became one of training stutterers to be conscious of the inappropriateness of the language they tended to use in talking about their problem. In group or individual discussions persons who came for treatment were taught to examine carefully what they meant when they referred to themselves as "stutterers" as though assuming that there was something about them which marked them as basically different from other people, or when they referred to what they did when they talked as their "stuttering" or "it" as though their problem was not what they did when they talked, but a thing inside of them which they needed to manage, stop, or control.

Finally, they were trained to set aside, at least temporarily, such words as "stuttering" in order to talk descriptively about their problem, with the expectation that, as they became aware that there was nothing to prevent them from going on except the things they themselves did when they talked, they would gradually become better able to talk without doing these things. On the basis of this sort of semantic reorientation, then, Johnson proceeded to place major emphasis on a great deal of actual speaking by stutterers—an increase both in speaking time and in the number of situations in which speech was attempted—with attention to "going ahead and talking" on the assumption that there were no basic physical or emotional reasons for not doing so.

Van Riper: Cancellations, Pull-outs, and Preparatory Sets

When Charles Van Riper left the University of Iowa in 1936 to establish a speech clinic at what is now Western Michigan University, it was with the determination to devote himself to finding more effective methods of treating stuttering. To accomplish his purpose he resolved that he would select a small group of severe stutterers each year, vary his therapy, keep careful records, and employ a five-year follow-up study to evaluate the results. His account of this activity is a remarkable record of therapeutic experimentation over a period of more than twenty years (see Van Riper, 1958). During this period he apparently tried almost every known and many unknown methods of treating stutterers and evolved a therapeutic program going considerably beyond that developed in the early years at Iowa. This program, however, may be regarded fundamentally as an extension of the Iowa concept of therapy since it stresses the reduction of anxiety about stuttering and the deliberate modification of the stuttering behavior based on analysis and understanding.

Although Van Riper has continually been concerned with the treatment of stutterers' fears and has developed a variety of original techniques for desensitizing stutterers to their difficulties and reducing their avoidances, perhaps his major contributions have been in relation to the problem of modifying the behavior itself. If there is a single term used by Van Riper that epitomizes his approach to this problem, it is the term *fluent stuttering*. From the beginning he regarded the stuttering block as in large part learned behavior. It appeared to him that whether the disorder had a neurological, neurotic, or any other type of origin it soon tended to become self-perpetuating, most of the abnormality consisting of anticipatory reactions for avoiding stuttering and reactions of frustration in response to the experience of becoming blocked. This suggested the possibility that one could learn to stutter with a minimum of abnormality. It was necessary to substitute for the habitual stuttering reactions a smooth, simple pattern of interruptions without struggle and free from the devices for avoidance, postponement, starting, and release that frequently complicated them. The goal, in short, was not to speak without stuttering, but to stutter "fluently."

As a substitute method of fluent stuttering, Van Riper first tried the simple repetitive pattern that Bryngelson had termed "voluntary stuttering," but soon found it unsatisfactory for this purpose, and retained it only in the form of "faking" or "pseudostuttering" on nonfeared words as a mental hygiene device. The pattern that seemed to fulfill his requirements as a method of stuttering more normally was a smooth prolongation of sound. He found that effective employment of this pattern made for an open, straightforward kind of stuttering, free from much of its usual complexity, and gave an ongoing, essentially "fluent" quality to stutterers' speech. The more skilled stutterers became at performing the pattern the more brief and effortless their blocks became and the closer their speech approached to normalcy.

This was true if stutterers did it effectively. Some appeared to manage it quite well. All too often, however, particularly under communicative stress, the smooth prolongations tended to give way to the tremors and spasmodic tensions of uncontrolled stuttering despite all that the stutterers could do to prevent this. Some method of teaching stutterers how to smooth out their blockages was evidently needed. As he worked on this problem, Van Riper noted that stutterers' abnormal attacks on feared words were due to the manner in which they behaved just *before* they said the word. During the period of anticipation prior to the word-attempt, there often appeared to be fragmentary silent rehearsals of the block that was about to occur. Stutterers seemed to place themselves in a particular kind of tense *preparatory set* when it was necessary for them to say what they thought was a difficult word. Apparently it was this set which gave rise to the block and which seemed to determine even the length and very form of the block.

As Van Riper studied the preparatory set, he discovered that it had several more or less distinct features. One was a tendency on the part of stutterers to tense the muscles of their speech organs as they readied themselves to say the word. A second was a peculiar inclination to say the first sound of a feared word with a fixed position of the articulators rather than as a normal movement leading smoothly into the next sound, a set that appeared to reflect the stutterer's characteristic tendency to think of the initial sound in isolation from the rest of the word as the principal obstacle to be hurdled. A third was a habit of "preforming" the first sound, or placing the articulators in position for the sound well in advance of the attempt to say it.

It is evident that, in the brief period of anticipation just prior to the attempt on the feared word, behavior took place that was of crucial importance in the precipitation of the block. The idea occurred to Van Riper that this period afforded the best opportunity to modify the stuttering. It was necessary to teach stutterers to react to their feeling of expectancy as a signal to assume certain new preparatory sets in place of the old ones. The new preparatory sets were, first, to begin the word with the articulators in a state of rest; second, to say the first sound as a movement leading into the next sound; and, third, to initiate voice or airflow immediately on the attempt to say the word. It is readily appreciated that these sets, if carried through with essential completeness, would result in normal speech. Van Riper's immediate goal was not normal speech, however. Altered preparatory sets were chiefly a means of helping stutterers to achieve their objective of learning to stutter "fluently."

The new preparatory sets served this purpose with marked success in some cases, but there were still some serious difficulties. The chief problem was that it was difficult for most stutterers to monitor their speech as painstakingly as this technique required them to and still communicate adequately. Van Riper found a partial solution to this problem in a device he termed "pull-outs." When stutterers were unable to change their preparatory sets effectively in their attempt on a given word and had begun to block on it in their usual way, they were trained to finish the word with a smooth, controlled, gliding prolongation. Since a large part of the abnormality of stuttering often consists of the frantic struggle to terminate the block, this tended to have the immediate effect of increasing fluency. Even more important, as stutterers learned to "pull out" of their blocks with greater ease, their altered behavior gradually came to be initiated progressively earlier in the course of the block until it began to reflect itself in changes in their preparatory sets.

Pull-outs seemed to work unusually well, far better than anything he had yet tried, but still Van Riper was not satisfied. Too often stutterers found that they had completed their blocks in the old manner before they had a chance to do anything about them. It was in the attempt to cope with this difficulty that Van Riper finally came to use a technique he referred to as "cancellation." When stutterers failed to use an easy prolongation or to pull out of the block successfully, they paused, studied their feelings and behavior, and immediately tried the word again. The object was not to say the word fluently on the second attempt, but to make some change for the better in their way of stuttering. Once stutterers had gained the ability to cancel their failures it was a relatively short step to more satisfactory pull-outs.

Together, preparatory set, pull-out, and cancellation proved to constitute a useful set of practical techniques for modifying stuttering. In teaching them to stutterers, Van Riper frequently began with cancellation and proceeded systematically to pull-out and then preparatory set. When all three had been mastered, stutterers employed them in reverse order on a given word, first attempting to manipulate their anticipatory set and using each in turn only as the others failed. As Van Riper viewed these procedures, they were not mere mechanical devices but in their deeper purpose a kind of psychotherapy. Cancellation, for example, may be seen as a basic form of therapeutic self-confrontation and, as stutterers make use of their blocks as opportunities to battle for control of their fears, malattitudes, and abnormal initiation and release of sounds, they may be compared with neurotic persons who gradually succeed in the course of the psychotherapeutic process in taking responsibility for their maladjustive behavior.

Among the important products of Van Riper's work were the findings of his five-year follow-up studies of small groups of stutterers whom he selected each year for eight months of intensive treatment (see Van Riper, 1958). They showed that about half the stutterers he treated had very fluent or essentially normal speech, were largely free from fear and avoidance, and were socially adequate five years after treatment. Many more were apparently much improved. The results, in short, were encouraging, although they indicated that much further progress remained to be made in the development of a satisfactory therapy for stutterers.

DRUG THERAPY

A variety of pharmaceutical agents have been used from time to time in the treatment of stuttering. Wide interest in such therapy, however, began in the 1950s with the introduction of tranquilizers because of the central role anxiety and tension have been assumed to play in the disorder. The results have been somewhat varied.[2] They have generally led to conclusions of restrained optimism about the use of tranquilizers as an adjunct to other therapy. A frequent report is that the drug has more effect on the complexity or severity of the blocks than on their frequency.

Since the introduction of haloperidol in 1960 a particularly large number of studies have been done of its effect on stuttering.[3] These studies, including some carefully designed double-blind investigations making use of objective measures of stuttering and placebo groups or conditions, appear to show that the drug has a real though limited effect. In addition to finding that many subjects have received little or no benefit, the studies reveal that a large proportion of subjects have tended to drop out of treatment because of the side effects of the drug, especially drowsiness. Both Andrews and Dozsa (1977) and Murray, Kelly, et al. (1977) reported that few of the subjects whose stuttering was reduced wished to continue the medication after the experiment.

The reason for the ameliorative influence of haloperidol on stuttering is not known. The drug is thought to block dopamine receptors in the central nervous system. Burns, Brady, and Kuruvilla (1978) reasoned that the administration of apomorphine might therefore increase stuttering by dopamine receptor stimulation. They found that it did not, although most of their subjects responded to haloperidol with reduced stuttering.

Favorable reports have also appeared about thiamin (Hale, 1951) and glutamic acid (Gutzmann, 1954), but information about their effectiveness is scanty. A survey by Kent (1961) of the use of carbon dioxide inhalation therapy with stutterers indicated varied and equivocal results. In a study by Bloch, Dalby, and Johannesen (1977) propanolol, which has been found effective against essential tremor, had no statistically significant effect on stuttering, although a number of subjects seemed to show improvement. Neither did oxprenolol, which has been found to improve skilled performance under stress (see Rustin, Kuhr, Cook, and James, 1981). Bethanecol chloride appeared to produce improvement in a study of two patients (Hays, 1987). Verapamil, which reduces calcium in smooth muscle cells, needed for muscle contraction, had no effect on stuttering in a study of 14 subjects by Brumfitt and Peake (1988).

---

[2]Winkelman (1954), Maxwell and Paterson (1958), Di Carlo, Katz, and Batkin (1959) Holliday (1959), Kent and Williams (1959), Burr and Mullendore (1960), Yannatos (1960) Fish and Bowling (1962), Fujita et al (1963), Kent (1963), Schilling (1963), Cacudi (1964), Aron (1965), Fish and Bowling (1965), Goldman and Guth (1965), Goldman (1966), Hommerich and Korzendorfer (1966), Leanderson and Levi (1967).

[3]Gattuso and Leocata (1962), Cozzo and Gabrielli (1965), Tapia (l969), Wells and Malcolm (1971), Quinn and Peachey (1973), Swift, Swift, and Arellano (1975), Rantala and Petri-Larmi (1976), Rosenberger, Wheelden, and Kalotkin (1976), Andrews and Dozsa (1977), Murray, Kelly, et al. (1977), Prins, Mandelkorn, and Cerf (1980).

BEHAVIOR THERAPY

An approach to stuttering therapy that has undergone rapid development since the 1960s is the use of so-called behavior modification techniques. This period has seen changes in thinking about the treatment of behavioral disorders generally. Accepted methods of psychotherapy, based to a large extent upon psychoanalysis, have been challenged by a growing number of workers who are skeptical of the effectiveness of these methods, the factual basis of their theoretical assumptions, and their medically oriented model of maladaptive behavior, which assumes that such behavior is a symptom of an underlying "neurosis." Instead, behavior therapists have attempted to view maladjustment conceptually as a matter of learned responses to demonstrable stimuli and to manipulate these responses by applying basic principles discovered by careful laboratory investigation of learning and behavior.

The learning-oriented discussions of stuttering by Wischner and Sheehan had done much to prepare a favorable reception for this outlook in the field of speech pathology, and stuttering therapy was not slow to begin experimenting with behavior modification. The outstanding effect of this development has been to encourage a spirit of innovation in the treatment of stuttering for which not even the emergence of Iowa therapy in the 1930s provides an adequate parallel.

As interest in behavior modification has grown, so has the number of different kinds of therapies to which the term has been applied, and it is difficult to give a simple definition of behavior therapy as used for stuttering. We will outline here essentially all of the principal procedures for treating stuttering which are generally referred to as behavior therapies. They include both classical and operant types of conditioning procedures as well as techniques that are not based primarily on conditioning at all.

Systematic Desensitization

Among the common maladaptive reactions with which people are troubled are many that involve irrational fears of identifiable things such as authority figures, high places, sexual inadequacy, spiders, or speech. Since fear is a classically conditioned response, an important place exists in behavior modification for classical conditioning techniques. Such a procedure, designed to extinguish fear responses, was designed by Wolpe (1958) and is referred to as reciprocal inhibition, or systematic desensitization. Wolpe noted that certain responses tended to inhibit anxiety—for example, relaxation, eating, motor activity, or assertive behavior. He found that if such responses could be made to occur in the presence of the stimulus that evoked the anxiety, its tendency to do so would be weakened. For example, a child might lose a fear of dogs if fed repeatedly in the vicinity of one.

Of course, the reverse might happen too. The child might lose all appetite for food in the presence of the dog. It was important to make sure that the fear did not overcome the response designed to inhibit it. Wolpe therefore introduced the concept of a hierarchy of fear-evoking stimuli varying progressively in strength. On the first occasion the dog may be tied up far enough from the child so that the eating response inhibits the fear. On successive occasions it may then be moved closer by degrees.

This would not be practical with thunderstorms, an impatient boss, or many other objects of irrational fear, however. For this reason Wolpe trained patients to fantasize their fears and applied his hierarchical concept of deconditioning to imagined rather than actual feared objects. This procedure has been widely used in the treatment of a large variety of phobic problems.

Wolpe's methods were first applied in stuttering therapy by Wolpe himself, Walton and Mather (1963), and Brutten and Shoemaker (1967), and have since been employed by others. They were developed in particular for use with stutterers by Brutten and Shoemaker (1967, Chap. 5) and are highly consistent with their viewpoint that the integral features of stuttering represent disruptions of speech by visceral fear reactions which have been classically conditioned to speech sounds, listeners, situations, or other neutral stimuli (see Chapter 2).

Brutten and Shoemaker make use of training in relaxation for this purpose. With the stutterer in a sufficiently relaxed condition to inhibit anxiety, fantasy is employed to present a hierarchy of feared speech situations repeatedly until they no longer serve as stimuli to fear.

For the elimination of the associated symptoms of stuttering, which they regard as instrumentally conditioned responses, they advocate the application of reactive inhibition through massed practice of such reactions. They refer to their therapy, in consequence, as a "two-process" one. On the basis of three years' experience with this approach they reported that, while not "universally" effective, it resulted in marked improvement for most of the stutterers with whom they had worked.

Operant Conditioning

A different type of conditioning therapy for stuttering is based on the methods developed by B. F. Skinner and his followers. These have lent themselves to use in clinical work with stutterers in a variety of ways.

Punishment of Stuttering

As we saw in Chapter 8, there have been a large number of laboratory demonstrations of temporary reduction in stuttering by contingent application of such stimuli as shock, noise, verbal disapproval, response-cost, and time-out from speaking, among others. Of these, only time-out has been put to repeated use in therapy.[4] Martin, Kuhl, and Haroldson (1972) reported its successful use with two preschool children. Each child had weekly conversations with Suzybelle, a puppet whose voice was provided by a speech clinician through an electronic connection from an adjoining room. During periods of time-out Suzybelle's illuminated glass case was darkened and she was silent for 10 seconds. For one child, time-out was made contingent on every stuttering block. In the other case, in which stuttering was very frequent, time-out was at first administered only for blocks that were at least 2 seconds in length until these disappeared. Both children improved markedly, and a one-year follow-up showed only a few stutterings in each case.

In a clinical application of verbal punishment Reed and Godden (1977) reduced the stuttering of two preschool children by using the words "slow down" as a contingent stimulus during twenty twice-weekly sessions. Tape recordings showed a decrease in stuttering at home.

Reinforcement of Fluency

In other clinical applications of operant conditioning procedures the stutterings have been ignored and reinforcement has been given for fluent utterances or stutter-free intervals of time. With a nine-year-old boy, Rickard and Mundy (1965) began by increasing his verbal output by verbal rewards or points earned for progressively longer utterances. They then reinforced his fluent verbalizations. The result was decreased stuttering, but a six-month follow-up showed that not all the improvement had lasted.

Leach (1969) tried something similar with a 12-year-old who stuttered severely. In the first 6 sessions the child earned two cents a minute for each minute of talking. Thereafter during half of each session he earned an extra cent for each 15-second period of fluent speech. After 42 sessions the stuttering was reduced to less than 2 per minute, and outside the clinic the speech was reported to be normal. A 2-month follow-up, however, showed a partial return of stuttering.

Shaw and Shrum (1972) administered reinforcement for fluency with 3 stutterers between the ages of 9 and 11 years. The immediate reinforcement, given for each 5 seconds of fluent speech in the case of one stutterer and for each 10 seconds of fluency in the other two cases, was a mark on a sheet of paper. A sufficient number of marks brought a reward in the shape of a toy or a piece of candy which the

---

[4]Haroldson, Martin, and Starr (1968), Martin and Haroldson (1969), Egolf, Shames, and Seltzer (1971), Martin, Kuhl, and Haroldson (1972), Costello (1975).

child had selected beforehand. In addition the children were informed at the start about the contingency. In the course of four 20-minute sessions on consecutive days there was a marked improvement in speech which carried over spontaneously into everyday situations and on last observation had apparently persisted for two months in one case and four months in another. The children had previously had other types of stuttering therapy for periods ranging from two months to three years without noticeable improvement.

Using essentially the same procedure with three children aged 6, 9, and 11 years, Manning, Trutna, and Shaw (1976) found that tangible rewards were not necessary. Verbal rewards chosen by the subjects (e.g., "good speech," or "You sounded real nice") proved as effective as the tangible ones.[5]

Token Economy

At the Prince Henry Hospital in Sydney, Australia, Ingham and Andrews and their co-workers treated stutterers in an experimental token economy program in which methods were varied systematically in order to test various clinical hypotheses.[6] Generally a small group of adult stutterers spent most of their waking hours together for three weeks. Periodically throughout the day counts were made of the percentage of stuttered syllables in their conversation, and tokens were either earned or lost in proportion to decreases or increases in their stuttering from session to session. Tokens were the only means by which they could buy food or other items such as cigarettes and magazines. Ingham and Andrews frequently combined this procedure with syllable-timed or "prolonged" speech patterns.

The three-week program generally resulted in fluent speech by the end of treatment. In one study (Andrews and Ingham, 1972a) a group of subjects who stuttered on a mean of about 18 percent of their syllables before treatment had almost no stuttering at the end of treatment and a mean of 7.8 percent on follow-up eighteen months later.

Modifying Thematic Content

In the applications of operant conditioning procedures we have touched on so far the target behavior has been either stuttering or fluency. In their attempts to achieve immediate fluency such applications are, of course, opposed in basic philosophy to Iowa therapy. Shames,

---

[5]A critical review of attempts to treat stuttering by reinforcement of fluency was contributed by Hegde (1978).

[6]Ingham, Andrews, and Winkler (1972), Andrews and Ingham (1972a, 1972b), Ingham and Andrews (1973a).

Egolf, and Rhodes (1969), however, described an operant conditioning program designed to modify stuttering symptoms in the gradual, stepwise manner of Iowa therapy. They also attempted to deal with the stutterer's assumptions and attitudes by conditioning the verbal behavior by which these are represented. The stutterer was systematically given approval such as "good" or "you're right" for positive verbal responses and disapproval such as "no" or "I don't agree" for negative verbal responses. Examples of positive responses were those that reflected the stutterers' insights into the nature of their speech difficulty ("I blink my eyes when I stutter"), expressed favorable feelings, or reported constructive actions or intentions ("I think I'll call him on the phone tonight"). Negative verbal responses included expressions of negative emotion ("Sometimes I hate everybody in the world"), or statements about stuttering that were not descriptive or reflected helplessness ("I can't get the word out").

Shames, Egolf, and Rhodes (1969) and Rhodes, Shames, and Egolf (1971) reported that positive verbal expressions tended to increase and negative ones tended to decrease as a result of this procedure. In addition, they found that a concomitant decrease in stuttering tended to take place even though the stuttering received no direct attention.

Even more frankly concerned with the stutterer's subjective experiences is the "cognitive conditioning therapy" described by Berecz (1973, 1976). Here stutterers vividly imagine a cognitive cue that usually triggers their stuttering (e.g., "They're all expecting me to speak" or "My throat is tense"). They then immediately self-administer a painful electric shock and substitute a more desirable cognition. Such an approach has strayed relatively far from Skinnerian behaviorism, of course, but Berecz asserted that "if emphasis . . . on overt behavioral analyses results in ignoring cognitive parameters, we are left with a 'black box' approach, which is necessary in the animal laboratory but hardly sufficient for human clients."

Artificial Speech Patterns

The term behavior therapy has often been extended to another broad approach to the modification of stuttering that is not based primarily on conditioning procedures in the usual sense, but on the use of various novel speech patterns for achieving immediate fluency. In much of this work the influence of operant conditioning has been evident. In some cases the clinical procedures have been systematically programmed and measurement of progress has been patterned on laboratory models. Procedures have sometimes been introduced for shaping unusual modes of speech by "successive approximations" in order to give them a more natural quality. Some workers have combined these therapeutic approaches with reinforcement. For these reasons the methods we are about to discuss have often been described as examples of operant conditioning. However, it is clarifying to distinguish them from therapies in which fluency is achieved directly through contingent consequences of the stutterer's speech behavior.

Delayed Auditory Feedback and Slow Speech

In Chapter 8 we saw that many stutterers can speak fluently under delayed auditory feedback, in large part because the delay forces them to speak more slowly. This expedient has been used widely in stuttering therapy, often with encouragement to the stutterer to fall into the slow, prolonged pattern to which the DAF is conducive.[7]

The first to use DAF in the context of operant conditioning was Goldiamond (1965). Goldiamond had been engaged in a program of laboratory research on stuttering as operant behavior in which he was using aversive stimuli such as loud tone to demonstrate punishment and negative reinforcement. In the course of this work he decided to test the effect of a brief period of delayed auditory feedback as an aversive stimulus. First he tried it as a punisher, turning it on each time the subject stuttered. The stuttering sharply diminished. The next step was to demonstrate its effectiveness as a negative reinforcer. The subject was now placed under continuous DAF, and the DAF was turned off for 10 seconds on the occurrence of every block. By all the rules of operant conditioning the stuttering should have increased in frequency. Instead something unexpected happened—speech was produced fluently in a slow, prolonged manner. The DAF was rarely turned off because the subject rarely stuttered.

Goldiamond saw an opportunity to devise a method for treating stutterers clinically. Using the facilities of the conditioning laboratory he developed a program in which a slow, prolonged pattern of fluent speech was first produced by the administration of DAF in the manner just described. Then the DAF was gradually attenuated until the stutterer was speaking in the same pattern without its help. Finally a normal rate of speech was gradually restored by machine control of successive displays of reading material. Goldiamond reported marked success with this method, including carry-over to outside situations in many cases.[8]

Goldiamond's reports of success received wide attention and considerably influenced others who were attracted by the operant model of behavior modification. Curlee and Perkins (1969) and Perkins (1973b)

---

[7]Nessel (1958), Adamczyk (1959, 1965), Lotzmann (1961), Goldiamond (1965), Zemeri (1966), Soderberg (1968, 1969b), Webster and Lubker (1968a), Curlee and Perkins (1969, 1973), Webster (1970), Ingham and Andrews (1971b), Perkins (1973b), Perkins, Rudas, Johnson, Michael, and Curlee (1974), Ryan and Van Kirk (1974).

[8]See Goldiamond (1965) and his personal communication cited by Soderberg (1968).

described a program of therapy in which slow, fluent speech was first established by DAF with a delay of 250 milliseconds, and the DAF was gradually faded out by reducing the interval of delay in 50-millisecond steps. Ingham and Andrews (1971b) used DAF in conjunction with their token economy program to aid in the establishment of fluency. They referred to the slow speech pattern that resulted from the prolongation of syllables as "prolonged speech." A study by Howie and Woods (1982) seemed to show that the syllable prolongation worked just as well without the tokens as with them. Ryan and Van Kirk (1974) made DAF the basis for programmed therapy in which systematic attention was given to transfer of the slow, fluent pattern of speech to a variety of situations outside the clinic and to the maintenance of normal speech once it was attained. They reported successful transfer to outside situations in a series of fifty cases. Workers employing DAF often expressed the belief that the use of a slow pattern of speech with prolongation of sounds or syllables in imitation of speech under DAF might be just as effective in producing fluency as DAF itself, and this was demonstrated by Ryan (1971) and by Watts (1971).

Muellerleile (1981) and Craven and Ryan (1984) described the use of portable delayed auditory feedback devices. At the present time the practice of a slow rate of speech through prolongation of syllables, with or without DAF, is one of the most widely used forms of behavior therapy.

Rhythmic or Metronome-Timed Speech

Like slow speech, rhythmic speech is a remedial method of the past that owes its rehabilitation both to the behavior modification development and to advances in electronic engineering. Most applications have employed a miniaturized electronic metronome device which the stutterer wears like a hearing aid.[9] The reports of Brady indicated that of 26 stutterers treated, 21 were able to speak with markedly increased fluency even without the device after several months of therapy, and of 20 cases followed up for periods ranging from 16 months to 4.5 years only 3 had had partial relapses.

Rhythmic speech can be learned and practiced without the use of a pacing device and will tend to eliminate stuttering as effectively. This has been amply demonstrated by Andrews and his co-workers in their use of syllable-timed speech, a form of speech that is produced one syllable at a time with even stress and timing.[10]

---

[9]Meyer and Mair (1963), Brady (1968, 1969, 1971), Horan (1968), Wohl (1968, 1970), Brady and Brady (1972), Trotter and Silverman (1974), Öst, Götestam, and Melin (1976), Silverman (1976b), Mallard (1977).

[10]Andrews and Harris (1964, Chap. 8), Ingham and Andrews (1971b), Andrews and Ingham (1972a, 1972b), Helps and Dalton (1979).

Since pacing words or syllables with a metronome tends to produce an unusual mode of speech, Silverman and Trotter (1973) made
an evaluation of the initial impression that was made on judges by
several stutterers using such a device. Although the observers consistently rated the stutterers more fluent with the aids than without
them, they did not necessarily have more favorable reactions. This
depended on the severity of the stuttering. Mallard and Meyer (1979)
found that naive listeners generally preferred the metronome-timed
speech of a moderate and severe stutterer to their stuttered speech.
Brady (1971) has tried to impart a degree of naturalness to metronome-timed speech by teaching the stutterer to time whole phrases to
the beat rather than just words or syllables.

Trotter and Silverman (1974) reported a series of probes to determine if the effectiveness of a miniature metronome would wear out
with continued use. In one test 3 adult subjects maintained their fluency in oral reading on each of 18 days. In a second study one schoolchild continued to benefit from the device through 14 sessions, of
reading and speaking, while another child benefitted through 26 sessions. In a third, an adult stutterer used a miniature metronome all
day for a period of 36 days with no diminution of the effect. Finally
one of the authors, a moderately severe stutterer, wore the device 12
to 16 hours a day for 16 months. While its effectiveness did not cease,
it was not as great at the end of this period as it had been during the
first three months. Subsequently Silverman (1976b) reported that he
had continued to use the same miniature metronome, for 3 years. Its
effectiveness diminished gradually until in the final 6-month period it
was of little benefit. "I found myself," Silverman wrote, "attending
less and less to the metronome beat while I spoke and becoming less
and less certain that using the device would have a significant impact
on the severity of my stuttering."

Other Speech Patterns

Still other approaches have been employed in behavior therapies
that seek immediate fluency through a change in the stutterer's manner
of speaking. Schwartz (1976) has given some prominence to a technique
known as *airflow*, in which the stutterer permits some breath to flow
out passively before initiating each utterance. Azrin and Nunn (1974)
offered a regulated breathing therapy. Peins, McGough, and Lee (1972,
1984) introduced the therapeutic use of legato speech, in which sounds,
syllables, and words are smoothly linked by continuous phonation and
flow of air. Webster (1974, 1979a) developed a program that emphasizes
gentle onsets of phonation. Weiner (1984c) described a treatment
method based essentially on training in good vocal usage, including
adequate breath support and optimal voice quality.

Masking Noise

As we saw in Chapter 8, loud masking noise is another condition that is likely to bring about immediate fluency for many stutterers. A number of attempts have been made to exploit this effect by designing portable masking noise generators for use in stuttering therapy.[11] The stutterer wears the unit in the manner of a binaural hearing aid and turns it on when blocking or anticipating a block. Trotter and Silverman (1973) reported clinical results showing that some stutterers may get some benefit from this technique over trial periods of weeks. One stutterer reported on by Trotter and Lesch (1967) was still being helped after 2.5 years. Some disadvantages discussed by Perkins and Curlee (1969) as a result of their experience with three cases were the conspicuousness of the double earplugs, the slight hearing loss they produced while they were being worn, and the fact that the device was of little help on the telephone. Some of these disadvantages have been minimized in the most recent models of a voice-activated unit known as the Edinburgh Masker,[12] which is available commercially and has been distributed fairly widely. Although it is not generally regarded as an adequate method of treatment in itself, clinical experience suggests that it may be a practical source of help in some cases.

Biofeedback

An approach whose potential has not been fully developed is the use of various forms of biofeedback. As yet, this has been largely confined to electromyographic (EMG) feedback, and its clinical applications have been limited in extent.

Guitar (1975) presented a laboratory model of EMG biofeedback therapy using the well-known device in which electrical potentials from surface electrodes over a muscle are converted into a steady low-frequency tone. When a threshold voltage, which may be selected by the therapist or experimenter, is exceeded, the frequency of the tone increases in proportion to the voltage and therefore to the tension in the muscle. With each of three subjects Guitar conducted successive experiments with the electrodes at the larynx, chin, upper lip, and, for purposes of control, the frontalis muscle. In each case the subject first remained at rest and tried to keep the tone at the lowest frequency. Successively lower threshold voltage levels were set until the subject had attained the lowest level possible. He now read a list

---

[11]Guttman (1960), Parker and Christopherson (1963), Derazne (1966), Trotter and Lesch (1967), Perkins and Curlee (1969), Donovan (1971), Trotter and Silverman (1973), Dewar, Dewar, and Barnes (1976), Kuppers and Wunschmann (1985).

[12]See Dewar, Dewar, and Barnes (1976) and Ingham, Southwood, and Horsburgh (1981).

of sentences containing his most difficult sounds in initial position, with instructions to keep the muscle potentials below threshold while awaiting the signal to say each sentence. Trials in which the subject received auditory feedback were alternated with trials in which he did not.

The procedure resulted in reductions of stuttering in all three cases. Training at the lip and larynx proved especially effective. Training at the frontalis muscle produced no effect. With an additional subject Guitar undertook a clinical program of biofeedback therapy consisting of five 40-minute sessions. In the first two sessions the stutterer was trained to reduce the muscle potentials at the site selected, the chin. The remaining three sessions were devoted to conversational speech during which the stutterer practiced reducing the voltage levels whenever he anticipated stuttering. In the first of the three speech sessions he received auditory feedback; in the last two he did not. The subject was successful in maintaining below-threshold voltage levels, and fluent speech, without feedback. He was then instructed to reduce levels during phone calls at work. After tape recordings of such calls demonstrated fluent speech for ten days, treatment was discontinued. Nine months later analysis of tape-recorded conversation and telephone calls showed that the subject was still speaking without stuttering.

A number of other workers have experimented with electromyographic biofeedback in what were for the most part laboratory studies for the purpose of developing treatment methodologies.[13] As we noted in Chapter 7, experiments have also been concerned with whether it is actually the muscle relaxation or some other factor that is responsible for the effect on stuttering.[14] Electromyographic feedback seems uniquely calculated to help stutterers eliminate the excessive tensions which appear to be the immediate underlying cause of so much of their speech difficulty. For this reason it may hold considerable promise both as a method in itself and as an adjunct to other therapies.

Dembrowski and Watson (1991a) described the use of combined plethysmographic, pneumotachographic, and electroglottographic biofeedback for the purpose of helping stutterers to maintain normal breathing, airflow, and phonation during speech.

Programmed Applications

The behavior therapies that have tended to have the most appeal for many speech clinicians are those in which stutterers progress by small,

---

[13]Aten and Blanchard (1974), Hanna, Wilfling, and McNeil (1975), Lanyon, Barrington, and Newman (1976), Lanyon (1977), Moore (1978), Gordon, Gordon, Gordon, Shapiro, Mentis, and Suchet (1981), Craig and Cleary (1982), St. Louis, Clausell, Thompson, and Rife (1982).

[14]Cross (1977), Moore (1978), Pachman, Oelschlaeger, Hughes, and Hughes (1978).

well-defined, easily attained steps in accordance with a highly structured program. We will describe here three of the best-known examples.

The Monterey Program

Devised by Ryan (1974, 1979), the program that has been in use at the Behavioral Sciences Institute at Monterey employs two alternative schedules for establishing fluency, GILCU (gradual increase in the length and complexity of utterances) and DAF. In the GILCU program a stutterer is instructed to begin by reading fluently one word at a time. Each fluent word is reinforced by the word "good" or a token. If the word is stuttered the clinician says, "Stop. Say it fluently." If necessary the stutterer may be shown how to say the word fluently in a slow, prolonged manner. After reading 10 consecutive fluent words the stutterer proceeds to read 2 words at a time to a criterion of 10 consecutive fluent pairs of words, then 3, 4, 5, and 6 words at a time in the same way; next one sentence at a time to a criterion of 5 consecutive fluent sentences; then successively 2, 3, and 4 sentences at a time. Now the stutterer is instructed to read continuously. Reinforcement is given first after 30 seconds of fluent reading, then at progressively longer intervals. After reading continuously for 5 minutes without stuttering, the client is considered to have established fluency in reading. The same steps are now repeated as the stutterer engages in monologues and later in conversation. In both cases the ultimate goal is 0.5 stuttered words or fewer per minute for 5 minutes.

Concurrently with this program for establishing fluency in the clinic, the stutterer is conducted through a program designed to transfer fluency to other situations and settings. This involves activities in the home, at school, at work, with strangers, on the telephone, and so forth, and is structured in considerable detail. Finally, there is a maintenance program in which the stutterer returns for reevaluation at progressively increasing intervals and may be recycled through those segments of the program for which performance does not satisfy specified criteria.

The DAF program is an alternative designed chiefly for older children and adults with relatively severe stuttering. It differs from the GILCU program in the method of establishing fluency. With the help of delayed auditory feedback the stutterer is trained to read and speak in a slow monotone in which all sounds are prolonged and articulation is slurred or deemphasized.

The Hollins Precision Fluency Shaping Program

Webster (1974, 1979a) designed an intensive three-week, all-day program in which fluency is achieved by training the stutterer to use gentle onsets of phonation. For this purpose the stutterer is first taught to use an exceedingly slow rate of speech. This is done in work directed in turn at so-called stretched-syllable, smooth-transition, slow-change, and full-breath targets, in which the stutterer learns to hold each syllable for 2 seconds, to eliminate breaks between and within syllables, and to avoid running out of breath when speaking in the resulting slow-motion manner.

After three days devoted to developing these skills the gentle onset target is introduced. The stutterer learns to initiate all voiced sounds very softly, increasing the intensity of the voice gradually from a barely audible to a normal level. All sounds are practiced individually and in syllables with the aid of a computerized voice monitoring instrument that flashes green or red to indicate correct or incorrect phonatory onsets. The speech sounds are worked on by groups. The stutterer is taught to articulate the voiced consonants by starting the gentle onset on the consonant itself, the voiceless fricatives and stop-plosives by starting the gentle onset on the vowel that follows.

By the end of the second week the stutterer has progressed to two-syllable words. In the third week the prolongation of syllables is gradually reduced and rate of speech is increased, more complex speech is introduced, the voice monitoring instrument is dispensed with, and the transfer is made to speeches, conversation, the telephone, and speech situations in shopping centers and elsewhere outside the treatment center.

Peters, Boves, and van Dielen (1986) described an instrument for detecting the abruptness of vocal onsets that offered some advantages over Webster's voice monitoring device. They also demonstrated that trained observers could make fairly reliable judgments about the abruptness of voice onsets, at least for isolated vowels.

Stutter-Free Speech

Shames and Florance (1980) combined techniques borrowed from operant conditioning, counseling, and psychotherapy in an innovative attempt to solve some of the problems encountered by behavior therapies for stuttering. The format for their program, which they call "Stutter-Free Speech," is a client-centered, nondirective interview session which is used in part to encourage the stutterer to explore and clarify feelings of anxiety, inadequacy, indecision, and resistance with regard to speech and therapy. In the course of these sessions the stutterer is trained with the aid of DAF to speak fluently at a slow rate with continuous phonation and airflow. From the beginning, the stutterer is taught to avoid the robotlike quality of this pattern by prolonging only on stressed words and aiming at normal inflection.

Once stutterers learn to monitor their speech to the degree that they can produce slow, fluent utterances without the aid of DAF, they are taught to self-reinforce this response by allowing themselves frequent brief intervals of spontaneous, unmonitored speech. Fluency is now transferred to the stutterer's daily life by means of written contracts that specify the times, places, and situations in which speech will be monitored, the target behaviors, and their reinforcements. The contract is negotiated by the stutterer and the clinician and is signed by them as well as by others, such as parents, when appropriate. The number of contracts is gradually increased until speech is being monitored throughout the day. When the stutterer's unmonitored speech begins to take on the slow, fluent quality of the monitored pattern, training in unmonitored speech begins. The brief intervals of reinforcement with unmonitored speech are now made longer and more frequent step by step until the stutterer is speaking spontaneously most of the time and monitoring infrequently. Therapy now enters a maintenance phase in which clinical contacts occur at progressively less frequent intervals.

TREATMENT IN EARLY CHILDHOOD

The remedial measures that have been discussed so far were developed chiefly for use with the adolescent, adult, or schoolchild whose stuttering is in its relatively developed form. Far less work has been done on the treatment of the earliest phase of the disorder. Until the 1930s almost all the therapy that was available for young children in the age range of two to six years consisted of the traditional parental injunctions to speak slowly, take a deep breath, think before speaking, or the like—a form of help now widely regarded as just as likely to intensify the problem as to alleviate it. With the growth of speech pathology as a profession a basic orientation with regard to the treatment of stuttering in early childhood was gradually established. This orientation emphasized alteration of the child's environment through parent counseling. It grew out of two main influences. One was the concept of primary and secondary stuttering advanced by Bluemel in 1932 and given wide currency by Van Riper (1939). Bluemel's theory held that "primary" stuttering would disappear of its own accord if the child were not helped or admonished for it. The other major influence was the diagnosogenic theory of Wendell Johnson. To some extent the parent counseling orientation also reflected the point of view that stuttering is an emotional disorder of childhood.

In recent years an increasing number of clinicians have begun to favor a more direct method of treatment of early stuttering than was afforded by the parent counseling programs of Johnson and Van

Riper. The result has been the application of modified forms of behavior therapy.

Parent Counseling

With the approach that has been in common use for many years, parents are persuaded to refrain from criticizing, correcting, or helping the child or from reacting negatively to the speech difficulties in any way and are advised to see that the speech interruptions are not brought to the child's attention by others.

Every opportunity is taken to improve the parent-child relationship. For some workers, for whom this is essentially the only important aspect of treatment, this means play therapy for the child and psychotherapy for the parents administered by qualified specialists. Others who consider this merely an adjunct to therapy advocate psychotherapy only in certain instances. In most cases their interest is primarily in making direct attempts to change some of the parents' child-training practices. In particular, the therapist is frequently concerned with helping parents to be less demanding, restrictive, or perfectionistic in their relationship with the stuttering child. This concern is based on the belief that an oppressive parental environment may increase disruption of fluency and foster anxieties about speech or fluency.

Attempts are also made to eliminate any factors or conditions that appear to increase speech hesitation. Careful observation indicates that children often have unusual difficulty when fatigued, excited, or speaking under pressure of some kind. Some immediate improvement in fluency may be achieved in some cases when the child is not compelled to speak to unresponsive listeners, to compete with others for the chance to talk, to confess guilt orally, or to speak when upset, tense, or excited for other reasons.

In some cases it is thought that parents unwittingly set unrealistic goals for the child by their own excessively rapid rate of speech or by the use of too much vocabulary that is over the child's head, and that they may need to be guided to speak more slowly and simply to the child. Measures of this kind may not be effective by themselves in eliminating the problem; but any change in the child's environment that serves to lessen the intensity of the stuttering probably helps in some measure to prevent the development of negative attitudes toward speech and consequently contributes to the likelihood that the child will in time "outgrow" the disorder.

Finally, everything possible is done to strengthen the child's anticipation of normal speech and self-assurance as a speaker. The chief method used is to give the child every opportunity to experience fluency and to gain a sense of enjoyment, adequacy, and success in speech situations. During periods of relatively fluent speech the child is encouraged to speak as much as possible. During episodes of unusual difficulty the parents may be trained to provide successful speaking experiences through the use of choral speaking, singing, recitation of nursery rhymes, rhythmic speaking, or puppetry. Similar techniques are frequently used by speech pathologists when they work directly with the young stutterer in conjunction with counseling of the parents.

In addition to these widely used measures a number of new procedures have been developed within the same orientation to early stuttering as essentially a problem of the parental environment. A unique method of dealing with environmental pressures that tend to increase the child's disfluency is the desensitization therapy which was described by Van Riper (1972, pp. 299, 300). This attempts to build up the child's tolerance for "fluency disruptors" by controlled exposure to speech pressures and frustrations administered by the speech pathologist during the clinical session.

Another example is the application of "filial therapy" to stuttering in children by Andronico and Blake (1971). This is a procedure for helping the parent to develop empathy with the child through training in the technique of play therapy.

Egolf, Shames, Johnson, and Kasprisin-Burrelli (1972) also described an experimental program in which the parent was directly involved in the therapy process. They first observed the interaction between parent and child in a waiting room situation and identified parental behavior, such as silence, verbal aggression, or interruption, which seemed calculated to maintain stuttering in the child. In a series of therapy sessions a clinician then interacted with the child in a contrasting manner. Later the parent was introduced to this situation and, with the clinician serving as a model, learned new ways of reacting to the child.

Within the same environmental orientation is the "message therapy" of Yovetich (1984), who trains parents of preschool stutterers to monitor the child's utterances as message units. The goal is to redirect the child's attention from the *how* of speaking to what he or she says.

Langlois and Long (1988) offered a program in which parents are taught to facilitate the child's language by such techniques as reflecting and expanding the child's utterances, self-talk, parallel talk, and slowing down their own speech.

In view of the frequency with which parents of young stutterers have been advised to decrease the rate of their own speech, some effort has been made to test the efficacy of this expedient, but the results are difficult to interpret, in part because of the marked tendency of early stuttering to show spontaneous ameliorations. (See Stephenson-Opsal and Ratner [1988] and Guitar, Schaefer, Donahue-

Kilburg, and Bond [1992].) Ratner (1992) could find no evidence that normal speaking children spoke more slowly when their mothers reduced their speech rates.

Behavior Therapy for Early Stuttering

Most behavior modification approaches for preschool stutterers teach a slow, smooth, relaxed pattern of speech by modeling.[15] The usual practice is to progress systematically from one- or two-word utterances to longer and more complex sentences. This has generally been combined with parent counseling.

Operant conditioning is another behavioral technique that has been advocated for early stuttering. Costello (1983) has developed a clinical program in which children receive social rewards or tokens for fluent utterances and are told to "stop" whenever they stutter. Johnson (1984) trains parents to eliminate all attending responses to stuttering and to increase attention to fluent utterances. Stocker and Gerstman (1983) described a program in which they reinforced reductions in stuttering with bits of candy or pennies. We have already mentioned use of the doll Suzybelle in a time-out procedure with two preschool stutterers by Martin, Kuhl, and Haroldson (1972).

Other methods that have been attempted in the direct treatment of early stuttering are rhythmic speech (Coppola and Yairi, 1982) and electromyographic biofeedback (St. Louis, Clausell, Thompson, and Rife, 1982). Riley and Riley (1984) include training in oral motor coordination, sentence formulation, and auditory processing in their program when the need for these appears to be indicated by diagnostic tests.

Reports of success in therapy with young stutterers based on virtually all approaches are common, and there appears to be a widely held belief among clinical workers that the disorder is usually easily treated in early childhood. Because of the transitory nature of so many cases of early stuttering, however, it is very difficult to assess the validity of such reports. In a study by Panelli, McFarlane, and Shipley (1978) 15 children who had been examined because of stuttering during their preschool years but not treated were reevaluated at age 7 to 14 years. Of the 15, 12 were judged to have recovered.

THE EFFECTIVENESS OF THERAPY

From this brief account of the subject of therapy it must be clear that we are as far as ever before in our history from any consensus about

---

[15]Guitar (1982), Wall (1982), Culp (1984), Gregory and Hill (1984), Shine (1984), Starkweather (1984).

the best way to treat stuttering. At the same time it is evident that we are able to offer many stutterers a considerable amount of help. It is a challenge to try to arrive at a realistic notion of our actual therapeutic capacity. Clinical lore tends to hand down two conflicting impressions about the effectiveness of treatment. One is that stuttering is a relatively difflcult problem to treat, at least in adults. The other is the impression that almost any kind of therapy is liable to work with stutterers. It is not a simple matter to reconcile these contradictory assumptions. Presumably there may be something useful to be learned from the reports of clinicians who have tried to evaluate the results of their efforts systematically. A distillation of such reports is given in the Appendix, where we have listed in table form the outcomes of clinical studies based on groups of at least five subjects.

The data presented in the Appendix must be interpreted with caution. To try to use them for comparing one method of treatment with another would be futile. The studies we have surveyed differed widely in their scientific rigor and sophistication. In order to present their results succinctly we have been compelled to leave out many details. Finally, the various terms used for significant improvement (we have given the investigators' own words as far as possible) are likely to have such different meanings for different workers that for that reason alone the percentages in the table can have only the roughest kind of comparability.

Despite this ambiguity, there is a remarkable message to be read in the table. It is unmistakable that a great variety of methods are capable of bringing about what a clinician may regard in good faith as a successful outcome of therapy in a large proportion of cases. Taking the table at face value one would be inclined to infer that substantial improvement, as defined in these studies, typically occurs as a result of almost any kind of therapy in about 60 to 80 percent of cases.

Furthermore, the variety of methods that have some potential for eliminating stuttering in individual cases is even greater than one could guess from the table alone. The reference list of this book would have been much longer if it had included the multitude of published reports of success with single cases, sometimes accompanied by accounts of satisfactory carry-over outside the clinic and persistence of fluency for relatively long periods after the termination of treatment. At a single congress of the International Society for Logopedics and Phoniatrics in 1965, for example, the techniques for which successes were claimed included gesturing, cluttering, phonation on inspiration, and the use of a foam rubber vibrator, among others. It is difficult to escape the impression that almost any number of similar methods that we could think of on the spur of the moment might have an equal chance of helping some stutterers. It would seem that therapy itself, apart from what is done in therapy, has considerable capacity for effecting change.

Why, then, is stuttering not universally regarded as the easiest of disorders to treat? We now come to the other side of the coin. The answer seems to be that few sophisticated clinicians of long experience are prepared to accept enthusiastic claims of success at face value. They have seen too many stutterers go from therapist to therapist achieving one ephemeral success after another. Many of them have also seen therapies once hailed for documented accomplishments fail to live up to their early promise and gradually fall into disuse. They would tend to be skeptical of many of the optimistic assertions about the outcome of therapy that we have gathered in the Appendix, and they would have a number of good reasons. For example, many of these reports are based on little more than subjective clinical impression. Most studies made little attempt to evaluate the stutterer's progress outside the clinic or to determine whether the benefits of treatment were lasting. Various pertinent aspects of improvement besides fluency were largely ignored. Attention was rarely given to the part that spontaneous recovery may play in stuttering, especially in children. (Note, for example, Daskalov's preschool group, who were doing much better two years after therapy than at the end of treatment.)

In short, the assessment of results of therapy is a process fraught with opportunities for error and self-delusion. The subject has been discussed extensively by Van Riper (1973, Chapter 7), Andrews and Ingham (1972a), Ingham and Andrews (1973b), Ingham (1984b, Chapter 12), and Sheehan (1984). We may summarize these and other discussions by enumerating twelve tests which a method of treating stuttering must meet before it can be considered successful:

1. The method must be shown to be effective with an ample and representative group of stutterers. The single-subject design has a place in scientific research. It has been widely misused, however, in the area of research on stuttering therapy, where most single cases written up for publication are apparently chosen for the precise reason that they were successes. This practice produces a distorted picture. In the end we learn little from it beyond what we already know —that somewhere, at some time, almost any therapy can achieve a remarkable result for some stutterers.

2. Results must be demonstrated by objective measures of speech behavior such as frequency of stuttering or rate of speech and by judges' ratings of severity. Such measurements should be made before, during, and after treatment by observers other than the experimenters themselves or without knowledge that might influence their judgment, and due account must be taken of the observers' reliability.

By themselves, subjective impressions of experimenters, stutterers, or family or friends of stutterers are inadequate because they may be colored by hopes, expectations, denial, or other psychological factors. The influences that affect subjective judgments may be subtle and difficult to predict. Lanyon, Lanyon, and Goldsworthy (1979), for example, found that clinicians' judgments of stutterers' success in mastering a biofeedback treatment procedure was significantly related to those stutterers' eagerness to present themselves in a favorable light as indicated by their K scores on the Minnesota Multiphasic Personality Inventory; yet the stutterers' K scores had little relationship to their progress as measured objectively.

3. Reports of therapeutic success must be based on repeated evaluations and adequate samples of speech. The great variability of stuttering from time to time and under different conditions is liable to result in assessments that are unrepresentative. F. H. Silverman (1975) tested fifty-one elementary school stutterers, thirty-nine secondary school stutterers, and twenty-five adult stutterers in a clinical situation. Only a third in each group said their stuttering had been typical of their usual stuttering.

4. Improvement must be shown to carry over to speaking situations outside the clinical setting. One of the best known and most frequently ignored facts about stuttering is that in the special environment of the speech clinic the speech of most stutterers is likely to become steadily more normal for reasons that have little to do with the effectiveness of the treatment. Such changes have been a frequent source of gratification to unsuspecting speech clinicians, and enthusiastic before-and-after tape recordings in these cases have sometimes created impressions of improvement that seemed little short of magical, although the stutterer had made few or modest gains outside the clinic.

5. The stability of the results must be demonstrated by long-term follow-up investigations. Any number of methods for making stuttering disappear have been known for many years; the great and persistent problem of stuttering therapy is how to keep the stutterer from relapsing.

A difficult question to answer is how long an interval we should allow to elapse between the end of treatment and the follow-up study. This is equivalent to asking how long a stutterer must talk normally or with improved speech before we can assume that the change is permanent. We do not know the answer to this question, but clinical experience prompts us to assert that a few months is not enough. Experienced clinicians can remember too many stutterers who relapsed after talking well for that long. For the same reason a year seems inadequate. Perhaps eighteen months to two years is the shortest interval after which most experienced clinicians would not feel unduly optimistic in hoping that the improvement was lasting.

The follow-up evaluation is likely to be biased if it is done in the same clinical environment in which the treatment was administered. Boberg and Sawyer (1977) demonstrated this experimentally when they retested stutterers by taking each one to a lounge on another part of the campus of their college, instructing the stutterer to engage in conversation with a confederate of the experimenters posing as a student. The clients stuttered more there than when speaking with a stranger in the familiar clinical surroundings. When not only the surroundings but also the persons conducting the follow-up study were associated with the stutterer's recovery, the results are even more likely to be misleading. One stutterer described to the author a follow-up evaluation he had received at a speech clinic that claimed a high rate of success with the form of therapy it employed. He had relapsed very considerably after treatment, but once back in the familiar clinical setting and finding that the person conducting the assessment was his former clinician, he spoke and read with little tendency to stutter.

Not only should the evaluation be conducted outside the clinic, but, with the subjects' prior permission, it is probably best done without the subjects' knowledge that their speech is being evaluated. The reason for this is that stutterers who are motivated to create a favorable impression of the benefit they have received may be able to muster better performance than usual for the purpose of an overt test. This was pointed out by Andrews and Ingham (1972a). At the end of intensive treatment of twenty-three adult stutterers by a token system combined with "prolonged" speech, their subjects' average percentage of stuttered syllables in a spontaneous speaking task had dropped from 16.41 to 0.11. In a similar test nine months later the mean percentage of stuttered syllables was still only 0.5. Eighteen months after treatment, however, recordings of the speech of seventeen of the subjects were obtained in their homes by a student who pretended to be interested in their responses to a personality test in order to fulfill a psychology course requirement. The average percentage of stuttered syllables had increased to 7.8.

In a later study Ingham (1975) compared overt and covert assessments made after the same interval of time following treatment and again found that the stutterers generally tended to speak more fluently when they knew that their progress was being evaluated. Howie, Woods, and Andrews (1982) even found a small but significant difference between overt and covert measurements immediately after treatment. On the other hand, Howie, Tanner, and Andrews (1981) found essentially no difference between overt and covert follow-up evaluations. Neither did Andrews and Craig (1982) for stutterers as a group, though they pointed out that differences appeared in individual cases. As yet, we do not know just how vital covert assessments are, but it is difficult to ignore the possibility that at least some stutterers may be apt to give misleading impressions of their fluency in long-term overt examinations. Precisely how stutterers manage this we do not know; but when treatment is based on a change of speech pattern such as slow or rhythmic speech, at least part of the explanation is not difficult to discern. The chances are that stutterers seldom use these patterns so long that their effectiveness literally"wears out." The writings of Andrews and Ingham, Perkins, and others who have described the results of such therapies with objectivity and candor suggest that when regression occurs it generally does so much earlier due to the stutterer's resistance to the embarrassment and bother of an unnatural way of speaking. If that is the case, it is a simple matter for stutterers to "turn on" their fluency again in the presence of their examiners. Curlee and Perkins (1973) evaluated their subjects' progress in conversational rate control therapy by sending them out to record their own speech on cassette recorders in outside situations. "On several chance meetings," Curlee and Perkins wrote, "clients were observed to be stuttering more than their tape recordings represent . . . Consequently, the measures of generalization reported in this study probably are best interpreted as being indicative of a client's ability to speak fluently when he chooses to maintain relatively stutter-free speech."

6. Suitable control groups or control conditions must be used to show that reductions in stuttering are the result of treatment. There are other variables besides adaptation to the clinician or clinical situation that may create a false impression of successful therapy. One is spontaneous recovery. Although this is especially common in children, degrees of spontaneous improvement are also found frequently in adults. A troublesome feature of the fluctuations in severity that occur over periods of time, as Hanna and Owen (1977) pointed out, is that stutterers (or their parents) have a natural tendency to seek help when the speech difficulty is extreme. As a result, the stuttering is likely to become less severe in time merely by virtue of "regression to the mean." Except in the case of preschool children, the effect is not likely to be large, however, as studies of stutterers who have been placed on waiting lists for treatment show.[16] Andrews estimated the average regression to be about 15 percent on the basis of data available in the literature. Another factor that must be taken into account is the temporary fluency that so often results from the stutterer's belief in the effectiveness of the therapy. In certain cases, as when testing the effects of drugs or biofeedback training, placebo treatments have been

---

[16]Andrews, Guitar, and Howie (1980), Ingham (1980), Andrews and Harvey (1981).

used to control for this effect. The necessity for this was strikingly demonstrated by Prins, Mandelkorn, and Cerf (1980) in their study of treatment by haloperidol when they found that a placebo had a measurable effect.

In many cases it is not feasible to administer a dummy treatment as a control. In such cases another method of therapy has sometimes been used as a basis for comparison. An alternative to a control group is a waiting list condition such as was employed by Andrews and Ingham (1972a). In this case the improvement, if any, that takes place in the stutterers' speech during a period of months prior to therapy serves as a basis of comparison for the change that occurs in the same subjects' stuttering during treatment.

7. The subjects' speech must sound natural and spontaneous to listeners. This is an especially important part of the evaluation of all therapies that teach stutterers to change their manner of speaking. Residual elements of slowness, monotony, or stereotypy in the subjects' speech may seem more peculiar to listeners than the stuttering itself. Stutterers are justified in rejecting such strangeness. In recent years an increasing number of researchers have been concerned with such questions as whether and how listeners can distinguish therapeutically derived fluency from normal speech and how to measure and enhance the naturalness of the stutterer's speech.[17]

8. The subjects must be free from the necessity to monitor their speech. Like unnaturalness, reduced automaticity of speech is a problem that plagues the most commonly used behavior therapies and is even more intractable. Yet fluency can hardly be considered normal as long as continual attention on the part of the speaker is required to maintain it.

9. Treatment must remove not only stuttering, but also the fears, the anticipations, and the person's self-concept as a stutterer. To judge the outcome of therapy solely on the basis of frequency counts of stuttering, ignoring the stutterer's perceptions and attitudes, is as extreme a procedure as relying solely on stutterers' accounts of their subjective

---

[17]Silverman and Trotter (1973), Perkins, Rudas, Johnson, Michael, and Curlee (1974), Frayne, Coates, and Marriner (1977), Ingham and Packman (1978), Runyan and Adams (1978, 1979), Mallard and Meyer (1979), Metz, Onufrak, and Ogburn (1979), Prosek and Runyan (1982,1983), Runyan, Hames, and Prosek (1982), Metz, Samar, and Sacco (1983), Iacono (1984), Martin, Haroldson, and Triden (1984), Ingham, Gow, and Costello (1985), Ingham, Martin, Haroldson, Onslow, and Leney (1985), Ingham and Onslow (1985), Mallard and Westbrook (1985), Robb, Lybolt, and Price (1985), Shenker and Finn (1985), Onslow and Ingham (1987), Ingham, Ingham, Onslow, and Finn (1989), Metz, Schiavetti, and Sacco (1990), Runyan, Bell, and Prosek (1990), Franken, Boves, Peters, and Webster (1991, 1992), Martin and Haroldson (1992), Onslow, Adams, and Ingham (1992), Onslow, Hayes, Hutchins, and Newman (1992), Onslow, van Doorn, and Newman (1992), Kalinowski, Noble, Armson, and Stuart (1994), Schiavetti, Martin, Haroldson, and Metz (1994).

impressions. This is particularly true when treatment has consisted of a change in the stutterer's accustomed manner of speaking. Sheehan (1984) put it incisively:

> A stutterer may feel miserable at the strain and vigilance required to keep an artificial pattern going. But the resulting monotone might dramatically lower the frequency count. Conversely, a stutterer might relax his suppressive vigilance enough to feel much freer and more open, even though the frequency count might be reported as higher by an objective observer. Which one feels better about himself? Who is ahead in a genuine therapeutic sense?

Howie and Andrews (1984), in their account of the Prince Henry "prolonged speech" program, wrote, "In general, while some clients are never heard to stutter, most still regard themselves as stutterers who are now able to speak fluently . . ." This has become a familiar comment in assessments of treatment programs.

In a number of studies the Erickson S-scale of communication attitudes or Woolf's Perceptions of Stuttering Inventory have been used in evaluating the outcome of therapy.[18] Silverman (1980a) developed an inventory for the specific purpose of measuring improvement in such dimensions as avoidance of words and situations, modification of attitudes and feelings about stuttering, modifications in the personal-social area, as well as changes in speaking behavior.

Andrews and Cutler (1974) observed that removal of symptoms by a behavior therapy brought only a partial improvement in subjects' attitudes toward speaking. These attitudes approximated those of normal speakers only after the subjects had completed a program of supervised speaking experience outside the speech clinic.

10. The success of a program of therapy should not be inflated by ignoring dropouts. The problem presented by stutterers who drop out of treatment has been pointed out by Martin (1981). Estimates of the amount of improvement during therapy are often based exclusively on those who complete the clinical program. On its face this practice may seem only reasonable, but stutterers may drop out because they are not benefitting, and when a considerable number of such dropouts are omitted in the final tabulation of results, a distorted picture of the effectiveness of the treatment is likely to be presented. The same applies to long-term follow-up studies; when they are limited to those subjects who respond to the invitation to appear for reassessment the findings may be severely biased.

---

[18]Andrews and Cutler (1974), Guitar (1976), Guitar and Bass (1978), Helps and Dalton (1979), Mallard and Kelly (1982).

11. The method must be shown to be effective in the hands of essentially any qualified clinician, including those without unusual status, prestige, or force of personality. Some studies have accomplished this by using a number of clinicians to administer the treatment.

12. The method must continue to be successful when it is no longer new and the initial wave of enthusiasm over it has died away. As we pointed but earlier in this chapter, there is reason to believe that such enthusiasm alone is capable of bringing about a large number of short-term recoveries from stuttering.

This is a formidable array of criteria. In view of our past history of failures and disappointments, however, it is perhaps not too demanding.

RELAPSE, PROGNOSIS, AND MAINTENANCE

Of all problems that limit the effectiveness of therapy, the one that has made the greatest claim on the attention of clinical researchers is relapse. In 1979 the problem of relapse in current programs of therapy was formally recognized by an international conference on the subject in Banff, Canada. In a paper reviewing objective studies of the long-term results of therapy, chiefly by some form of behavior modification, Martin concluded that roughly a third of stutterers appeared to achieve lasting fluency, about a third relapsed significantly after treatment, and about a third either dropped out of therapy before completing it or were not available for follow-up evaluation (Martin, 1981).

Relatively little is known about the subject of relapse. The nature of the process and its causes may well differ with the type of treatment used, and we may not understand relapse well until we better understand why different kinds of therapy bring about reductions in stuttering in the first place. Although relapse plagues all forms of treatment, it is particularly distressing in the case of today's most commonly used behavior therapies, partly because these appear to remove stuttering so rapidly and completely. Detractors argue that relapse is inevitable with such therapies. They assert that it is unreasonable to expect a lifelong problem such as stuttering to be permanently eradicated in the short time it takes to learn to speak fluently in a slow manner by prolonging syllables, and they doubt that the stutterer has in any basic sense learned to speak normally in these cases.[19] Advocates sometimes lay the blame on what they regard as the stutterer's inherent proneness to disfluency. Thus Andrews (1984b): "Stuttering is a chronic disorder and many adults can only remain fluent by dint of constant effort." Perkins (1979) suggested that for

_____
[19]See Sheehan (1984) and Sheehan and Sheehan (1984).

some stutterers the problem of maintaining fluency is largely one of identity. "When fluent, they feel like unwelcome strangers to themselves. . . . They wish to feel like themselves, and stuttering is part of that self-image." In a long-term follow-up of stutterers who had undergone "smooth speech" therapy, Craig and Calver (1991) found that the majority of those who had suffered a relapse related it to feeling under pressure to talk faster. Many others imputed it to embarrassment about the speech pattern.

Investigations of prognosis in stuttering therapy have been concerned chiefly with the influence of personality facters.[20] Although the results of these studies have been conflicting, a possible relationship has emerged between outcome of treatment and a measure of "locus of control of behavior," the extent to which individuals perceive what happens to them to be a consequence of their own behavior (Craig and Andrews, 1985; Madison, Budd, and Itzkowitz, 1986). Studies by Guitar (1976), Guitar and Bass (1978), and Helps and Dalton (1979) seemed to show that stutterers with less favorable speech attitudes were less likely to obtain long-term benefit from a behavior therapy employing rate control techniques.[21]

Whatever factors underly the relapse that dogs the use of artificial speech patterns, so seldom do such techniques result in genuinely spontaneous and automatic fluency that some advocates have come to believe the techniques should be taught essentially as an option for the stutterer to use on occasions when normal-sounding speech is demanded.[22]

An increasing number of behavior therapy programs in recent years have incorporated so-called maintenance procedures in an effort to cope with the possibility of relapse following treatment. Examples of such procedures are periodic clinical contacts after the termination of treatment,[23] self-therapy assignments, and work on speech attitudes. Ingham (1980, 1982) conducted research on specific maintenance procedures. Boberg, Howie, and Woods (1979) reviewed the literature on the subject, and Ingham (1984a) offered a systematic description and classification of maintenance techniques. Many clinical workers have come to believe that therapeutic gains are not likely

---

[20]Shames (1952), Sheehan, Frederick, Rosevear, and Spiegelman (1954), Prins and Miller (1973), Perkins, Rudas, Johnson, Michael, and Curlee (1974), Helps and Dalton (1979), Lanyon, Lanyon, and Goldsworthy (1979), Craig and Howie (1982), Craig, Franklin, and Andrews (1984), Craig and Andrews (1985), Madison, Budd, and Itzkowitz (1986), Kraaimaat, Janssen, and Brutten (1988).

[21]Controversy developed over the interpretation of the Guitar and Bass findings. See Young (198I) and Ulliana and Ingham (1984).

[22]Perkins (undated), Starkweather (1984).

[23]The term follow-up is sometimes used to refer to such contacts. They should not be confused with follow-up assessments some time after the termination of therapy.

to be maintained without changes in some of the stutterer's feelings and attitudes. The number of writers advocating attempts to combine behavior therapy with attention to speech attitudes indicates that such programs constitute a dominant trend for the immediate future.[24]

SUMMARY AND CONCLUSIONS

The earliest methods for treating stuttering were based on suggestion, relaxation, and unusual modes of speaking such as slow speech, rhythmic speech, or endless varieties of articulation, inflection, or phrasing. Since virtually all of these techniques tended to give effective and immediate relief from stuttering, they had undergone a long era of use by the earliest decades of the twentieth century. Relapse proved to be so frequent, however, that many professional workers became disenchanted with the indiscriminate use of any measure that brought about immediate fluency—sometimes referred to disparagingly as "empirical" methods.

The first reaction against these old forms of therapy came in the shape of the psychoanalytic approach to stuttering. As is usual with initial reactions, it was extreme. Those who hoped to help stutterers were adjured to ignore the speech entirely and to give their attention to the "whole personality." A second wave of reaction produced what we have referred to in this book as Iowa therapy, shortly after the beginning of professional speech and language pathology in the United States. In fact, much of the impetus for the development of the new profession and scientific discipline came from growing opposition to outworn methods of treating stutterers in use by commercial speech "specialists" and well-meaning professionals with little knowledge of speech disorders. To the inventors of Iowa therapy it seemed that the trouble was not that it was so hard to help stutterers, but that it was so easy to help them. These workers based their approach on a distrust of quick achievement of fluency. It seemed to them axiomatic that in the case of a problem such as stuttering any gains so cheaply won were unlikely to be lasting. Consequently, they advocated gradual modification of the symptoms on the basis of the speakers' understanding of what they did when they stuttered and in the context of work designed to decrease their anxiety about stuttering.

Proponents of Iowa therapy believed it tended to achieve more stable gains than did the older methods. It also had certain limitations that the older methods did not. It tended to make relatively heavy demands on the time, skill, patience, and insight of both the stutterer

---

[24]Perkins (1979), Guitar and Peters (1980), Shames and Florance (1980), Cooper (1984), Curlee (1984), Weiner (1984c), Evesham and Fransella (1985), Boberg (1984), Starkweather (1984).

and the clinician. In the hands of a poorly trained therapist it could degenerate into little more than an attempt to teach stutterers to live with their speech difficulty. At best, it almost never resulted in normal fluency.

By the 1960s these limitations had become quite evident. Moreover the professional climate of the 1930s had been all but forgotten. The time was ripe for a new development, and it came in the form of behavior therapies for stuttering. Some of these were based on conditioning, though not everyone agreed that all of their effects on stuttering were bona fide examples of conditioning. Behavior modification also lent a new respectability to slow speech, rhythmic speech, and other old devices. These emerged from the commercial "stammering schools" where, in the United States at least, they had been confined for thirty years and were taken up enthusiastically by new practitioners, often with the help of conditioning principles and electronic aids.

As a result of this development the outcome of therapy with stutterers began to be reported in more optimistic terms than it had been for some decades. At the same time, considerable skepticism was voiced by those to whom such claims seemed overenthusiastic and ill-informed. The soundness of methods that achieved quick fluency had hardly been an issue since these methods were challenged by Iowa therapy in the 1930s. Now it became an issue once more, with the roles of challenger and challenged reversed.

More time will have to elapse before this issue is resolved. At this writing it is possible to make some reasonable claims for either side. On the one hand those who argued so vehemently against attempts at quick cures in the 1930s may have left an exaggerated impression of their futility on the generation of speech clinicians they trained to be wary of them. The old methods certainly had their share of successes. On the other hand, some of the more extreme optimism about such methods of some years ago has proved to be short-lived. It is interesting to note the assessment by Perkins (1973a) of eight years of clinical experience with behavior therapy based chiefly on rate control with the aid of DAF. He estimated that while 70 percent of those treated acquired normal speech during therapy, more than half subsequently relapsed. Moreover, all felt they were still stutterers. "What became increasingly apparent," Perkins observed, "was that achievement of fluency was relatively easy, but that this was not tantamount to achieving normal speech."

The most recent development in the treatment of stuttering is the attempt to integrate aspects of Iowa therapy with elements of the behavioral or "fluency shaping" approach. In part, this means a return to preoccupation with the stutterer's fears and avoidances from which there had been a broad retreat in the 1970s. In addition, a growing number of speech clinicians are equipping stutterers both with techniques for acquiring immediate fluency and with methods of modifying stuttering in the Iowa tradition. Having learned both controlled fluency and acceptable stuttering, in the terminology of Peters and Guitar (1991), stutterers may proceed in several ways. They may use acceptable stuttering for every day and keep controlled fluency in reserve for special occasions. Or they may use acceptable stuttering when controlled fluency fails. Or they may use either, depending on what they feel most comfortable with in a given situation.

Finally, the growth of the stutterers' self-help movement in recent years has added a new dimension to the outlook for the betterment of stutterers' lives. Support groups for stutterers have grown in number worldwide, and there are now national organizations of such groups in the United States, Canada, Australia, Japan, and some fourteen European countries. In the United States the national organization is the National Stuttering Project, based in San Francisco. The NSP establishes local self-help groups in all parts of the country, holds regional and national conferences, disseminates information, functions as a consumer advocate when issues affecting stutterers arise within the speech and hearing profession, and serves as an ombudsman for stutterers, whether they are discriminated against as individuals in the workplace or denigrated as a class in the entertainment media. For the speech clinician the local self-help group, when one is available, is an invaluable resource. Self-help organizations encourage members to give up the struggle to hide their stuttering and to assert the right to speak without fear even though they stutter. And they generate the group spirit that provides the strength to do so. Speech clinicians possess nothing as powerful for changing stutterers' fearful and avoidant speech attitudes. When participation in a self-help group is not a realistic possibility for the stutterer, a good alternative is the reading of the NSP's monthly publication, *Letting Go*, or the book-length gleanings from that periodical,[25] or the publication for children, *Letting Go, Jr.*

THE NATURE OF RECOVERY

When we have said all that we must about the limitations of current therapies and the hazards that often make recovery more apparent than real, one fact of fundamental importance remains. It is that stuttering is remediable. We see evidence of this partly in the great number of children who recover from stuttering and partly in the observa-

---

[25]Ahlbach, J., and Benson, V. (eds.), *To Say What is Ours.* San Francisco: National Stuttering Project (1994).

tion that adults, too, make recoveries that meet all criteria for genuineness, although complete recovery in adulthood is far less common. Also, while no known therapy will help all stutterers, virtually all therapies, as we have seen, have the power to help some.

Recovery is a fact. It is the underlying nature of the recovery process that we do not yet fully understand. What is the necessary and irreducible factor that is common to all recoveries? Without the answer to this question we are at a considerable disadvantage in our efforts to find a solution to the problem of therapy. Recognizing that it is a controversial question, we venture to suggest an answer. It is that the ultimate basis for essentially all true recovery from stuttering is to be found in the observation that if stutterers could forget that they were stutterers, and in so doing forget to do all of the things that stutterers think they have to do in order to talk, they would have no further difficulty with their speech.

In an important sense this is what virtually all therapies appear to accomplish when they are successful. The hypnotist does it cheaply by a simple appeal to stutterers to believe that they will not stutter. Many other therapists do much the same thing, more effectively on the whole by imbuing stutterers with faith in a method. Some therapies make stutterers forget about their speech difficulty by the use of bizarre speech patterns that compel them to masquerade as someone they are not. Others attempt it by measures for eliminating anxiety about stuttering. The chances are that permanent recovery can be plucked from any therapy if stutterers become convinced that they will not stutter any more and have no need to be concerned about their speech.

Unfortunately, none of these methods is likely to accomplish this fully and permanently with adult stutterers in a very large proportion of cases. To forget, for all practical purposes, that one is a stutterer in the face of every reminder is an extraordinarily difficult thing to do, especially when the problem is fully developed. Certain conditions seem to have great power to bring this about, but they are not always found in ordinary methods of therapy as we now know them. They are to be found in experiences so overwhelming that they shake people to their psychological roots. For example, one stutterer, according to a reliable report, recovered from stuttering after surviving an airplane crash. In a similar case related by Tawadros (1957) a young man got over his stuttering when his hand was battered in a machine-shop accident that almost cost him his life. The incident was said to have made his old problems and anxieties seem like trifles.

The lesson in these examples appears to be that recovery from stuttering may come from vicissitudes which recreate the stutterer's system of personal values so radically that fears or pressures involving speech no longer have a high priority. There are certainly other examples besides narrow escapes from death. Intense mystical or religious experiences appear to have this potentiality. A young woman of the author's acquaintance stopped stuttering after she became a Christian Scientist. For a few stutterers the potential for such vicissitudes is to be found in psychotherapy. For many it may exist in personal development and maturation. It is quite possible that what we call spontaneous recovery in children has, at least in part, a somewhat similar basis. That is, for many persons, the attitudes that underlie stuttering, to the extent that there are such, may belong to an essentially childhood system of values and may be put aside along with a belief in the bogie man as the attitudes and values of greater maturity are achieved.

It is possible to summarize these inferences adequately by saying that the basic therapeutic problem posed by stuttering may represent the kind and degree of difficulty involved in rooting out a superstition, dogma, or prejudice. We may be fairly confident that essentially any adult members of the most inaccessible New Guinea mountain tribe, no matter how isolated from our culture, could without excessive difficulty be taught to drive an automobile or operate an electronic computer. To liberate them from some of their superstitions in exchange for a few baseless beliefs of our own, however, would in all probability be a far more troublesome matter. Perhaps the ultimate advances in our ability to cope with stuttering must await more adequate scientific theories of learning and cognition that will enable us to deal better with the commonplace irrationalities of everyday living.

Suggested Readings

Boberg, E. (ed.), *Maintenance of Fluency: Proceedings of the Banff Conference.* New York: Elsevier North-Holland (1981).

Boberg, E., and Kully, D., *Comprehensive Stuttering Program.* San Diego: College-Hill Press (1985).

Brady, J. P., The pharmacology of stuttering: A critical review. *Amer. J. Psychiatry*, 148, 1309–16 (1991).

Brutten, E. J., and Shoemaker, D. J., *The Modification of Stuttering.* Englewood Cliffs, N.J.: Prentice-Hall (1967), Chap. 5.

Conture, E. G., *Stuttering.* Englewood Cliffs, N.J.: Prentice-Hall (1982).

Dalton, P. (ed.), *Approaches to the Treatment of Stuttering.* London: Croom Helm (1983).

Eisenson, J. (ed.), *Stuttering: A Second Symposium.* New York: Harper & Row (1975).

Gray, B. B., and England, G. (eds.), *Stuttering and the Conditioning Therapies.* Monterey, Calif.: Monterey Inst. Speech and Hearing (1969).

Gregory, H. H. (ed.), *Learning Theory and Stuttering Therapy.* Evanston, Ill.: Northwestern Univ. Press (1968).

Gregory, H. H. (ed.), *Controversies About Stuttering Therapy.* Baltimore: Univ. Park Press (1979).

Gronhovd, K. D., and Zermer, A. A., Anxiety in stutterers: Rationale and procedures for management. In Lass, N. J. (ed.), *Speech and Language: Advances in Basic Research and Practice, Vol. 8.* New York: Academic Press (1982).

Ham, R., *Techniques of Stuttering Therapy*. Englewood Cliffs, N.J.: Prentice-Hall (1986).

Ham, R., *Therapy of Stuttering, Preschool Through Adolescence*. Englewood Cliffs, N.J.: Prentice-Hall (1990).

Hulit, L. M., *Stuttering Therapy: A Guide to the Charles Van Riper Approach*. Springfield, Ill.: Charles C Thomas (1985).

Ingham, R. J., *Stuttering and Behavior Therapy*. San Diego: College-Hill Press (1984).

Ingham, R. J., and Onslow, M., Generalization and maintenance of treatment benefits for children who stutter. *Seminars in Speech and Language*, 8, 303–26: (1987).

Johnson, W., et al, *Speech Handicapped School Children, 3rd ed.* New York: Harper & Row (1967), pp. 286–329.

Leith, W. R., *Handbook of Stuttering Therapy for the School Clinician*. San Diego: College-Hill Press (1984).

Luper, H. L., and Mulder, R. L., *Stuttering. Therapy for Children*. Englewood Cliffs, N.J.: Prentice-Hall (1964).

Peins, M., Conternporary *Approaches in Stuttering Therapy*. Boston: Little, Brown (1984).

Perkins, W. H. (ed.), *Stuttering Disorders*. New York: Thieme-Stratton (1984).

Perkins, W. H., *Stuttering Prevented*. San Diego: Singular Publishing Group (1992).

Peters, T. J., and Guitar, B., *Stuttering: An Integrated Approach to Its Nature and Treatment*. Baltimore: Williams & Wilkins (1991).

Prins, D., and Ingham, R. J., *Treatment of Stuttering in Early Childhood: Methods and Issues*. San Diego: College-Hill Press (1983).

Proceedings of the NIDCD workshop on treatment efficacy research in stuttering. *J. Fluency Dis., 18,* 121–361:(1993).

Rustin, L., Purser, H., and Rowley, D. (eds.), *Progress in the Treatment of Fluency Disorders*. London: Taylor and Francis; San Diego, Singular Publishing Group (1987).

Ryan, B. P., *Programmed Therapy for Stuttering in Children and Adults*. Springfield, Ill.: Charles C Thomas (1974).

St. Louis, K. O. (ed.), *The Atypical Stutterer: Principles and Practices of Rehabilitation*. Orlando, Fl.: Academic Press (1986).

Shames, G. H., and Egolf, D. B., *Operant Conditioning and the Management of Stuttering: A Book for Clinicians*. Englewood Cliffs, NJ.: Prentice-Hall (1976).

Shames, G. H., and Florance, C. L., *Stutter-Free Speech: A Goal for Therapy*. Columbus: Merrill (1980).

Shames, G. H., and Rubin, H. (eds.), *Stuttering Then and Now, Part III*. Columbus: Merrill (1986).

Silverman, F. H., Relapse following stuttering therapy. In Lass, N. J. (ed.), *Speech and Language: Advances in Basic Research and Practice, Vol. 5*. New York: Academic Press (1981).

Speech Foundation of America, Publications 1-20. Memphis, Tenn.

Van Riper, C., Experiments in stuttering therapy. In Eisenson, J. (ed.), *Stuttering: A Symposium*. New York: Harper & Row (1958).

Van Riper, C., *The Treatrnent of Stuttering*. Englewood Cliffs, N.J.: Prentice-Hall (1973)

Wall, M. J., and Meyers, F. L., *Clinical Management of Childhood Stuttering*. Baltimore: University Park Press (1984).

Williams, D. E., Stuttering therapy for children. In Travis, L. E. (ed.), *Handbook of Speech Pathology and Audiology*. New York: Appleton-Century-Crofts (1971).

APPENDIX[a]

Results of Treatment

	Method	N	Age	Duration of Treatment	Results of Treatment	Follow-Up Interval	Results on Follow-Up[b]
Cherry, Sayers, and Marland (1955)	Shadowing	5	Adults	2-4 weeks	100% showed striking improvement		
Kelham and McHale (1966)	Shadowing	38	4-43	5-70 sessions	74% improved or much improved		
Kondas (1967)	Shadowing	17	8-20	3 weeks (?) - 9 months	71% much improved or cured	1-5 years	59% much improved or cured
Peins, McGough, and Lee (1972)	Slow, legato speech	12	Mean 21	6 months	92% showed reduction in severity	2½ years	Of 7 cases, 6 had maintained improvement.[c]
Checiek (1983)	Hand-movement-timed speech	60	7-18	3-4 months	Positive results in 75%		
Andrews and Harris (1964)	Syllable-timed speech	10	21-30	11 weeks	100% stuttering inhibited for at least a few days	12 months	10% improved
Andrews and Harris (1964)	Syllable-timed speech and discussions of stuttering	10	19-44	11 weeks	100% stuttering inhibited for at least a few days	6 months	30% improved
Andrews and Harris (1964)	Syllable-timed speech	10	16-19	11 weeks	100% stuttering inhibited for at least a few days	9 months	20% improved
Andrews and Harris (1964)	Syllable-timed speech	5	11	11 weeks	100% stuttering inhibited for at least a few days	9 months	60% improved

APPENDIX[a] (continued)

	Method	N	Age	Duration of Treatment	Results of Treatment	Follow-Up Interval	Results on Follow-Up[b]
Brandon and Harris (1964)	Syllable-timed speech	28			64% successful		
Helps and Dalton (1979)	Syllable-timed speech	21	18-47	4 weeks	Mean percent of stuttered words fell from 20.7 to 11.7 in conversation	1 year	Mean percent of stuttered words was 15.2 in conversation
Ingham, Andrews, and Winkler (1972)	Syllable-timed speech and group psychotherapy	20	Adults	2 weeks	Mean percent of stuttered syllables reduced from 22.4 to 7.5		
Wohl (1968)	Electronic metronome	146	15-68	Up to 1 year	63% greatly improved or fluent		
Brady and Brady (1972)	Electronic metronome	26	12-53	Several months	81% showed substantial improvement	16-54 months	85% maintained increased fluency
Öst et al (1976)	Shadowing or electronic metronome	15	14-46	3 months	Metronome group showed significant mean reduction in stuttering	14 months	Improvement was maintained
Mallard (1977)	Electronic metronome	5	Adults	1 month	Reduction of stuttering in 80%		
Adamczyk (1959)	Delayed auditory feedback	15	6-28	2-3 months	87% showed significant improvement		
Adamczyk (1965)	Delayed auditory feedback	60	6-45	4 months	60% showed significant or complete improvement		

Study	Method	N	Age	Duration	Results	Follow-up	Follow-up results
Gross and Nathanson[d]	Delayed auditory feedback	8		4 weeks	100% significantly reduced stuttering	6 months	All maintained minimal stuttering in oral reading
Curlee and Perkins (1969)	Delayed auditory feedback	14	Adolescents and adults	30 hours	All achieved normal conversational speech		
Webster (1970)	Delayed auditory feedback	8	15-47	10-40 hours	Stuttering reduced essentially to zero in all subjects	10 months	The fluency had persisted in all subjects
Perkins et al. (1974)	Delayed auditory feedback	27	12-52	90 hours	In 70% of subjects stuttering was reduced by at least 85%	6 months	In 30% of subjects stuttering was reduced by at least 85%
Perkins et al. (1974)	Delayed auditory feedback and speech training	17	19-51	91-184 hours	In 71% of subjects stuttering was reduced by at least 85%	6 months	In 53% of subjects stuttering was reduced by at least 85%
Ryan and Van Kirk (1974)	Delayed auditory feedback	50	9-66	Approx. 20 hours	Stuttered words per minute reduced from 9 to 0.1 on the average	Mean of 4.8 years	Sample of 11 subjects had mean of 1.7 words per minute[e]
Spencer (1976)	Smooth motion speech	5	Adults and children[f]	4 months	Stuttering was reduced to less than 1% of syllables		
Boberg (1976)	Prolonged speech	21	17-44	3 weeks	Stuttering decreased from mean of 21% of syllables stuttered to 1.3%	6-24 months	Sample of 13 subjects showed mean relapse of 22%[g]

APPENDIX[a] (continued)

	Method	N	Age	Duration of Treatment	Results of Treatment	Follow-Up Interval	Results on Follow-Up[b]
Resick et al. (1978)	Prolonged speech	6	Adults	2 weeks		6 months	Improvement persisted in reading and conversation but not on the telephone
Helps and Dalton (1979)	Prolonged speech	44	18-43	4 weeks	Mean percent of stuttered words fell from 24.3 to 7.8 in sample of conversation	1 year	Mean percent of stuttered words was 7.1 in conversation
Franck (1980)	Prolonged speech	68	Mean of 20.2 years	1 year	93% increased fluency by 60% or more	6 months or more	Of 45 subjects, 55% maintained improvement of 60% or more
Boberg (1981)	Prolonged speech	16	16-46	3 weeks[h]	Mean percent stuttered syllables decreased from 16.55 to 1.41	12 months	Mean percent stuttered syllables of 8 subjects was 1.53 at end of 12-month maintenance period
Boberg (1981)	Prolonged speech	6		3 weeks	Mean percent stuttered syllables decreased from 29.89 to 2.33	2 years	Mean percent stuttered syllables of 3 subjects was 17.68; no maintenance was provided
Howie, Tanner, and Andrews (1981)	Prolonged speech	36	Adults	3 weeks[h]	Stuttering was virtually eliminated	2 months	After 2 months in maintenance program there was little significant deterioration

Study	Treatment	N	Age	Length	Outcome	Follow-up	Follow-up outcome
Howie, Tanner, and Andrews (1981)	Prolonged speech	43	Adults	3 weeks[h]		12-18 months	Of 43 subjects, 21 were at least 85% improved
Evesham and Huddleston (1983)	Prolonged speech	47	Adults	2 weeks	91% stuttered on less than 1% of syllables		
Boberg (1984)	Prolonged speech	12	18-47	3 weeks[h]	Mean percent of stuttered syllables decreased from 18.9 to 0.9		
Evesham and Fransella (1985)	Prolonged speech	23	Adults	2 weeks[h]		18 months	Of 22 subjects, 21 were improved
Evesham and Fransella (1985)	Prolonged speech and personal construct therapy	24	Adults	2 weeks[h]		18 months	Of 22 subjects, all were improved; relapse was less than in the prolonged-speech-only group
Webster (1974)	Gentle phonatory onsets	20	8-52	3 weeks		4-33 months	45% stuttered on 1% of words or less in conversation
Webster (1975)	Gentle phonatory onsets	56	8-59	3 weeks	Significant differences in pre- and post-treatment measures of stuttering	2 years	70% retained significant gains in fluency
Schwartz and Webster (1977)	Gentle phonatory onsets	29	9-over 50	3 months	97% improved; 72% stuttered on 6% or less of words	Minimum of 45 days	Of 8 subjects followed up, 4 retained their gains or were improved
Webster (1979a)	Gentle phonatory onsets	200		3 weeks	Stuttering was reduced to a mean of 1.3% of words	Mean of 10 months	78% stuttered on 3% of words or less

APPENDIX[a] (continued)

	Method	N	Age	Duration of Treatment	Results of Treatment	Follow-Up Interval	Results on Follow-Up[b]
Webster (1980)	Gentle phonatory onsets	200		3 weeks	Mean percent of stuttered words decreased from 15.1 to 1.3	Mean of 10 months	Mean percent of stuttered words was 3.2
Mallard and Kelley (1982)	Gentle phonatory onsets	50	14-50	3 weeks	Mean percent of stuttered words fell from 20.05 to 2.92	At least 6 months	Mean percent of stuttered words for 28 subjects was 9.74
Heller, Shulman, and Teryek (1983)	Gentle phonatory onsets	85	6-65	6 weeks	84% achieved normal or near-normal fluency in conversation	6 months-5 years	80% maintained their post-treatment fluency levels
Franklin et al. (1992)	Gentle phonatory onsets	32	15-46	4 weeks	Mean % of stuttered syllables declined from 25.7 to 5.8	6 months	Mean % of stuttered syllables was 16.3
Hasbrouck et al. (1987)	Airflow, relaxation	6	10-16	4 weeks	Mean % of stuttered words declined from 9.7 to 0.2	6-7 months	Mean % of stuttered words was 3.5
Hasbrouck and Lowry (1989)	Airflow, relaxation	24	19-38	5 weeks	All had 1% or fewer stuttered words	1-24 months	70% had 1% or fewer stuttered words
Andrews and Tanner (1982b)	Airflow	6	Adults	5 days	Mean reduction in stuttering was 90%	12 months	Stuttering no longer differed significantly from level at intake
Azrin and Nunn (1974)	Regulated breathing	14	4-67	12-hour session[i]	All had at least 93% reduction in stuttering		

Study	Procedure	N	Age	Treatment time	Results	Follow-up	Follow-up results
Azrin, Nunn, and Frantz (1979)	Regulated breathing	21	Adults	1 or 2 sessions[j]	Stuttering decreased by mean of 94%	16 months	11 subjects contacted reported a mean reduction in stuttering of 79%
Ladouceur, Boudreau, and Théberge (1981)	Regulated breathing	16	15-47	2 hours	Reduction in stuttering averaged 50%	1 month	Reduction in stuttering averaged 50%
Côté and Ladouceur (1982)	Regulated breathing	16	Adults	3 ½-hour sessions	Subjects stuttered significantly less	6 months	Changes in stuttering were maintained
Greenberg and Marks (1982)	Regulated breathing	15	Adults	12 hours		6 months	Of 10 subjects, 8 were much, 1 slightly improved
Andrews and Tanner (1982a)	Regulated breathing	6	Adults	2 6-hour sessions	4 subjects who completed therapy reduced stuttering about 45%	3 months	Only 1 subject showed significant improvement
Ladouceur, Côté, Leblond, and Bouchard (1982)	Regulated breathing	12	17-74	2 90-minute sessions	Average stuttering decreased from 11.5% to 5.6% of syllables	2 months	Average stuttering increased to 8.4% of syllables
Ladouceur and Martineau (1982)	Regulated breathing	15	5-16	3 45-minute sessions		1 month	Average stuttering decreased 50% from baseline to follow-up, but did not differ from that of a control group
Kuhr and Rustin (1985)	Relaxation and regulated breathing	8	22-54	3 weeks[h]	Average stuttering fell from 14.3% to 2.4% of syllables	25-61 months	Average stuttering was 5.9% of syllables

APPENDIX[a] (continued)

Study	Treatment	N	Age	Duration	Outcome	Follow-up	Notes
Weiner (1984c)	Vocal training	27		14-156 sessions	All achieved high levels of fluency	0-6 years	18 responding to questionnaire reported fluency of 80% to 100%, 60% to 100% under stress
MacCulloch, Eaton, and Long (1970)	Auditory masking	8		24 weeks	100% improved		
Dewar, Dewar, Austin, and Brash (1979)	Edinburgh masker	195	Adults		89% responded well	6-28 months	Of 67 tested, 82% reported great or considerable benefit
Adams (1972)	Systematic desensitization	12	7-28	10-70 weeks	75% made at least some improvement	6 months-over 2 years	No loss of improvement
Gray and England (1972)	Systematic desensitization	30	14-45	1 year	50% of 15 who remained in therapy were improved, greatly improved, or cured		
Boudreau and Jeffrey (1973)	Systematic desensitization	8	16-22	2-3 months	5 subjects showed marked improvement	20 months	The 3 subjects who received no other speech therapy or home practice retained their gains
Burgraff (1974)	Systematic desensitization	9	Adults	7-8 weeks	Mean reduction in stuttering of 35 to 40%		

Study	Treatment	N	Age	Duration	Outcome	Follow-up	Follow-up result
Andrews and Ingham (1972a)	Token economy and prolonged or syllable-timed speech	23	Adults	20 days	Mean percent of stuttered syllables reduced from 16.4 to 0.1	18 months	Mean percent of stuttered syllables was 7.8
Ingham, Andrews, and Winkler (1972)	Token economy	9	Adults	2 weeks	Mean percent of stuttered syllables reduced from 18.2 to 6.7		
Ingham, Andrews, and Winkler (1972)	Token economy, syllable-timed speech, and group psychotherapy	9	Adults	2 weeks	Mean percent of stuttered syllables reduced from 17.4 to 0.2		
Guitar and Bass (1978)	Token economy and prolonged speech	20	Adults	3 weeks	Mean percent of stuttered syllables reduced from 10 to 0	1 year	Mean percent of stuttered syllables was 2.6
Elliott and Williamson (1973)	Token reward	10	Adolescents	12 days	100% improved markedly	6 months	Significant improvement in 7 of 8 cases
Mowrer (1975)	Reinforcement of fluency	20	8-43	3½-46½ hours	Mean percent of stuttered words reduced from 11.7 to 2.4		
Stocker and Gerstman (1983)	Reinforcement of fluency	24	Mean of 6.9	Mean of 7.4 months	75% were rated fluent or exceptionally fluent		
Ryan (1981)	Various programmed therapies	40	7-16	Mean of 15.6 hours	Mean stuttered words per minute fell from 8.2 to 0.3*	Mean of 12.5 months	Average stuttered words per minute for the 13 subjects followed up was 0.8
Rustin, Ryan, and Ryan (1987)	Verbal reward and punishment, DAF	107	6-45	Mean of 2.6 months	Mean stuttered words per minute decreased from 10.9 to 0.2		

APPENDIX[a] (continued)

Study	Treatment	N	Age/Grade	Duration	Outcome	Follow-up	Follow-up outcome
Mallard and Westbrook (1988)	Token and verbal reward and punishment	20	Grades K to 5	9 months	Mean % of stuttered syllables declined from 12.0 to 9.0	4 months	Mean % of stuttered syllables was 7.0
Craig and Andrews (1985)	Smooth, slow speech	17	Adults	3 weeks	Mean % stuttered syllables declined from 12.9 to 0.9	10 months	Mean % of stuttered syllables was 1.9
Andrews and Feyer (1985)	Smooth, slow speech	37	21–60	3 weeks	Mean % of stuttered syllables declined from 14.0 to 0.1	10-15 months	Mean % of stuttered syllables was 1.1
Jehle and Boberg (1987)	Slow speech, gentle onsets of phonation	8	17–30	3 weeks	Mean % of stuttered syllables declined from 18.0 to 0.7		
Jehle and Boberg (1987)	Slow speech, gentle onsets of phonation	7	13–16	3 weeks	Mean % of stuttered syllables declined from 21.6 to 4.1		
Boberg and Kully (1985)	Slow speech, gentle onsets of phonation	17	14–38	3 weeks	Mean % of stuttered syllables declined from 25.1 to 1.0		
Randoll (1988)	Slow speech	7	4–9	Mean of 6 months for most cases	In 4 cases, improvement in stuttered words per minute		
Stang (1984)	Composite behavior therapy	78	8–17	4 to 6 months	49% were stutter-free, 19% usually fluent	22-64 months	Of 69 subjects, 17% were stutter-free, 48% usually fluent

Study	Treatment	N	Ages	Duration	Outcome	Follow-up	Follow-up outcome
Ladouceur and Saint-Laurent (1986)	Composite therapy	8	18-36	4 weeks	Percent of stuttered syllables was significantly reduced	6 months	Percent of disfluent syllables did not differ significantly from that of 8 nonstutterers
Maxwell (1982)	Cognitive and behavioral self-control therapy	23	Mean of 24	12 months	Overall ratings fell from moderate to mild		
Purser and Rustin (1983)	Cognitive-behavioral therapy	32		10 weeks	The subjects were clearly improved, but did not differ from a control group		
Johnson (1955a)	Parent counseling	46	2-9	5-51 months	72% had normal or nearly normal speech		
Johnson and Associates (1959)	Parent counseling	74	2-8	—		Mean 28.5 months	45% had no problem[m]
Neaves (1970)	Child guidance clinic	93	8-12			1-3 years	44% responded successfully
Neaves (1970)	Child guidance clinic	72	13-17			1-3 years	60% responded successfully
Wyatt and Herzan (1962)	Psychotherapy with mother and child	12	2-6	4-12 months	83% showed marked improvement		
Wyatt and Herzan (1962)	Psychotherapy with mother and child	8	7-15	4-12 months	63% showed marked improvement		
Wyatt (1969)	Psychotherapy with parent and child	28	2-13	3-91 weeks	79% had improved or normal speech	3-11 years	58% had no stuttering

APPENDIX[a] (continued)

Study	Drug	N	Age	Duration	Results		
Winkelman (1954)	Chlorpromazine	5		2-8 months	40% had moderate or marked improvement		
Hackett et al[n]	Chlorpromazine	7	9-16	24 weeks	71% greatly improved[o]		
Mitchell[p]	Reserpine and speech therapy	16	Adults	8 weeks	0% showed decreased frequency or severity of stuttering		
Hollister[n]	Reserpine and speech therapy	8	Adults	60 days	50% improved[q]		
Glasner[n]	Reserpine	7	4-8	7 weeks	43% increased smoothness of speech pattern		
Maxwell and Paterson (1958)	Meprobamate and speech therapy	18	18-50	8 months	78% showed good or very good improvement		
Kent and Williams (1959)	Meprobamate and speech therapy	8	18-29	99 days	38% much improved[r]	4 months	38% much improved
Di Carlo, Katz, and Batkin (1959)	Meprobamate	30	15-45	6 weeks	In the drug group (N = 10) a substantial reduction occurred in stuttering in oral reading. Stuttering increased in the placebo group and showed no change in the no medication group		
Holliday (1959)	Meprobamate	20	Adults	3 weeks	Neither the drug nor the placebo group showed a significant change in		

Study	Drug	N	Age	Duration	Results	Follow-up	Follow-up results
					frequency of stuttering, but clinicians' ratings of tension showed a decrease for the drug group		
Gattuso and Leocata (1962)	Haloperidol	50	5-12	1 month	80% of the children aged 5-8 had no symptoms; the remaining 20% improved		
Tapia (1969)	Haloperidol	12	8-16		2 subjects improved by count of stuttering		
Wells and Malcolm (1971)	Haloperidol	36	15-60	8 weeks	Of 12 in the drug group, 83% showed considerable improvement	3 years	"Fluency" remained improved, but repetitions and interjections not significantly[s]
Quinn and Peachey (1973)	Haloperidol	18	15-39	3 weeks	22% showed more than a 50% decrease of stuttering in spontaneous speech		
Swift, Swift, and Arellano (1975)	Haloperidol	22	23-50	3 weeks	Of 7 in drug group who completed treatment 6 showed improvement		
Plath and Caspers[t]	Haloperidol and speech therapy	90	5-33	6 months	Substantial improvement and in some cases cures occurred	6 months	Among the successfully treated cases only one relapsed
Rantala and Petri-Larmi	Haloperidol	58	Adults and children	8 weeks	"Spasms" decreased more under drug than		

APPENDIX[a] (continued)

	Drug	N	Age	Duration	Results
(1976)					under placebo; decrease in repetitions was not significant
Rosenberger, Wheelden, and Kalotkin (1976)	Haloperidol	8	20-32	6-12 weeks	No significant effect on mean frequency of stuttering; percent of time disfluent in spontaneous speech was less in the drug condition
Andrews and Dozsa (1977)	Haloperidol	15	19-29	At least 20 days	40% of subjects reduced their stuttering by at least half
Andrews and Dozsa (1977)	Haloperidol	15	16-46	At least 20 days	20% reduced stuttering by at least half; mean frequency of stuttering was not significantly less than under placebo
Murray, Kelly, et al. (1977)	Haloperidol	18	Adolescents and adults	3 months	61% were more improved on drug than on placebo
Prins, Mandelkorn, and Cerf (1980)	Haloperidol	14	7-41	8 weeks	The drug had a relatively small effect
Cozzo and Gabrielli (1965)	Haloperidol and Triperidol	48	4-14		33% showed marked improvement
Schilling (1963)	Bellergal	61	Children and adults	2-3 months	52% showed good or very good improvement

Study	Drug	N	Age	Duration	Results		
Aron (1965)	Trifluoperazine and amylobarbitone	46	Adults	3 weeks	80% showed varying degrees of improvement in speech	3 weeks	No carry-over of effects of drug
Fish and Bowling (1965)	D-amphetamine and trifluoperazine	28	10-59	1-2 months	79% showed improvement		
Fish and Bowling (1962)	Dexadrine	11	11-60	3 months	45% had dramatic improvement or no stuttering		
Fujita et al. (1963)	Chlordiaze-poxide	23	Children and adults		There was marked or moderate improvement in 65%		
Hommerich and Korzendorfer (1966)	Chlordiaze-poxide	46	8 years-adulthood	3 months	74% were improved or cured[u]		
Goldman and Guth (1965)	Thioridazine and chlordiazepoxide	8		6 weeks	75% were rated milder on thioridazine		
Cacudi (1964)	Thioridazine	21	4-14	2 months	Cure or marked improvement seen in 67%		
Goldman (1966)	Thioridazine and speech therapy	20	10-52	4 months	Drug group was rated less severe, but mean frequency of stuttering did not change		
Leanderson and Levi (1967)	Opipramol or diazepam	44	Adults	54 days	Neither drug had a marked effect; Opipramol reduced stuttering moderately		

APPENDIX[a] (continued)

Study	Treatment	N	Age	Duration	Results
Hale (1951)	Thiamin		2-8	1 month	55% had observable improvement
Bloch et al. (1977)	Propanolol	26	Adults and children		There was no significant effect on the frequency of stuttering, but improvement was reported in individual cases
Rustin, Kuhr, Cook, and James (1981)	Oxprenolol and speech therapy	31	18-55	12 weeks	The drug had no effect, but speech therapy (slow rate and relaxation) resulted in a highly significant improvement
Arthurs et al. (1954)	Carbon dioxide inhalation	14	21-36	30-70 administrations	0% showed improvement in fluency
Smith (1953)	Carbon dioxide inhalation	33	20-55	10-36 weeks	48% showed 50 to 100% improvement
Donath (1928)	Hypnosis	48	5-36		71% were improved or cured
Lockhart and Robertson (1977)	Hypnosis	7	18-62	4-6 weeks	All achieved fluency
Lockhart and Robertson (1977)	Hypnosis and speech therapy	23	15-43	12-54 weeks	10 achieved fluency; 8 were still in therapy
Bryngelson[v]	Handedness change	127	6-16	16 months	90% had marked improvement or normal speech

Study	Technique	N	Age	Duration	Outcome	Follow-up	Follow-up results
Fishman (1937)	Negative practice	5	12-20	1 month	60% showed definite improvement		
Petkov and Iosifov (1960)	Composite therapy	50	Grades 3-9	45 days	96% had significant improvement or recovery		
Jones-Prus (1980)	Slow rate, rhythmic speech	5	4-8	2-9 months	Subjects improved from moderate or severe to mild or very mild	7-18 months	Only 1 subject showed a mild regression
Culp (1984)	Easy speech	14	2-5	15-70 hours	All had fluency within normal limits	2 years	Of 7 children, all but 1 had fluency within normal limits
Shine (1984)	Easy speaking voice	18	2-8	1-28 months	All were fluent	14-64 months	Of 14 children, 13 had maintained fluency
Riley and Riley (1984)	Component based therapy	44	3-12	Mean of 47.9 hours	82% had no or mild stuttering	2-4 years	Of 37 children, 81% had no or mild stuttering
Riley and Riley (1986)	Oral motor training	9	3-6	8-22 hours	Improvement % ranged from 19 to 100, with a mean of 62		
Onslow, Costa, and Rue (1990)	Verbal reward and punishment	4	3-5	4-10 weeks	All subjects showed significant reductions in stuttering	9 months	All showed significant reductions in stuttering
Runyan and Runyan (1986)	Slow rate, light contacts, continuous, phonation	9	3-7	1 year	Number of stuttered words per minute decreased from 10-74 to 1.7-5	2 years	The 5 subjects evaluated stuttered on a mean of 1.7 to 3 words per minute

APPENDIX[a] (continued)

Daskalov (1962)	Speech exercises, improvement of home environment	123	Preschool	3-6 months or longer	69% greatly improved or cured	2 years	88% greatly improved or cured
Daskalov (1962)	Speech exercises, metronome practice	260	School-children		84% greatly improved or cured	2 years	43% greatly improved or cured
Daskalov (1962)	Composite therapy	440	Adults		74% greatly improved or cured	2 years	54% greatly improved or cured
Kurth and Schmidt (1964)	Speech therapy and psychotherapy	32	6-13		67% significantly improved or cured		
Zaliouk and Zaliouk (1965)	Relaxation, breathing and speech exercises	58	6-15	Mean of 6 months	81% had full recovery		
Lepsova (1965)	Speech training at summer camp	72	School-children	3-4 weeks	60% showed significant or very good improvement		51% showed significant or very good improvement in following school year
Novák (1975)	Composite therapy	25	17-35	6-8 weeks	Considerable improvement in practically 100%	2 years	Improvement in 44%

Fransella (1970)	Personal construct therapy	20	17-49	2 years	74% improved	9 months-3 years	Of 9 followed up, 8 maintained or bettered their improvement[w]
Dalali and Sheehan (1974)	Assertion training	8	Adults	6 hours	No change in severity of stuttering		
Dalali and Sheehan (1974)	Feeling clarification	8	Adults	6 hours	No change in severity of stuttering		
Dalali and Sheehan (1974)	Avoidance reduction	8	Adults	6 hours	No change in severity of stuttering		
Haskell and Larr (1974)	Role training	6	Adults	11 hours	All improved considerably		
Moleski and Tosi (1976)	Rational-emotive therapy or systematic desensitization	20	Adults	8 sessions	Rational-emotive therapy was more effective than systematic desensitization		
Gendelman (1977)	Confrontation	40	Adolescents	20 or more sessions	90% were normally fluent or improved	2 months-3 years	Prior level of fluency was maintained by 81% of 27 followed up
Rubin and Culatta (1971)	Commitment to fluency	15	13-40	½-18 months	60% had normal fluency outside the clinic		
Irwin (1972)	Easy stammering	26	17-52	1-4 years	96% had good to complete improvement		
Peins, McGough, and Lee (1972)	Iowa therapy after Van Riper	12	Mean 22	6 months	67% showed a reduction in severity of stuttering		

APPENDIX[a] (continued)

Study	Treatment	N	Age	Duration	Results	Follow-up	Outcome
Prins (1970)	Residential Iowa therapy program	94	8-21	8 weeks		6 months-3½ years	77% perceived themselves as making much or complete improvement
Gregory (1972)	Iowa therapy and relaxation	17	Mean of 28	9 months	There was a significant reduction in stuttering to a mild to moderate level of severity	9 months	A slight regressive trend was not statistically significant
Burgraff (1974)	Iowa therapy after Van Riper	9	Adults	7-8 weeks	Mean reduction in stuttering of 35-40%		
Mallard and Westbrook (1988)	Van Riper therapy	20	Grades K to 5	9 months	Mean % of stuttered syllables declined from 12.0 to 1.0	4 months	Mean % of stuttered syllables was 7.0
Prins and Nichols (1974)	Iowa therapy	9	11-15	6 weeks		5 months	48% perceived themselves as making much or complete improvement
Prins (1976)	Modified Iowa therapy	9	10-16	6 weeks		5 months	69% perceived themselves as making much or complete improvement

[a]The assistance of Joseph Grossman with portions of this survey is gratefully acknowledged.
[b]Follow-up refers to reevaluation a specified time after termination of therapy.
[c]Follow-up data from Peins, McGough, and Lee (1984).
[d]Cited by Soderberg (1969b).
[e]Follow-up data from Ryan (1981).
[f]Members of the same family.
[g]Follow-up reported by Boberg and Sawyer (1977).
[h]Plus maintenance.
[i]Supplemented by 1-8 months of contacts by telephone.
[j]Supplemented by 3 months of contacts by telephone.
[k]For the 13 subjects who were followed up.
[l]Varied from a single interview to a program of unspecified duration.
[m]This compared with 23% of those whose parents received no counseling.
[n]Cited by Kent (1963).
[o]Of 6 stutterers in a placebo group 50% were greatly improved.
[p]Cited by Burr and Mullendore (1960).
[q]25% improved on placebo and speech therapy.
[r]By judges' ratings. Other measures failed to show any improvement.
[s]Follow-up reported by Cookson and Wells (1973).
[t]Cited by Wertenbroch (1976).
[u]77% of a placebo group were reported improved or cured.
[v]Cited by Travis (1931, p. 191).
[w]Follow-up data from Fransella (1972).

REFERENCES

Abbott, J. A., Repressed hostility as a factor in adult stuttering. *J. Speech Dis.*, *12*, 428–30 (1947).

Accordi, M., Bianchi, R., Consolaro, C., Tronchin, F., DeFilippi, R., Pasqualon, L., Ugo, E., and Croatto, L., L'Eziopatogenesi della balbuzie: Studio stadstico su 2802 casi. *Acta Phoniatrica Latina*, *5*,171–80 (1983).

Adamczyk, B., Anwendung des Apparates für die Erzeugung von künstlichem Widerhall bei der Behandlung des Stotterns. *Folia Phoniat*, *11*, 216–18 (1959).

Adamczyk, B., Die Ergebnisse der Behandlung des Stotterns durch das Telephonechosystem. *De Therapia Vocis et Loquelae, Vol. 1.* XIII Congr. Int. Soc. Logoped. Phoniat., (1965).

Adamczyk, B. and Kuniszyk-Józkowiak, W., Effect of echo and reverberation of a restricted information capacity on the speech process. *Folia Phoniat.*, *39*, 9–17 (1987).

Adamczyk, B., Kuniszyk-Józkowiak, W., and Smolka, E., Influence of echo and reverberation on the speech process. *Folia Phoniat*, *31*, 70–81 (1979).

Adamczyk, B., Sadowska, E., and Kuniszyk-Józkowiak, W., Influence of reverberation on stuttering. *Folia Phoniat.*, *27*, 1–6 (1975).

Adams, L. H., A comparison of certain sound wave characteristics of stutterers and nonstutterers. In Johnson, W., and Leutenegger, R. R (eds.), *Stuttering in Children and Adults.* Minneapolis: Univ. Minn. Press (1955).

Adams, M. R., The use of reciprocal inhibition procedures in the treatment of stuttering. *J. Communic. Dis.*, *5*, 59–66 (1972).

Adams, M. R., A physiologic and aerodynamic interpretation of fluent and stuttered speech. *J. Fluency Dis.*, *1*, 35–47 (1974).

Adams, M. R., Voice onsets and segment durations of normal speakers and beginning stutterers. *J. Fluency Dis.*, *12*, 133–39 (1987).

Adams, M. R., The demands and capacities model: I. Theoretical elaborations. *J. Fluency Dis.*, *15*, 135–41 (1990).

Adams, M. R., and Brutten, G. J., An exploratory study of some learning-based procedures for modifying stuttering. *J. Communic. Dis.*, *3*, 123–32 (1970).

Adams, M. R., and Dietze, D. A., A comparison of the reaction times of stutterers and nonstutterers to items on a word association test. *J. Speech Hearing Res. 8*, 195–202 (1965).

Adams, M. R., and Hayden, P., The ability of stutterers and nonstutterers to initiate and terminate phonation during production of an isolated vowel. *J. Speech Hearing Res.*, *19*, 290–96 (1976).

Adams, M. R., and Hutchinson, J., The effects of three levels of auditory masking on selected vocal characterisdcs and the frequency of disfluency of adult stutterers. *J. Speech Hearing Res.*, *17*, 682–88 (1974).

Adams, M. R., Lewis, J. I., and Besozzi, T. E., The effect of reduced reading rate on stuttering frequency. *J. Speech Hearing Res., 16,* 671–75 (1973).

Adams, M. R., and Moore, W. H., Jr., The effects of auditory masking on the anxiety level, frequency of dysfluency, and selected vocal characterisdcs of stutterers. *J. Speech Hearing Res., 15,* 572–78 (1972).

Adams, M. R., and Popelka, G., The influence of "time-out" on stutterers and their dysfluency. *Behav. Ther., 2,* 334–39 (1971).

Adams, M. R, and Ramig, P., Vocal characteristics of normal speakers and stutterers during choral reading. *J. Speech Hearing Res., 23,* 457–69 (1980).

Adams, M. R., and Reis, R., The influence of the onset of phonation on the frequency of stuttering. *J. Speech Hearing Res., 14,* 639–44 (1971).

Adams, M. R., and Reis, R, Influence of the onset of phonation on the frequency of stuttering: A replication and reevaluation. *J. Speech Hearing Res., 17,* 752–54 (1974).

Adams, M. R., and Reis, R., A reply to Martin Young. *J. Speech Hearing Res., 18,* 602–05 (1975).

Adams, M. R, Riemenschneider, S., Metz, D., and Conture, E., Voice onset and articulatory constriction requirements in a speech segment and their relation to the amount of stuttering adaptation. *J. Fluency Dis., 1,* 23–29 (1975).

Adams, M. R., and Runyan, C. M., Stuttering and fluency: Exclusive events or points on a continuum? *J. Fluency Dis., 6,* 197–218 (1981).

Adams, M. R., Runyan, C., and Mallard, A. R., Air flow characteristics of the speech of stutterers and nonstutterers. *J. Fluency Dis., 1,* 4–12 (1975).

Adams, M. R., Sears, R. L., and Ramig, P. R., Vocal changes in stutterers and nonstutterers during monotoned speech. *J. Fluency Dis., 7,* 21–25 (1982) .

Adams, S., A study of the growth of language between two and four years. *J. Juv. Res., 16,* 269–77 (1932).

Adler, J. B., and Starkweather, C. W., Oral and laryngeal reaction times in stutterers. *Asha, 21,* 769 (1979). Abstract.

Agnello, J., The effects of manifest anxiety and stuttering adaptation: Implications for treatment. *Asha, 4,* 377 (1962). Abstract.

Agnello, J. G., Voice onset and voice termination features of stutterers. In Webster, L. M., and Furst, L. C. (eds.), *Vocal Tract Dynamics and Dysfluency.* New York: Speech and Hearing Inst. (1975).

Ahlbach, J., and Benson, V. (eds.), *To Say What is Ours.* San Francisco: National Stuttering Project (1994).

Aimard, P., Plantier, A., and Wittling, M., Le bégaiement: Contribution a l'étude de l'audition et l'intégration phonétique. *Rev. Laryng. Otol.-Rhinol., 87,* 254–56 (1966).

Ainsworth, S., Studies in the psychology of stuttering: XII. Empathetic breathing of auditors while listening to stuttering speech. *J. Speech Dis., 4,* 149–56 (1939).

Allen, A V., The role of the Rh blood factor in the etiology of certain speech disorders. *Speech Monogr., 15,* 202–03 (1948). Abstract.

Allen, C. P., and Daly, D. A., Effects of transcendental meditation and EMG biofeedback relaxation on stuttering. *Asha, 20,* 730 (1978). Abstract.

Altrows, I. F., and Bryden, M. P., Temporal factors in the effects of masking noise on fluency of stutterers. *J. Communic. Dis., 10,* 315–29 (1977).

Ambrose, N. G., Yairi, E., and Cox, N., Genetic aspects of early childhood stuttering. *J. Speech Hearing Res., 36,* 701–06 (1993).

Amirov, R. Z., Daloneishie rezultaty izuchenia vysshei nervnoi deiatel'nosti pri zaikanii. *dsh Abstr.*, *2*, 74–75 (1962).

Ammons, R., and Johnson, W., Studies in the psychology of stuttering: XVIII. The construction and application of a test ot attitude toward stuttering. *J. Speech Dis.*, *9*, 39–49 (1944).

Anderson, J. M., Hood, 5. B., and Sellers, D. E., Central auditory processing abilities of adolescent and preadolescent stuttering and nonstuttering children. *J. Fluency Dis.*, *13*, 199–214 (1988).

Anderson, J., and Whealdon, M. L., A study of the blood group distribution among stutterers. *J. Speech Dis.*, *6*, 23–28 (1941).

Anderson, L. O., Stuttering and allied disorders. Compar. *Psychol. Monogr.*, *Vol. 1* (1923).

Andrews, G., Epidemiology of stuttering. In Curlee, R. F., and Perkins, W. H. (eds.), *Nature and Treatment of Stuttering: New Directions*. San Diego: College–Hill Press (1984a).

Andrews, G., Evaluation of the benefits of treatment. In Perkins, W. H. (ed.), *Stuttering Disorders*. New York: Thieme–Stratton (1984b).

Andrews, G., and Craig, A., Stuttering: Overt and covert measurement of the speech of treated subjects. *J. Speech Hearing Dis.*, *47*, 96–99 (1982).

Andrews, G., Craig, A., Feyer, A.-M., Hoddinott, S., Howie, P., and Neilson, M., Stuttering: A review of research findings and theories circa 1982. *J. Speech Hearing Dis.*, *48*, 226–46 (1983).

Andrews, G., and Cutler, J., Stuttering therapy: The relation between changes in symptom level and attitudes. *J. Speech Hearing Dis.*, *39*, 312–19 (1974).

Andrews, G., and Dozsa, M., Haloperidol and the treatment of stuttering. *J. Fluency Dis.*, *2*, 217–24 (1977) .

Andrews, G., and Feyer, A.-M., Does behavior therapy still work when the experimenters depart? An analysis of a behavioral treatment program for stutterers . *Behavior Modification*, *9*, 443–57 (1985).

Andrews, G., Guitar, B., and Howie, P., Meta–analysis of the effects of stuttering treatment. *J. Speech Hearing Dis.*, *45*, 287–307 (1980).

Andrews, G., and Harris, M., *The Syndrome of Stuttering*. Clinics in Developmental Med., No. 17. London: Spastics Society Medical Education and Information Unit in association with Wm. Heinemann Medical Books (1964).

Andrews, G., and Harvey, R., Regression to the mean in pretreatment measures of stuttering. *J. Speech Hearing Dis.*, *46*, 204–07 (1981).

Andrews, G., Howie, P. M., Dozsa, M., and Guitar, B. E., Stuttering: Speech pattern characteristics under fluency-inducing conditions. *J. Speech Hearing Res.*, *25*, 208–16 (1982).

Andrews, G., and Ingham, R. J., An approach to the evaluation of stuttering therapy. *J. Speech Hearing Res.*, *15*, 296–302 (1972a).

Andrews, G., and Ingham, R. J., Stuttering: An evaluation of follow-up procedures for syllable-timed speech/token system therapy. *J. Communic. Dis.*, *5*, 307–19 (1972b).

Andrews, G., and Quinn, P. T., Stuttering and cerebral dominance. *J. Communic. Dis.*, *5*, 212 (1972).

Andrews, G., Quinn, P. T., and Sorby, W. A., Stuttering: An investigation into cerebral dominance for speech. *J. Neurol. Neurosurg. Psychiat.*, *35*, 414–18 (1972).

Andrews, G., and Tanner, S., Stuttering treatment: An attempt to replicate the regulated breathing method. *J. Speech Hearing Dis., 47*, 138–40 (l982a).

Andrews, G., and Tanner, S., Stuttering: The results of 5 days treatment with an airflow technique. *J. Speech Hearing Dis., 47*, 427–29 (1982b).

Andrews, M. L., and Smith, R. G., Perceptions of auditory components of stuttered speech. *J. Communic. Dis., 9*, 121–28 (1976).

Andronico, M. P., and Blake, I., The application of filial therapy to young children with stuttering problems. *J. Speech Hearing Dis., 36*, 377–81 (1971).

Ardila, A., Bateman, J. C., Niño, C. R., Pulido, Rivera, D. B., and Vanegas, C. J., An epedemiologic study of stuttering. *J. Communic. Dis., 27*, 37–48 (1994) .

Ardila, A., and Lopez, M. V., Severe stuttering associated with right hemisphere lesion. *Brain Lang., 7*, 239–46 (1986) .

Arend, R., Handzel, L., and Weiss, B., Dysphatic stuttering. *Folia Phoniat., 14*, 55–66 (1962).

Arends, N., Povel, D.-J., and Kolk, H., Stuttering as an attentional phenomenon. *J. Fluency Dis., 13*, 141–51 (1988).

Armson, J., and Kalinowski, J., Interpreting results of the fluent speech paradigm in stuttering research. Difficulties in separating cause from effect. *J. Speech Hearing Res., 37*, 69–82 (1994).

Arnold, G. E. Special features and new viewpoint of phoniatric practice in New York. *Folia Phoniat., 10*, 96–111 (1958).

Aron, M L., The nature and incidence of stuttering among a Bantu group of school-going children. *J. Speech Hearing Dis., 27*, 116–28 (1962).

Aron, M. L., The effects of the combination of trifluoperazine and amylobarbitone on adult stutterers. *Med. Proc. So. Afr. J. Advancement Med. Sci., 11*, 227–33 (1965).

Aron, M. L., The relationships between measurements of stuttering behavior. *J. So. Afr. Logoped. Soc., 14*, 15–34 (1967).

Arthurs, R. G. S., Cappon, D., Douglass, E., and Quarrington, B., Carbon dioxide therapy with stutterers. *Dis. Nerv. System, 15*, 123–26 (1954).

Asp, C. W., Time–intensity trade and lateralized localization of interaural intensity differences by stutterers and non–stutterers. *Speech Monogr., 35*, 316–17 (1968).

Aten, J. L., and Blanchard, S., EMG biofeedback in the treatment of stuttering: Selected case studies. *Asha, 16*, 555 (1974). Abstract.

Atkins, C. P., Perceptions of speakers with minimal eye contact: Implications for stutterers. *J. Fluency Dis., 13*, 429–36 (1988).

Avari, D. N., and Bloodstein, O., Adjacency and prediction in school-age stutterers. *J. Speech Hearing Res., 17*, 33–40 (1974).

Azrin, N., Jones, R. J., and Flye, B., A synchronization effect and its application to stuttering by a portable apparatus. *J. App. Behav. Anal., 1*, 283–95 (1968).

Azrin, N. H., and Nunn, R. G., A rapid method of eliminating stuttering by a regulated breathing approach. *Behav. Res. Ther., 12*, 279–86 (1974).

Azrin, N. H., Nunn, R. G., and Frantz, S. E., Comparison of regulated breathing versus abbreviated desensitization on reported stuttering episodes. *J. Speech Hearing Dis., 44*, 331–39 (1979).

Backus, O., Incidence of stuttering among the deaf. *Ann. Otol. Rhinol. Laryngol., 47,* 632–35 (1938).

Baken, R J, McManus; D. A., and Cavallo, S. A., Prephonatory chest wall posturing in stutterers. *J. Speech Hearing Res., 26,* 444–50 (1983).

Bakker, K., and Brutten, G. J., Labial and laryngeal reaction times of stutterers and nonstutterers. In Peters, H. F. M., and Hulstijn, W. (eds.), *Speech Motor Dynamics in Stuttering.* New York: Springer (1987).

Bakker, K., and Brutten, G. J., A comparative investigation of the laryngeal premotor, adjustment, and reaction times of stutterers and nonstutterers. *J. Speech Hearing Res., 32,* 239–44 (1989).

Bakker, K., Brutten, G. J., Janssen, P., and van der Meulen, S., An eyemarking study of anticipation and dysfluency among elementary school stutterers. *J. Fluency Dis., 16,* 25–33 (1991).

Ballard, P. B., Sinistrality and speech. *J. Exper. Ped., 1,* 298–310 (1912).

Bar, A., Effects of listening instructions on attention to manner and content of stutterers' speech. *J. Speech Hearing Pes., 10,* 87–92 (1967).

Bar, A., Analyses of roles, stuttering and interaction processes during interviews with stutterers. *J. Communic. Dis., 2,* 126–40 (1969).

Bar, A., and Jakab, I., Graphic identification of the stuttering episode as experienced by stutterers. In Jakab, I. (ed.), *Art Interpretation and Art Therapy. Psychiatry and Art, Vol. 2.* V Int. Coll. Psychopathol. Expression. Basel: Karger (1969).

Bar, A., Singer, J., and Feldman, R. G., Subvocal muscle activity during stuttering and fluent speech: A comparison, *J. So. Afr. Logoped. Soc., 16,* 9–14 (1969).

Baratz, R., and Mesulam, M.-M., Adult-onset stuttering treated with anticonvulsants. *Arch. Neurol., 38,* 132 (1981).

Barbara, D. A., A psychosomatic approach to the problem of stuttering in psychotics. *Amer. J. Psychiat., 103,* 188–95 (1946).

Barbara, D. A., *Stuttering: A Psychodynamic Approach to Its Understanding and Treatment.* New York: Julian Press (1954).

Barber, V., Studies in the psychology of stuttering: XV. Chorus reading as a distraction in stuttering. *J. Speech Dis., 4,* 371–83 (1939).

Barber, V., Studies in the psychology of stuttering: XVI. Rhythm as a distraction in stuttering. *J. Speech Dis;, 5,* 29–42 (1940).

Barr, D. F., and Carmel; N. R., Stuttering inhibition with high frequency narrow-band masking noise. *J. Aud. Res., 9,* 40–44 (1969).

Barr, H., A quantitative study of the specific phenomena observed in stuttering. *J. Speech Dis., 5,* 277–80 (1940).

Barrett, K. H., Keith, R. W., Agnello, J. G., and Weiler, E. M., Central auditory processing of stutterers and nonstutterers. *Asha, 21,* 769 (1979). Abstract.

Barrett, R. S., and Stoeckel, C. M., Unilateral eyelid movement control in stutterers and nonstutterers. *Asha, 21,* 769 (1979). Abstract.

Bastijens, P., Brutten, G. J., and Stes, R., The effect of punishment and reinforcement procedures on a stutterer's factor two avoidance response. *J. Fluency Dis., 3,* 77–85 (1978).

Baumgartner, J. M., and Brutten, G. J., Expectancy and heart rate as predictors of the speech performance of stutterers. *J. Speech Hearing Pes., 26,* 383–88 (1983).

Bearss, L. M., An investigation of conflict in stutterers and non-stutterers. *Speech Monogr.*, *18*, 237–38 (1951). Abstract.

Bearss, M. L., An investigation of the effect of penalty on the expectancy and frequency of stuttering. *Speech Monogr.*, *19*, 189–90 (1952). Abstract.

Bebout, L., and Bradford, A., Cross–cultural attitudes toward speech disorders. *J. Speech Hearing Res.*, *35*, 5–52 (1992).

Beech, H. R., and Fransella, F., *Research and Experiment in Stuttering*. New York: Pergamon (1968).

Belyakova, L. I., Sravintelnaya kharakteristika elektromyogramm bolnikh s zaikaniem na fone organicheskovo porazhenia tsentralnoi nervnoi sistemi i nevroticheskikh reaktsii. *Zh. Nevropatol. Psikhiat.*, *73*, 715–20 (1973).

Bender, J. F., *The Personality Structure of Stuttering*. New York: Pitman Publishing Corp. (1939).

Bender, J. F., and Kleinfeld, V. M., *Principles and Practices of Speech Correction*. New York: Pitman Publishing Corp. (1938).

Bente, D., Schönhärl, E., and Krump, J., Elektroencephalographische Befunde bei Stotterem und ihre Bedeutung für die medikamentöse Therapie. *Arch. Ohr.-Nas.-Kehlk. Heilk.*, *169*, 513–19 (1956).

Berecz, J. M., The treatment of stuttering through precision punishment and cognitive arousal. *J. Speech Hearing Dis.*, *38*, 256–67 (1973).

Berecz, J. M., Cognitive conditioning therapy in the treatment of stuttering. *J. Communic. Dis.*, *9*, 301–15 (1976).

Berger, E. M., The relation between expressed acceptance of self and expressed acceptance of others. *J. Abnorm. Soc. Psychol.*, *47*, 778–82 (1952).

Bergmann, G., Studies in stuttering as a prosodic disturbance. *J. Speech Hearing Res.*, *29*, 290–300 (1986).

Bergmann, G., Stuttering as a prosodic disturbance: A link between speech execution and emotional processes. In Peters, H. F. M., and Hulstijn, W., (eds.), *Speech Motor Dynamics in Stuttering*. New York: Springer (1987).

Berlin, A. J., An exploratory attempt to isolate types of stuttering. *Speech Monogr.*, *22*, 196–97 (1955). Abstract.

Berlini C. I, Parents' diagnoses of stuttering. *J. Speech Hearing Res.*, *3*, 372–79

Berlinsky, S. L., A comparison of stutterers and non-stutterers in four conditions of induced anxiety. *Speech Monogr.*, *22*, 197 (1955). Abstract.

Bernhardt, R. B., Personality conflict and the act of stuttering. *Dissert. Abstr.*, *14*, 709 (1954).

Bernstein, N. E., Are there constraints on childhood disfluency? *J. Fluency Dis.* *6*, 341–50 (1981).

Berry, M. F., *The Medical History of Stuttering Children*. Ph.D. Dissert., Univ. Wis. (1937a).

Berry, M. F., Twinning in stuttering families. *Human Biol.*, *9*, 329–46 (1937b).

Berry, M. F., A common denominator in twinning and stuttering. *J. Speech Dis.*, *3*, 51–57 (1938a).

Berry, M. F., Developmental history of stuttering children. *J. Pediat.*, *12*, 209–17 (1938b).

Berry, M. F., A study of the medical history of stuttering children. *Speech Monogr.*, *5*, 97–114 (1938c).

Berry, M. F., and Eisenson, J., *Speech Disorders*. New York: Appleton-Century Crofts (1956).

Berry, R. C., and Silverman, F. H., Equality of intervals on the Lewis-Sherman-scale of stuttering severity. *J. Speech Hearing Res.*, *15*, 185–88 (1972).

Berryman, J. D., and Kools, J. A., Disfluency of nonstuttering children in relation to specific measures of language, reading, and mental maturity. *J. Fluency Dis.*, *1*, 18–24 (1975).

Berwick, N. H., Stuttering in response to photographs of selected listeners. In Johnson, W., and Leutenegger, R. R. (eds.), *Stuttering in Children and Adults*. Minneapolis: Univ. Minn. Press (1955).

Besozzi, T. E., and Adams, M. R., The influence of prosody on stuttering adaptation. *J. Speech Hearing Res.*, *12*, 818–24 (1969).

Biggs, B., and Sheehan, J., Punishment or distraction? Operant stuttering revisited. *J. Abnorm. Psychol.*, *74*, 256–62 (1969).

Bills, A. G., The relation of stuttering to mental fatigue. *J. Exper. Psychol.*, *17*, 574–84 (1934).

Bilto, E. W., A comparative study of certain physical abilities of children with speech defects and children with normal speech. *J. Speech Dis.*, *6*, 187–203 (1941).

Bishop, D. V. M., Is there a link between handedness and hypersensitivity? *Cortex*, *22*, 289–96 (1986).

Bishop, J. H., Williams, H. G., and Cooper, W. A., Age and task complexity variables in motor performance of stuttering and nonstuttering children. *J. Fluency Dis.*, *16*, 207–17 (1991a).

Bishop, J. H., Williams, H. G., and Cooper, W. A., Age and task complexity variables in motor performance of children with articulation-disordered, stuttering, and normal speech. *J. Fluency Dis.*, *16*, 219–28 (1991b).

Bjerkan, B., Word fragmentations and repetitions in the spontaneous speech of 2-6-year-old children. *J. Fluency Dis.*, *5*, 137–48 (1980).

Black, J. A., A comparative study of the perception of freedom-in-leisure between stuttering and nonstuttering individuals. *J. Fluency Dis.*, *12*, 239–43 (1937).

Blackburn, B., Voluntary movements of the organs of speech in stutterers and non-stutterers. *Psychol. Monogr.*, *41*, 1–13 (1931).

Blankenship, J., "Stuttering" in normal speech. *J. Speech Hearing Res.*, *7*, 95–96 (1964).

Blankenship J., and Kay, C., Hesitation phenomena in English speech: A study in distribution. *Word*, *20*, 360–72 (1964).

Blanton, S., A survey of speech defects. *J. Educ. Psychol.*, *7*, 581–92 (1916).

Blanton, S., Stuttering. *Mental Hygiene*, *15*, 271–82 (1931).

Blanton, S., and Blanton, M. G., *For Stutterers*. New York: D. Appleton-Century (1936).

Bloch, E. L., and Goodstein, L. D., Functional speech disorders and personality: A decade of research. *J. Speech Hearing Dis.*, *36*, 295–314 (1971).

Bloch, V., Dalby, M., and Johannesen, E., Effekten af propanolol (inderal) på stammen. *dsh Abstr.*, *17*, 226 (1977).

Blood, G. W., Laterality differences in child stutterers: Heterogeneity, severity levels, and statistical treatments. *J. Speech Hearing Dis.*, *50*, 66–72 (1985) .

Blood, G. W., and Blood, I. M., Central auditory function in young stutterers. *Percept. Mot. Skills*, *59*, 699–705 (1984).

Blood, G. W., and Blood, I. M., Laterality preferences in adult female and male stutterers. *J. Fluency Dis., 14*, 1–10 (1989a).

Blood, G. W., and Blood, I. M., Multiple data analysis of dichotic listening advantages of stutterers. *J. Fluency Dis., 14*, 97–107 (1989b).

Blood, G. W., Blood, I. M., and Hood, S. B., The development of ear preferences in stuttering and nonstuttering children: A longitudinal study. *J. Fluency Dis., 12*, 119–31 (1987).

Blood, G. W., and Hood, S. B., Elementary school-aged stutterers' disfluencies during oral reading and spontaneous speech. *J. Fluency Dis., 3*, 155–65 (1978).

Blood, G. W., and Seider, R., The concomitant problems of young stutterers. *J. Speech Hearing Dis., 46*, 31–33 (1981).

Blood, I. M., and Blood, G. W., Relationship between stuttering severity and brainstem-evoked response testing. *Percept. Mot. Skills, 59*, 935–38 (1984).

Blood, I. M., and Blood, G. W., Relationship between disfluency variables and dichotic listening in stutterers. *Percept. Mot. Skills, 62*, 37–38 (1986).

Bloodstein, O., Studies in the psychology of stuttering: XIX. The relationship between oral reading rate and severity of stuttering. *J. Speech Dis., 9*, 161–73 (1944).

Bloodstein, O., Conditions under which stuttering is reduced or absent: A review of literature. *J. Speech Hearing Dis., 14*, 295–302 (1949).

Bloodstein, O., Hypothetical conditions under which stuttering is reduced or absent. *J. Speech Hearing Dis., 15*, 142–53 (1950a).

Bloodstein, O., A rating scale study of conditions under which stuttering is reduced or absent. *J. Speech Hearing Dis., 15*, 29–36 (1950b).

Bloodstein, O., Stuttering as an anticipatory struggle reaction. In Eisenson, J. (ed.), *Stuttering: A Symposium*. New York: Harper & Row (1958).

Bloodstein, O., The development of stuttering: I. Changes in nine basic features. *J. Speech Hearing Dis., 25*, 219–37 (1960a).

Bloodstein, O., The development of stuttering: II. Developmental phases. *J. Speech Hearing Dis., 25*, 366–76 (1960b).

Bloodstein, O., The development of stuttering: III. Theoretical and clinical implications. *J. Speech Hearing Dis., 26*, 67–82 (1961a).

Bloodstein, O., Stuttering in families of adopted stutterers. *J. Speech Hearing Dis., 26*, 395–96 (1961b).

Bloodstein, O., Stuttering and normal nonfluency—A continuity hypothesis. *Brit. J. Dis. Communic., 5*, 30–39 (1970).

Bloodstein, O., The anticipatory struggle hypothesis; Implications of research on the variability of stuttering. *J. Speech Hearing Res., 15*, 487–99 (1972).

Bloodstein, O., The rules of early stuttering. *J. Speech Hearing Dis., 39*, 379–94 (1974)

Bloodstein, O., Stuttering as tension and fragmentation. In Eisenson, J. (ed.), *Stuttering: A Second Symposium*. New York: Harper & Row (1975).

Bloodstein, O., Stuttering as an anticipatory struggle disorder. In Curlee, R. F., and Perkins, W. H. (eds.), *Nature and Treatment of Stuttering: New Directions*. San Diego: College–Hill Press (1984).

Bloodstein, O., *Stuttering: The Search for a Cause and Cure*. Boston: Allyn & Bacon (1993).

Bloodstein, O., Alper, J., and Zisk, P. K., Stuttering as an outgrowth of normal disfluency. In Barbara, D. A; (ed.), *New Directions in Stuttering*. Springfield, Ill.: Charles C Thomas (1965).

Bloodstein, O., and Bloodstein, A., Interpretations of facial reactions to stuttering. *J. Speech Hearing Dis., 20,* 148–55 (1955).

Bloodstein, O., and Gantwerk, B. F., Grammatical function in relation to stuttering in young children. *J. Speech Hearing Res., 10,* 786–89 (1967).

Bloodstein, O., and Grossman, M., Early stutterings: Some aspects of their form and distribution. *J. Speech Hearing Res., 24,* 298–302 (1981).

Bloodstein, O., Jaeger, W., and Tureen, J., A study of the diagnosis of stuttering by parents of stutterers and non-stutterers. *J. Speech Hearing Dis., 17,* 308–15 (1952).

Bloodstein, O., and Schreiber, L.R., Obsessive-compulsive reactions in stutterers. *J. Speech Hearing Dis. 22,* 33–39 (1957).

Bloodstein, O., and Shogan, R.L., Some clinical notes on forced stuttering. *J. Speech Hearing Disc., 37,* 177–86 (1972).

Bloodstein, O., and Smith, S. M., A study of the diagnosis of stuttering with special reference to the sex ratio. *J. Speech Hearing Dis., 19,* 459–66 (1954).

Bloom, C. M., and Silverman, F. H., Do all stutterers adapt? *J. Speech Hearing Res., 16,* 518–21 (1973).

Bloom, C., and Silverman, F., Stability of performances of individual stutterers on oral reading adptation tasks. *J. Fluency Dis., 4,* 39–44 (1979).

Bloom, J., Child training and stuttering. *Speech Monogr., 26,* 132–33 (1959). Abstract.

Bloom, L., Notes for a history of speech pathology. *Psychoanal. Rev., 65,* 433–63 (1978).

Bluemel, C. S., Primary and secondary stammering. *Quart. J. Speech, 18,* 187–200 (1932).

Bluemel, C. S., The dominant gradient in stuttering. *Quart. J. Speech, 19,* 233–42 (1933).

Bluemel, C. S., *Stammering and Allied Disorders*. New York: Macmillan (1935).

Bluemel, C. S., *The Riddle of Stuttering*. Danville, Ill.: Interstate Publishing Co. (1957).

Blum, G. S., and Hunt, H. F., The validity of the Blacky Pictures. *Psychol. Bull., 49,* 238–50 (1952).

Boberg, E., Intensive group therapy program for stutterers. *Human Communic., 1,* 29–42 (1976).

Boberg, E., Maintenance of fluency: An experimental program. In Boberg, E. (ed.), *Maintenance of Fluency: Proceedings of the Banff Conference*. New York: Elsevier (1981).

Boberg, E., Intensive adult/teen therapy program. In Perkins, W. H. (ed.), *Stuttering Disorders*. New York: Thieme-Stratton (1984).

Boberg, E. (ed.), *Neuropsychology of Stuttering*. Edmonton, Alberta: Univ. Alberta Press (1993).

Boberg, E., Ewart, B., Mason, G., Lindsay, K., and Wynn, S., Stuttering in the retarded: II. Prevalence of stuttering in EMR and TMR children. *Ment. Retardation Bull., 6,* 67–76 (1978).

Boberg, E., Howie, P., and Woods, L., Maintenance of fluency: A review. *J. Fluency Dis., 4,* 93–116 (1979).

Boberg, E., and Kully, D., *Comprehensive Stuttering Program*. San Diego: College-Hill Press (1985).

Boberg, E., and Sawyer, L., The maintenance of fluency following intensive therapy. *Human Communic.*, 2, 21–28 (1977).

Boberg, E., Yeudall, L. T., Schopflocher, D., and Bo-Lassen, P., The effect of an intensive behavioral program on the distribution of EEG alpha power in stutterers during the processing of verbal and visuospatial information. *J. Fluency Dis.*, 8, 245–63 (1983).

Boehmler, R. M., Listener responses to non-fluencies. *J. Speech Hearing Res.*, 1, 132–41 (1958).

Böhme, G., Stammering and cerebral lesions in early childhood. Examinations of 802 children and adults with cerebral lesions. *Folia Phoniat.*, 20, 239–49 (1968).

Boland, J. L., An investigation of certain birth factors as they relate to stuttering. *Speech Monogr.*, 17, 287 (1950). Abstract.

Boland, J. L., Type of birth as related to stuttering. *J. Speech Hearing Dis.*, 16, 40–43 (1951).

Boland, J. L., A comparison of stutterers and non-stutterers on several measures of anxiety. *Speech Monogr.*, 20, 144 (1953). Abstract.

Bonfanti, B. H., and Culatta, R., An analysis of the fluency patterns of institutionalized retarded adults. *J. Fluency Dis.*, 10, 291–300 (1985).

Bonin, B., Ramig, P., and Prescott, T., Performance differences between stuttering and nonstuttering subjects on a sound fusion task. J. Fluency Dis., 10, 291–300 (1985).

Boome, E. J., and Richardson, M. A., *The Nature and Treatment of Stuttering*. London: Methuen (1931).

Borack, S. A., *A Study of Disfluency in Children with Articulation Defects*. M. S. Thesis, Brooklyn Coll. (1969).

Borden, G. J., Initiation versus execution time during manual and oral counting by stutterers. *J. Speech Hearing Res.*, 26, 389–96 (1983).

Borden, G., J., Baer, T., and Kenney, M. K., Onset of voicing in stuttered and fluent utterances. *J. Speech Hearing Res.*, 28, 363–72 (1985).

Borden, G. J., Dorman, M. F., Freeman, F. J., and Raphael, L. J., Electromyographic changes with delayed auditory feedback of speech. *J. Phonetics*, 5, 1–8 (1977).

Borden, G. J., Kim., D. H., and Spiegler, K., Acoustics of stop consonant-vowel relationships during fluent and stuttered utterances. *J. Fluency Dis.*, 12, 175–84 (1987).

Bosshardt, H.-G., Subvocalization and reading rate differences between stuttering and nonstuttering children and adults. *J. Speech Hearing Res.*, 33, 776–85 (1990).

Bosshardt, H.-G., Differences between stutterers' and nonstutterers' short-term recall and recognition performance. *J. Speech Hearing Res.*, 36, 286–93 (1993).

Bosshardt, H.-G., and Nandyal, I., Reading rates of stutterers and nonstutterers during silent and oral reading. *J. Fluency Dis.*, 13, 407–20 (1988).

Boudreau, L. A., and Jeffrey, C. J., Stuttering treated by desensitization. *J. Behav. Ther. Exp. Psychol.*, 4, 209–12 (1973).

Bourdon, K. H., and Silber, D. E., Perceived parental behavior among stutterers and nonstutterers. *J. Abnorm. Psychol.*, 75, 93–97 (1970).

Boysen, A. E., and Cullinan, W. L., Object-naming latency in stuttering and nonstuttering children. *J. Speech Hearing Res.*, 14, 728–38 (1971).

Brady, J. P., A behavioral approach to the treatment of stuttering, *Amer. J. Psychiat., 125*, 843–48 (1968).

Brady, J. P., Studies on the metronome effect on stuttering. *Behav. Res. Ther., 7*, 197–204 (1969).

Brady, J. P., Metronome-conditioned speech retraining for stuttering. *Behav. Ther., 2*, 129–50 (1971).

Brady, J. P., The pharmacology of stuttering: A critical review. *Amer. J. Psychiatry, 148*, 1309–16 (1991).

Brady, J. P., and Berson, J., Stuttering, dichotic listening, and cerebral dominance. *Arch. Gen. Psychiat., 32*, 1449–52 (1975).

Brady, J. P., and Brady, C. N., Behavior therapy of stuttering. *Folia Phoniat., 24*, 355–59 (1972).

Brady, W. A., and Hall, D. E., The prevalence of stuttering among school-age children. *Lang. Speech Hearing Serv. Schools, 7*, 75–81 (1976).

Brady, W. A., Sommers, R. K., and Moore, W. H., Jr., Cerebral speech processing in stuttering children and adults. *Asha, 15*, 472 (1973). Abstract.

Brandon, S., and Harris, M., Stammering—An experimental treatment programme using syllable-timed speech. *Brit. J. Dis. Commun., 2*, 64–68 (1967).

Brandt, D. E., and wilde, G. J. S., A technique for controlling speech disfluencies induced by delayed auditory feedback. *J. Fluency Dis., 2*, 149–56 (1977).

Brankel, O., Pneumotachographische Studien bei Stotterern. *Folia Phoniat., 13*, 136–43 (1961).

Brankel, O., Die Bedeutung der synchronen Erfassung von akustischen, pneumotachographischen, myographischen und elektromyographischen Symptomenbildern beim Stottern. *Folia Phoniat., 15*, 177–88 (1963).

Branscom, M. E., Hughes, J., and Oxtoby, E. T., Studies of nonfluency in the speech of preschool children. In Johnson, W., and Leutenegger, R. R. (eds.), *Stuttering in Children and Adults*. Minneapolis: Univ. Minn. Press (1955).

Braun, O., Probleme and Möglichkeiten der Lernmotivierung sprachbehinderte Kinder in Unterricht und Therapie in Schulen für Sprachbehinderte. *Sprachheilarbeit, 19*, 47–62 (1974).

Brayton, E. R., and Conture, E. G., Effects of noise and rhythmic stimulation on the speech of stutterers. *J. Speech Hearing Res., 21*, 285–94 (1978).

Brenner, N. C., Perkins, W. H., and Soderberg, G. A., The effect of rehearsal on frequency of stuttering. *J. Speech Hearing Res., 15*, 483–86 (1972).

Bright, C. M., The development of a test of listening ability of stutterers. *Speech Monogr., 15*, 214–15 (1948). Abstract.

Brill, A. A., Speech disturbances in nervous and mental diseases. *Quart. J. Speech Educ., 9*, 129–35 (1923).

Brindle, B. R., and Dunster, J. R., Prevalence of communication disorders in an institutionalized mentally retarded population. *Human Communication, 8*, 72–80 (1984).

Broida, H., An empirical study of sex-role identification and sex-role preference in stuttering. *Speech Monogr., 30*, 242–43 (1963). Abstract.

Brookshire, R. H., Effects of random and response contingent noise upon disfluencies of normal speakers. *J. Speech Hearing Res., 12*, 126–34 (1969).

Brookshire, R. H., and Eveslage, R. A., Verbal punishment of disfluency following augmentation of disfluency by random delivery of aversive stimuli. *J. Speech Hearing Res., 12*, 383–88 (1969).

Brookshire, R. H., and Martin, R. R., The differential effects of three verbal punishers on the disfluencies of normal speakers. *J. Speech Hearing Res., 10*, 496–505 (1967).

Brown, C. J., Zimmermann, G. N., Linville, R. N., and Hegmann, J. P., Variations in self-paced behaviors in stutterers and nonstutterers. *J. Speech Hearing Res., 33*, 317–23 (1990).

Brown, S. F., The influence of grammatical function on the incidence of stuttering. *J. Speech Dis., 2*, 207–15 (1937).

Brown, S. F., A further study of stuttering in relation to various speech sounds. *Quart. J. Speech, 24*, 390–97 (1938a).

Brown, S. F., Stuttering with relation to word accent and word position. *J. Abnorm. Soc. Psychol., 33*, 112–20 (1938b).

Brown, S. F., The theoretical importance of certain factors influencing the incidence of stuttering. *J. Speech Dis., 3*, 223–30 (1938c).

Brown, S. F., The loci of stutterings in the speech sequence. *J. Speech Dis., 10*, 181–92 (1945).

Brown, S. F., and Hull, H. C., A study of some social attitudes of a group of 59 stutterers. *J. Speech Dis., 7*, 323–24 (1942).

Brown, S. F., and Moren, A., The frequency of stuttering in relation to word length during oral reading. *J. Speech Dis., 7*, 153–59 (1942).

Brown, S. F., and Shulman, E. E., Intramuscular pressure in stutterers and non-stutterers. *Speech Monogr., 7*, 63–74 (1940).

Brown, S. L., and Colcord, R. D., Perceptual comparisons of adolescent stutterers' and nonstutterers' fluent speech. *J. Fluency Dis., 12*, 419–27 (1987).

Bruce, M. C., and Adams, M. R., Effects of two types of motor practice on stuttering adaptation. *J. Speech Hearing Res., 21*, 421–28 (1978).

Brumfitt, S. M., and Peake, M. D., A double-blind study of verapamil in the treatment of stuttering. *Brit. J. Dis. Communic., 23*, 35–40 (1988).

Brunner, W., and Frank, F., Vergleichende pulstelemetrische Undersuchungen an Stotterern. *Folia Phoniat., 27*, 325–36 (1975).

Brunner, W., and Frank, F., Das pulstelemetrische Verhalten von Stotterern, geheilten Stotterern und Sprachgesunden. *Folia Phoniat., 28*, 174–81 (1976).

Bruno, G. Camarda, V., and Curi, L., Contributo allo studio dei fattori causali organici nella patogenesi della balbuzie. *Bol. Mal. Or. Gola Naso, 83*, 753–58 (1965).

Brutten, E. J., *Anxiety as a Personality Factor Among Stutterers*. M. A. Thesis, Brooklyn Coll. (1951).

Brutten, E. J., Colorimetric measurement of anxiety: A clinical and experimental procedure. *Speech Monogr., 26*, 282–87 (1959).

Brutten, E. J., Palmar sweat investigation of disfluency and expectancy adaptation. *J. Speech Hearing Res., 6*, 40–48 (1963).

Brutten, E. J., and Gray, B. B., Effect of word cue removal on adaptation and adjacency: A clinical paradigm. *J. Speech Hearing Dis., 26*, 385–89 (1961).

Brutten, E. J., and Shoemaker, D. J., *The Modification of Stuttering*. Englewood Cliffs, N.J.: Prentice-Hall (1967).

Brutten, G. J., Stuttering: Topography, assessment and behavior change strategies. In Eisenson, J. (ed.), *Stuttering: A Second Symposium*. New York: Harper & Row (1975).

Brutten, G. J., The effect of punishment on a Factor I stuttering behavior. *J. Fluency Dis., 5*, 77–85 (1980).

Brutten, G. J., Bakker, K., Janssen, P., and van der Meulen, S., Eye movements of stuttering and nonstuttering children during silent reading. *J. Speech Hearing Res., 27*, 562–66 (1984).

Brutten, G. J., and Dancer, J. E., Stuttering adptation under distributed and massed conditions. *J. Fluency Dis., 5*, 1–10 (1980).

Brutten, G. J., and Dunham, S. L., The Communication Attitude Test: A normative study of grade school children. *J. Fluency Dis., 14*, 371–77 (1989).

Brutten, G. J., and Janssen, P., An eye-marking investigation of anticipated and observed stuttering. *J. Speech Hearing Res., 22*, 20–28 (1979).

Brutten, G. J., and Janssen, P., A normative and factor analysis study of the responses of Dutch and American stutterers to the Speech Situations Checklist. *Proc. 18th Cong. Int. Assoc. Logoped. Phoniat.* Washington, D.C.: Amer. Speech-Lang.-Hearing Assoc. (1981).

Brutten, G. J., and Miller, R., The disfluencies of normally fluent black first graders. *J. Fluency Dis., 13*, 291–99 (1988).

Brutten, G. J., and Shoemaker, D. J., Stuttering: The disintegration of speech due to conditioned negative emotion. In Gray, B. B., and England, G. (eds), *Stuttering and the Conditioning Therapies*. Monterey, Calif.: Monterey Inst. Speech Hearing (1969).

Brutten, G. J., and Trotter, A. C., Hemispheric interference: A dual-task investigation of youngsters who stutter. *J. Fluency Dis., 10*, 77–85 (1985).

Brutten, G. J., and Trotter, A. C., A dual-task investigation of young stutterers and nonstutterers. *J. Fluency Dis., 11*, 275–84 (1986).

Bryngelson, B., A photophonographic analysis of the vocal disturbances in stuttering. *Psychol. Monogr., 43*, 1–30 (1932).

Bryngelson, B., Sidedness as an etiological facgtor in stuttering. *J. Genet. Psychol., 47*, 204–17 (1935).

Bryngelson, B., A study of laterality of stutterers and normal speakers. *J. Speech Dis., 4*, 231–34 (1939).

Bryngelson, B., and Brown, S. F., Season of birth of speech defectives in Minnesota. *J. Speech Dis., 4*, 319–22 (1939).

Bryngelson, B., and Rutherford, B., A comparative study of laterality of stutterers and non-stutterers. *J. Speech Dis., 2*, 15–16 (1937).

Bullen, A. K., A cross-cultural approach to the problem of stuttering. *Child Dev., 16*, 1–88 (1945).

Burdin, L. G., A survey of speech defectives in the Indianapolis primary grades. *J. Speech Dis., 5*, 247–58 (1940).

Burgraff, R. I., The efficacy of systematic desensitization via imagery as a therapeutic technique with stutterers. *Brit. J. Dis. Communic., 9*, 134–39 (1974).

Burke, B. D. Reduced auditory feedback and stuttering. *Behav. Res. Ther., 7*, 303–08 (1969).

Burke, B. D., Variables affecting stutterers' initial reactions to delayed auditory feedback. *J. Communic. Dis., 8*, 141–55 (1975).

Burleson, D. E., A personality study of fourth, fifth and sixth grade stutterers and non-stutterers based on the Bender Visual Motor Gestalt Test. *Speech Monogr., 18,* 238 (1951). Abstract.

Burley, P. M., and Morely, R., Self-monitoring processes in stutterers. *J. Fluency Dis., 12,* 71–8 (1987).

Burley, P. M., and Rinaldi, W., Effects of sex of listener and of stutterer on ratings of stuttering speakers. *J. Fluency Dis., 11,* 329–33 (1986).

Burns, D., Brady, J. P., and Kuruvilla, K., The acute effect of haloperidol and apomorphine on the severity of stuttering. *Biolog. Psychiat., 13,* 255–64 (1978).

Burr, H. G., and Mullendore, J. M., Recent investigations on tranquilizers and stuttering. *J. Speech Hearing Dis., 25,* 33–37 (1960).

Buscaglia, L. F., An experimental study of the Sarbin-Hardyck Test as indexes of role perception for adolescent stutterers. *Speech Monogr., 30,* 243 (1963). Abstract.

Busse, E. W., and Clark, R. M., The use of the electroencephalogram in diagnosing speech disorders in children. *Folia Phoniat., 9,* 182–87 (1957).

Byrd, K., and Cooper, E. B., Apraxic speech characteristics in stuttering, developmentally apraxic, and normal speaking children. *J. Fluency Dis., 14,* 215–29 (1989a).

Byrd, K., and Cooper, E. B., Expressive and receptive language skills in stuttering children. *J. Fluency Dis., 14,* 121–26 (1989b).

Cabañas, R., Some findings in speech and voice therapy among mentally deficient children. *Folia Phoniat., 6,* 34–39 (1954).

Cacudi, G., Effeti di un psicofarmaco (tioridazina) nella practica pedopsichiatrica. Turbe funzionali del linguaggio. *Infanz. Anorm., 60,* 861–68 (1964).

Cali, G., Pisana, F., and Tagliareni, F., Balbuzie e rilievi elettroencefalografici. *Clin. ORL, 17,* 316–28 (1965).

Canter, G. J., Observations on neurogenic stuttering: A contribution to differential diagnosis. *Brit. J. Dis. Communic., 6,* 139–43 (1971).

Caplan, L., An investigation of some aspects of stuttering-like speech in adult dysphasic subjects. *J. So. Afr. Speech Hearing Assoc., 19,* 52–66 (1972).

Card, R. E., A study of allergy in relation to stuttering. *J. Speech Dis., 4,* 223–30 (1939).

Carlson, J. J., Psychosomatic study of fifty stuttering children: III. Analysis of responses on the Revised Stanford-Binet. *Amer. J. Orthopsychiat., 16,* 120–26 (1946).

Carp, F. M., Psychosexual development of stutterers. *J. Project. Techniques, 26,* 388–91 (1962).

Carpenter, M., and Sommers, R. K., Unisensory and bisensory perceptual and memory processing in stuttering adults and normal speakers. *J. Fluency Dis., 12,* 291–304 (1987).

Caruso, A. J., Abbs, J. H., and Gracco, V. L., Kinematic analysis of multiple movement coordination during speech in stutterers. *Brain, 111,* 439–55 (1988).

Caruso, A. J., Conture, E. G., and Colton, R. H., Selected temporal parameters of coordination associated with stuttering in children. *J. Fluency Dis., 13,* 57–82 (1988).

Caruso, A. J., Gracco, V. L., and Abbs, J. H., A speech motor control perspective on stuttering: Preliminary observations. In Peters, H. F. M., and Hulstijn, W. (eds.), *Speech Motor Dynamics in Stuttering*. New York: Springer (1987).

Castellini, V., Salami, A., and Ottoboni, A., Ricerche elettronistagmografiche in soggetti balbuzienti. *Minerva ORL, 22*, 119–25 (1972).

Cecconi, C. P., Hood, S. B., and Tucker, R. K., Influence of reading level difficulty on the disfluencies of normal children. *J. Speech Hearing Res., 20*, 475–84 (1977).

Cerf, A., and Prins, D., Stutterers' ear preference for dichotic syllables. *Asha, 16*, 566–67 (1974). Abstract.

Chaney, C. F., Loci of disfluencies in the speech of nonstutterers. *J. Speech Hearing Res., 12*, 667–68 (1969).

Chapman, A. H., and Cooper, E. B., Nature of stuttering in a mentally retarded population. *Amer. J. Ment. Defic., 78*, 153–57 (1973).

Chase, R. A., Effect of delayed auditory feedback on the repetition of speech sounds. *J. Speech Hearing Dis., 23*, 583–90 (1958).

Chase, R. A., and Sutton, S., Reply to: "Masking of auditory feedback in stutterers' speech." *J. Speech Hearing Res., 11*, 222–23 (1968).

Chase, R. A., Sutton, S., and Rapin, I. Sensory feedback influences on motor performance. *J. Aud. Res., 1*, 212–23 (1961).

Checiek, M. S., Ergebnisse der psychophysiologischen Therapiemethode bei stotternden Kindern und Jugendlicen im Alter von 7-18 Jahren. *Folia Phoniat., 35*, 115 (1983). Abstract.

Cherry, C., and Sayers, B., Experiments upon the total inhibition of stammering by external control and some clinical results. *J. Psychosomat. Res., 1*, 233–46 (1956).

Cherry, C., Sayers, B., and Marland, P. M., Experiments on the complete suppression of stammering. *Nature, 176*, 874–75 (1955).

Chmelová, A., Kujalová, V., Sedláčková, E., and Zelený, A., Neurohumorale Reaktionen bei Stotterern und Polterern. *Folia Phoniat., 27*, 283–86 (1975).

Christensen, A. H., A quantitative study of personality dynamics in stuttering and nonstuttering siblings. *Speech Monogr., 19*, 144–145 (1952). Abstract.

Christensen, J. E., and Lingwall, J. B., Verbal contingent stimulation of stuttering in laboratory and home settings. *J. Fluency Dis., 7*, 359–68 (1982).

Christensen, J. E., and Lingwall, J. B., The relationship between treatment exposure times and changes in stuttering frequency during contingent stimulation. *J. Fluency Dis., 8*, 275–81 (1983).

Chworowski, C. R., A comparative study of the diadochokinetic rates of stutterers and nonstutterers in speech related and non-speech related movements. *Speech Monogr., 19*, 192 (1952). Abstract.

Ciambrone, S. W., Adams, M. R., and Berkowitz, M. A correlational study of stutterers' adaptation and voice initiation times. *J. Fluency Dis., 8*, 29–37 (1983).

Cimorell-Strong, J. M., Gilbert, H. R., and Frick, J. V., Dichotic speech perception: A comparison between stuttering and nonstuttering children. *J. Fluency Dis., 8*, 77–91 (1983).

Clifford, S., Twitchell, M., and Hull, R. H., Stuttering in South Dakota Indians. *Central States Speech J., 16*, 59–60 (1965).

Cohen, E., A comparison of oral [reading] and spontaneous speech of stutterers with special reference to the adaptation and consistency effects. *Speech Monogr., 20*, 144–45 (1953). Abstract.

Cohen, L. R., Thompson, P. F., Ruppel, R. W., and Flaherty, R. P., Assertive training: An adjunct to fluency shaping. *J. Fluency Dis., 1*, 10–25 (1975).

Cohen, M. S., and Hanson, M. L., Intersensory processing efficiency of fluent speakers and stutterers. *Brit. J. Dis. Communic., 10*, 111–22 (1975).

Colburn, N., Clustering of disfluency in nonstuttering children's early utterances. *J. Fluency Dis., 10*, 51–58 (1985).

Colburn, N., and Mysak, E. D., Developmental disfluency and emerging grammar. I. Disfluency characteristics in early syntactic utterances. *J. Speech Hearing Res., 25*, 414–20 (1982a).

Colburn, N., and Mysak, E. D., Developmental disfluency and emerging grammar. II. Co-occurrence of disfluency with specified semantic-syntactic structures. *J. Speech Hearing Res., 25*, 421–27 (1982b).

Colcord, R. D., and Adams, M. R., Voicing duration and vocal SPL changes associated with stuttering reduction during singing. *J. Speech Hearing Res., 22*, 468–79 (1979).

Colcord, R. D., and Gregory, H. H., Perceptual analyses of stuttering and nonstuttering children's fluent speech productions. *J. Fluency Dis., 12*, 185–95 (1987).

Collins, C. R., and Blood, G. W., Acknowledgment and severity of stuttering as factors influencing nonstutterers' perceptions of stuttering. *J. Speech Hearing Dis., 55*, 75–81 (1990).

Comas, R. C., Tartamudez o espasmofemia funcional. Relato y aportes conceptuales. *Rev. Cubana Pediat., 46*, 595–605 (1974).

Comas, R. C., Incidencia de espasmofemia functional (tartamudez) durante la rehabilitación del fisurado palatino. *dsh Abstr., 15*, 393 (1975).

Commodore, R. W., Communicative stress and stuttering frequency during normal, whispered and articulation-without-phonation speech modes: A further study. *Human Communic., 5*, 143–50 (1980).

Commodore, R. W., and Cooper, E. B., Communicative stress and stuttering frequency during normal, whispered, and articulation-without-phonation speech modes. *J. Fluency Dis., 3*, 1–12 (1978).

Connett, M. H., Experimentally induced changes in the relative frequency of stuttering on a specified speech sound. In Johnson, W., and Leutenneger, R. R. (eds.), *Stuttering in Children and Adults*. Minneapolis: Univ. Minn. Press (1955).

Conradi, E., Psychology and pathology of speech development in the child. *Pedagog. Sem., 11*, 328–80 (1904).

Conradi, E., Speech defects and intellectual progress. *J. Educ. Psychol., 3*, 35–38 (1912).

Conture, E. G., Some effects of noise on the speaking behavior of stutterers. *J. Speech Hearing Res., 17*, 714–23 (1974).

Conture, E. G., and Brayton, E. R., The influence of noise on stutterers' different disfluency types. *J. Speech Hearing Res., 18*, 381–84 (1975).

Conture, E. G., Colton, R. H., and Gleason, J. R., Selected temporal aspects of coordination during fluent speech of young stutterers. *J. Speech Hearing Res., 31,* 640–53 (1988).

Conture, E. G., and Kelly, E. M., Young stutterers' nonspeech behavior during stuttering. *J. Speech Hearing Res., 34,* 1041–56 (1991).

Conture, E. G., McCall, G. N., and Brewer, D. W., Laryngeal behavior during stuttering. *J. Speech Hearing Res., 20,* 661–68 (1977).

Conture, E. G., Rothenberg, M., and Molitar, R. D., Electroglottographic observations of young stutterers' fluency. *J. Speech Hearing Res., 29,* 384–93 (1986).

Conture, E. G., Schwartz, H. D., and Brewer, D. W., Laryngeal behavior during stuttering: A further study. *J. Speech Hearing Res., 28,* 233–40 (1985).

Conture, E. G., and van Naerssen, E., Reading abilities of school-age stutterers. *J. Fluency Dis., 2,* 295–300 (1977).

Conway, J. K., and Quarrington, B., Positional effects in the stuttering of contextually organized verbal material. *J. Abnorm. Soc. Psychol., 67,* 299–303 (1963).

Cookson, I. B., and Wells, P. G., Haloperidol in the treatment of stutterers. *Brit. J. Psychiat., 123,* 491 (1973).

Cooper, C. S., and Cooper, E. B., Variations in adult stutterer attitudes towards clinicians during therapy. *J. Communic. Dis., 2,* 141–53 (12969).

Cooper, E. B., Client-clinician relationships and concomitant factors in stuttering therapy. *J. Speech Hearing Res., 9,* 194–207 (1966).

Cooper, E. B., A therapy process for the adult stutterer. *J. Speech Hearing Dis., 33,* 246–60 (1968).

Cooper, E. B., Integrating behavior therapy and traditional insight treatment procedures with stutterers. *J. Communic. Dis., 4,* 40–43 (1971).

Cooper, E. B., Recovery from stuttering in a junior and senior high school population. *J. Speech Hearing Res., 15,* 632–38 (1972).

Cooper, E. B., Personalized fluency control therapy: A status report. In Peins, M. (ed.), *Contemporary Approaches in Stuttering Therapy.* Boston: Little, Brown (1984).

Cooper, E. B., Cady, B. B., and Robbins, C. J., The effect of the verbal stimulus words wrong, right, and tree on the disfluency rates of stutterers and nonstutterers. *J. Speech Hearing Res., 13,* 239–44 (1970).

Cooper, E. B., Parris, R., and Wells, M. T., Prevalence of and recovery from speech disorders in a group of freshmen at the University of Alabama. *Asha, 16,* 359–60 (1974). Abstract.

Cooper, M. H., and Allen, G. D., Timing control accuracy in stutterers and non-stutterers. *J. Speech Hearing Res., 20,* 55–71 (1977).

Coppa, A., and Bar, A., Use of questions to elicit adaptation in the spontaneous speech of stutterers and nonstutterers. *Folia Phoniat., 26,* 378–88 (1974).

Coppola, V. A., and Yairi, E., Rhythmic speech training with preschool stuttering children: An experimental study. *J. Fluency Dis., 7,* 447–57 (1982).

Corcoran, J. A., Jr., Effects of neutral and positive stimuli on stuttering: "Calling attention to stuttering" revisited. *J. Fluency Dis., 5,* 99–114 (1980).

Cordes, A. K., Ingham, R. J., Frank, P., and Costello Ingham, J. Time-interval analysis of interjudge and intrajudge agreement for stuttering event judgments. *J. Speech Hearing Res., 35*, 483–94 (1992).

Cords, T., Untersuchung der lautdauer innerhalb eines Satzes bei Stottern mit Hilfe der kymographischen Aufnahme. *Vox, 22*, 70–75 (1936).

Coriat, I. H., Stammering. A psychoanalytic interpretation. *Nerv. Ment. Dis. Monogr., Ser. No. 47*, 1–68 (1928).

Coriat, I. H., The psychoanalytic conception of stammering. *Nerv. Child, 2*, 167–71 (1943).

Costello, J., The establishment of fluency with time-out procedures: Three case studies. *J. Speech Hearing Dis., 409*, 216–31 (1975).

Costello, J. M., Current behavioral treatments for children. In Prins, D., and Ingham, R. J. (eds.), *Treatment of Stuttering in Early Childhood*. San Diego: College-Hill Press (1983).

Costello, J. M., and Hurst, M. R., An analysis of the relationship among stuttering behaviors. *J. Speech Hearing Res., 24*, 247–56 (1981).

Côté, C., and Ladouceur, R., Effects of social aids and the regulated breathing method in the treatment of stutterers. *J. Consult. Clin. Psychol., 50*, 450 (1982).

Cox, M. D., The stutterer and stuttering: Neuropsychological correlates. *J. Fluency Dis., 7*, 129–40 (1982).

Cox, N. J., and Kidd, K. K., Can recovery from stuttering be considered a genetically milder subtype of stuttering? *Behavior Genetics, 13*, 129–39 (1983).

Cox, N. J., Kramer, P. L., and Kidd, K. K., Segregation analyses of stuttering. *Genetic Epidemiol., 1*, 245–53 (1984).

Cox, N. J., Seider, R. A., and Kidd, K. K., Some environmental factors and hypotheses for stuttering in families with several stutterers. *J. Speech Hearing Res., 27*, 543–48 (1984).

Coyle, M. M., and Mallard, A. R., Word-by-word analysis of observer agreement utilizing audio and audiovisual techniques. *J. Fluency Dis., 4*, 23–28 (1979).

Cozzo, G., and Gabrielli, L., La therapie du begayement avec les butyrophenones. *De Therapia Vocis et Loquelae, Vol. I.* XIII Congr. Int. Soc. Logoped. Phoniat. (1965)

Craig, A., An investigation into the relationship between anxiety and stuttering. *J. Speech Hearing Dis., 55*, 290–94 (1990).

Craig, A., and Andrews, G., The prediction and prevention of relapse in stuttering. The value of self-control techniques and locus of control measures. *Behav. Modification, 9*, 427–42 (1985).

Craig, A. R., and Calver, P., Following up on treated stutterers: Studies of perceptions of fluency and job status. *J. Speech Hearing Res., 34*, 279–84 (1991).

Craig, A. R., and Cleary, P. J., Reduction of stuttering by young male stutterers using EMG feedback. *Biofeedback and Self-Regulation, 7*, 241–55 (1982).

Craig, A. R., Franklin, J. A., and Andrews, G., A scale to measure locus of control behavior. *Brit. J. Med. Psychol., 57*, 173–80 (1984).

Craig, A. R., and Howie, P. M., Locus of control and maintenance of behavioral therapy skills. *Brit. J. Clin. Psychol., 21*, 65–66 (1982).

Craven, D. C., and Ryan, B. P., The use of a portable delayed auditory feed-back unit in stuttering therapy. *J. Fluency Dis.*, *9*, 237–43 (1984).

Cross, D. E., Effects of false increasing, decreasing, and true electromyographic biofeedback on the frequency of stuttering. *J. Fluency Dis.*, *2*, 109–16 (1977).

Cross, D. E., Finger reaction time of stuttering and nonstuttering children and adults. *Asha*, *20*, 730 (1978). Abstract.

Cross, D. E., Comparison of reaction time and accuracy measures of laterality for stutterers and normal speakers. *J. Fluency Dis.*, *12*, 271–86 (1987).

Cross, D. E., and Cooper, E. B., Self-versus investigator-administered presumed fluency reinforcing stimuli. *J. Speech Hearing Res.*, *19*, 241–46 (1976).

Cross, D. E., and Luper, H. L., Voice reaction time of stuttering and nonstuttering children and adults. *J. Fluency Dis.*, *4*, 59–77 (1979).

Cross, D. E., and Luper, H. L., Relation between finger reaction time and voice reactikon time in stuttering and nonstuttering children and adults. *J. Speech Hearing Res.*, *26*, 356–61 (1983).

Cross, D. E., and Olson, P. L., Articulatory-laryngeal interaction in stutterers and normal speakers: Effects of a bite-block on rapid voice initiation. *J. Fluency Dis.*, *12*, 407–18 (1987a).

Cross, D. E., and Olson, P., Interaction between jaw kinematics and voice onset for stutterers and nonstutterers in a VRT task. *J. Fluency Dis.*, *12*, 367–80 (1987b).

Cross, D. E., Shadden, B. B., and Luperr, H. L., Effects of stimulus ear presentation on the voice reaction time of adult stutterers and nonstutterers. *J. Fluency Dis.*, *4*, 45–58 (1979).

Cross, H. M., The motor capacities of stutterers. *Arch. Speech*, *7*, 112–32 (1936).

Cross, J., and Cooke, P. A., Vocal and manual reaction times of adult stutterers and nonstutterers. *Asha*, *21*, 693 (1979). Abstract.

Crowe, K. M., and Kroll, R. M., Response latency and response class for stutterers and nonstutterers as measured by a word-association task. *J. Fluency Dis.*, *16*, 35–54 (1991).

Crowe, T. A., and Cooper, E. B., Parental attitudes toward and knowlege of stuttering. *J. Communic. Dis.*, 10, 343–57 (1977).

Crowe, T. A., and Walton, J. H., Teacher attitudes toward stuttering. *J. Fluency Dis.*, *6*, 163–74 (1981).

Culatta, R., Bader, J., McCaslin, A., and Thomason, N., Primary-school stutterers: Have attitudes changed? *J. Fluency Dis.*, *10*, 87–91 (1985).

Culatta, R., and Sloan, A., The acquisition of the label "stuttering" by primary level schoolchildren. *J. Fluency Dis.*, *2*, 29–34 (1977).

Cullinan, W. L., Stability of adaptation in the oral performance of stutterers. *J. Speech Hearing Res.*, *6*, 70–83 (1963a).

Cullinan, W. L., Stability of consistency measures in stuttering. *J. Speech Hearing Res.*, *6*, 134–38 (1963b).

Cullinan, W. L., Consistency measures revisited. *J. Fluency Dis.*, *13*, 1–9 (1988).

Cullinan, W. L., and Prather, E. M., Reliability of "live" ratings of the speech of stutterers. *Percept. Mot. Skills*, *27*, 403–09 (1968).

Cullinan, W. L., Prather, E. M., and Williams, D. E., Comparison of procedures for scaling severity of stuttering. *J. Speech Hearing Res.*, *6*, 187–94 (1963).

Cullinan, W. L., and Springer, M. T., Voice initiation times in stuttering and nonstuttering children. *J. Speech Hearing Res., 23,* 344–60 (1980).

Culp, D. M., The preschool fluency development program: Assessment and treatment. In Peins, M. (ed.), *Contemporary Approaches in Stuttering Therapy.* Boston: Little, Brown (1984).

Culton, G. L., Speech disorders among college freshmen: A 13-year survey. *J. Speech Hearing Dis., 51,* 3–7 (1986).

Curlee, R. F., Observer agreement on disfluency and stuttering. *J. Speech Hearing Res., 24,* 595–600 (1981).

Curlee, R. F., Counseling with adults who stutter. In Perkins, W. H. (ed.), *Stuttering Disorders.* New York: Thieme-Stratton (1984).

Curlee, R. F., and Perkins, W. H., The effect of punishment of expectancy to stutter on the frequencies of subsequent expectancies and stuttering. *J. Speech Hearing Res., 11,* 787–95 (1968).

Curlee, R. F., and Perkins, W. H., Conversational rate control therapy for stuttering. *J. Speech Hearing Dis., 34,* 245–50 (1969).

Curlee, R. F., and Perkins, W. H., Effectiveness of a DAF conditioning program for adolescent and adult stutterers, *Behav. Res. Ther., 11,* 395–401 (1973).

Curran, M. F., and Hood, S. B., The effect of instructional bias on listener ratings of specific disfluency types in children. *J. Fluency Dis., 2,* 99–107 (1977a).

Curran, M. F., and Hood, S. B., Listener ratings of severity for specific disfluency types in children. *J. Fluency Dis., 2,* 87–97 (1977b).

Curry, F. K. W., and Gregory, H. H., The performance of stutterers on dichotic listening tasks thought to reflect cerebral dominance. *J. Speech Hearing Res., 12,* 73–82 (1969).

Curtis, J. F., A study of the effect of muscular exercise upon stuttering. *Speech Monogr., 9,* 61–74 (1942).

Curtis, J. F., Disorders of articulation. In Johnson, W., Brown, S. F., Curtis, J. F., Edney, C. W., and Keaster, J., *Speech Handicapped School Children, 3rd ed.* New York: Harper & Row (1967).

Cypreansen, L., Group therapy for adult stutterers. *J. Speech Hearing Dis., 13,* 313–19 (1948).

Cyprus, S., Hezel, R. T., Rossi, D., and Adams, M. R., Effects of simulated stuttering on listener recall. *J. Fluency Dis., 9,* 191–97 (1984).

Dabul, B., and Perkins, W. H., The effects of stuttering on systolic blood pressure. *J. Speech Hearing Res., 16,* 586–91 (1973).

Dahlstrom, W. G., and Craven, D. D., The MMPI and stuttering phenomena in young adults. *Amer. Psychol., 7,* 341 (1952). Abstract.

Dalali, I. D., and Sheehan, J. G., Stuttering and assertion training. *J. Communic. Dis., 7,* 97–111 (1974).

Dale, P., Factors related to dysfluent speech in bilingual Cuban-American adolescents. *J. Fluency Dis., 2,* 311–13 (1977).

Daly, D. A., and Cooper, E. B., Rate of stuttering adaptation under two electroshock conditions. *Behav. Res. Ther., 5,* 49–54 (1967).

Daly, D.A., and Frick, J. V., The effects of punishing stuttering expectations and stuttering utterances: A comparative study. *Behav. Ther., 1,* 228–39 (1970).

Daly, D. A., and Kimbarow, M. L., Stuttering as operant behavior: Effects of the verbal stimuli *wrong, right,* and *tree* on the disfluency rates of school-age stutterers and nonstutterers. *J. Speech Hearing Res., 21,* 589–97 (1978).

Daniels, E. M., An analysis of the relation between handedness and stuttering with special reference to the Orton-Travis theory of cerebral dominance. *J. Speech Dis., 5,* 309–26 (1940).

Danzger, M., and Halpern, H., Relation of stuttering to word abstraction, part of speech, word length, and word frequency. *Percept. Mot. Skills, 37,* 959–62 (1973).

Darley, F. L., *A Normative Study of Oral Reading Rate.* M. A. Thesis, Univ. Iowa (1940).

Darley, F. L., The relationship of parental atitudes and adjustments to the development of stuttering. In Johnson, W., and Leutenegger, R. R. (eds.), *Stuttering in Children and Adults.* Minneapolis: Univ. Minn. Press (1955).

Darley, F. L., and Spriesterbach, D. C., *Diagnostic Methods in Speech Pathology, 2nd ed.* New York: Harper & Row (1978).

Daskalov, D. D., K voprosu ob osnovnikh printsipakh i metodakh preduprezhdenia lechenia zaikania. Zh. Nevropatol. *Psikhiat., 62,* 1047–52 (1962).

Davenport, R. W., Dichotic listening in four severity levels of stuttering. *Asha, 21,* 769 (1979). Abstract.

Davis, D. M., The relation of repetitions in the speech of young children to certain measures of language maturity and situational factors: Part I. *J. Speech Dis., 4,* 303–18 (1939).

Davis, D. M., The relation of repetitions in the speech of young children to certain measures of language maturity and situational factors: Parts II & III. *J. Speech Dis., 5,* 235–46 (1940).

Deal, J. L., Sudden onset of stuttering: A case report. *J. Speech Hearing Dis., 47,* 301–03 (1982).

Dean, C. R., and Brown, R. A., A more recent look at the prevalence of stuttering in the United States. *J. Fluency Dis., 2,* 157–66 (1977).

Decker, T. N., Healey, E. C., and Howe, S. W., Brainstem auditory electrical response characteristics of stutterers and nonstutterers: A preliminary report. *J. Fluency Dis., 7,* 385–401 (1982).

DeJoy, D. A., and Gregory, H. H., The relationship of children's disfluencies to the syntax, length, and vocabulary of their sentences. *Asha, 15,* 472 (1973). Abstract.

DeJoy, D. A., and Gregory, H. H., The relationship of preschoolers' syntactic maturity to the frequency of specific disfluency types in their spontaneous speech. *Folia Phoniat., 28,* 219–20 (1976). Abstract.

DeJoy, D. A., and Gregory, H. H., The relationship between age and frequency of disfluency in preschool children. *J. Fluency Dis., 10,* 107–22 (1985).

DeJoy, D. A., and Jordan, W. J., Listener reactions to interjections in oral reading versus spontaneous speech. *J. Fluency Dis., 13,* 11–25 (1988).

Delaney, C. M., The function of the middle ear muscles in stuttering. *So. Afr. J. Communic. Dis., 26,* 20–34 (1979).

Dembrowski, J., and Watson, B. C., An instrumented method for assessment and remediation of stuttering: A single-subject case study. *J. Fluency Dis., 16,* 241–73 (1991a).

Dembrowski, J., and Watson, B. C., Preparation time and response complexity effects on stutterers' and nonstutterers' acoustic LRT. *J. Speech Hearing Res., 34,* 49–59 (1991b).

Dempsey, G. L., and Granich, M., Hypno-behavioral therapy in the case of a traumatic stutterer: A case study. *Int. J. Clin. Exper. Hypnosis, 26*, 125–33 (1978).

De Nil, L. F., and Abbs, J. H., Kinaesthetic acuity of stutterers and nonstutterers for oral and non-oral movements. *Brain, 114*, 2145–58 (1991).

De Nil, L., and Brutten, G. J., Stutterers and nonstutterers: A preliminary investigation of children's speech-associated attitudes. *Tijdschrift voor Logopedie en Audiologie, 16*, 85–90 (1986).

De Nil, L. F., and Brutten, G. J., Speech-associated attitudes of stuttering and nonstuttering children. *J. Speech Hearing Res., 34*, 60–66, (1991a).

De Nil, L. F., and Brutten, G. J., Voice onset times of stuttering and nonstuttering children: The influence of externally and linguistically imposed time pressure. *J. Fluency Dis., 16*, 143–58 (1991b).

Denny, M., and Smith, A., Gradations in a pattern of neuromuscular activity associated with stuttering. *J. Speech Hearing Res., 35*, 1216–29 (1992).

DePlatero, D. M., La prueba del dibujo de la figura humana en el niño tardamudo. *dsh Abstr. ,9*, 94–95 (1969).

Derazne, J., Speech pathology in the U.S.S.R. In Rieber, R. W., and Brubaker, R. S. (eds.), *Speech Pathology*. Amsterdam: North Holland (1966).

Despert, J. L., Psychosomatic study of fifty stuttering children: I. Social, physical and psychiatric findings. *Amer. J. Orthopsychiat., 16*, 100–13 (1946).

Devore, J. E., Nandur, M. S., and Manning, W. H., Projective drawings and children who stutter. *J. Fluency Dis., 9*, 217–26 (1984).

Dewar, A., Dewar, A. D., and Anthony, J. F. K., The effect of auditory feedback masking on concomitants of stammering. *Brit J. Dis. Communic., 11*, 95–102 (1976).

Dewar, A., Dewar, A. D., Austin, W. T. S., and Brash, H. M., The long term use of an automatically triggered auditory feedback masking device in the treatment of stammering. *Brit. J. Dis. Communic., 14*, 219–29 (1979).

Dewar, A., Dewar, A. D., and Barnes, H. E., Automatic triggering of auditory feedback masking in stammering and cluttering. *Brit. J. Dis. Communic., 11*, 19–26 (1976).

Di Carlo, L. M., Katz, J., and Batkin, S., An exploratory investigation of the effect of meprobamate on stuttering behavior. *J. Nerv. Ment. Dis., 128*, 558–61 (1959).

Dickson, S., *An Application of the Blacky Test of a Study of the Psychosexual Development of Stutterers*. M. A. Thesis, Brooklyn Coll. (1954).

Dickson, S., Incipient stuttering and spontaneous remission of stuttered speech. *J. Communic. Dis., 4*, 99–110 (1971).

Dinnan, J. A., McGuiness, E., and Perrin, L., Auditory feedback—Stutterers versus nonstutterers. *J. Learn. Disabil., 3*, 209–13 (1970).

Di Simoni, F. G., Preliminary study of certain timing relationships in the speech of stutterers. *J. Acoust. Soc. Amer., 56*, 695–96 (1974).

Dixon, C. C., Stuttering adaptation in relation to assumed level of anxiety. In Johnson, W., and Leutenegger, R. R. (eds.), *Stuttering in Children and Adults*. Minneapolis: Univ. Minn. Press (1955).

Dixon, C. C., The effect of interjected nonpropositional verbalization during oral reading on stuttering frequency. *J. Educ. Res., 51*, 153–55 (1957).

Doms, M. C., and Lissens, D., Stuttering and the laryngectomee. In Lebrun, Y., and Hoops, R. (eds.), *Neurolinguistic Approaches to Stuttering*. The Hague: Mouton (1973).

Donath, J., Heilung des Stotterns mittels Hypnose. *Med. Welt, 2*, 1532–33 (1928).

Donnan, G. A., Stuttering as a manifestation of stroke. *Med. J. Australia, 66*, 44–45 (1979).

Donohue, I. R., Stuttering adaptation during three hours of continuous oral reading. In Johnson, W., and Leutenegger, R. R. (eds.), *Stuttering in Children and Adults*. Minneapolis: Univ. Minn. Press (1955).

Donovan, G., A new device for the treatment of stammering. *Brit. J. Dis. Communic., 6*, 86–88 (1971).

Doody, I., Kalinowski, J., Armson, J., and Stuart, A., Stereotypes of stutterers and nonstutterers in three rural communities in Newfoundland. *J. Fluency Dis., 18*, 363–73 (1993).

Dorman, M. F., and Porter, R. J., Jr., Hemispheric lateralization for speech perception in stutterers. *Cortext, 11*, 181–85 (1975).

Douglass, E., and Quarrington, B., The differentiation of interiorized and exteriorized secondary stuttering. *J. Speech Hearing Dis., 17*, 377–85 (1952).

Douglass, L. C., A study of bilaterally recorded electroencephalograms of adult stutterers. *J. Exper. Psychol., 32*, 247–65 (1943).

Douglass, R. L., An experimental electroencephalographic study of stimulus reaction in stutterers. *Speech Monogr., 19*, 146 (1952). Abstract.

Duffy, R. J., Hunt, M. F., Jr., and Giolas, T. G., Effects of four types of disfluency on listener reactions. *Folia Phoniat., 27*, 106–15 (1975).

Duncan, M. H., Home adjustment of stutterers versus nonstutterers. *J. Speech Hearing Dis., 14*, 255–59 (1949).

Dunlap, K., Habits: Their Making and Unmaking. New York: Liveright (1932).

Edgren, B., Leanderson, R., and Levi, L., A research programme on stuttering and stress. *Acta Otolaryngol., Suppl. No. 263*, 113–18 (1970).

Egland, G. O., Repetitions and prolongations in the speech of stuttering and nonstuttering children. In Johnson, W., and Leutenegger, R. R. (eds.), *Stuttering in Children and Adults*. Minneapolis: Univ. Minn. Press (1955).

Egolf, D. B., Shames, G. H., Johnson, P. R., and Kasprisin-Burelli, A., The use of parent-child interaction patterns in therapy for young stutterers. *J. Speech Hearing Dis., 37*, 222–32 (1972).

Egolf, D. B., Shames, G. H., and Seltzer, H. N., The effects of time-out on the fluency of stutterers in group therapy. *J. Communic. Dis., 4*, 111–18 (1971).

Eisenson, J. Some characteristics of the written speech of stutterers. *Pedagog. Sem., 50*, 457–58 (1937).

Eisenson, J., A perseverative theory of stuttering. In Eisenson, J. (ed.), *Stuttering: A Symposium*. New York: Harper & Row (1958).

Eisenson, J., Observations of the incidence of stuttering in a special culture. *Asha, 8*, 391–94 (1966).

Eisenson, J., Stuttering as perseverative behavior. In Eisenson, J. (ed.), *Stuttering: A Second Symposium*. New York: Harper & Row (1975).

Eisenson, J., and Horowitz, E. The influence of propositionality on stuttering. *J. Speech Dis., 10*, 193–97 (1945).

Eisenson, J., and Pastel, E., A study of the perseverating tendency in stutterers. *Quart. J. Speech, 22*, 626–31 (1936).

Eisenson, J., and Wells, C., A study of the influence of communicative responsibility in a choral speech situation for stutterers. *J. Speech Dis., 7*, 259–62 (1942).

Eisenson, J., and Winslow, C. N., The perseverating tendency in stutterers in a perceptual function. *J. Speech Dis., 3*, 195–98 (1938).

Elliott, S., and Williamson, C., An evaluation of a token reward system in the treatment of adolescent stammerers. *dsh Abstr., 13*, 296 (1973).

Emerick, L. L., Extensional definition and attitude toward stuttering. *J. Speech Hearing Res., 3*, 181–86 (1960).

Enger, N. C., Hood, S. B., and Shulman, B. B., Language and fluency variables in the conversational speech of linguistically advanced preschool and school-aged children. *J. Fluency Dis., 13*, 173–98 (1988).

Erickson, R. L., Assessing communication attitudes among stutterers. *J. Speech Hearing Res., 12*, 711–24 (1969).

Everhart, R. W., An investigation of stuttering in an individual as related to genetically transmitted factors. *Speech Monogr., 16*, 316 (1949). Abstract.

Evesham, M., and Fransella, F., Stuttering relapse: The effect of a combined speech and psychological reconstruction programme. *Brit. J. Dis. Communic., 20*, 237–48 (1985).

Evesham, M., and Huddleston, A. Teaching stutterers the skill of fluent speech as a preliminary to the study of relapse. *Brit. J. Dis. Communic., 18*, 31–38 (1983).

Fagan, L. B., The relation of dextral training to the onset of stuttering. *Quart. J. Speech, 17*, 73–76 (1931).

Fagan, L. B., A clinico-experimental approach to the reeducation of the speech of stutterers. *Psychol. Monogr., 43*, 53–66 (1932).

Fairbanks, G., Some correlates of sound difficulty in stuttering. *Quart. J. Speech, 23*, 67–69 (1937).

Fairbanks, G., Systematic research in experimental phonetics: 1. A theory of the speech mechanism as a servosystem. *J. Speech Hearing Dis., 19*, 133–39 (1954).

Fairbanks, G., Selective vocal effects of delayed auditory feedback. *J. Speech Hearing Dis., 20*, 333–46 (1955).

Fairbanks, G., and Guttman, N., Effects of delayed auditory feedback upon articulation. *J. Speech Hearing Res., 1*, 12–22 (1958).

Falck, F. J., Interrelationships among certain behavioral characteristics, age, sex, and duration of therapy in a group of stutterers. *Speech Monogr., 23*, 141–42 (1956). Abstract.

Falck, F. J., Lawler, P. S., and Yonovitz, A., Effects of stuttering on fundamental frequency. *J. Fluency Dis., 10*, 123–35 (1985).

Farber, S., *Identical Twins Reared Apart: A Reanalysis*. New York: Basic books (1981).

Farmer, A., and Brayton, E. R., Speech characteristics of fluent and dysfluent Down's syndrome adults. *Folia Phoniat., 31*, 284–90 (1979).

Fein, L. I., Stuttering as a cue related to the precipitation of moments of stuttering. *Asha, 12*, 456 (1970). Abstract.

Feldman, R. L., Self-disclosure in parents of stuttering children. *J. Communic. Dis., 9*, 227–34 (1976).

Felstein, J., Language analysis of stutterers. *Speech Monogr., 17*, 290 (1950). Abstract.

Fenichel, O., *The Psychoanalytic Theory of Neurosis.* New York: W. W. Norton (1945).

Ferrand, C. T., Gilbert, H. R., and Blood, G. W., Selected aspects of central processing and vocal motor function in stutterers and nonstutterers. *J. Fluency Dis., 16*, 101–15 (1991).

Few, L. R., and Lingwall, J. B., A further analysis of fluency within stuttered speech. *J. Speech Hearing Res., 15*, 356–63 (1972).

Fiedler, F. E., and Wepman, J. M., An exploratory investigation of the self-concept of stutterers. *J. Speech Hearing Dis., 16*, 110–14 (1951).

Fierman, E. Y., The roles of cues in stuttering adaptation. In Johnson, W., and Leutenegger, R. R. (eds.), *Stuttering in Children and Adults.* Minneapolis: Univ. Minn. Press (1955).

Finitzo, T., Pool, K. D., Freeman, F. J., Devous, M. D., and Watson, B. C., Cortical dysfunction in developmental stutterers. In Peters, H. F. M., Hulstijn, W., and Starkweather, C. W. (eds.), *Speech Motor Control and Stuttering.* Amsterdam: Elsevier (1991).

Finkelstein, P., and Weisberger, S. E., The motor proficiency of stutterers. *J. Speech Hearing Dis., 19*, 52–589 (1954).

Fish, C. H., and Bowling, E., Effect of amphetamines on speech defects in the mentally retarded. *Calif. Med., 96*, 109–11 (1962).

Fish, C. H., and Bowling, E., Stuttering: The effect of treatment with d-amphetamine and a tranquilizing agent, trifluoperazine. A preliminary report on an uncontrolled study. *Calif. Med., 103*, 337–39 (1965).

Fisher, M. N., Stuttering: A psychoanalytic view. *J. Contemporary Psychother., 2*, 124–27 (1970).

Fisher, M. S., Language patterns of pre-school children. *J. Exper. Educ., 1*, 70–85 (1932).

Fishman, H. C., A study of the efficacy of negative practice as a corrective for stammering. *J. Speech Dis., 2*, 67–72 (1937).

Fitch, J. L., and Batson, E. A., Hemispheric asymmetry of alpha wave suppression in stutterers and nonstutterers. *J. Fluency Dis., 14*, 47–55 (1989).

Fitzgerald, H. E., Cooke, P. A., and Greiner, J. R., Speech and bimanual hand organization in adult stutterers and nonstutterers. *J. Fluency Dis., 9*, 51–65 (1984).

Fitzpatrick, J. A., An investigation of the body image in secondary stutterers revealed through self-drawings. *Speech Monogr., 27*, 240 (1960). Abstract.

Flanagan, B., Goldiamond, I., and Azrin, N., Operant stuttering: The control of stuttering behavior through response-contingent consequences. *J. Exper. Anal. Behav., 1*, 173–77 (1958).

Flanagan, B., Goldiamond, I., and Azrin, N. H., Instatement of stuttering in normally fluent individuals through operant procedures. *Science, 130*, 979–81 (1959).

Fleischman, B. L., Stuttering and delinquency. *Speech Monogr., 13*, 110–11 (1946). Abstract.

Fletcher, J. M., An experimental study of stuttering. *Amer. J. Psychol., 25,* 201–55 (1914).

Floyd, S., and Perkins, W. H., Early syllable dysfluency in stutterers and non-stutterers: A preliminary report. *J. Communic. Dis., 7,* 279–82 (1974).

Flügel, F., Erhebungen von Persönlichekitsmerkmalen an Müttern stotternder Kinder und Jugendlicher. *dsh Abstr., 19,* 226 (1979).

Font, M. M., A comparison of the free associations of stutterers and nonstutters. In Johnson, W., and Leutenegger, R. R. (eds.), *Stuttering in Children and Adults.* Minneapolis: Univ. Minn. Press (1955).

Forster, D. C., and Webster, W. G., Concurrent task interference in stutterers: dissociating hemispheric specialization and activation. *Canad. J. Psychol., 45,* 321–35 (1991).

Forte, M., and Schlesinger, I. M., Stuttering as a function of time of expectation. *J. Communic. Dis., 5,* 347–58 (1972).

Fossler, H. R., Disturbances in breathing during stuttering. *Psychol. Monogr., 40,* 1–32 (1930).

Fowlie, G. M., and Cooper, E. B., Traits attributed to stuttering and nonstuttering children by their mothers. *J. Fluency Dis., 3,* 233–46 (1978).

Fox, D. R., Electroencephalographic analysis during stuttering and nonstuttering. *J. Speech Hearing Res., 9,* 488–97 (1966).

Franck, R., Integration of an intensive program for stutterers within the normal activities of a major acute hospital. *Aust. J. Human Communic. Dis., 8,* 4–15 (1980).

Frank, A., and Bloodstein, O., Frequency of stuttering following repeated unison readings. *J. Speech Hearing Res., 14,* 519–24 (1971).

Franke, U., Geschlechter Verhältnis und Geschwisterposition bei sprachaufälligen Kindern. *Sprachheilarb., 28,* 8–16 (1983).

Franken, M. C., Boves, L., Peters, H. F. M., and Webster, R. L. Prosodic features in the speech of post-therapy stutterers compared with the speech of nonstutterers. In Peters, H. F. M., Hulstijn, W., and Starkweather, C. W. (eds.), *Speech Motor Control and Stuttering.* Amsterdam: Elsevier (1991).

Franken, M. C., Boves, L., Peters, H. F. M., and Webster, R. L., Perceptual evaluation of the speech before and after fluency shaping stuttering therapy. *J. Fluency Dis., 17,* 223–41 (1992).

Fransella, F., An experimental evaluation of the speech correction semantic differential. *Speech Monogr., 32,* 488–51 (1965).

Fransella, F., Rhythm as a distractor in the modification of stuttering. *Behav. Res. Ther., 5,* 253–55 (1967).

Fransella, F., Self concepts and the stutterer. *Brit. J. Psychiat., 114,* 1531–35 (1968).

Fransella, F., Stuttering: Not a symptom but a way of life. *Brit. J. Dis. Communic., 5,* 22–29 (1970).

Fransella, F., The "rhythm effect" in stuttering as a function of predictability of utterance. *Behav. Res. Ther., 9,* 265–71 (1971).

Fransella, F., Personal Change and Reconstruction. London: Academic (1972).

Fransella, F., and Beech, H. R., An experimental analysis of the effect of rhythm on the speech of stutterers. *Behav. Res. Ther., 3,* 195–201 (1965).

Frasier, J., An exploration of stutterers' theories of their own stuttering. In Johnson, W., and Leutenegger, R. R. (eds.), *Stuttering in Children and Adults.* Minneapolis: Univ. Minn. Press (1955).

Frayne, H., Coates, S., and Marriner, N., Evaluation of post treatment fluency by naive subjects. Aust. *J. Human Communic. Dis., 5,* 48–54 (1977).

Freeman, F. J., Phonation in stuttering: A review of current research. *J. Fluency Dis., 4,* 78–89 (1979).

Freeman, F. J., Laryngeal muscle activity of stutterers. In Curlee, R. F., and Perkins, W. H. (eds.), *Nature and Treatment of Stuttering: New Directions.* San Diego: College-Hill Press (1984).

Freeman, F. J., and Rosenfield, D. B., "Source" in dysfluency. *J. Fluency Dis., 7,* 295–96 (1982).

Freeman, F. J., and Ushijima, T., Laryngeal activity accompanying the moment of stuttering: A preliminary report of EMG investigations. *J. Fluency Dis., 1,* 36–45 (1975).

Freeman, F. J., and Ushijima, T., Laryngeal muscle activity during stuttering. *J. Speech Hearing Res., 21,* 538–62 (1978).

Freestone, N. W., An electroencephalographic study on the moment of stuttering. *Speech Monogr., 9,* 28–60 (1942).

Freund, H., Über inneres Stottern. Zeitschr. *Ges. Neurol. Psychiat., 151,* 585–98 (1934a).

Freund, H., Zur Frage der Beziehungen zwischen Stottern und Poltern. Monatsschr. Ohrenheilk. *Laryngol. Rhinol., 68,* 1446–57 (1934b).

Freund, H., Psychosis and stuttering. J. Nerv. Ment. Dis., 122, 161–72 (1955).

Freund, H., *Psychopathology and the Problems of Stuttering.* Springfield, Ill.: Charles C. Thomas (1966).

Frick, J. V., *An Exploratory Study of the Effect of Punishment (Electric Shock) Upon Stuttering Behavior.* Ph.D. Dissert., Univ. Iowa (1951).

Frick, J. V., Spontaneous recovery of the stuttering response as a function of the degree of adaptation. In Johnson, W., and Leutenegger, R. R. (eds.), *Stuttering in Children and Adults.* Minneapolis: Univ. Minn. Press (1955).

Frick, J. V., Evaluation of motor planning techniques for the treatment of stuttering. Asha, 7, 377 (1965). Abstract.

Friedman, S., *Diadochocinesis of the Breathing Mechanism of Stutterers and Nonstutterers.* M. A. Thesis, Brooklyn Coll. (1955).

Fritzell, B., The prognosis of stuttering in schoolchildren: A 10-year longitudinal study. In *Proc. XVI Congr. Int. Soc. Logoped. Phoniat.* Basel: Karger (1976).

Fritzell, B., Petersén, I., and Selldén, U., An EEG study of stuttering and nonstuttering school children. *De Therapia Vocis et Loquelae, Vol. I.* XIII Congr. Int. Soc. Logoped. Phoniat. (1965).

Froeschels, E., Beitrage zur Symptomatologie des Stotterns. *Monatsschr. Ohrenheilk., 55,* 1109–12 (1921).

Froeschels, E., Pathology and therapy of stuttering. *Nerv. Child, 2,* 148–61 (1943).

Froeschels, E., A technique for stutterers—"ventriloquism." *J. Speech Hearing Dis., 15,* 336–37 (1950).

Froeschels, E., and Rieber, R. W., The problem of auditory and visual imperceptivity in stutterers. *Folia Phoniat., 15,* 13–20 (1963).

Fruewald, E., Intelligence rating of severe college stutterers compared with that of others entering universities. *J. Speech Dis., 1,* 47–51 (1936).

Fucci, D., Petrosino, L., Gorman, P., and Harris, D., Vibrotactile magnitude production scaling: A method for studying sensory-perceptual responses of stutterers and fluent speakers. *J. Fluency Dis.*, *10*, 69–75 (1985).

Fujita, K., Eguchi, C., Hirose, H., Shigeki, S., and Sakai, Y. [Clinical and experimental studies on the effectiveness of chlordiazepoxide in speech disorders.] *Otolaryngol.* (Tokyo), 35, 89–97 (1963). English abstract.

Fukawa, T., Yoshioka, H., Ozawa, E., and Yoshida, S., Difference of susceptibility to delayed auditory feedback between stutterers and nonstutterers. *J. Speech Hearing Res.*, *31*, 475–79 (1988).

Gaines, N. D., Runyan, C. M., and Meyers, S. C., A comparison of young stutterers' fluent versus stuttered utterances on measures of length and complexity. *J. Speech Hearing Res.*, *34*, 37–42 (1991).

Galamon, T., Szulc-Kuberska, J., and Tronczyńska, J., The disturbances of histidine metabolism in hereditary stammering. *Folia Phoniat.*, *21*, 449–53 (1969).

Garber, S. F., and Martin, R. R., The effects of white noise on the frequency of stuttering. *J. SpeechHearing Res.*, *17*, 73–79 (1974).

Garber, S. F., and Martin, R. R., Effects of noise and increased vocal intensity on stuttering. *J. Speech Hearing Res.*, *20*, 233–40 (1977).

Gardner, W. H., Study of the pupillary reflex with special reference to stuttering. *Psychol. Monogr.*, *49*, 1–31 (1937).

Gately, W. G., The effects of generalized anxiety on listeners' responses to dysfluent speech. *Speech Monogr.*, *34*, 302–03 (1967). Abstract.

Gattuso, R., and Leocata, A., L'Haloperidol nella terapia della balbuzie. *Clin. ORL*, *14*, 227–34 (1962).

Gautheron, B., Liorzou, A., Even, C., and Valencien, B., The role of the larynx in stuttering. In Lebrun, Y., and Hoops, R. (eds.), *Neurolinguistic Approaches to Stuttering*. The Hague: Mouton (1973).

Gemelli, R. J., Classification of child stuttering: Part I. Transient developmental, neurogenic acquired, and persistent child stuttering. *Child Psychiat. Human Dev.*, *12*, 220–53 (1982a).

Gemelli, R. J., Classification of child stuttering: Part II. Persistent late onset male stuttering, and treatment issues for persistent stutterers—psychotherapy or speech therapy, or both? *Child Psychiat. Human Dev.*, *13*, 3–34 (1982b).

Gendelman, E. G., Confrontation in the treatment of stuttering. *J. Speech Hearing Dis.*, *42*, 85–89 (1977).

Geniesse, H., Stuttering. *Science*, *82*, 518 (1935).

Gens, G. W., Correlation of neurological findings, psychological analyses and speech disorders among institutionalized epileptics. *Train. Sch. Bull.*, *47*, 3–18 (1950).

Geschwind, N., and Behan, P., Left-handedness: Association with immune disease, migraine, and developmental learning disorder. *Proc. Natl. Acad. Sci.*, *79*, 5097–100 (1982).

Geschwind, N., and Behan, P. O., Laterality, hormones, and immunity. In Geschwind, N., and Galaburda, A. M. (eds.), *Cerebral Dominance: The Biological Foundations*. Cambridge, Mass.: Harvard Univ. Press (1984).

Geschwind, N., and Galaburda, A. M., Cerebral lateralization: Biological mechanisms, associations, and pathology: I. A hypothesis and a program for research. *Arch. Neurol.*, *42*, 429–59 (1985).

Gibney, N. J., Delayed auditory feedback: Changes in the volume intensity and the delay interval as variables affecting the fluency of stutterers' speech. *Brit. J. Psychol., 64*, 55–63 (1973).

Gifford, M. F., *Correcting Nervous Speech Disorders.* New York: Prentice-Hall (1940).

Gildston, P., *Stuttering and Delinquency: A Study of the Possible Relationship Between Repressed Hostility and Stuttering.* M. A. Thesis, Queens Coll. (1959).

Gildston, P., Stutterers' self-acceptance and perceived parental acceptance. *J. Abnorm. Psychol., 72*, 59–64 (1967).

Gillespie, S. K., and Cooper, E. B., Prevalence of speech problems in junior and senior high schools. *J. Speech Hearing Res., 16*, 739–43 (1973).

Giolas, T. G., and Williams, D. E., Children's reactions to nonfluencies in adult speech. *J. Speech Hearing Res., 1*, 86–93 (1958).

Girone, D., and Bruno, G., Some characteristics of the glycemic curve in stutterers. *Folia Phoniat., 9*, 87–91 (1957).

Gladstien, K. L., Seider, R. A., and Kidd, K. K., Analysis of the sibship patterns of stutterers. *J. Speech Hearing Res., 24*, 460–62 (1981).

Glasner, P. J., and Rosenthal, D., Parental diagnosis of stuttering in young chidren. *J. Speech Hearing Dis., 22*, 288–95 (1957).

Glassmann, D. M., *Personality Characteristics of the Stutterer As Revealed Through Projective Figure Drawings.* M. A. Thesis, Brooklyn Coll. (1967).

Glauber, I. P., *The psychoanalysis of stuttering.* In Eisenson, J. (ed.), Stuttering: A symposium. New York: Harper & Row (1958).

Glogowski, K., 1st das Stottern erbbedingt? *Folia Phoniat., 28*, 235–36 (1976). Abstract.

Godai, U., Tatarelli, R., and Bonanni, G., Stuttering and tics in twins. *Acta Geneticae Medicae et Gemellologiae, 25*, 369–75 (1976).

Gold, C., *Frequency of Stuttering Following Repeated Unison Readings: A Replication of Frank and Bloodstein (1971).* M.A. Project, Univ. Minn. (1994).

Goldiamond, I., Stuttering and fluency as manipulatable operant response classes. In Krasner, L., and Ullmann, L. P. (eds.), *Research in Behavior Modification.* New York: Holt, Rinehart & Winston (1965).

Goldman, R., The use of Mellaril as an adjunct to the treatment of stuttering. *Excerpta Medica Int. Congr. Series No. 150.* Proc. IV World Congr. Psychiat. (1966).

Goldman, R., Cultural influences on the sex ratio in the incidence of stuttering. *Amer. Anthropologist, 69*, 78–81 (1967).

Goldman, R., and Guth, P., The effects of psychotherapeutic drugs on stuttering. *De Therapia Vocis et Loquelae, Vol. I.* XIII Congr. Int. Soc. Logoped. Phoniat. (1965).

Goldman, R., and Shames, G. H., Comparisons of the goals that parents of stutterers and parents of nonstutterers set for their children. *J. Speech Hearing Dis., 29*, 381–89 (1964a).

Goldman, R., and Shames, G. H., A study of goal-setting behavior of parents of stutterers and parents of nonstutterers. *J. Speech Hearing Dis., 29*, 192–94 (1964b).

Goldman-Eisler, F., The predictability of words in context and the length of pauses in speech. *Lang. Speech, 1*, 226–31 (1958a)

Goldman-Eisler, F., Speech production and the predictability of words in context. *Quart. J. Exper. Psychol., 10*, 96–106 (1958b).

Goldman-Eisler, F., A comparative study of two hesitation phenomena. *Lang. Speech, 4*, 18–26 (1961).

Goldsand, J. G., Sensory perseveration in stutterers and nonstutterers. *J. Speech Dis., 9*, 180 (1944). Abstract.

Golub, A., The cumulative effect of constant and varying reading material on stuttering adaptation. In Johnson, W., and Leutenegger, R. R. (eds.), *Stuttering in Children and Adults*. Minneapolis: Univ. Minn. Press (1955).

Golub, A. J., The heart rates of stutterers and nonstutterers in relation to frequency of stuttering during a series of oral readings. *Speech Monogr., 20*, 146–47 (1953). Abstract.

Goodall, H. B., and Brobby, G. W., Stuttering, sickling, and cerebral malaria: A possible organic basis for stuttering. *Lancet, 1* (8284), 1279–81 (1982).

Goodstein, L. D., MMPI profiles of stutterers' parents: A follow-up study. *J. Speech Hearing Dis., 21*, 430–35 (1956).

Goodstein, L. D., Functional speech disorders and personality: A survey of the research. *J. Speech Hearing Res., 1*, 359–76 (1958).

Goodstein, L. D., and Dahlstrom, W. G., MMPI differences between parents of stuttering and nonstuttering children. *J. Consult. Psychol., 20*, 365–70 (1956). Reproduced, with editorial adaptations, as Chapter 7 in Johnson, W. and Associates, *The Onset of Stuttering*. Minneapolis: Univ. Minn. Press (1959).

Gordon, E., Gordon, A., Gordon, L., Shapiro, M., Mentis, M., and Suchet, M., Biofeedback and stuttering. *So. Afr. J. Communic. Dis., 28*, 105–12 (1981).

Gordon, I., Allergy, enuresis, and stammering. *Brit. Med. J.*, Mar. 14, 357–58 (1942).

Gordon, P. A., Language task effects: A comparison of stuttering and nonstuttering children. *J. Fluency Dis., 16*, 275–87 (1991).

Gordon, P. A., and Luper, H. L., Speech disfluencies in nonstutterers: Syntactic complexity and production task effects. *J. Fluency Dis., 14*, 429–45 (1989).

Gordon, P. A., Luper, H. L., and Peterson, H. A., The effects of syntactic complexity on the occurrence of disfluencies in 5 year old stutterers. *J. Fluency Dis., 11*, 151–64 (1986).

Goss, A. E., Stuttering behavior and anxiety theory: I. Stuttering behavior and anxiety as a function of the duration of stimulus words. *J. Abnorm. Soc. Psychol., 47*, 38–50 (1952).

Goss, A. E., Stuttering behavior and anxiety as a function of experimental taining. *J. Speech Hearing Dis., 21*, 343–51 (1956).

Gottsleben, R. H., The incidence of stuttering in a group of mongoloids. *Train. Sch. Bull., 51*, 209–18 (1955).

Gould, E., and Sheehan, J., Effect of silence on stuttering. *J. Abnorm. Psychol., 72*, 441–45 (1967).

Gow, M. L., and Ingham, R. J., Modifying electroglottograph-identified intervals of phonation: The effect on stuttering. *J. Speech Hearing Res., 35*, 495–511 (1992).

Graf, O. I., Incidence of stuttering among twins. IN Johnson, W., and Leutenegger, r. R. (eds.), *Stuttering in Children and Adults*. Minneapolis: Univ. Minn. Press (1955).

Graham, J. K., A neurologic and electroencephalographic study of adult stutterers and matched normal speakers. *Speech Monogr., 33*, 290 (1966). Abstract.

Gray, B. B., Theoretical approximations of stuttering adaptation. *Behav. Res. Ther., 3*, 171–85 (1965a).

Gray, B., Theoretical approximations of stuttering adaptation: Statement of predictive accuracy. *Behav. Res. Ther., 3*, 221–27 (1965b).

Gray, B. B., and Brutten, E. J., The relationship between anxiety, fatigue and spontaneous recovery in stuttering. *Behav. Res. Ther., 2*, 251–59 (1965).

Gray, B. B., and England, G., Some effects of anxiety deconditioning upon stuttering frequency. J. *Speech Hearing Res., 15*, 114–22 (1972).

Gray, B. B., and Karmen, J. L., The relationship between nonverbal anxiety and stuttering adaptation. J. *Communic. Dis., 1*, 141–51 (1967).

Gray, K. C., and Williams, D. E., Anticipation and stuttering: A pupillographic study. J. *Speech Hearing Res., 12*, 833–39 (1969).

Gray, M., The X family: A clinical and laboratory study of a "stuttering" family. J. *Speech Dis., 5*, 343–48 (1940).

Greenberg, D., and Marks, I., Behavioural psychotherapy of uncommon referrals. *Brit. J. Psychiat., 141*, 148–53 (1982).

Greenberg, J. B., The effect of a metronome on the speech of young stutterers. *Behav. Ther., 1*, 240–44 (1970).

Greene, J. S., and Small, S. M., Psychosomatic factors in stuttering. *Med. Clinics North Amer., 28*, 615–28 (1944).

Gregory, H. H., Stuttering and auditory central nervous system disorder. J. *Speech Hearing Res., 7*, 335–41 (1964).

Gregory, H. H., An assessment of the results of stuttering therapy. J. *Communic. Dis., 5*, 320–34 (1972).

Gregory, H. H., and Hill, D., Stuttering therapy for children. In Perkins, W. H. (ed.), *Stuttering Disorders*. New York: Thieme-Stratton (1984).

Gregory, H. H., and Mangan, J., Auditory processes in stutterers. In Lass, N. J. (ed.), *Speech and Language: Advances in Basic Research and Practice, Vol. 7*. New York: Academic Press (1982).

Greiner, J. R., Fitzgerald, H. E., and Cooke, P. A., Bimanual hand writing in right-handed and left-handed stutterers and nonstutterers. *Neuropsychologia, 24*, 441–47 (1986a).

Greiner, J. R., Fitzgerald, H. E., and Cooke, P. A., Speech fluency and hand performance on a sequential tapping task in left- and right-handed stutterers and nonstutterers. J. *Fluency Dis., 11*, 55–69 (1986b).

Greiner, J. R., Fitzgerald, H. E., Cooke, P. A., and Djurdić, S. D., Assessment of sensitivity to interpersonal stress in stutterers and nonstutterers. J. *Communic. Dis., 18*, 215–25 (1985).

Griggs, S., and Still, A. W., An analysis of individual differences in words stutterered. J. *Speech Hearing Res. 22*, 572–80 (1979).

Gronhovd, K. D., A comparison of the fluent oral reading rates of stutterers and nonstutterers. J. *Fluency Dis., 2*, 247–52 (1977).

Gross, M. S., A study of the effects of punishment and reinforcement on the dysfluencies of stutterers. *Speech Monogr., 36*, 281 (1969). Abstract.

Gross, M. S., and Holland, A. L., The effects of response contingent electroshock upon stuttering. *Asha, 7*, 376 (1965). Abstract.

Grossman, D. J., A study of the parents of stuttering and non-stuttering children using the Minnesota Multiphasic Personality Inventory and the Minnesota Scale of Parents' Opinions. *Speech Monogr., 19*, 193–94 (1952). Abstract.

Gruber, L., and Powell, R. L., responses of stuttering and nonstuttering children to a dichotic listening task. *Percept. Mot. Skills, 38*, 263–64 (1974).

Guitar, B., Reduction of stuttering frequency using analog electromyographic feedback. *J. Speech Hearing Res., 18*, 672–85 (1975).

Guitar, B., Pretreatment factors associated with the outcome of stuttering therapy. *J. Speech Hearing Res., 19*, 590–60 (1976).

Guitar, B., Fluency shaping with young stutterers. *J. Childhood Communic. Dis., 6*, 50–59 (1982).

Guitar, B., and Bass, C., Stuttering therapy: The relation between attitude change and long-term outcome. *J. Speech Hearing Dis., 43*, 392–400 (1978).

Guitar, B., and Grims, S., Assessing attitudes of children who stutter. *Asha, 21*, 763 (1979). Abstract.

Guitar, B., Guitar, C., Neilson, P., O'Dwyer, N., and Andrews, G., Onset sequencing of selected lip muscles in stutterers and nonstutterers. *J. Speech Hearing Res., 31*, 28–35 (1988).

Guitar, B., and Peters, T. J., *Stuttering: An Integration of Contemporary Therapies.* Memphis: Speech Foundation of America (1980).

Guitar, B., Schaefer, H. K., Donahue-Kilburg, G., and Bond, L., Parent verbal interactions and speech rate: A case study in stuttering. *J. Speech Hearing Res., 35*, 742–54 (1992).

Guttman, N., Speech correction in the U.S.S.R. *J. Speech Hearing Dis., 25*, 306 (1960).

Gutzmann, H., *Das Stottern.* Frankfurt am Main: J. Rosenheim (1898).

Gutzmann, H., Die Atembewegung in ihrer Beziehung zu dem Sprachstörungen. Monatsschr. *Sprachheilk., 18*, 179–201 (1908).

Gutzmann, H., Versuche mit Glutamin-Behandlung bei Sprachstörungen aller Art. *Folia Phoniat., 6*, 1–8 (1954).

Hafford, J., A comparative study of the salivary pH of the normal speaker and stutterer. *J. Speech Dis., 6*, 173–84 (1941).

Hageman, C. F., and Greene, P. N., Auditory comprehension of stutterers on a competing message task. *J. Fluency Dis., 14*, 109–20 (1989).

Hahn, E. F., A study of the relationship between the social complexity of the oral reading situation and the severity of stuttering. *J. Speech Dis., 5*, 5–14 (1940).

Hahn, E. F., A study of the relationship between stuttering occurrence and grammatical factors in oral reading. *J. Speech Dis., 7*, 329–35 (1942a).

Hahn, E. F., A study of the relationship between stuttering occurrence and phonetic factors in oral reading. *J. Speech Dis., 7*, 143–51 (1942b).

Hale, L. L., A consideration of thiamin supplement in prevention of stuttering in preschool children. *J. Speech Hearing Dis., 16*, 327–33 (1951).

Hall, J. W., and Jerger, J., Central auditory function in stutterers. *J. Speech Hearing Res., 21,* 324–37 (1978).

Hall, K. D., and Yairi, E., Fundamental frequency, jitter, and shimmer in preschoolers who stutter. *J. Speech Hearing Res., 35,* 1002–8 (1992).

Hall, P. K., The occurrence of disfluencies in language-disordered school-age children. *J. Speech Hearing Dis., 42,* 364–69 (1977).

Halle, F., Über Störungen der Atmung bei Stotterern. Monatsschr. *Sprachheilk., 10,* 225–36 (1900).

Halvorson, J. A., The effects on stuttering frequency of pairing punishment (response cost) with reinforcement. *J. Speech Hearing Res., 14,* 356–64 (1971).

Ham, R., *Techniques of Stuttering Therapy.* Englewood Cliffs, N.J.: Prentice-Hall (1986).

Ham, R., Clinician preparation: Experiences with pseudostuttering. *J. Fluency Dis., 15,* 305–15 (1990a).

Ham, R. E., *Therapy of Stuttering, Preschool Through Adolescence.* Englewood Cliffs, N.J.: Prentice-Hall (1990b).

Ham, R. E., What is stuttering: Variations and stereotypes. *J. Fluency Dis., 15,* 259–73 (1990c).

Ham, R., and Steer, M. D., Certain effects of alterations in auditory feedback. *Folia Phoniat., 19,* 53–62 (1967).

Hamilton, P. G., *The Visual Characteristics of Stutterers During Silent Reading.* Ph.D. Dissert., Columbia Univ. Teachers Coll. (1940).

Hamre, C. E., and Wingate, M. E., Stuttering consistency in varied contexts. *J. Speech Hearing Res., 16,* 238–47 (1973).

Hand, C. R., and Haynes, W. O., Linguistic processing and reaction time differences in stutterers and nonstutterers. *J. Speech Hearing Res., 26,* 181–85 (1983).

Hanna, R., and Morris, S., Stuttering, speech rate, and the metronome effect. *Percept. Mot. Skills, 44,* 452–54 (1977).

Hanna, R., and Owen, N., Facilitating transfer and maintenance of fluency in stuttering therapy. *J. Speech Hearing Dis., 42,* 65–76 (1977).

Hanna, R., Wilfling, F., and McNeil, B., A biofeedback treatment for stuttering. *J. Speech Hearing Dis., 40,* 270–73 (1975).

Hannah, E. P., and Gardner, J. G., A note on syntactic relationships in nonfluency. *J. Speech Hearing Res., 11,* 853–60 (1968).

Hannley, M., and Dorman, M. F., Some observations on auditory function and stuttering. *J. Fluency Dis., 7,* 93–108 (1982).

Hansen, H. P., The effect of a measured audience reaction on stuttering behavior patterns. *Speech Monogr., 23,* 144 (1956). Abstract.

Hansen, K., Objektive Untersuchungen über Atembewegungen bei stotternden Schulkindern. *Vox, 13,* 25–29 (1927).

Hanson, B. R., The effects of a contingent light-flash on stuttering and attention to stuttering. *J. Communic. Dis., 11,* 451–58 (1978).

Hanson, B. R., Gronhovd, K. D., and Rice, P. L., A shortened version of the Southern Illinois University Speech Situation Checklist for the identification of speech-related anxiety. *J. Fluency Dis., 6,* 351–60 (1981).

Hardin, C. B., Pindzola, R. H., and Haynes, W. O., A tachistoscopic study of hemispheric processing in stuttering and nonstuttering children. *J. Fluency Dis., 17,* 265–81 (1992).

Harms, M. A., and Malone, J. Y., The relationship of hearing acuity to stammering. *J. Speech Dis.*, 4, 363–70 (1939).

Haroldson, S. K., Martin, R. R., and Starr, C. D., Time-out as a punishment for stuttering. *J. Speech Hearing Res.*, 11, 560–66 (1968).

Harrington, J., Coarticulation and stuttering: An acoustic and electropalatographic study. In Peters, H. F. M., and Hulstijn, W. (eds.), *Speech Motor Dynamics in Stuttering*. New York: Springer (1987).

Harrington, J., Stuttering, delayed auditory feedback, and linguistic rhythm. *J. Speech Hearing Res.*, 31, 36–47 (1988).

Harris, C. M., Martin, R. R., and Haroldson, S. K., Punishment of expectancy responses by stutterers. *J. Speech Hearing Res.*, 14, 710–17 (1971).

Harris, D., Fucci, D., and Petrosino, L., Magnitude estimation and crossmodal matching of auditory and lingual vibrotactile sensation by normal speakers and stutterers. *J. Speech Hearing Res.*, 34, 177–82 (1991).

Harris, R., *The Effect of Amplification of the Stutterer's Voice on the Frequency of Stuttering*. M. A. Thesis, Brooklyn Coll. (1955).

Harris, W. E., Studies in the psychology of stuttering: XVII. A study of the transfer of the adaptation effect in stuttering. *J. Speech Dis.*, 7, 209–21 (1942).

Harrison, H. S., A study of the speech of sixty institutionalized epileptics. *Speech Monogr.*, 14, 210 (1947). Abstract.

Hartwell, E. M., Application of the laws of physical training for the prevention and cure of stuttering. *Proc. Int. Congr. Educ. of the World's Columbian Expos.*, 739–49 (1893).

Hartz, G., Zur Frage des Zusammenhangs zwischen Intelligenz und Stottern. *Sprachheilarb.*, 15, 109–16 (1970).

Hasbrouck, J. M., Doherty, J., Mehlmann, M. A., Nelson, R., Randle, B., and Whitaker, R., Intensive stuttering therapy in a public school setting. *Lang. Speech Hearing Services in Schools*, 18, 330–43 (1987).

Hasbrouck, J. M., Graham, N. L., and Brooks, R. S., The effect of manipulation of speech disfluency on stuttering frequency. *Asha*, 18, 610 (1976). Abstract.

Hasbrouck, J. M., and Lowry, F., Elimination of stuttering and maintenance of fluency by means of airflow, tension reduction, and discrimination stimulus control procedures. *J. Fluency Dis.*, 14, 165–83 (1989).

Hasbrouck, J. M., and Martin, R. R., Further comparison of two different schedules of time-out for disfluency. *Asha*, 16, 514 (1974). Abstract.

Haskell, R. J., and Larr, A. L., Psychodramatic role training with stutterers. Group Psychother. *Psychodrama*, 27, 30–36 (1974).

Hawkins, R. T., and Brutten, E. J., The effect of stimulus strength on stuttering adjacency. *Asha*, 6, 416 (1964). Abstract.

Hayden, P. A., Adams M. R., and Jordahl, N., The effects of pacing and masking on stutterers' and nonstutterers' speech initiation times. *J. Fluency Dis.*, 7, 9–19 (1982).

Hayden, P. A., Jordahl, N., and Adams, M. R., Stutterers' voice initiation times during conditions of novel stimulation. *J. Fluency Dis.*, 7, 1–7 (1982).

Hayden, P. A., Scott, D. A., and Addicott, J., The effects of delayed auditory feedback on the overt behaviors of stutterers. *J. Fluency Dis.*, 2, 235–46 (1977).

Haynes, W. O., and Hood, S. B., Language and disfluency variables in normal speaking children from discrete chronological age groups. *J. Fluency Dis.*, 2, 57–74 (1977).

Haynes, W. O., and Hood, S. B., Disfluency changes in children as a function of the systematic modification of linguistic complexity. *J. Communic. Dis.*, 11, 79–93 (1978).

Hays, P., Bethanecol chloride in treatment of stuttering. *Lancet*, Jan. 31; (8527) : 271 (1987).

Haywood, H. C., Differential effects of delayed auditory feedback on palmar sweating, heart rate, pulse pressure. *J. Speech Hearing Res.*, 6, 181–86 (1963).

Healey, E. C., Speaking fundamental frequency characteristics of stutterers and nonstutterers. *J. Communic. Dis.*, 15, 21–29 (1982).

Healey, E. C., Fundamental frequency contours of stutterers' vowels following fluent stop consonant productions. *Folia Phoniat.*, 36, 145–51 (1984).

Healey, E. C., and Adams, M. R., Speech timing skills of normally fluent and stuttering children and adults. *J. Fluency Dis.*, 6, 233–46 (1981).

Healey, E. C., and Bernstein, B., Acoustic analyses of young stutterers' and nonstutterers' disfluencies. In Peters, H. F. M., Hulstijn, W., and Starkweather, C. W. (eds.), *Speech Motor Control and Stuttering*. Amsterdam: Elsevier (1991).

Healey, E. C., and Gutkin, B., Analysis of stutterers' voice onset times and fundamental frequency contours during fluency. *J. Speech Hearing Res.*, 27, 219–25 (1984).

Healey, E. C., and Howe, S. W., Speech shadowing characteristics of stutterers under diotic and dichotic conditions. *J. Communic. Dis.*, 20, 493–506 (1987).

Healey, E. C., Mallard, A. R. III, and Adams, M. R., Factors contributing to the reduction of stuttering during singing. *J. speech Hearing Res.*, 19, 475–80 (1976).

Healey, E. C., and Ramig, P. R., Acoustic measures of stutterers' and nonstutterers' fluency in two speech contexts. *J. Speech Hearing Res.*, 29, 325–31 (1986).

Hegde, M. N., Propositional speech and stuttering. *J. All India Inst. Speech Hearing*, 1, 21–24 (1970).

Hegde, M. N., The effect of shock on stuttering. *J. All India Inst. Speech Hearing*, 2, 104–10 (1971a).

Hegde, M. N., The short and long term effects of contingent aversive noise on stuttering. *J. All India Inst. Speech Hearing*, 2, 7–14 (1971b).

Hegde, M. N., Stuttering adaptation, reactive inhibition and spontaneous recovery. *J. All India Inst. Speech Hearing*, 2, 40–47 (1971c).

Hegde, M. N., Stuttering, neuroticism and extraversion. *Behav. Res. Ther.*, 10, 395–97 (1972).

Hegde, M. N., Fluency and fluency disorders: Their definition, measurement, and modification. *J. Fluency Dis.*, 3, 51–71 (1978).

Hegde, M. N., Antecedents of fluent and dysfluent oral reading: A descriptive analysis. *J. Fluency Dis.*, 7, 323–41 (1982).

Hegde, M. N., and Brutten, G. J., Reinforcing fluency in stutterers: An experimental study. *J. Fluency Dis.*, 2, 315–28 (1977).

Hegde, M. N., and Hartman, D. E., Factors affecting judgments of fluency: I. Interjections. *J. Fluency Dis.*, 4, 1–11 (1979a).

Hegde, M. N., and Hartman, D. E., Factors affecting judgments of fluency: II. Word repetitions. *J. Fluency Dis., 4,* 13–22 (1979b).

Heinzel, J., and Ubricht, W., Untersuchung zur intellektuellen Struktur stotternder Kinder. *Sprachheilarb., 28,* 229–33 (1983).

Hejna, R. F., *A Study of the Loci of Stuttering in Spontaneous Speech.* Ph.D. Dissert., Northwestern Univ. (1955).

Hejna, R. F., Stuttering frequency in relation to word frequency usage. *Asha, 5,* 781 (1963). Abstract.

Hejna, R. F., The relationship between accent or stress and stuttering during spontaneous speech. *Asha, 14,* 479 (1972). Abstract.

Heller, J. C., Shulman, A. T., and Teryek, J., Short- and long-term outcome of intensive stuttering therapy: Factors affecting results. *Folia Phoniat., 34,* 133–34 (1983). Abstract.

Helm, N. A., and Butler, R. B., Transcutaneous nerve stimulation in acquired speech disorders. *Lancet,* No. 8049, Vol. II, 1177–78 (1977).

Helm, N. A., Butler, R. B., and Benson, D. F., Acquired stuttering. *Neurol., 28,* 1159–65 (1978).

Helm, N. A., Butler, R. B., and Canter, G. J., Neurogenic acquired stuttering. *J. Fluency Dis., 5,* 269–79 (1980).

Helmreich, H. G., and Bloodstein, O., The grammatical factor in childhood disfluency in relation to the continuity hypothesis. *J. Speech Hearing Res., 16,* 731–38 (1973).

Helps, R., and Dalton, P., The effectiveness of an intensive group speech therapy programme for adult stammerers. *Brit. J. Dis. Communic., 14,* 17–30 (1979).

Heltman, H. J., *First Aid for Stutterers.* New York: Expression Co. (1943).

Heltman, H. J., and Peacher, G. M., Misarticulation and diadokokinesis in the spastic paralytic. *J. Speech Dis., 8,* 137–45 (1943).

Hendel, D., and Bloodstein, O., Consistency in relation to inter-subject congruity in the loci of stutterings. *J. Communic. Dis., 6,* 37–43 (1973).

Henrikson, E. H., Simultaneously recorded breathing and vocal disturbances of stutterers. *Arch. Speech, 1,* 133–49 (1936).

Herndon, G. Y., A study of the time discrimination abilities of stutterers and nonstutterers. Speech Monogr., 34, 303–04 (1967).

Herren, R. Y., The effect of stuttering on voluntary movement. *J. Exper. Psychol., 14,* 289–98 (1931).

Herren, R. Y., The relation of stuttering and alcohol to certain tremor rates. *J. Exper. Psychol., 15,* 87–96 (1932).

Hertzman, J., High school mental hygiene survey. *Amer. J. Orthopsychiat., 18,* 238–56 (1948).

Hill, H., Stuttering: I. A critical review and evaluation of biochemical investigations. *J. Speech Dis., 9,* 245–61 (1944a).

Hill, H., Stuttering: II. A review and integration of physiological data. *J. Speech Dis., 9,* 289–324 (1944b).

Hill, H. E., An experimental study of disorganization of speech and manual responses in normal subjects. *J. Speech Hearing Dis., 19,* 295–305 (1954).

Hillman, R. E., and Gilbert, H. R., Voice onset time for voiceless stop consonants in the fluent reading of stutterers and nonstutterers. *J. Acoust. Soc. Amer., 61,* 610–11 (1977).

Hirschberg, J., A dadogásról. *Orvosi Hetilap, 106,* 780–84 (1965).

Hogewind, F., Medical treatment of stuttering. *J. Speech Dis., 5,* 203–08 (1940).

Hohmeier, J., Zur beruflichen Situation von Stotternden. *Sprachheilarb., 32,* 25–31 (1987).

Holliday, A. R., Effect of meprobamate on stuttering. *Northwest Med., 58,* 837–41 (1959).

Hommerich, K. W., and Korzendorfer, M., Untersuchung über die Anwendung von Chlordiazepoxyd (Librium) in der Stottertherapie. *HNO, 14,* 211–18 (1966).

Homzie, M. J., Lindsay, J. S., Simpson, J., and Hasenstab, S. Concomitant speech, language, and learning problems in adult stutterers and in members of their families. *J. Fluency Dis., 13,* 261–77 (1988).

Hood, S. B., Effect of communicative stress on the frequency and form-types of disfluent behavior in adult stutterers. *J. Fluency Dis., 1,* 36–47 (1975).

Hoops, R., and Wilkinson, P., Group ratings of stuttering severity. In Lebrun, Y., and Hoops, R. (eds.), *Neurolinguistic Approaches to Stuttering.* The Hague: Mouton (1973).

Horan, M. C., An improved device for inducing rhythmic speech in stutterers. *Austral. Psychol., 3,* 19–25 (1968).

Horii, Y., and Ramig, P. R., Pause and utterance durations and fundamental frequency characteristics of repeated oral readings by stutterers and non-stutterers. *J. Fluency Dis., 12,* 257–70 (1987).

Horlick,. R. S., and Miller, M. H., A comparative personality study of a group of stutterers and hard of hearing patients. *J. Gen. Psychol., 63,* 259–66 (1960).

Horner, J., and Massey, W., Progressive dysfluency associated with right hemisphere disease. *Brain and Language, 18,* 71–85 (1983).

Horovitz, L. J., Johnson, S. B., Pearlman, R. C., Schaffer, E. J., and Hedin, A. K., Stapedial reflex and anxiety in fluent and disfluent speakers. *J. Speech Hearing Res., 21,* 762–67 (1978).

Horowitz, E., Effects of parental criticism of defective articulation. *De Therapia Vocis et Loquelae, Vol. I.* XIII Congr. Int. Soc. Logoped. Phoniat. (1965).

Horsely, I. A., and Fitzgibbon, C. T., Stuttering children: investigation of a stereotype. *Brit. J. Dis. Communic., 22,* 19–35 (1987).

Howell, P., Changes in voice level caused by several forms of altered feedback in fluent speakers and stutterers. *Lang. Speech, 33,* 325–38 (1990).

Howell, P., and El-Yaniv, N., The effects of presenting a click in syllable-initial position on the speech of stutterers: Comparison with a metronome click. *J. Fluency Dis., 12,* 249–56 (1987).

Howell, P., El-Yaniv, N., and Powell, D. J., Factors affecting fluency in stutterers when speaking under altered auditory feedback. In Peters, H. F. M., and Hulstijn, W. (eds.), *Speech Motor Dynamics in Stuttering.* New York: Springer (1987).

Howell, P., Marchbanks, R. J., and El-Yaniv, N., Middle ear muscle activity during vocalization in normal speakers and stutterers. *Acta Oto-Laryngologica, 102,* 396–402 (1986).

Howell, P., and Vause, L., Acoustic analysis and perception of vowels in stuttererd speech. *J. Acoust. Soc. Amer., 79,* 1571–79 (1986).

Howell, P., and Williams, M., The contribution of the excitatory source to the perception of neutral vowels in stuttered speech. *J. Acoust. Soc. Amer., 84,* 80–89 (1988).

Howell, P., and Williams, M., Acoustic analysis and perception of vowels in children's and teenagers' stuttered speech. *J. Acoust. Soc. Amer., 91,* 1697–1706 (1992).

Howell, P., Williams, M., and Vause, L., Acoustic analysis of repetitions in stutterers' speech. In Peters, H. F. M., and Hulstijn, W. (eds.), *Speech Motor Dynamics in Stuttering.* New York: Springer (1987).

Howell, P., Williams. M., and Young, K. Production of vowels by stuttering children and teenagers. In Peters, H. F. M., Hulstijn, W., and Starkweather, C. W. (eds.), *Speech Motor Control and Stuttering.* Amsterdam: Elsevier (1991).

Howell, P., and Wingfield, T., Perceptual and acoustic evidence for reduced fluency in the vicinity of stuttering episodes. *Lang. Speech, 33,* 31–46 (1990).

Howie, P., The identification of genetic components in speech disorders. *Aust. J. Human Communic. Dis., 4,* 155–63 (1976).

Howie, P. M., Concordance for stuttering in monozygotic and dizygotic twin pairs. *J. Speech Hearing Res., 24,* 317–21 (1981a).

Howie, P. M., Intrapair similarity in frequency of disfluency in monozygotic and dizygotic twin pairs containing stutterers. *Behav. Genet., 11,* 227–37 (1981b).

Howie, P., and Andrews, G., Treatment of adult stutterers: Managing fluency. In Curlee, R. F., and Perkins, W. H. (eds.), *Nature and Treatment of Stuttering: New Directions.* San Diego: College-Hill Press (1984).

Howie, P. M., Tanner, S., and Andrews, G., Short- and long-term outcome in an intensive treatment program for adult stutterers. *J. Speech Hearing Dis., 46,* 104–09 (1981).

Howie, P. M., and Woods, C. L., Token reinforcement during the instatement and shaping of fluency in the treatment of stuttering. *J. Appl. Behav. Anal., 15,* 55–64 (1982).

Howie, P. M., Woods, C. L., and Andrews, G., Relationship between covert and overt speech measures immediately before and immediately after stuttering treatment. *J. Speech Hearing Dis., 47,* 419–22 (1982).

Hubbard, C. P., and Yairi, E., Clustering of disfluencies in the speech of stuttering and nonstuttering preschool children. *J. Speech Hearing Res., 31,* 228–33 (1988).

Huffman, E. S., and Perkins, W. H., Dysfluency characteristics identified by listeners as "stuttering" and "stutterer." *J. Communic. Dis., 7,* 89–96 (1974).

Hugo, R, 'n Kommunikatiefgefundeerde ondersoek na bepaalde waarnemingsverskynsels by disfemie. *J. So. Afr. Speech Hearing Assoc., 19,* 39–51 (1972).

Hulit, L. M., Effects of nonfluencies on comprehension. *Percept. Mot. Skills, 42,* 1119–22 (1976).

Hull, F. M., *National Speech and Hearing Survey.* U.S. Dept. Health, Educ., Welfare, Project No. 50978, Grant No. OE-32-15-0050-5010 (1969).

Hunsley, Y. L., Dysintegration in the speech musculature of stutterers during the production of a non-vocal temporal pattern. *Psychol. Monogr., 49,* 32–49 (1937).

Hurford, D. P., and Webster, R. L., Decreases in simple reaction time as a function of stutterers' participation in a behavioral therapy. *J. Fluency Dis., 10,* 301–10 (1985).

Hurst, M. A., and Cooper, E. B., Vocational rehabilitation counselors' attitudes toward stuttering. *J. Fluency Dis., 8,* 13–27 (1983).

Hurst, M. I., and Cooper, E. B., Employer attitudes toward stuttering. *J. Fluency Dis., 8,* 1–12 (1983).

Hutchinson, E. C., and Mackay, G. R., Conditioning speech nonfluencies through the use of an aversive stimulus. *Folia Phoniat., 25,* 373–82 (1973).

Hutchinson, J. M., Aerodynamic patterns of stuttered speech. In Webster, L. M., and Furst, L. C. (eds.), *Vocal Tract Dynamics and Dysfluency.* New York: Speech and Hearing Inst. (1975).

Hutchinson, J. M., and Brown, D., The Adams and Reis observations revisited. *J. Fluency Dis., 3,* 149–54 (1978).

Hutchinson, J. M., and Burk, K. W., An investigation of the effects of temporal alterations in auditory feedback upon stutterers and clutterers. *J. Communic. Dis., 6,* 193–205 (1973).

Hutchinson, J. M., and Navarre, B. M., The effect of metronome pacing on selected aerodynamic patterns of stuttered speech: Some preliminary observations and interpretations. *J. Fluency Dis., 2,* 189–204 (1977).

Hutchinson, J. M., and Norris, G. M., The differential effect of three auditory stimuli on the frequency of stuttering behaviors. *J. Fluency Dis., 2,* 283–93 (1977).

Hutchinson, J. M., and Ringel, R. L., The effect of oral sensory deprivation on stuttering behavior. *J. Communic. Dis., 8,* 249–58 (1975).

Hutchinson, J. M., and Watkins, K. L., A preliminary investigation of lip and jaw coarticulation in stutterers. *Asha, 16,* 533 (1974). Abstract.

Hutchinson, J. M., and Watkin, K. L., Jaw mechanics during release of the stuttering moment: Some initial observations and interpretations. *J. Communic. Dis., 9,* 269–79 (1976).

Iacono, T. A., The effect of pre-information on naive listeners' judgements of post treatment stutterers. *Aust. J. Human Communic. Dis., 12,* 25–34 (1984).

Ickes, W. K., A palmar sweat measure of the effect of drugs on stuttering behavior. *J. Fluency Dis., 1,* 2–9 (1975).

Ickes, W. K., and Pierce, S., The stuttering moment: A plethysmographic study. *J. Communic. Dis., 6,* 155–64 (1973).

Ilg, F., Learned, J., Lockwood, A., and Ames, L. B., The three-and-a-half-year old. *J. Genet. Psychol., 75,* 21–31 (1949).

Ingebregtsen, E., Some experimental contributions to the psychology and psychopathology of stutterers. *Amer. J. Orthopsychiat., 6,* 630–50 (1936).

Ingham, R. J., A comparison of covert and overt assessment procedures in stuttering therapy outcome evaluation. *J. Speech Hearing Res., 18,* 346–54 (1975).

Ingham, R. J., Onset, prevalence, and recovery from stuttering: A reassessment of findings from the Andrews and Harris study. *J. Speech Hearing Dis., 41,* 280–81 (1976).

Ingham, R. J., Modification of maintenance and generalization during stuttering treatment. *J. Speech Hearing Res., 23,* 732–45 (1980).

Ingham, R. J., The effects of self-evaluation training on maintenance and generalization during stuttering treatment. *J. Speech Hearing Dis.*, 47, 271–80 (1982).

Ingham, R. J., Generalization and maintenance of treatment. In Curlee, R. F., and Perkins, W. H. (eds.), *Nature and Treatment of Stuttering: New Directions.* San Diego: College-Hill Press (1984a).

Ingham, R. J., *Stuttering and Behavior Therapy.* San Diego: College-Hill Press (1984b).

Ingham, R. J., and Andrews, G., The relation between anxiety reduction and treatment. *J. Communic. Dis.*, 4, 289–301 (1971a).

Ingham, R. J., and Andrews, G., Stuttering: The quality of fluency after treatment. *J. Communic. Dis.*, 4, 279–88 (1971b).

Ingham, R. J., and Andrews, G., An analysis of a token economy in stuttering therapy. *J. Appl. Behav. Anal.*, 6, 219–29 (1973a).

Ingham, R. J., and Andrews, G., Behavior therapy and stuttering: A review. *J. Speech Hearing Dis.*, 38, 405–41 (1973b).

Ingham, R. J., Andrews, G., and Winkler, R., Stuttering; A comparative evaluation of the shortterm effectiveness of four treatment techniques. *J. Communic. Dis.*, 5, 91–117 (1972).

Ingham, R. J., and Carroll, P. J., Listener judgment of differences in stutterers' nonstuttered speech during chorus- and nonchorus-reading conditions. *J. Speech Hearing Res.*, 20, 293–302 (1977).

Ingham, R. J., and Cordes, A. K., Interclinic differences in stuttering-event counts. *J. Fluency Dis.*, 17, 171–76 (1992).

Ingham, R. J., Cordes, A. K., and Finn, P., Time-interval measurement of stuttering: Systematic replication of Ingham, Cordes, and Gow (1993). *J. Speech Hearing Res.*, 36, 1168–76 (1993).

Ingham, R. J., Cordes, A. K., and Gow, M. L., Time-interval measurement of stuttering: Modifying interjudge agreement. *J. Speech Hearing Res.*, 36, 503–15 (1993).

Ingham, R. J., Gow, M., and Costello, J. M., Stuttering and speech naturalness: Some additional data. *J. Speech Hearing Dis.*, 50, 217–19 (1985).

Ingham, R. J., Ingham, J. C., Onslow, M., and Finn, P., Stutterers' self-ratings of speech naturalness: Assessing effects and reliability. *J. Speech Hearing Res.*, 32, 419–31 (1989).

Ingham, R. J., Martin, R. R., Haroldson, S. K., Onslow, M., and Leney, M., Modification of listener-judged naturalness in the speech of stutterers. *J. Speech Hearing Res.*, 28, 495–504 (1985).

Ingham, R. J., Martin, R. R., and Kuhl, P., Modification and control of rate of speaking by stutterers. *J. Speech Hearing Res.*, 17, 489–96 (1974).

Ingham, R. J., Montgomery, J., and Ulliana, L., The effect of manipulating phonation duration on stuttering. *J. Speech Hearing Res.*, 26, 579–87 (1983).

Ingham, R. J., and Onslow, M., Measurement and modification of speech naturalness during stuttering therapy. *J. Speech Hearing Dis.*, 50, 261–18 (1985).

Ingham, R. J., and Onslow, M., Generalization and maintenance of treatment benefits of children who stutter. *Seminars Speech Lang.*, 8, 303–26 (1987).

Ingham, R. J., and Packman, A. C., Perceptual assessment of normalcy of speech following stuttering therapy. *J. Speech Hearing Res.*, 21, 63–73 (1978).

Ingham, R. J., and Packman, A., A further evaluation of the speech of stutterers during chorus-and nonchorus reading conditions. *J. Speech Hearing Res., 22,* 784–93 (1979).

Ingham, R. J., Southwood, H., and Horsburgh, G., Some effects of the Edinburgh masker on stuttering during oral reading and spontaneous speech. *J. Fluency Dis., 6,* 135–54 (1981).

Inglis, A. L., Neurological stammer—A case study. *Aust. J. Human Communic. Dis., 7,* 58–62 (1979).

Irving, R. W., and Webb, M. W., Teaching esophageal speech to a pre-operative severe stutterer. *Ann. Otol. Rhinol. Laryngol., 70,* 1069–79 (1961).

Irwin, A., The treatment and results of "easy-stammering." *Brit. J. Dis. Communic., 7,* 151–56 (1972).

Ito, T., Speech dysfluency and acquisition of syntax in children 2–6 years old. *Folia Phoniat., 38,* 310 (1986). Abstract.

Jacoby, B., An investigation of the carotid sinus reflex in stutterers. *Speech Monogr., 14,* 201–02 (1947). Abstract.

Jakobovits, L. A., Utilization of semantic satiation in stuttering: A theoretical analysis. *J. Speech Hearing Dis., 31,* 105–14 (1966).

James, J. E., The influence of duration on the effects of time-out from speaking. *J. Speech Hearing Res., 19,* 206–15 (1976).

James, J. E., Punishment of stuttering: Contingency and stimulus parameters. *J. Communic. Dis., 14,* 375–86 (1981a).

James, J. E., Self-monitoring of stuttering: Reactivity and accuracy. *Behav. Res. Ther., 19,* 291–96 (1981b).

James, J. E., Parameters of the influence of self-initiated time-out from speaking on stuttering. *J. Communic. Dis., 16,* 123–32 (1983).

James, J. E., and Ingham, R. J., The influence of stutterers' expectancies of improvement upon response to time-out. *J. Speech Hearing Res., 17,* 86–93 (1974).

James, J. E., Ricciardelli, L. A., Rogers, P., and Hunter, C. E., A preliminary analysis of the ameliorative effects of time-out from speaking on stuttering. *J. Speech Hearing Res., 32,* 604–10 (1989).

Jamison, D. J., Spontaneous recovery of the stuttering response as a function of the time following adaptation. In Johnson, W., and Leutenegger, R. R. (eds.), *Stuttering in Children and Adults.* Minneapolis: Univ. Minn. Press (1955).

Jäncke, L., The 'audio-phoniatric coupling' in stuttering and nonstuttering adults: Experimental contributions. In Peters, H. F. M., Hulstijn, W., and Starkweather, C. W. (eds.), *Speech Motor Control and Stuttering.* Amsterdam: Elsevier (1991).

Jäncke, L., Variability and duration of voice onset time and phonation in stuttering and nonstuttering adults. *J. Fluency Dis., 19,* 21–37 (1994).

Janssen, P., and Brutten, G. J., The differential effects of punishment of oral prolongations. In Lebrun, Y., and Hoops, R. (eds.), *Neurolinguistic Approaches to Stuttering.* The Hague: Mouton (1973).

Janssen, P., and Brutten, G. J., Pupillometric responses of young stutterers. *Proc. 18th Congr. Int. Assoc. Logoped. Phoniat.* Washington, D. C.: Amer. Speech-Lang.-Hearing Assoc. (1981).

Janssen, P., and Kraaimaat, F., Disfluency and anxiety in stuttering and non-stuttering adolescents. *Behav. Anal. Modific.*, *4*, 116–26 (1980).

Janssen, P., and Kraamaat, F., Onset and termination of accessory facial movements during stuttering. *Percept. Mot. Skills*, *63*, 11–17 (1986).

Janssen, P., Kraamaat, F., and Brutten, G., Relationship between stutterers' genetic history and speech associated variables. *J. Fluency Dis.*, *15*, 39–48 (1990).

Janssen, P., Kraamaat, F., and van der Meulen, S., Reading ability and disfluency in stuttering and nonstuttering elementary school children. *J. Fluency Dis.*, *8*, 39–53 (1983).

Janssen, P., and Wieneke, G., The effects of fluency inducing conditions on the variability in the duration of laryngeal movements during stutterers' fluent speech. In Peters, H. F. M., and Hulstijn, W. (eds.), *Speech Motor Dynamics in Stuttering*. New York: Springer (1987).

Janssen P., Wieneke, G., and Vaane, E., Variability in the initiation of articulatory movements in the speech of stutterers and normal speakers. *J. Fluency Dis.*, *8*, 341–58 (1983).

Jasper, H. H., A laboratory study of diagnostic indices of bilateral neuromuscular organization in stutterers and normal speakers. *Psychol. Monogr.*, *43*, 72–1744 (1932).

Jasper, H. H., and Murray, E., A study of the eye-movements of stutterers during oral reading. *J. Exper. Psychol.*, *15*, 528–38 (1932).

Jayaram, M., Grammatical factors in stuttering in monolingual and bilingual stutterers. *J. Communic. Dis.*, *16*, 287–97 (1983).

Jayaram, M., Distribution of stuttering in sentences: Relationship to sentence length and clause position. *J. Speech Hearing Res.*, *27*, 338–41 (1984).

Jehle, P., and Boberg, E., Intensivbehandlung für jugendliche und erwachsene Stotternde von Boberg und Kully. *Folia Phoniat.*, *39*, 256–68 (1987).

Jehle, P., Kühn, T., and Renner, J. A., Einstellungen Stotternder und Nicht-Stotternder zur Kommunikation: Einige Ergebnisse aus der Anwendung der Skala "S24" von Erickson und Andrews/Cutler. *Sprachheilarb.*, *34*, 121–28 (1989).

Jensen, P. J., Markel, N. N., and Beverung, J. W., Evidence of conversational disrhythmia in stutterers. *J. Fluency Dis.*, *11*, 183–200 (1986).

Jensen, P. J., Sheehan, J. G., Williams, W. N., and LaPointe, L. L., Oral sensory-perceptual integrity of stutterers. *Folia Phoniat.*, *27*, 38–45 (1975).

Jerger, J., Diagnostic audiometry. In Jerger, J. (ed.), *Modern Developments in Audiology*, *2nd ed*. New York: Academic (1973).

Jerger, J., Diagnostic use of impedance measures. In Jerger, J. (ed.), *Manual of Impedance Audiometry*. New York: American Electromedics (1975).

Johannsen, H. S., and Victor, C., Visual information processing in the left and right hemispheres during unilateral tachistoscopic stimulation of stutterers. *J. Fluency Dis.*, *11*, 285–91 (1986).

Johnson, L., Facilitating parental involvement in therapy of the preschool difluent child. In Perkins, W. H. (ed.), *Stuttering Disorders*. New York: Thieme-Stratton (1984).

Johnson, W., *The Influence of Stuttering on the Personality*. Univ. Iowa Studies in Child Welfare, Vol. 5, No. 5. Iowa City: Univ. Iowa (1932).

Johnson, W., An interpretation of stuttering. *Quart. J. Speech*, 19, 70–76 (1933).

Johnson, W., The influence of stuttering on the attitudes and adaptations of the stutterer. *J. Soc. Psychol.*, *5*, 415–20 (1934a).

Johnson, W., Stutterers' attitudes toward stuttering. *J. Abnorm. Soc. Psychol.*, *29*, 32–44 (1934b).

Johnson, W., The dominant thumb in relation to stuttering, eyedness and handedness. *Amer. J. Psychol.*, *49*, 293–97 (1937).

Johnson, W., The role of evaluation in stuttering behavior. *J. Speech Dis.*, *3*, 85–89 (1938).

Johnson, W., The Indians have no word for it. I. Stuttering in children. *Quart. J. Speech*, *30*, 330–37 (1944).

Johnson, W., A study of the onset and development of stuttering. In Johnson, W., and Leutenegger, R. R. (eds.), *Stuttering in Children and Adults*. Minneapolis: Univ. Minn. Press (1955a).

Johnson, W., The time, the place, and the problem. In Johnson, W., and Leutenegger, R. R. (eds.), *Stuttering in Children and Adults*. Minneapolis: Univ. Minn. Press (1955b).

Johnson, W., Measurements of oral reading and speaking rate and disfluency of adult male and female stutterers and nonstutterers. *J. Speech Hearing Dis., Monogr. Suppl. No. 7*, 1–20 (1961a).

Johnson, W., *Stuttering and What You Can Do about It*. Minneapolis: Univ. Minn. Press (1961b).

Johnson, W., and Ainsworth, S., Studies in the psychology of stuttering: X. Constancy of loci of expectancy of stuttering. *J. Speech Dis.*, *3*, 101–04 (1938).

Johnson, W., et al, a study of the onset and development of stuttering. *J. Speech Dis.*, *7*, 251–57 (1942). (Published in more complete form in Johnson, 1955a.)

Johnson, W., et al, *Speech Handicapped School Children, rev. ed.* New York: Harper & Bros. (1956).

Johnson, W., et al, *Speech Handicapped School Children, 3rd ed.* New York: Harper & Row (1967).

Johnson, W. and Associates, *The Onset of Stuttering*. Minneapolis: Univ. Minn. Press (1959).

Johnson, W., and Brown, S. F., Stuttering in relation to various speech sounds. *Quart. J. Speech*, *21*, 481–96 (1935).

Johnson, W., and Colley, W. H., The relationship between frequency and duration of moments of stuttering. *J. Speech Dis.*, *10*, 35–38 (1945).

Johnson, W., Darley, F. L., and Spriestersbach, D. C., *Diagnostic Methods in Speech Pathology*. New York: Harper & Row (1963).

Johnson, W., and Innes, M., Studies in the psychology of stuttering: XIII. A statistical analysis of the adaptation and consistency effects in relation to stuttering. *J. Speech Dis.*, *4*, 79–86 (1939).

Johnson, W., and King, A., An angle board and hand usage study of stutterers and non-stutterers. *J. Exper. Psychol.*, *31*, 293–311 (1942).

Johnson, W., and Knott, J. R., The moment of stuttering. *J. Genet. Psychol.*, *48*, 475–79 (1936).

Johnson, W., and Knott, J. R., Studies in the psychology of stuttering: I. The distribution of moments of stuttering in successive readings of the same material. *J. Speech Dis.*, *2*, 17–19 (1937).

Johnson, W., Larson, R. P., and Knott, J. R., Studies in the psychology of stuttering: VI. The role of cues representative of stuttering moments during oral reading. *J. Speech Dis., 2,* 101–04 (1937).

Johnson, W., and Millsapps, L. S., Studies in the psychology of stuttering: VI. The role of cues representative of stuttering moments during oral reading. *J. Speech Dis., 2,* 101–04 (1937).

Johnson, W., and Rosen, L., Studies in the psychology of stuttering: VII. Effect of certain changes in speech pattern upon frequency of stuttering. *J. Speech Dis., 2,* 105–09 (1937).

Johnson, W., and Sinn, A., Studies in the psychology of stuttering: V. Frequency of stuttering with expectation of stuttering controlled. *J. Speech Dis., 2,* 98–100 (1937).

Johnson, W., and Solomon, A., Studies in the psychology of stuttering: IV. A quantitative study of expectation of stuttering as a process involving a low degree of consciousness. *J. Speech Dis., 2,* 95–97 (1937).

Johnson, W., Stearns, G., and Warweg, E., Chemical factors and the stuttering spasm. *Quart. J. Speech, 19,* 409–15 (1933).

Johnson, W., Young, M. A., Sahs, A. L., and Bedell, G. N., Effects of hyperventilation and tetany on the speech fluency of stutterers and nonstutterers. *J. Speech Hearing Res., 2,* 203–15 (1959).

Jones, E. L., Explorations of experimental extinction and spontaneous recovery in stuttering. In Johnson, W., and Leutenegger, R. R. (eds.), *Stuttering in Children and Adults.* Minneapolis: Univ. Minn. Press (1955).

Jones, M. J., An electroencephalographic study of stutterers and normal speakers during silence. *Speech Monogr., 16,* 310–11 (1949). Abstract.

Jones, R. J., and Azrin, N. H., Behavioral engineering: Stuttering as a function of stimulus duration during speech synchronization. *J. Appl. Behav. Anal., 2,* 223–29 (1969).

Jones, R. K., Observations on stammering after localized cerebral injury. *J. Neurol. Neurosurg. Psychiat., 29,* 192–95 (1966).

Jones-Prus, D., Training fluency as a motor skill in the treatment of dysfluent children. *Human Communic., 5,* 75–86 (1980).

Kaasin, K., and Bjerkan, B., Critical words and the locus of stuttering in speech. *J. Fluency Dis., 7,* 433–46 (1982).

Kadi-Hanifi, K., and Howell, P., Syntactic analysis of the spontaneous speech of normally fluent and stuttering children. *J. Fluency Dis., 17,* 151–70 (1992).

Kalinowski, J., Armson, J., Roland-Mieszkowski, M., Stuart, A., and Gracco, V. L., Effects of alterations in auditory feedback and speech rate on stuttering frequency. *Lang. Speech, 36,* 1–16 (1993).

Kalinowski, J. S., Lerman, J. W., and Watt, J., A Preliminary examination of the perceptions of self and others in stutterers and others. *J. Fluency Dis., 12,* 317–31 (1987).

Kalinowski, J., Noble, S., Armson, J., and Stuart, A., Pretreatment and post-treatment speech naturalness ratings of adults with mild and severe stuttering. *Amer. J. Speech-Lang. Pathol., 3,* 61–66 (1994).

Kalotkin, M., Manschreck, T., and O'Brien, D., Electromyographic tension levels in stutterers and normal speakers. *Percep. Mot. Skills, 49,* 109–10 (1979).

Kamhi, A. G., Lee, R. F., and Nelson, L. K., Word, syllable, and sound awareness in language-disordered children. *J. Speech Hearing Dis., 50,* 207–12 (1985).

Kamhi, A. G., and McOsker, T. G., Attention and stuttering: Do stutterers think too much about speech? *J. Fluency Dis., 7,* 309–21 (1982).

Kamiyama, G., A comparative study of stutterers and nonstutterers in respect to critical flicker frequency and sound localization. *Speech Monogr., 31,* 291 (1964). Abstract.

Kapos, E., and Standlee, L. S., Behavioral rigidity in adult stutterers. *J. Speech Hearing Res., 1,* 294–96 (1958).

Karlin, I. W., and Sobel, A. E., A comparative study of the blood chemistry of stutterers and nonstutterers. *Speech Monogr., 7,* 75–84 (1940).

Karlin, I. W., and Strazzulla, M., Speech and language problems of mentally deficient children. *J. Speech Hearing Dis., 17,* 286–94 (1952).

Karr, G. M., The performance of stutterers on central auditory tests. *So. Afr. J. Communic. Dis., 24,* 100–09 (1977).

Kasprisin-Burrelli, A., Egolf, D. B., and Shames, G. H., A comparison of parental verbal behavior with stuttering and nonstuttering children. *J. Communic. Dis., 5,* 335–46 (1972).

Katz, J., The use of staggered spondiac words for assessing the integrity of the central auditory nervous system. *J. Aud. Res., 2,* 327–37 (1962).

Katz, L., *Dependency and Immaturity in Stuttering Children.* M. A. Thesis, Brooklyn Coll. (1966).

Kazdin, A. E., The effect of response cost and aversive stimulation in suppressing punished and nonpunished speech disfluencies. *Behav. Ther., 4,* 73–82 (1973).

Keane, V. E., The incidence of speech and language problems in the mentally retarded. *Ment. Retard., 10,* 3–8 (1972).

Keele, S. W., Attention demands of memory retrieval. *J. Exper. Psychol., 93,* 245–48 (1972).

Keese, A., and Fischer, U., Das Zielsetzungsverhalten stotternder Schüler. *Sprachheilarb., 21,* 39–47 (1976).

Keisman, I. B., *Stuttering and Anal Fixation.* Ph.D. Dissert., N.Y. Univ. (1958).

Kelham, R., and McHale, A., The application of learning theory to the treatment of stammering. *Brit. J. Dis. Communic., 1,* 114–18 (1966).

Kelly, E. M., and Conture, E. G., Acoustic and perceptual correlates of adult stutterers' typical and imitated stuttering. *J. Fluency Dis., 13,* 233–52 (1988).

Kelly, E. M., and Conture, E. G., Speaking rates, response time latencies, and interrupting behaviors of young stutterers, nonstutterers, and their mothers. *J. Speech Hearing Res., 35,* 1256–67 (1992).

Kelly, G. A., Some common factors in reading and speech disabilities. *Psychol. Monogr. 43,* 175–201 (1932).

Kelly, J. C., *A Study of the Suggestibility of Stammerers and Normals.* M. A. Thesis, Northwestern Univ. (1935).

Kennedy, A. M., and Williams, D. A., Association of stammering and the allergic diathesis. *Brit. Med. J., Dec. 24, No. 4068,* 1306–09 (1938).

Kent, L. R., Carbon dioxide therapy as a medical treatment for stuttering. *J. Speech Hearing Dis., 26,* 268–71 (1961).

Kent, L. R., The use of tranquilizers in the treatment of stuttering. *J. Speech Hearing Dis., 28*, 288–94 (1963).

Kent, L. R., and Williams, D. E., Use of meprobamate as an adjunct to stuttering therapy. *J. Speech Hearing Dis., 24*, 64–69 (1959).

Kent, L. R., and Williams, D. E., Alleged former stutterers in grade two. *Asha, 5*, 772 (1963). Abstract.

Kent, R. D., Stuttering as a temporal programming disorder. In Curlee, R. F., and Perkins, W. H. (eds.), *Nature and Treatment of Stuttering: New Directions.* San Diego: College-Hill Press (1984).

Kenyon, E. L., The etiology of stammering: Fundamentally a wrong psychophysiologic habit in the control of the vocal cords for the production of an individual speech sound. *J. Speech Dis., 7*, 97–104 (1942).

Kern, A., Der Einfluss des Hörens auf das Stottern. *Arch. Psychiat. Nervenk., 97*, 429–50 (1932).

Kerr, S. H., Phonatory adjustment times in stutterers and nonstutterers. *Asha, 18*, 664 (1976). Abstract.

Kidd, K. K., A genetic perspective on stuttering. *J. Fluency Dis., 2*, 259–69 (1977).

Kidd, K. K., Heimbuch, R. C., and Records, M. A., Vertical transmission of susceptibility to stuttering with sex-modified expression. *Proc. Natl. Acad. Sci, 78*, 606–10 (1981).

Kidd, K. K., Heimbuch, R. C., Records, M. A., Oehlert, G., and Webster, R. L., Familial stuttering patterns are not related to one measure of severity. *J. Speech Hearing Res., 23*, 539–45 (1980).

Kidd, K. K., Kidd, J. R., and Records, M. A., The possible causes of the sex ratio in stuttering and its implications. *J. Fluency Dis., 3*, 13–23 (1978).

Kidd, K. K., Reich, T., and Kessler, S., *Genetics, 74*, No. 2, Part 2: s137 (1973).

Kidd, K. K., Reich, T., and Kessler, S., Genetic analyses of stuttering. Unpublished manuscript (1974).

Kiehn, E., Untersuchungen über die Fähigkeit zu feinabgemessenen Bewegungen (Feinmotorick) bei stammelnden, stotternden und normalen Volksschülern. *Vox, 21*, 32–35 (1935).

Kimmell, M., Studies in the psychology of stuttering: IX. The nature and effect of stutterers' avoidance reactions. *J. Speech Dis., 3*, 95–100 (1938).

King, P. T., Perseveration in stutterers and nonstutterers. *J. Speech Hearing Res., 4*, 346–57 (1961).

Kinstler, D. B., Covert and overt maternal rejection in stuttering. *J. Speech Hearing Dis., 26*, 145–55 (1961).

Kirk, L., Stuttering and quasi-stuttering in Ga. J. Communic. *Dis., 10*, 109–26 (1977). Reprinted in Rieber, R. W. (ed.), The Problem of Stuttering: Theory and Therapy. New York: Elsevier North-Holland (1977).

Klich, R. J., and May, G. M., Spectrographic study of vowels in stutterers' fluent speech. *J. Speech Hearing Res., 25*, 364–70 (1982).

Kline, D. F., An experimental study of the frequency of stuttering in relation to certain goal-activity drives in basic human behavior. *Speech Monogr., 26*, 137 (1959). Abstract.

Kline, M. L., and Starkweather, C. W., Receptive and expressive language performance in young stutterers. *Asha, 21*, 797 (1979). Abstract.

Klouda, G. V., and Cooper, W. E., Syntactic clause boundaries, speech timing, and stuttering frequency in adult stutterers. *Lang. Speech, 30,* 263–76 (1987).

Klouda, G. V., and Cooper, W. E., Contrastive stress, intonation, and stuttering frequency. *Lang. Speech, 31,* 3–20 (1988).

Knabe, J. M., Nelson, L. A., and Williams, F., Some general characteristics of linguistic output: Stutterers versus nonstutterers. *J. Speech Hearing Dis., 31,* 178–82 (1966).

Knepflar, K. J., Speaking fluency in the parents of stutterers and nonstutterers. *Asha, 7,* 391 (1965). Abstract.

Knott, J. R., A study of stutterers' stuttering and nonstuttering experiences on the basis of pleasantness and unpleasantness. *Quart. J. Speech, 21,* 328–31 (1935).

Knott, J. R., Correll, R. E., and Shephard, J. N., Frequency analysis of electroencephalograms of stutterers and nonstutterers. *J. Speech Hearing Res., 2,* 74–80 (1959).

Knott, J. R., and Johnson, W., The factor of attention in relation to the moment of stuttering. *J. Genet. Psychol., 48,* 479–80 (1936).

Knott, J. R., Johnson, W., and Webster, M. J., Studies in the psychology of stuttering: II. A quantitative evaluation of expectation of stuttering in relation to the occurrence of stuttering. *J. Speech Dis., 2,* 20–22 (1937).

Knott, J. R., and Tjossem, T. D., Bilateral electroencephalograms from normal speakers and stutterers. *J. Exper. Psychol., 32,* 357–62 (1943).

Knower, F. H., A study of speech attitudes and adjustments. *Speech Monogr., 5,* 130–203 (1938).

Knox, J. A., Acoustic analysis of stuttering behavior within the context of fluent speech. *Dissert. Abs. Int., Sect. B, Vol. 36, No. 12,* Part I (1976).

Knudsen, T. A., A study of the oral recitation problems of stutterers. *J. Speech Dis., 4,* 235–39 (1939).

Knura, G., Experimentelle Untersuchung des Lernerfolgs bei stotternden und nichtstotternden Volksschulkindern. *Sprachheilarb., 15,* 1–12 (1970).

Koller, W. C. Dysfluency (stuttering) in extrapyramidal disease. *Arch. Neurol., 40,* 175–77 (1983).

Kondas, O., The treatment of stammering in children by the shadow method. *Behav. Res. Ther., 5,* 325–29 (1967).

Kondas, O., Experiment of the shadowing method with children stammerers. *dsh Abstr., 11,* 338 (1971).

Kools, J. A., and Berryman, J. D., Differences in disfluency behavior between male and female nonstuttering children. *J. Speech Hearing Res., 14,* 125–30 (1971).

Koopmans, M., Slis, I., and Rietveld, T., The influence of word position and word type on the incidence of stuttering. In Peters, H. F. M., Hulstijn, W., and Starkweather, C. W. (eds.), *Speech Motor Control and Stuttering.* Amsterdam: Elsevier (1991).

Kopp, G. A., Metabolic studies of stutterers: I. Biochemical study of blood composition. *Speech Monogr., 1,* 117–32 (1934).

Kopp, H., Psychosomatic study of fifty stuttering children: II. Ozeretzky tests. *Amer. J. Orthopsychiat., 16,* 114–19 (1946).

Kopp, H. G., Eye movements in reading as related to speech dysfunction in male stutterers. *Speech Monogr., 30*, 248 (1963). Abstract.

Korzybski, A., *Science and Sanity: An Introduction to Non-Aristotelian Systems and General Semantics, 2nd ed.* New York: Int. Non-Aristotelian Library Publishing Co. (1941).

Kraaimaat, F., and Janssen, P., Relation between specific types of dysfluencies and autonomic and cognitive indices of anxiety in stuttering and nonstutering adolescents. *Proc. 18th Congr. Int. Assoc. Logoped. Phoniat.* Washington, D.C.: Amer. Speech-Lang.-Hearing Assoc. (1981).

Kraamaat, F., and Janssen, P., Are the accessory facial movements of the stutterer learned behaviors? *Percept. Mot. Skills, 60*, 11–17 (1985).

Kraamaat, F., Janssen, P., and Brutten, G. J., The relationship between stutterers' cognitive and autonomic anxiety and therapy outcome. *J. Fluency Dis., 13*, 107–13 (1988).

Kraamaat, F. L., Janssen, P., and van Dam-Boggen, R., Social anxiety and stuttering. *Percept. Mot. Skills, 72*, 766, (1991).

Kramer, M. B., Green, D., and Guitar, B., A comparison of stutterers and nonstutterers on masking level differences and synthetic sentence identification tasks. *J. Communic. Dis., 20*, 379–90 (1987).

Krause, R., Nonverbales interaktives Verhalten von Stotterern und ihren Gesprächspartnern. *Schweiz. Zeitschr. Psychol. Anwend., 37*, 177–201 (1978).

Krause, R., A social psychological approach to the study of stuttering. In Fraser, C., and Scherer, K. R. (eds.), *Advances in the Social Psychology of Language*. Maison des Sciences de l'Homme and Cambridge Univ. Press (1982).

Krikorian, C. M., and Runyan, C. M., A perceptual comparison: Stuttering and nonstuttering children's nonstuttered speech. *J. Fluency Dis., 8*, 283–90 (1983).

Kroll, R. M., and Hood, S. B., Differences in stuttering adaptation between oral reading and spontaneous speech. *J. Communic. Dis., 7*, 227–37 (1974).

Kroll, R. M., and Hood, S. B., The influence of task presentation and information load on the adaptation effect in stutterers and normal speakers. *J. Communic. Dis., 9*, 95–110 (1976).

Kroll, R. M., and O'Keefe, B. M., Molecular self-analysis of stuttered speech via speech time expansion. *J. Fluency Dis., 10*, 93–105 (1985).

Krugman, M., Psychosomatic study of fifty stuttering children: IV. Rorschach study. *Amer. J. Orthopsychiat., 16*, 127–33 (1946).

Kuhr, A., and Rustin, L., The maintenance of fluency after intensive in-patient therapy: Long-term follow-up. *J. Fluency Dis., 10*, 229–36 (1985).

Kully, D., and Boberg, E., An investigation of interclinic agreement in the identification of fluent and stuttered syllables. *J. Fluency Dis., 13*, 309–18 (1988).

Küppers, B., and Wüunschmann, G., Neue Entwicklungen auf dem Gebiet Elektroakustischer Sprech- and Therapiehilfen für Stotterer. *Sprachheilarb., 30*, 261–72 (1985).

Kurshev, V. A., Emotsionalnye reaktsii pri zaikanii po dannym pletizmografii. *Zh. Vyssh. Nerv. Deiatel., 18*, 517–18 (1968a).

Kurshev, V. A., Issledovanie vnerechenovo dykhaniya u zaikayuschikhsya. *Zh. Nevropatol. Psikhiat., 68*, 1840–41 (1968b).

Kurshev, V. A., O neosoznannykh reaktsiyakh u zaikayuschikhsya. *Zh. Nevropatol. Psikhiat.*, *69*, 1075–77 (1960).

Kurth, E., and Schmidt, E., Mehrdimensionale Untersuchungen an stotternden Kindern. *Probleme Ergebnisse Psychol.*, *12*, 49–58 (1964).

LaCroix, Z. E., Management of disfluent speech through self-recording procedures. *J. Speech Hearing Dis.*, *38*, 272–74 (1973).

Laczkowska, M., Painting in stuttering children. *De Therapia Vocis et Loquelae, Vol. I.* XIII Congr. Int. Soc. Logoped. Phoniat. (1965).

Laczkowski, A., Urine investigations in children with speech defects. *De Therapia Vocis et Loquelae, Vol. I.* XIII Congr. Int. Soc. Logoped. Phoniat. (1965).

Ladouceur, R., Boudreau, L., and Théberge, S., Awareness training and regulated-breathing method in modification of stuttering. *Percept. Mot. Skills*, *53*, 187–94 (1981).

Ladouceur, R., Côté, C., Leblond, G., and Bouchard, L., Evaluation of regulated-breathing method and awareness training in the treatment of stuttering. *J. Speech Hearing Dis.*, *47*, 422–26 (1982).

Ladouceur, R., and Martineau, G., Evaluation of regulated-breathing method with and without parental assistance in the treatment of child stutterers. *J. Behav. Ther. Exp. Psychiat.*, *13*, 301–06 (1982).

Ladouceur, R., and Saint-Laurent, L., Stuttering: A multidimensional treatment and evaluation package. *J. Fluency Dis.*, *11*, 93–103 (1986).

LaFollette, A. C., Parental environment of stuttering children. *J. Speech Hearing Dis.*, *21*, 202–07 (1956).

Lambeck, A., Objektive Untersuchungen an Stotterern zur Festellung der Beziehungen der Mitbewegung zur Sprechatmung. *Vox*, *11*, 25–26 (1925).

Langer, R. M., A clinical study of the reactions of preschool children to stuttered and non-stuttered speech in another child. *Speech Monogr.*, *36*, 286 (1969). Abstract.

Langlois, A., Hanrahan, L. L., and Inouye, L. L., A comparison of interactions between stuttering children, nonstuttering children, and their mothers. *J. Fluency Dis.*, *11*, 263–73 (1986).

Langlois, A., and Long, S. H., A model for teaching parents to facilitate fluent speech. *J. Fluency Dis.*, *13*, 163–72 (1988).

Langová, J., and Morávek, M., Some results of experimental examinations among stutterers and clutterers. *Folia Phoniat.*, *16*, 290–96 (1964).

Langová, J., Morávek, M., Novák, A., and Petřík, M., Experimental interference with auditory feedback. *Folia Phoniat.*, *22*, 191–96 (1970).

Langová, J., Morávek, M., Široký, A., and Šváb, L., Einfluss der Sprechaktivität auf den evozierten Vestibularnystagmus bei Stotterern. *Folia Phoniat.*, *27*, 287–91 (1975).

Langová, J., Siroký, A., Šváb, L., and Morávek, M., Odraz neuróz řečive funkci vestibulárniĥo ústroji. *dsh Absdtr.*, *19*, 490 (1979).

Langová, J., and Šváb, L., Reduction of stuttering under experimental social isolation. The role of the adaptation effect. *Folia Phoniat.*, *25*, 17–22 (1973).

Lankford, S. D., and Cooper, E. B., Recovery from stuttering as viewed by parents of self-diagnosed recovered stutterers. *J. Communic. Dis.*, *7*, 171–80 (1974).

Lanyon, R. I., The relationship of adaptation and consistency to improvement in stuttering therapy. *J. Speech Hearing Res.*, *8*, 263–69 (1965).

Lanyon, R. I., The measurement of stuttering severity. *J. Speech Hearing Res.*, *10*, 836–43 (1967).

Lanyon, R. I., Some characteristics of nonfluency in normal speakers and stutterers. *J. Abnorm. Psychol.*, *73*, 550–55 (1968).

Lanyon, R. I., Effect of biofeedback-based relaxation on stuttering during reading and spontaneous speech. *J. Consult. Clin. Psychol.*, *45*, 860–66 (1977).

Lanyon, R. I., and Barocas, V. S., Effects of contingent events on stuttering and fluency. *J. Consult. Clin. Psychol.*, *43*, 786–93 (1975).

Lanyon, R. I., Barrington, C. C., and Newman, A. C., Modification of stuttering through EMG biofeedback: A preliminary study. *Behav. Ther.*, *7*, 96–103 (1976).

Lanyon, R. I., and Duprez, D. A., Nonfluency, information, and word length. *J. Abnorm. Psychol.*, *76*, 93–97 (1970).

Lanyon, R. I., Goldsworthy, R. J., and Lanyon, B. P., Dimensions of stuttering and relationship to psychopathology. *J. Fluency Dis.*, *3*, 103–13 (1978).

Lanyon, R. I., Lanyon, B. P., and Goldsworthy, R. J., Outcome predictors in the behavioral treatment of stuttering. *J. Fluency Dis.*, *4*, 131–39 (1979).

Lasalle, L. R., and Conture, E. G., Eye contact between young stutterers and their mothers. *J. Fluency Dis.*, *16*, 173–99 (1991).

Lass, N. J., Ruscello, D. M., Pannbacker, M. D., Schmitt, J. F., and Everly-Myers, D. S., Speech-language pathologists' perceptions of child and adult female and male stutterers. *J. Fluency Dis.*, *14*, 127–34 (1989).

Laštovka, M., The monosynaptic spinal cord reflex activity changes in stuttering. *Folia Phoniat.*, *22*, 129–38 (1970).

Laštovka, M., Tetanická pohotovost u koktavých a brebtavých. *dsh Abstr.*, *18*, 464 (1978).

Laštovka, M., Influence of some psychopharmaca on the increase of the amplitude of electrically induced monosynaptic spinal cord reflex during the paroxysm of stuttering: 1. Effect of diazepam. *Folia Phoniat.*, *31*, 15–20 (1979a).

Laštovka, M., Influence of some psychopharmaca on the increase of the amplitude of electrically induced monosynaptic spinal cord reflex during the paroxysm of stuttering: 2. Effect of chlorpromazine. *Folia Phoniat.*, *31*, 21–26 (1979b).

Laštovka, M., Pokus o sledováni cásti motorické zpetná vazby u koktavých pomoci elektricky evokavané inervacni pauzy [tzv. silent period]. *dsh Abstr.*, *19*, 490 (1979c).

Leach, E., Stuttering: Clinical application of response-contingent procedures. In Gray, B. B., and England, G. (eds.), *Stuttering and the Conditioning Therapies*. Monterey, Calif.: Monterey Inst. Speech Hearing (1969).

Leanderson, R., and Levi, L., A new approach to the experimental study of stuttering and stress. *Acta Oto-Laryngol.*, *Suppl. 224*, 311–16 (1967).

Leavitt, R. R., *The Puerto Ricans: Culture Change and Language Deviance*. Tucson: Univ. Arizona Press (1974).

Lebrun, Y., Bijleveld, H., and Rousseau, J.-J., A case of persistent neurogenic stuttering following a missile wound. *J. Fluency Dis.*, *15*, 251–85 (1990).

Lebrun, Y., and Leleux, C., Acquired stuttering following right brain damage in dextrals. *J. Fluency Dis.*, *10*, 137–41 (1985).

Lebrun, Y., Leleux, C., Rousseau, J.-J., and Devreaux, F., Acquired stuttering. *J. Fluency Dis., 8,* 323–30 (1983).

Lebrun, Y., Rétif, J., and Kaiser, G., Acquired stuttering as a forerunner of motorneuron disease. *J. Fluency Dis., 8,* 161–67 (1983).

Lechner, B. K., The effects of delayed auditory feedback and masking on the fundamental frequency of stutterers and nonstutterers. *J. Speech Hearing Res., 22,* 343–53 (1979).

Lee, B. S., Some effects of side-tone delay. *J. Acoust. Soc. Amer., 22,* 639–40 (1950a).

Lee, B. S., Effects of delayed speech feedback. *J. Acoust. Soc. Amer., 22,* 824–26 (1950b).

Lee, B. S., Artificial stutter. *J. Speech Hearing Dis., 16,* 53–55 (1951).

Lees, R. M., The effect of foreperiod length on the acoustic voice reaction times of stutterers. *J. Fluency Dis., 13,* 157–62 (1988).

Leith, W. R., and Mims, H. A., Cultural influences in the development and treatment of stuttering: A preliminary report on the black stutterer. *J. Speech Hearing Dis., 40,* 459–66 (1975).

Leith, W. R., and Timmons, J. L., The stutterer's reaction to the telephone as a speaking situation. *J. Fluency Dis., 8,* 233–43 (1983).

Lemert, E. M., Some Indians who stutter. *J. Speech Hearing Dis., 18,* 168–74 (1953).

Lemert, E. M., Stuttering and social structure in two Pacific societies. *J. Speech Hearing Disc., 27,* 3–10 (1962).

Lepsova, M., Ein Ferienlager für stotternde Kinder. *De Therapia Vocis et Loquelae, Vol. I.* XIII Congr. Int. Soc. Logoped. Phoniat. (1965).

Lerea, L., An exploratory study of the effects of experimentally induced success and falure upon the oral reading performances and the levels of aspiration of stutterers. *Speech Monogr., 22,* 202–03 (1955). Abstrct.

Lerman, J. W., Powers, G. R., and Rigrodsky, S., Stuttering patterns observed in a sample of mentally retarded individuals. *Train. Sch. Bull., 62,* 27–32 (1965).

Lerman, J. W., and Shames, G. H., The effect of situational difficulty difficulty on stuttering. *J. Speech Hearing Res., 8,* 271–80 (1965).

Leske, M. C., Prevalence estimates of communicative disorders in the U.S.: Speech disorders. *Asha, 23,* 217–25 (1981).

Leutenegger, R. R., Adaptation and recovery in the oral reading of stutterers. *J. Speech Hearing Dis., 22,* 276–87 (1957).

Lewis, D., and Sherman, D., Measuring the severity of stuttering. *J. Speech Hearing Dis., 16,* 320–26 (1951).

Lewis, J. I., Ingham, R. J., and Gervens, A., Voice initiation and termination times in stutterers and normal speakers. *Asha, 21,* 693 (1979). Abstract.

Lewis, K. E., The structure of disfluency behaviors in the speech of adult stutterers. *J. Speech Hearing Res., 34,* 492–500 (1991).

Liebetrau, R. M., and Daly, D. A., Auditory processing and perceptual abilities of "organic" and "functional" stutterers. *J. Fluency Dis., 6,* 219–31 (1981).

Lightfoot, C., Serial identification of colors by stutterers. *J. Speech Hearing Dis., 13,* 193–208 (1948).

Lindsley, D. B., Bilateral differences in brain potentials from the two cerebral Hemispheres in relation to laterality and stuttering. *J. Exper. Psychol., 26,* 211–25 (1940).

Lingwall, J. B., and Bergstrand, G. G., Perceptual boundaries for judgments of "normal," "abnormal" and "stuttered" prolongations. *Asha, 21,* 733 (1979). Abstract.

Lockhart, M. S., and Robertson, A. W., Hypnosis and speech therapy as a combined therapeutic approach to the problem of stammering: A study of thirty patients. *Brit. J. Dis. Communic., 12,* 97–108 (1977).

Long, K. M., and Pindzola, R. H., Manual reaction time to linguistic stimuli in child stutterers and nonstutterers. *J. Fluency Dis., 10,* 143–49 (1985).

Lotzmann, G., Zur Anwendung variierter Verzögerungszeiten bei Balbuties. *Folia Phoniat., 13,* 276–312 (1961).

Louko, L. J., Edwards, M. L., and Conture, E. G., Phonological characteristics of young stutterers and their normally fluent peers: Preliminary observations. *J. Fluency Dis. 15,* 191–210.

Lounsbury, F. G., Pausal, juncture and hesitation phenomena. In Osgood, C. E., and Sebeok, T. A. (eds.), *Psycholinguistics: A Survey of Theory and Research.* Baltimore: Waverly Press (1954).

Louttit, C. M., and Halls, E. C., Survey of speech defects among public school children of Indiana. *J. Speech Dis., 1,* 73–80 (1936).

Love, L. R., and Jeffress, L. A., Identification of brief pauses in the fluent speech of stutterers and nonstutterers. *J. Speech Hearing Res., 14,* 229–40 (1971).

Love, W. R., The effect of pentobarbital sodium (Nembutal) and amphetamine sulphate (Benzedrine) on the severity of stuttering. In Johnson, W., and Leutenegger, R. R. (eds.), *Stuttering in Children and Adults.* Minneapolis: Univ. Minn. Press (1955).

Lovett Doust, J. W., Stress and psychopathology in stutterers. Can. *J. Psychol., 10,* 31–37 (1956).

Lovett Doust, J. W., and Coleman, L. I. M., The psychophysics of communication: III. Discriminatory awareness in stutterers and its measurement by the critical flicker fusion threshold. *Arch. Neurol. Psychiat., 74,* 650–52 (1955).

Lowinger, L., The psychodynamics of stuttering: An evaluation of the factors of aggression and guilt feelings in a group of institutionalized children. *Dissert. Abstr., 12,* 725 (1952).

Lubman, C. G., Speech program for severely retarded children. *Amer. J. Ment. Defic., 60,* 297–300 (1955).

Luchsinger, R., Untersuchungen des vegetativen Nervensystems bei Stotterern. *Schweiz. Med. Wochenschr., 73,* 868–;70 (1943).

Luchsinger, R., Gibt es organisch bedingte Stottererfälle? *Arch. Ohr.-Nas.-Kehlk. Heilk., 165,* 612–18 (1954).

Luchsinger, R., Die Vererbung von Spach- und Stimmstörungen. *Folia Phoniat., 11,* 7–64 (1959).

Luchsinger, R., and Dubois, C., Ein Vergleich der Sprachmelodie- und Lautstärkekurve bei Normalen, Gehirnkranken und Stotterern. *Folia Phoniat., 15,* 21–41 (1963).

Luchsinger, R., and Landolt, H. Über das Poltern, das sogenannte "Stottern mit Polterkomponente," und deren Beziehung zu den Aphasien. *Folia Phoniat., 7,* 12–43 (1955).

Luessenhop, A. J., Boggs, J. S., LaBorwit, L. J., and Walle, E. L., Cerebral dominance in stutterers determined by Wada testing. *Neurol., 23,* 1190–92 (1973).

Luperr, H. ZL., Consistency of stuttering in relation to the goal gradient hypothesis. *J. Speech Hearing Dis., 21,* 336–42 (1956).

Luper, H. L., and Chambers, J. L., An analysis of stutterers' responses to the Picture Identification Test. *Asha, 4,* 377 (1962). Abstract.

Lybolt, J. T., Language disability and dysfluent speech in elementary school children. *Folia Phoniat., 38,* 326–27 (1986). Abstract.

MacCulloch, M. J., and Eaton, R., A note on reduced auditory pain threshold in 44 stuttering children. *Brit. J. Dis. Communic., 6,* 148–53 (1971).

MacCulloch, M. J., Eaton, R., and Long, E., The long term effect of auditory masking on young stutterers. *Brit. J. Dis. Communic., 5,* 165–73 (1970).

MacDonald, J. D., and Martin, R. R., Stuttering and disfluency as two reliable and unambiguous response classes. *J. Speech Hearing Res., 16,* 691–99 (1973).

MacFarlane, W. B., Hanson, M., Walton, W., and Mellon, C. D., Stuttering in five generations of a single family. *J. Fluency Dis., 16,* 117–23 (1991).

Macioszek, G., Die verzögerte akustische Rückmeldung bei Stotterern mit unterschiedlichem Ausmass der Störung. *Zeitschr. für Klinische Psychol., 2,* 278–99 (1973).

MacKay, D. G., Effects of ambiguity on stuttering: Towards a theory of speech production at the semantic level. *Kybernetik, 5,* 195–208 (1969).

MacKay, D. G., and MacDonald, M. C., Stuttering as a sequencing and timing disorder. In Curlee, R. F., and Perkins, W. H. (eds.), *Nature and Treatment of Stuttering: New Directions.* San Diego: College-Hill Press (1984).

Maclay, H., and Osgood, C. E., Hesitation phenomena in spontaneous English speech. *Word, 15,* 19–44 (1959).

Maddox, J., Studies in the psychology of stuttering: VIII. The role of visual cues in the precipitation of moments of stuttering. *J. Speech Dis., 3,* 90–94 (1938).

Madison, L. S., Budd, K. S., and Itzkowitz, J. S., Changes in stuttering in relation to children's locus of control. *J. Genet. Psychol., 147,* 233–40 (1986).

Madison, L., and Norman, R. D., A comparison of the performance of stutterers and nonstutterers on the Rosenzweig Picture Frustration Test. *J. Clin. Psychol., 8,* 179–83 (1952).

Mahl, G. F., Disturbances and silences in the patient's speech in psychotherapy. *J. Abnorm. Soc. Psychol., 53,* 1–15 (1956).

Mahl, G. F., Measures of two expressive aspects of a patient's speech in two psychotherapeutic interviews. In Gottschalk, L. A. (ed.), *Comparative Psycholinguistic Analysis of Two Psychotherapeutic Interviews.* New York: Int. Univ. Press (1961).

Mahr, G., and Leith, W., Psychogenic stuttering of adult onset. *J. Speech Hearing Res., 35,* 283–86 (1992).

Mallard, A. R., The effects of syllable-timed speech on stuttering behavior: An audiovisual analysis. *Behav. Ther., 8,* 947–52 (1977).

Mallard, A. R., Hicks, D. M., and Riggs, D. E., A comparison of stutterers and nonstutterers in a task of controlled voice onset. *J. Speech Hearing Res., 25,* 287–90 (1982).

Mallard, A. R., and Kelley, J. S., The precision fluency shaping program: Replication and evaluation. *J. Fluency Dis., 7*, 287–94 (1982).

Mallard, A. R., and Meyer, L. A., Listener preferences for stuttered and syllable-timed speech production. *J. Fluency Dis., 4*, 117–21 (1979).

Mallard, A. R., and Webb, W. G., The effects of auditory and visual "distractors" on the frequency of stuttering. *J. Communic. Dis., 13*, 207–12 (1980).

Mallard, A. R., and Westbrook, J. B., Vowel duration in stutterers participating in Precision Fluency Shaping. *J. Fluency Dis., 10*, 221–28 (1985).

Mallard, A. R., and Westbrook, J. B., Variables affecting stuttering therapy in school settings. *Lang. Speech Hearing Services Schools, 19*, 362–70 (1988).

Mann, M. B., Nonfluencies in the oral reading of stutterers and nonstutterers of elementary school age. In Johnson, W., and Leutenegger, R. R. (eds.), *Stuttering in Children and Adults*. Minneapolis: Univ. Minn. Press (1955).

Manning, W. H., and Cooper, E. B., Variations in attitudes of the adult stutterer toward his clinician related to progress in therapy. *J. Communic. Dis., 2*, 154–62 (1969).

Manning, W. H., and Coufal, K. J., The frequency of disfluencies during phonatory transitions in stuttered and nonstuttered speech. *J. Communic. Dis., 9*, 75–81 (1976).

Manning, W. H., Dailey, D., and Wallace, S., Attitude and personality characteristics of older stutterers. *J. Fluency Dis., 9*, 207–15 (1984).

Manning, W. H., Lee, B. A., and Lass, N. J., The use of time-expanded speech in the identification of part-word repetitions of stutterers. *J. Communic. Dis., 11*, 11–15 (1978).

Manning, W. H., and Riensche, L., Auditory assembly abilities of stuttering and nonstuttering children. *J. Speech Hearing Res., 19*, 77–83 (1976).

Manning, W. H., Trutna, P. A., and Shaw, C. K., Verbal versus tangible reward for children who stutter. *J. Speech Hearing Dis., 41*, 52–62 (1976).

Maraist, J. A., and Hutton, C., Effects of auditory masking upon the speech of stutterers. *J. Speech Hearing Dis., 22*, 385–89 (1957).

Market, K. E., Montague, J. C., Jr., Buffalo, M.D., and Drummond, S. S., Acquired stuttering: Descriptive data and treatment outcome. *J. Fluency Dis., 15*, 21–33 (1990).

Marshall, R. C., and Neuburger, S. I., Effects of delayed auditory feedback on acquired stuttering following head injury. *J. Fluency Dis., 12*, 355–65 (1987).

Martens, C. F., and Engel, D. C., Measurement of the sound-based word avoidance of persons who stutter. *J. Fluency Dis., 11*, 241–50 (1986).

Martin, R. R., Stuttering and perseveration in children. *J. Speech Hearing Res., 5*, 332–39 (1962).

Martin, R. R., Direct magnitude-estimation judgments of stuttering severity using audible and audible-visible speech samples. *Speech Monogr., 32*, 169–77 (1965).

Martin, R. R., Introduction and perspective: Review of published studies. In Boberg, E. (ed.), *Maintenance of Fluency: Proceedings of the Banff Conference*. New York: Elsevier North-Holland (1981).

Martin, R., and Gaviser, J., Time-out as a punishment for button pushing. *J. Speech Hearing Res., 14*, 144–48 (1971).

Martin, R. R., and Haroldson, S. K., The relationship between anticipation and consistency of stutterered words. *J. Speech Hearing Res., 10,* 323–27 (1967).

Martin, R. R., and Haroldson, S. K., The effects of two treatment procedures on stuttering. *J. Communic. Dis., 2,* 115–25 (1969).

Martin, R. R., and Haroldson, S. K., Time-out as a punishment for stuttering during conversation. *J. Communic. Dis., 4,* 15–19 (1971).

Martin, R. R., and Haroldson, S. K., Disfluencies of young children in private speech and in conversation. *Human Communic., 3,* 21–25 (1975).

Martin, R., and Haroldson, S., Effect of vicarious punishment on stuttering frequency. *J. Speech Hearing Res., 20,* 21–26 (1977).

Martin, R., and Haroldson, S. K., Effects of five experimental treatments on stuttering. *J. Speech Hearing Res., 22,* 132–46 (1979).

Martin, R. R., and Haroldson, S. K., Stuttering identification: Standard definition and moment of stuttering. *J. Speech Hearing Res., 24,* 59–63 (1981).

Martin, R. R., and Haroldson, S. K., Contingent self-stimulation for stuttering. *J. Speech Hearing Dis., 47,* 407–13 (1982).

Martin, R. R., and Haroldson, S. K., An experimental increase in stuttering frequency. *J. Speech Hearing Res., 31,* 272–74 (1988).

Martin, R. R., and Haroldson, S. K., Stuttering and speech naturalness: Audio and audiovisual judgments. *J. Speech Hearing Res., 35,* 521–28 (1992).

Martin, R. R., Haroldson, S. K., and Kuhl, P., Disfluencies in child-child and child-mother speaking situations. *J. Speech Hearing Res., 15,* 753–56 (1972a).

Martin, R. R., Haroldson, S. K., and Kuhl, P., Disfluencies of young children in two speaking situations. *J. Speech Hearing Res., 15,* 831–36 (1972b).

Martin, R., Haroldson, S. K., and Triden, K. A., Stuttering and speech naturalness. *J. Speech Hearing Res., 49,* 53–58 (1984).

Martin, R. R., Haroldson, S. K., and Woessner, G. L., Perceptual scaling of stuttering severity. *J. Fluency Dis., 13,* 27–47 (1988).

Martin, R. R., Johnson, L. J., Siegel, G. M., and Haroldson, S. K., Auditory stimulation, rhythm, and stuttering, *J. Speech Hearing Res., 28,* 487–95 (1985).

Martin, R. R., Kuhl, P., and Haroldson, S., An experimental treatment with two preschool stuttering children. *J. Speech Hearing Res., 15,* 743–52 (1972).

Martin, R. R., Lawrence, B. A., Haroldson, S. K., and Gunderson, D., Stuttering and oral stereognosis. *Percept. Mot. Skills, 53,* 155–62 (1981).

Martin, R., Parlour, S. F., and Haroldson, S., Stuttering and level of linguistic demand: The Stocker Probe. *J. Fluency Dis., 15,* 93–106 (1990).

Martin, R., St. Louis, K., Haroldson, S., and Hasbrouck, J., Punishment and negative reinforcement of stuttering using electric shock. *J. Speech Hearing Res., 18,* 478–90 (1975).

Martin, R. R., and Siegel, G. M., The effects of response contingent shock on stuttering. *J. Speech Hearing Res., 9,* 340–52 (1966a).

Martin, R. R., and Siegel, G. M., The effects of simultaneously punishing stuttering and rewarding fluency. *J. Speech Hearing Res., 9,* 466–75 (1966b).

Martin, R. R., and Siegel, G. M., The effects of a neutral stimulus (buzzer) on motor responses and disfluencies in normal speakers. *J. Speech Hearing Res., 12,* 179–84 (1969).

Martin, R. R., Siegel, G. M., Johnson, L. J., and Haroldson, S. K., Sidetone amplification, noise, and stuttering. *J. Speech Hearing Res., 276*, 518–27 (1984).

Martyn, M. M., and Sheehan, J., Onset of stuttering and recovery. *Behav. Res. Ther., 6*, 295–307 (1968).

Martyn, M. M., Sheehan, J., and Slutz, K., Incidence of stuttering and other speech disorders among the retarded. *Amer. J. Ment. Defic., 74*, 206–11 (1969).

Mast, V. R., Level of aspiration as a method of studying the personality of adult stutterers. *Speech Monogr., 19*, 196 (1952). Abstract.

Mattingly, S. C., The performance of stutterers and nonstutterers on two tasks of dichotic listening. *Asha, 12*, 427 (1970). Abstrct.

Maxwell, D. L., Social and vocational attitudes toward stuttering. *Proc. 18th Congr. Int. Assoc. Logoped. Phoniat.* Washington, D. C.: Amer. Speech-Lang.-Hearing Assoc. (1981).

Maxwell, D. L., Cognitive and behavioral self-control strategies: Applications for the clinical management of adult stutterers. *J. Fluency Dis., 7*, 403–32 (1982).

Maxwell, R. D. H., and Paterson, J. W., Meprobamate in the treatment of stuttering. *Brit. Med. J., No. 5075, Apr.*, 873–74 (1958).

May, A. E., and Hackwood, A., Some effects of masking and eliminating low frequency feedback on the speech of stammerers. *Behav. Res. Ther., 6*, 219–23 (1968).

Mazzucchi, A., Moretti, G., Carpeggiani, P., Parma, M., and Paini, P., Clinical observations on acquired stuttering. *Brit. J. Dis. Communic., 16*, 19–30 (1981).

McAllister, A. H., *Clinical Studies in Speech Therapy.* London: Univ. London Press (1937).

McClean, M. D., Surface recording of the perioral reflexes: Preliminary observations on stutterers and nonstutterers. *J. Speech Hearing Res., 30*, 283–87 (1987).

McClean, M., Goldsmith, H., and Cerf, A., Lower-lip EMG and displacement during bilabial disfluencies in adult stutterers. *J. Speech Hearing Res., 27*, 342–49 (1984).

McClean, M. D., Kroll, R. M., and Loftus, N. S., Kinematic analysis of lip closure in stutterers' fluent speech. *J. Speech Hearing Res., 33*, 755–60 (1990).

McClean, M. D., Kroll, R. M., and Loftus, N. S., Correlation of stuttering severity and kinematics of lip closure. In Peters, H. F. M., Hulstijn, W., and Starkweather, C. W. (eds.), *Speech Motor Control and Stuttering.* Amsterdam: Elsevier (1991).

McClean, M.D., and McLean, A., Jr., Case report of stuttering acquired in association with phenytoin use for post-head-injury seizures. *J. Fluency Dis., 10*, 241–55 (1985).

McCroskey, R. L., Effect of speech on metabolism: A comparison between stutterers and nonstutterers. *J. Speech Hearing Dis., 22*, 46–52 (1957).

McDearmon, J. R., Primary stuttering at the onset of stuttering: A reexamination of data. *J. Speech Hearing Res., 11*, 631–37 (1968).

Mcdonald, E. T., and Frick, J. V., Store clerks' reaction to stuttering. *J. Speech Hearing Dis., 19*, 306–11 (1954).

McDonough, A. N., and Quesal, R. W., Locus of control orientation of stutterers and nonstutterers. *J. Fluency Dis.*, *13*, 97–106 (1988).

McDowell, E. D., *The Educational and Emotional Adjustments of Stuttering Children*. New York: Columbia Univ. Teachers Coll. (1928).

McFarland, D. H., Smith, A., Moore, C. A., and Weber, C. M., Relationship between amplitude of tremor and reflex responses of the human jaw-closing system. *Brain Res.*, *366*, 272–78 (1986).

McFarlane, S. C., and Lavorato, A. S., relationship between voice reaction time and stuttering severity. *Asha*, *25*, 102 (1983). Abstract.

McFarlane, S. C., and Prins, D., Neural response time of stutterers and nonstutterers in selected oral motor tasks. *J. Speech Hearing Res.*, *21*, 768–78 (1978).

McFarlane, S. C., and Shipley, K. G., Latency of vocalization onset for stutterers and nonstutterers under conditions of auditory and visual cuing. *J. Speech Hearing Dis.*, *46*, 307–12 (1981).

McGee, S. R., Hutchinson, J. M., and Deputy, P. N., The influence of the onset of phonation on the frequency of disfluency among children who stutter. *J. Speech Hearing Res.*, *24*, 269–72 (1981).

McGuire, R. A., Loren, C., and Rastatter, M. P., Naming reaction times to tachistoscopically presented pictures: Some evidence for right hemisphere encoding capacity. *Percept. Mot. Skills*, *62*, 303–06 (1986).

McHale, A., An investigation of personality attributes of stammering, enuretic and school-phobic children. *Brit. J. Educ. Psychol.*, *37*, 400–03 (1967).

McIntyre, M. E., Silverman, F. H., and Trotter, W. D., Transcendental meditation and stuttering: A preliminary report. *Percept. Mot. Skills*, *39*, 294 (1974).

McKinnon, S. L., Hess, C. W., and Landry, R. G., Reactions of college students to speech disorders. *J. Communic. Dis.*, *19*, 75–82 (1986).

McKnight, R. C., and Cullinan, W. L., Subgroups of stuttering children: Speech and voice reaction times, segmental durations, and naming latencies. *J. Fluency Dis.*, *12*, 217–33 (1987).

McLaughlin, S. F., and Cullinan, W. L., Disfluencies, utterance length, and linguistic complexity in nonstuttering children. *J. Fluency Dis.*, *14*, 17–36 (1989).

McLean, A. E., and Cooper, E. B., Electromyographic indications of laryngeal-area activity during stuttering expectancy. *J. Fluency Dis.*, *3*, 205–19 (1978).

McLean-Muse, A., Larson, C. R., and Gregory, H. H., Stutterers' and nonstutterers' voice fundamental frequency changes in response to auditory stimuli. *J. Speech Hearing Res.*, *31*, 549–55 (1988).

McLelland, J. K., and Cooper, E. B., Fluency-related behaviors and attitudes of 178 young stutterers. *J. Fluency Dis.*, *3*, 253–63 (1978).

McMillan, M. O., and Pindzola, R. H., Temporal disruptions in the 'accurate' speech of articulatory defective speakers and stutterers. *J. Mot. Behav.*, *18*, 179–86 (1986).

Meltzer, A., Horn stuttering. *J. Fluency Dis.*, *17*, 257–64 (1992).

Meltzer, H., Personality differences among stutterers as indicated by the Rorschach Test. *Amer. J. Orthopsychiat.*, *4*, 262–80 (1934).

Meltzer, H., Talkativeness in stuttering and nonstuttering children. *J. Genet. Psychol.*, *46*, 371–90 (1935).

Meltzer, H., Personality differences between stuttering and nonstuttering children as indicatd by the Rorschach Test. *J. Psychol.*, *17*, 39–59 (1944).

Merits-Patterson, R., and Reed, C. G., Disfluencies in the speech of language-delayed children. *J. Speech Hearing Res., 24,* 55–58 (1981).

Metfessel, M., and Warren, N. D., Overcompensation by the non-preferred hand in an action-current study of simultaneous movements of the fingers. *J. Exper. Psychol., 17,* 246–56 (1934).

Métraux, R. W., Speech profiles of the pre-school child 18 to 54 months. *J. Speech Hearing Dis., 15,* 37–53 (1950).

Metz, D. E., Conture, E. G., and Colton, R. H., Temporal relations between the respiratory and laryngeal systems prior to stuttered disfluencies. *Asha, 18,* 664 (1976). Abstract.

Metz, D. E., Onufrak, J. A., and Ogburn, R. S., An acoustical analysis of stutterers' speech prior to and at the termination of speech therapy. *J. Fluency Dis., 4,* 249–54 (1979).

Metz, D. E., Samar, V. J., and Sacco, P. R., Acoustic analysis of stutterers' fluent speech before and after therapy. *J. Speech Hearing Res., 26,* 531–36 (1983).

Metz, D. E., Schiavetti, N., and Sacco, P. R., Acoustic and psychopohysical dimensions of the perc;eived speech naturalness of nonstutterers and postreatment stutterers. *J. Speech Hearing Dis., 55,* 516–25 (1990).

Meyer, B. C., Psychosomatic aspects of stuttering. *J. Nerv. Ment. Dis., 101,* 127–57 (1945).

Meyer, V., and Mair, J. M. M., A new technique to control stammering: A preliminary report. *Behav. Res. Ther., 1,* 251–54 (1963).

Meyers, S. C., Qualitative and quantitative differences and patterns of variability in disfluencies emitted by preschool stutterers and nonstutterers during dyadic conversations. *J. Fluency Dis., 11,* 293–306 (1986).

Meyers, S. C., Nonfluencies of preschool stutterers and conversational partners: Observing reciprocal relatioinships. *J. Speech Hearing Dis., 54,* 106–12 (1989).

Meyers, S. C., Verbal behaviors of preschool stutterers and conversational partners: Observing reciprocal relationships. *J. Speech Hearing Dis., 55,* 706–12 (1990).

Meyers, S. C., and Freeman, F. J., Are mothers of stutterers different? An investigation of social-communicative interaction. *J. Fluency Dis., 10,* 193–209 (1985a).

Meyers, S. C., and Freeman, F. J., Interruptions as a variable in stuttering and disfluency. *J. Speech Hearing Res., 28,* 428–35 (1985b).

Meyers, S. C., and Freeman, F. J., Mother and child speech rates as a variable in stuttering and disfluency. *J. Speech Hearing Res., 28,* 436–44 (1985c).

Meyers, S. C., Hall, N. E., and Aram, D. M., Fluency and language recovery in a child with a left-hemisphere lesion. *J. Fluency Dis., 15,* 159–73 (1990).

Meyers, S. C., Hughes, L. F., and Schoeny, Z. G., Temporal-phonemic processing skills in adult stutterers and nonstutterers. *J. Speech Hearing Res., 32,* 274–80 (1989).

Milisen, R., Expectancy reactions in stutterers. *Abstr. Proc. Amer. Speech Correct. Assn., 7,* 52–55 (1937).

Milisen, R., Frequency of stuttering with anticipation of stuttering controlled. *J. Speech Dis., 3,* 2097–14 (1938).

Milisen, R., and Johnson, W., A comparative study of stutterers, former stutterers and normal speakers whose handedness has been changed. *Arch. Speech, 1,* 61–86 (1936).

Miller, J. A., and Miller, T. W., Adaptation effect in nonfluent speech behavior of controlled stutterers and nonstutterers. *J. Fluency Dis.*, *2*, 305–10 (1977).

Miller, N. E., Experimental studies of conflict. In Hunt, J. McV. (ed.), *Personality and the Behavior Disorders*. New York: Ronald Press (1944).

Miller, S., and Watson, B. C., The relationship between communication attitude, anxiety, and depression in stutterers and nonstutterers. *J. Speech Hearing Res.*, *35*, 789–98 (1992).

Mills, A. W., and Streit, H., Report of a speech survey. Holyoke, Massachusetts. *J. Speech Dis.*, *7*, 161–67 (1942).

Minifie, F. D., and Cooker, H. S., A disfluency index. *J. Speech Hearing Dis.*, *29*, 189–92 (1964).

Moleski, R., and Tosi, D. J., Comparative psychotherapy: Rational-emotive therapy versus systematic desensitization in the treatment of stuttering. *J. Consult. Clin. Psychol.*, *44*, 309–11 (1976).

Molt, L. F., Selected acoustic and physiologic measures of speech motor coordination in stuttering and nonstuttering children. In Peters, H. F. M., Hulstijn, W., and Starkweather, C. W. (eds.), *Speech Motor Control and Stuttering*. Amsterdam: Elsevier (1991).

Molt, L. F., and Guilford, A. M., Auditory processing and anxiety in stutterers. *J. Fluency Dis.*, *4*, 255–67 (1979),

Molt, L. F., and Luper, H. L., Latency of slow cortical auditory evoked responses in stutterers. *Asha*, *25*, 164 (1983a). Abstract.

Moncur, J. P., Parental domination in stuttering. *J. Speech Hearing Dis.*, *17*, 155–65 (1952).

Moncur, J. P., Symptoms of maladjustment differentiating young stutterers from nonstutterers. *Child Dev.*, *26*, 91–96 (1955).

Montgomery, A. A., and Cooke, P. A., Perceptual and acoustic analysis of repetitions in stutterered speech. *J. Communic. Dis.*, *9*, 317–30 (1976).

Montgomery, B. M., and Fitch, J. L., The prevalence of stuttering in the hearing-impaired school age population. *J. Speech Hearing Dis.*, *53*, 131–35 (1988).

Moore, M. A. S., and Adams, M. R., The Edinburgh masker: A clinical analog study. *J. Fluency Dis.*, *10*, 281–90 (1985).

Moore, S. E., and Perkins, W. H., Validity and reliability of judgments of authentic and simulated stuttering. *J. Speech Hearing Dis.*, *55*, 383–91 (1990).

Moore, W. E., A conditioned reflex study of stuttering. *J. Speech Dis.*, *3*, 163–83 (1938).

Moore, W. E., Hypnosis in a system of therapy for stutterers. *J. Speech Dis.*, *11*, 117–22 (1946).

Moore, W. E., Relations of stuttering in spontaneous speech to speech content and to adaptation. *J. Speech Hearing Dis.*, *19*, 208–16 (1954).

Moore, W. E., A study of the blood chemistry of stutterers under two hypnotic conditions. *Speech Monogr.*, *26*, 64–68 (1959).

Moore, W. E., Soderberg, G., and Powell, D., Relations of stuttering in spontaneous speech to speech content and verbal output. *J. Speech Hearing Dis.*, *17* 371–76 (1952).

Moore, W. H., Jr., Bilateral tachistoscopic word perception of stutterers and normal subjects. *Brain Lang.*, *3*, 434–42 (1976).

Moore, W. H., Jr., Some effects of progressively lowering electromyographic levels with feedback procedures on the frequency of stuttered verbal behaviors. *J. Fluency Dis., 3*, 127–38 (1978).

Moore, W. H., Jr., Central nervous system characteristics of stutterers. In Curlee, R. F., and Perkins, W. H., *Nature and Treatment of Stuttering: New Directions*. San Diego: College-Hill (1984a).

Moore, W. H., Jr., Hemispheric alpha asymmetries during an electromyographic biofeedback procedure for stuttering: A single-subject experimental design. *J. Fluency Dis., 9*, 143–62 (1984b).

Moore, W. H., Jr., Hemispheric alpha asymmetries of stutterers and nonstutterers for the recall and recognition of words and connected reading passages: Some relationships to severity of stuttering. *J. Fluency Dis., 11*, 71–89 (1986).

Moore, W. H., Jr., and Boberg, E., Hemispheric processing and stuttering. In Rustin, L., Purser, H., and Rowley, D. (eds.), *Progress in the Treatment of Fluency Disorders*. London: Taylor and Francis (1987).

Moore, W. H., Jr., Craven, D. C., and Faber, M. M., Hemispheric alpha asymmetries of words with positive, negative, and neutral arousal values preceding tasks of recall and recognition: Electrophysiological and behavioral results from stuttering males and nonstuttering males and females. *Brain Lang., 17*, 211–24 (1982).

Moore, W. H., Jr., Cunko, C., and Flowers, P., Cumulative integrated electromyographic activity of selected speech-related muscle groups of nonstutterers during massed oral readings. *J. Fluency Dis., 4*, 149–61 (1979).

Moore, W. H., Jr., Flowers, P., and Cunko, C., Some relationships between adptation and electromyographic activity at laryngeal and masseter sites in stutterers. *J. Fluency Dis., 6*, 81–94 (1981).

Moore, W. H., Jr., and Haynes, W. O., Alpha hemispheric asymmetry and stuttering: Some support for a segmentation dysfunction hypothesis. *J. Speech Hearing Res., 23*, 229–47 (1980).

Moore, W. H., Jr., and Lang, M. K., Alpha asymmetry over the right and left hemispheres of stutterers and control subjects preceding massed oral readings: A preliminary investigation. *Percept. Mot. Skills, 44*, 223–30 (1977).

Moore, W. H., Jr., and Lorendo, L. C., Hemispheric alpha asymmetries of stuttering males and nonstuttering males and females for words of high and low imagery. *J. Fluency Dis., 5*, 11–26 (19890).

Moore, W. H., Jr., and Ritterman, S. I., The effects of response contingent reinforcement and response contingent punishment upon the frequency of stuttered verbal behavior. *Behav. Res. Ther., 11*, 43–48 (1973).

Morávek, M., and Langová, J., Some electrophysiological findings among stutterers and clutterers. *Folia Phoniat., 14*, 305–16 (1962).

Morávek, M., and Langová, J., Problem of the development of the initial tonus in stuttering. *Folia Phoniat., 19*, 109–16 (1967).

Morgenstern, J. J., *Psychological and Social Factors in Children's Stammering*. Ph.D. Dissert., Univ. Edinburgh (1953).

Morgenstern, J. J., Socio-economic factors in stuttering. *J. Speech Hearing Dis., 21*, 25–33 (1956).

Morley, A., An analysis of associated and predisposing factors in the symptomatology of stuttering. *Psychol. Monogr., 49*, 50–107 (1937).

Morley, M. E., A ten-year survey of speech disorders among university students. *J. Speech Hearing Dis., 17*, 25–31 (1952).

Morley, M. E., *The Development and Disorders of Speech in Childhood*. Edinburgh: Livingstone (1957).

Morris, D. W., Position as a factor of attentional clearness in relation to stuttering. *J. Speech Dis., 3*, 141–58 (1938).

Moser, H. M., A qualitative analysis of eye-movements during stuttering. *J. Speech Dis., 3*, 131–39 (1938).

Moss, S. E., The influence of varying degrees of voicing on the adaptation effect in the repeated oral readings of stutterers. *Aust. J. Human Communic. Dis., 4*, 127–32 (1976).

Mowrer, D., An instructional program ot increase fluent speech of stutterers. *J. Fluency Dis., 1*, 25–35 (1975).

Mowrer, D. E., Effect of audience reaction upon fluency rates of six stutterers. *J. Fluency Dis., 3*, 193–203 (1978).

Muellerleile, S., Portable delayed auditory feedback device: A preliminary report. *J. Fluency Dis., 6*, 361–63 (1981).

Muma, J. R., Syntax of preschool fluent and disfluent speech: A transformational analysis. *J. Speech Hearing Res., 14*, 428–41 (1971).

Murphy, A. T., An electroencephalographic study of frustration in stutterers. *Speech Monogr., 20*, 148–49 (1953). Abstract.

Murphy, A. T., and FitzSimons, R. M., *Stuttering and Personality Dynamics*. New York: Ronald Press (1960).

Murphy, M. and Baumgartner, J. M., Voice initiation and termination time in stuttering and nonstuttering children. *J. Fluency Dis., 6*, 257–64 (1981).

Murray, E., Dysintegration of breathing and eye-movements in stutterers during silent reading and reasoning. *Psychol. Monogr., 43*, 218–75 (1932).

Murray, F. P., An investigation of variably induced white noise upon moments of stuttering. *J. Communic. Dis., 2*, 109–14 (1969).

Murray, H. L., and Reed, C. G., Language abilities of preschool stuttering children. *J. Fluency Dis., 2*, 171—76 (1977).

Murray, K. S., Empson, J. A. C., and Weaver, S. M., Rehearsal and preparation for speech in stutterers: A psychophysiological study. *Brit. J. Dis. Communic., 22*, 145–50 (1987).

Murray, T. J., Kelly, P., Campbell, L., and Stefanik, K., haloperidol in the treatment of stuttering. *Brit. J. Psychiat., 130*, 370–73 (1977).

Myers, F. L., Relationship between eight physiological variables and severity of stuttering. *J. Fluency Dis., 3*, 181–91 (1978).

Mysak, E. D., Servo theory and stuttering. *J. Speech Hearing Dis., 25*, 188–95 (1960).

Mysak, E. D., *Speech Pathology and Feedback Theory*. Springfield, Ill.: Charles C Thomas (1966).

Nagafuchi, M., and Saso, S., Stuttering following stroke. *Folia Phoniat., 38*, 333 (1986). Abstract.

Naylor, R. V., A comparative study of methods of estimating the severity of stuttering. *J. Speech Hearing Dis., 18*, 30–37 (1953).

Neaves, A. I., To establish a basis for prognosis in stammering. *Brit J. Dis. Communic.*, *5*, 46–58 (1970).

Neelley, J. N., A study of the speech behavior of stutterers and nonstutterers under normal and delayed auditory feedback. *J. Speech Hearing Dis., Monogr. Suppl. 7*, 63–82 (1961).

Neelley, J. N., and Timmons, R. J., Adaptation and consistency in the disfluent speech behavior of young stutterers and nonstutterers. *J. Speech Hearing Res., 10*, 250–56 (1967).

Neilson, M. D., and Neilson, P. D., Systems analysis of tracking performance in stutterers and normals. *Asha, 21*, 770 (1979). Abstract.

Neilson, P. D., Andrews, G., Guitar, B. E., and Quinn, P. T., Tonic Stretch reflexes in lip, tongue, and Jaw muscles. *Brain Res., 178*, 311–27 (1979).

Neilson, P. D., Quinn, P. T., and Neilson, M. D., Auditory tracking measures of hemispheric asymmetry in normals and stutterers. *Aust. J. Human Communic. Dis., 4*, 121–26 (1976).

Nelson, S. E., Personal contact as a factor in the transfer of stuttering. Human Biol., 11, 393–401 (1939).

Nelson, S. E., Hunter, N., and Walter, M., Stuttering in twin types. *J. Speech Dis., 10*, 335–43 (1945).

Nessel, E., Die verzögerte Sprachrückkopplung (Lee Effekt) bei Stotterern. *Folia Phoniat., 10*, 199–204 (1958).

Newman, L. L., and Smit, A. B., Some effects of variations in response time latency on speech rate, interruptions, and fluency in children's speech. J. *Speech Hearing Res., 32*, 635–44 (1989).

Newman, P. W., A study of adaptation and recovery of the stuttering response in self-formulated speech. *J. Speech Hearing Dis., 19*, 450–58 (1954).

Newman, P. W., Adaptation performances of individual stutterers: Implications for research. *J. Speech Hearing Res.., 6*, 293–94 (1963).

Newman, P. W., Bunderson, K., and Brey, R. H., Brain stem electrical responses of stutterers and normals by sex, ears, and recovery. *J. Fluency Dis., 10*, 59–67 (1985).

Newman, P. W., Channell, R., and Palmer, M. L., A comparative study of the independence of unilateral ocular motor control in stutterers and nonstutterers. *J. Fluency Dis., 11*, 105–16 (1986).

Newman, P. W., Fawcett, K. D., and Russon, K. V., Cognitive processing in stuttering as related to translating slurvian. *J. Fluency Dis., 11*, 251–56 (1986).

Newman, P. W., Harris, R. W., and Hilton, L. M., Vocal jitter and shimmer in stuttering. *J. Fluency Dis., 14*, 87–95 (1989).

Newton, K. R., Blood, G. W., and Blood, I. M., Simultaneous and staggered dichotic word and digit tests with stutterers and nonstutterers. *J. Fluency Dis., 11*, 201–16 (1986).

Nippold, M. A., Schwarz, I. E., and Jescheniak, J.-D., Narrative ability in school-age stuttering boys: A preliminary investigation. *J. Fluency Dis., 16*, 289–308 (1991).

Norbut, C. A., Perception of specific disfluency types by normal-speaking children. *Asha, 18*, 631 (1976). Abstract.

Norcross, K., and Andrews, G., Instruments for measuring stuttering. *Aust. J. Human Communic. Dis., 1*, 47–49 (1973).

Norman, D. A., and Waugh, N. C., Stimulus and response interference in recognition memory experiments. *J. Exper. Psychol.*, *78*, 551–59 (1968).

Novák, A. Results of the treatment of severe forms of stuttering in adults. *Folia Phoniat.*, *27*, 278–82 (1975).

Novák, A., The influence of delayed auditory feedback in stutterers. *Folia Phoniat.*, *30*, 278–85 (1978).

Nowack, W. J., and Stone, R. E., Acquired stuttering and bilateral cerebral disease. *J. Fluency Dis.*, *12*, 141–46 (1987).

Nuck, M. E., Blood, G. W., and Blood, I. M., Fluent and disfluent normal speakers' responses on a synthetic sentence identification (SSI) task. *J. Communic. Dis.*, *20*, 161–69 (1987).

Nudelman, H. B., Herbrich, K. E., Hoyt, B. D., and Rosenfield, D. B., Dynamic characteristics of vocal frequency tracking in stutterers and nonstutterers. In Peters, H. F. M., and Hulstijn, W. (eds.), *Speech Motor Dynamics in Stuttering*. New York: Springer (1987).

Nudelman, H. B., Herbrich, K. E., Hoyt, B. D., and Rosenfield, D. B., A neuroscience model of stuttering. *J. Fluency Dis.*, *14*, 399–427 (1989).

Nutall, E. C., and Scheidel, T. M., Stutterers' estimates of normal apprehensiveness toward speaking. *Speech Monogr.*, *32*, 455–57 (1965).

Nwokah, E. E., The imbalance of stuttering behavior in bilingual speakers. *J. Fluency Dis.*, *13*, 357–73 (1988).

Oelschlaeger, M. L., and Brutten, G. J., Response-contingent positive stimulation of the part-word repetitions displayed by four stutterers. *J. Fluency Dis.*, *1*, 10–17 (1975).

Oelschlaeger, M. L., and Brutten, G. J., The effect of instructional stimulation on the frequency of repetitions, interjections, and words spoken during the spontaneous speech of four stutterers. *Behav. Ther.*, *7*, 37–46 (1976).

Okasha, A., Bishry, Z., Kamel, M., and Hassan, A. H., Psychosocial study of stammering in Egyptian children. *Brit. J. Psychiat.*, *124*, 531–33 (1974).

Okasha, A., Moneim, S. A., Bishry, Z., Kamel, M., and Moustafa, M., Electroencephalographic study of stammering. *Brit. J. Psychiat.*, *124*, 534–35 (1974).

O'Keefe, B. M., and Kroll, R. M., Clinicians' molar and molecular stuttering analyses of expanded and nonexpanded speech. *J. Fluency Dis.*, *5*, 43–54 (1980).

Onslow, M., Adams, R., and Ingham, R., Reliability of speech naturalness ratings of stuttererd speech during treatment. *J. Speech Hearing Res.*, *35*, 994–1001 (1992).

Onslow, M., Costa, L., and Rue, S. Direct early intervention with stuttering: Some preliminary data. *J. Speech Hearing Dis.*, *55*, 405–16 (1990).

Onslow, M., Gardner, K., Bryant, K. M., Stuckings, C. L., and Knight, T., Stutterered and normal speech events in early childhood: The validity of a behavioral data language. *J. Speech Hearing Res.*, *35*, 79–87 (1992).

Onslow, M., Hayes, B., Hutchins, L., and Newman, D., Speech naturalness and prolonged-speech treatments for stuttering: Further variables and data. *J. Speech Hearing Res.*, *35*, 274–82 (1992).

Onslow, M., and Ingham, R. J., Speech quality measurement and the management of stuttering. *J. Speech Hearing Dis.*, *52*, 2–17 (1987).

Onslow, M., van Doorn, J., and Newman, D., Variability of acoustic segment durations after prolonged-speech treatment for stuttering. *J. Speech Hearing Res., 35*, 529-36 (1992).

Ornstein, A. F., and Manning, W. H., Self-efficacy scaling by adult stutterers. *J. Communic. Dis., 18*, 313–20 (1985).

Orton, S., and Travis, L. E., Studies in stuttering: IV. Studies of action currents in stutterers. *Arch. Neurol. Psychiat., 21*, 61–68 (1929).

Öst, L.-G., Götestam, K. G., and Melin, L., A controlled study of two behavioral methods in the treatment of stuttering. *Behav. Ther., 7*, 587–92 (1976).

Otto, F. M., and Yairi, E, An analysis of speech disfluencies in Down's syndrome and in normally intelligent subjects. *J. Fluency Dis., 1*, 26–32 (1975).

Oxtoby, E. T., Frequency of stuttering in relation to induced modification following expectancy of stuttering. In Johnson, W., and Leutenegger, R. R. (eds.), *Stuttering in Children and Adults*. Minneapolis: Univ. Minn. Press (1955).

Pachman, J. S., Oelschlaeger, M. L., Hughes, A., and Hughes, H., Toward identifying effective agents in use of biofeedback to decelerate stuttering behavior. *Percept. Mot. Skills, 46*, 1006 (1978).

Palen, C., and Peterson, J. M., Word frequency and children's stuttering: The relationship to sentence structure. *J. Fluency Dis., 7*, 55–62 (1982).

Palmer, M. F., and Gillette, A. M., Sex differences in the cardiac rhythms of stutterers. *J. Speech Dis., 3*, 3–12 (1938).

Palmer, M. F., and Gillette, A. M., Respiratory cardiac arrhythmia in stuttering. *J. Speech Dis., 4*, 133–40 (1939).

Palmer, M. F., and Osborn, C. D. A study of tongue pressures of speech defective and normal speaking individuals. *J. Speech Dis., 5*, 133–40 (1940).

Panconcelli-Calzia, G., Die Bedingtheit des Lombardschen Versuches in der Stimm-und-Sprachheilkunde, *Acta Otolaryngol., 45*, 244–51 (1955).

Panelli, C. A., McFarlane, S. C., and Shipley, K. G., Implications of evaluating and intervening with incipient stutterers. *J. Fluency Dis., 3*, 41–50 (1978).

Parker, C. S., and Christopherson, F., Electronic aid in the treatment of stammer. *Med. Electron. Biol. Engng., 1*, 121–25 (1963).

Parker, H. T., *Defects of Speech in School Children*. Educational Research Series No. 15. Melbourne, Australia: Melbourne Univ. Press (1932).

Parson, B. S., *Lefthandedness*. New York: Macmillan (1924).

Patterson, J., and Pring, T., Listener attitudes to stuttering speakers: No evidence for a gender difference. *J. Fluency Dis., 16*, 201–05 (1991).

Pattie, F. A., and Knight, B. B., Why does the speech of stutterers improve in chorus reading? *J. Abnorm. Soc. Psychol., 39*, 362–67 (1944).

Patty, J., and Quarrington, B., The effects of reward on types of stuttering. *J. Communic. Dis., 7*, 65–77 (1974).

Peacher, W. G., and Harris, W. E., Speech disorders in World War II: VIII. Stuttering. *J. Speech Dis., 11*, 303–08 (1946).

Pearl, S. Z., and Bernthal, J. E., The effect of grammatical complexity upon disfluency behavior of nonstuttering preschool children. *J. Fluency Dis., 5*, 55–68 (1980).

Peins, M., Adaptation effect and spontaneous recovery in stuttering expectancy. *J. Speech Hearing Res., 4*, 91–99 (1961a).

Peins, M., Consistency effect in stuttering expectancy. *J. Speech Hearing Res.*, *4*, 397–98 (1961b).

Peins, M., McGough, W. E., and Lee, B. S., Double tape recorder therapy for stutterers. In Peins, M. (ed.), *Contemporary Approaches in Stuttering Therapy*. Boston: Little, Brown (1984).

Perkins, D., An item by item compilation and comparison of the scores of 75 young adult stutterers on the California Test of Personality. *Speech Monogr.*, *14*, 211 (1947). Abstract.

Perkins, W. H., Stuttering as approach-avoidance behavior: A preliminary investigation. *Speech Monogr.*, *20*, 149–50 (1953). Abstract.

Perkins, W. H., Stuttering and discriminative awareness (SRS Research Grant RD-2275-S, Final Report). Washington, D. C.: Div. of Res. and Demonstration Grants, Social and Rehab. Serv., Dept. of Health, Educ., and Welfare (1969).

Perkins, W. H., Replacement of stuttering with normal speech: I. Rationale. *J. Speech Hearing Dis.*, *38*, 283–94 (1973a).

Perkins, W. H., Replacement of stuttering with normal speech: II. Clinical procedures. *J. Speech Hearing Dis.*, *38*, 295–303 (1973b).

Perkins, W. H., From psychoanalysis to discoordination. In Gregory, H. H. (ed.), *Controversies About Stuttering Therapy*. Baltimore: Univ. Park Press (1979).

Perkins, W. H., *Stuttering Prevented*. San Diego: Singular Publishing Group (1992).

Perkins, W. H., An alternative to automatic fluency. In Gruss, J. F. (ed.), *Stuttering Therapy: Transfer and Maintenance*. Memphis: Speech Foundation of America (undated).

Perkins, W. H., Bell, J., Johnson, L., and Stocks, J., Phone rate and the effective planning time hypothesis of stuttering. *J. Speech Hearing Res.*, *22*, 747–55 (1979).

Perkins, W. H., and Curlee, R. F., Clinical impressions of portable masking unit effects in stuttering. *J. Speech Hearing Dis.*, *34*, 360–62 (1969).

Perkins, W. H., and Hagen, C., The relation between frequency of stuttering and open expressions of agression. *Asha*, *7*, 391 (1965). Abstract.

Perkins, W. H., Kent, R. D., and Curlee, R. F., A theory of neuropsycholinguistic function in stuttering. *J. Speech Hearing Res.*, *34*, 734–52 (1991).

Perkins, W., Rudas, J., Johnson, L., and Bell, J., Stuttering: Discoordination of phonation with articulation and respiration. *J. Speech Hearing Res.*, *19*, 509–22 (1976).

Perkins, W. H., Rudas, J., Johnson, L., Michael, W. B., and Curlee, R. F., Replacement of stuttering wtih normal speech: III. Clinical effectiveness. *J. Speech Hearing Dis.*, *39*, 416–28 (1974).

Perozzi, J. A., Phonetic skill (sound-mindedness) of stuttering children. *J. Communic. Dis.*, *3*, 207–10 (1970).

Perozzi, J. A., and Kunze, L. H., Language abilities of stuttering children. *Folia Phoniat.*, *21*, 386–92 (1969).

Perrin, K. L., and Eisenson, J., An examination of ear preference for speech and nonspeech stimuli in a stuttering population. *Asha*, *12*, 427 (1970). Abstract.

Peters, C. A., A study of mirror reading in speech defectives and normal speakers. *Arch. Speech*, *1*, 48–60 (1936).

Peters, H. F. M., and Boves, L., Aerodynamic functions in fluent speech utterances of stutterers and nonstutterers in different speech conditions. In Peters, H. F. M., and Hulstijn, W. (eds.), *Speech Motor Dynamics in Stuttering*. New York: Springer (1987).

Peters, H. F. M., and Boves, L., Coordination of aerodynamic and phonatory processes in fluent speech utterances of stutterers. *J. Speech Hearing Res., 31*, 352–61 (1988).

Peters, H. F. M., Boves, L., and van Dielen, I. C. H., Perceptual judgment of abruptness of voice onset in vowels as a function of the amplitude envelope. *J. Speech Hearing Dis., 51*, 299–308 (1986).

Peters, H. F. M., and Hulstijn, W., Stuttering and anxiety: The difference between stutterers and nonstutterers in verbal apprehension and physiologic arousal during the anticipation of speech and non-speech tasks. *J. Fluency Dis., 9*, 67–84 (1984).

Peters, H. F. M., and Hulstijn, W., Programming and initiation of speech utterances in stuttering. In Peters, H. F. M., and Hulstijn, W. (eds.), *Speech Motor Dynamics in Stuttering*. New York: Springer (1987).

Peters, H. F. M., and Hulstijn, W. (eds.), *Speech Motor Dynamics in Stuttering*. New York: Springer (1987).

Peters, H. F. M., Hulstijn, W., and Starkweather, C. W., Acoustic and physiological reaction times of stutterers and nonstutterers. *J. Speech Hearing Res., 32*, 668–80 (1989).

Peters, H. F. M., Hulstijn, W., and Starkweather, C. W. (eds.), *Speech Motor Control and Stuttering*. Amsterdam: Elsevier (1991).

Peters, R. W., Love, L., Otto, D., Wood, T., and Benignus, V., Cerebral processing of speech and non-speech signals by stutterers. *Proc. XVI Congr. Int. Soc. Logoped. Phoniat.* Basel: Karger (1976).

Peters, R. W., and Simonson, W. E., Generalization of stuttering behavior through associative learning. *J. Speech Hearing Res., 3*, 9–14 (1960).

Peters, T. J., Oral language skills of children who stutter. *Speech Monogr., 35*, 325 (1968). Abstract.

Peters, T. J., and Guitar, B., *Stuttering: An Integrated Approach to Its Nature and Treatment*. Baltimore: Williams & Wilkins (1991).

Peterson, H. A., Affective meaning of words as rated by stuttering and nonstuttering readers. *J. Speech Hearing Res., 12*, 337–43 (1969).

Peterson, H. A., Rieck, M. B., and Hoff, R. K., A test of satiation as a function of adaptation in stuttering. *J. Speech Hearing Res., 12*, 110–17 (1969).

Petkov, D., and Iosifov, I., Nash opti lechenia zaikania v obstanovke ozdorovitelnio-logopedichskovo lageria. *Zh. Nevropatol. Psikhiat., 60*, 903–04 (1960).

Petrosino, L., Fucci, D., Gorman, P., and Harris, D., Midline and off-midline tongue and right- and left-hand vibrotactile thresholds of stutterers and normal-speaking individuals. *Percept. Mot. Skills, 65*, 253–54 (1987).

Phillips, P. P., and Myers, C. D., Peer-group social status of children who stutter. *Asha, 20*, 735 (1978). Abstract.

Pienaar, W. D., Body awareness in certain types of speech defective individuals. *J. Proj. Tech. Person. Assess., 32*, 537–41 (1968).

Pierce, C. M., and Lipcon, H. H., Stuttering: Clinical and electroencephalographic findings. *Military Med., 124*, 511–19 (1959).

Pindzola, R. H., Acoustic evidence of aberrant velocities in stutterers' fluent speech. *Percept. Mot. Skills, 62*, 399–405 (1986).

Pindzola, R. H., Durational characteristics of the fluent speech of stutterers and nonstutterers. *Folia phoniat., 39*, 90–97 (1987).

Pinsky, S. D., and McAdam, D. W., Electroencephalographic and dichotic indices of cerebral laterality in stutterers. *Brain, Lang., 11*, 374–97 (1980).

Pitluk, N., Aspects of the expressive language of cluttering and stuttering children. *So. Afr. J. Communic. Dis., 29*, 77–84 (1982).

Pitrelli, F. R., Psychosomatic and Rorschach aspects of stuttering. *Psychiat. Quart., 22*, 175–94 (1948).

Pittenger, K., A study of the duration of temporal intervals between successive moments of stuttering. *J. Speech Dis., 5*, 333–41 (1940).

Pizzat, F. J., A personality study of college stutterers. *Speech Monogr., 18*, 240–41 (1951). Abstract.

Platt, L. J., and Basili, A., Jaw tremor during stuttering block: An electromyographic study. *J. Communic. Dis., 6*, 102–09 (1973).

Platzky, R., and Girson, J., Indigenous healers and stuttering. *So. Afr. J. Communic. Dis., 40*, 43–48 (1993).

Podolskaya, O. V., and Shklovsky, V. M., Ob osobennostyakh nefermentativnoi fibrinolitichkoi aktivnosti i obrazovania kompleksov adrenalin-geparin i noradrenalin-geparin v krovi bolnikh logonervozom. *Zh. Nevropatol. Psikhiat., 73*, 711–15 (1973).

Ponsford, R. E., Brown, W. S., Marsh, J. T., and Travis, L. E., Evoked potential correlates of cerebral dominance for speech perception in stutterers and nonstutterers. Electroencephalogr. *Clin. Neurophysiol., 39*, 434 (1975). Abstract.

Pool, K. D., Devous, M.D., Freeman, F. J., Watson, B. C., and Finitzo, T., Regional cerebral blood flow in developmental stutterers. *Arch. Neurol., 48*, 509–12 (1991).

Porfert, A. R., and Rosenfield, D. B., Prevalence of stuttering. *J. Neurol. Neurosurg. Psychiat., 41*, 954–56 (1978).

Porter, H. V. K., Studies in the psychology of stuttering: XIV. Stuttering phenomena in relation to size and personnel of audience. *J. Speech Dis., 4*, 323–33 (1939).

Porterfield, C. L., Adaptive mechanisms of young disadvantaged stutterers and nonstutterers. *J. Proj. Tech. Person. Assess., 33*, 371–75 (1969).

Postma, A., and Kolk, H., Speech errors, disfluencies, and self-repairs of stutterers in two accuracy conditions. *J. Fluency Dis., 15*, 291–303 (1990).

Postma, A., and Kolk, H., Manual reaction times and error rates in stutterers. *Percept. Mot. Skills, 72*, 627–30 (1991).

Postma, A., and Kolk, H., Error monitoring in people who stutter: Evidence against auditory feedback theories. *J. Speech Hearing Res., 35*, 1024–32 (1992).

Postma, A., Kolk, H., and Povel, D.-J., Speech planning and execution in stutterers. *J. Fluency Dis., 15*, 49–59 (1990).

Poulos, M. G., and Webster, W. G., Family history as a basis for subgrouping people who stutter. *J. Speech Hearing Res., 34*, 5–10 (1991).

Prescott, J., Event-related potential indices of speech motor programming in stutterers and nonstutterers. *Biol. Psychol., 27*, 259–73 (1988).

Prescott, J., and Andrews, G., Early and late components of the contingent negative variation prior to manual and speech responses in stutterers and nonstutterers. *Int. J. Psychophysiol., 2,* 121–30 (1984).

Preus, A., Stuttering in Down's syndrome. Scand. *J. Educ. Res., 16,* 89–104 (1972).

Preus, A., *Identifying Subgroups of Stutterers.* Oslo: Universitetsforlaget (1981).

Preus, A., Nevrogen og psykogen stamming. Nord. Tidsskr. Logoped. *Foniat., 8,* 49–60 (1983).

Preus, A., Gullikstad, L., Grøtterød, H., Erlandsen, O., and Halland, J., En undersøkelse over forekomst av stamming i en lest tekst. *Norsk Tidsskr. Logoped., 16,* 11–18, 22 (1970).

Prins, D., Pre-therapy adaptation of stuttering and its relation to speech meaures of therapy progress. *J. Speech Hearing Res., 11,* 740–46 (1968).

Prins, D., Improvement and regression in stutterers following short-term intensive therapy. *J. Speech Hearing Dis., 35,* 123–35 (1970).

Prins, D., Personalıty, stuttering severity, and age. *J. Speech Hearing Res., 15,* 148–54 (1972).

Prins, D., Stutterers' perceptions of therapy improvement and of posttherapy regression: Effects of certain program modifications. *J. Speech Hearing Dis., 41,* 452–63 (1976).

Prins, D., Continuity, fragmentation, and tension: Hypotheses applied to evaluation and intervention with preschool disfluent children. In Prins, D., and Ingham, R. J. (eds.), *Treatment of Stuttering in Early Childhood.* San Diego: College-Hill Press (1983).

Prins, D., and Beaudet, R., Defense preference and stutterers' speech disfluencies: Implications for the nature of the disorder. *J. Speech Hearing Res., 23,* 757–68 (1980).

Prins, D., and Hubbard, C. P., Response contingent stimuli and stuttering: Issues and implications. *J. Speech Hearing Res., 31,* 696–709 (1988).

Prins, D., and Hubbard, C. P., Acoustical durations of speech segments during stuttering adaptation. *J. Speech Hearing Res., 33,* 494–504 (1990).

Prins, D., and Hubbard, C. P., Constancy of interstress intervals in the fluent speech of people who stutter during adaptation trials. *J. Speech Hearing Res., 35,* 799–804 (1992).

Prins, D., Hubbard, C. P., and Krause, M., Syllabic stress and the occurrence of stuttering. *J. Speech Hearing Res., 34,* 1011–16 (1991).

Prins, D., and Lohr, F., Behavioral dimensions of stuttered speech. *J. Speech Hearing Res., 15,* 61–71 (1972).

Prins, D., Mandelkorn, T., and Cerf, F. A., Principal and differential effects of haloperidol and placebo treatments upon speech disfluencies in stutterers. *J. Speech Hearing Res., 23,* 614–29 (1980).

Prins, D., and McQuiston, B., Differential analysis of pre-therapy adaptation in stutterers and its relation to selected indicies of therapy progress. *Asha, 6,* 401 (1964). Abstract.

Prins, D., and Miller, M., Personality, improvement, and regression in stuttering therapy. *J. Speech Hearing Res., 16,* 685–90 (1973).

Prins, D., and Nichols, A., Client impressions of the effectiveness of stuttering therapy. A comparison of two programs. *Brit. J. Dis. Communic., 9,* 123–33 (1974).

Proceedings of the NIDCD Workshop on Treaatment Efficacy Research in Stuttering, Sept. 21–22, 1992. *J. Fluency Dis., 18*, 121–361 (1993).

Prosek, R. A., Montgomery, A. A., and Walden, B. E., Constancy of relative timing for stutterers and nonstutterers. *J. Speech Hearing Res., 31*, 654–58 (1988).

Prosek, R. A., Montgomery, A. A., Walden, B. E., and Hawkins, D. B., Formant frequencies of stuttered and fluent vowels. *J. Speech Hearing Res., 30*, 301–05 (1987).

Prosek, R. A., Montgomery, A. A., Walden, B. E., and Schwartz, D. M., Reaction-time measures of stutterers and nonstutterers. *J. Fluency Dis., 4*, 269–78 (1979).

Prosek, R. A., and Runyan, C. M., Temporal characteristics related to the discrimination of stutterers' and nonstutterers' speech samples. *J. Speech Hearing Res., 25*, 29–33 (1982).

Prosek, R. A., and Runyan, C. M., Effects of segment and pause manipulations on the identification of treated stutterers. *J. Speech Hearing Res., 26*, 510–16 (1983).

Prosek, R. A., Walden, B. E., Montgomery, A. A., and Schwartz, D. M., Some correlates of stuttering severity judgments. *J. Fluency Dis., 4*, 215–22 (1979).

Pukačová, M., Psychologické charakteristiky balbutikov. dsh Abstr., 14, 308 (1974).

Purser, H., and Rustin, L., The psychology of treatment evaluation: Cognitive-behavioural treatment of adult dysfluency. *Folia Phoniat., 34*, 165–66 (1983). Abstract.

Putney, W. W., *Characteristics of Creative Drawings for Stutterers*. Ph.D. Dissert., Penn. State Univ. (1955).

Quarrington, B., The performance of stutterers on the Rosenzweig Picture-Frustration Test. *J. Clin. Psychol., 9*, 189–92 (1953).

Quarrington, B., Cyclical variation in stuttering frequency and some related forms of variation. *Canad. J. Psychol., 10*, 179–84 (1956).

Quarrington, B., Measures of stuttering adaptation. *J. Speech Hearing Res., 2*, 105–12 (1959).

Quarrington, B., Some psychological aspects of the adaptation phenomenon in stuttering. *dsh Abstr., 2*, 355 (1962).

Quarrington, B., Stuttering as a function of the information value and sentence positoin of words. *J. Abnorm. Psychol., 70*, 221–24 (1965).

Quarrington, B., The parents of stuttering children: The literature re-examined. *Canad. Psychiatric Assoc. J., 19*, 103–10 (1974).

Quarrington, B., Conway, J., and Siegel, N., An experimental study of some properties of stuttered words. *J. Speech Hearing Res., 5*, 387–94 (1962).

Quarrington, B., and Douglass, E., Audibility avoidance in nonvocalized stutterers. *J. Speech Hearing Dis., 25*, 358–65 (1960).

Quarrington, B., Seligman, J., and Kosower, E., Goal setting behavior of parents of beginning stutterers and parents of nonstuttering children. *J. Speech Hearing Res., 12*, 435–42 (1969).

Quesal, R. W., and Shank, K. H., Stutterers and others: A comparison of communication attitudes. *J. Fluency Dis., 3*, 247–52 (1978).

Quinan, C., Sinistrality in relation to high blood pressure and defects of speech. *Arch. Int. Med.*, *27*, 255–61 (1921).

Quinn, P. T., Stuttering: Some observations on speaking when alone. *J. Aust. Coll. Speech Ther.*, *21*, 92–94 (1971).

Quinn, P. T., Stuttering: Cerebral dominance and the dichotic word test. *Med. J. Aust.*, *2*, 639–43 (1972).

Quinn, P. T., Cortical localization of speech in normals and stutterers. *Aust. J. Human Communic. Dis.*, *4*, 118–20 (1976).

Quinn, P. T., and Andrews, G., Speech-related middle ear muscle activity in normal speakers and stutterers. *Aust. J. Human Communic. Dis.*, *4*, 117 (1976).

Quinn, P. T., and Andrews, G., Neurological stuttering—A clinical entity? *J. Neurol. Neurosurg. Psychiat.*, *40*, 699–701 (1977).

Quinn, P. T., and Peachey, E. C., Haloperidol in the treatment of stutterers. *Brit. J. Psychiat.*, *123*, 247–48 (1973).

Quist, R. W., and Martin, R. R., The effect of response contingent verbal punishment on stuttering. *J. Speech Hearing Res.*, *10*, 795–800 (1967).

Ragsdale, J. D., and Ashby, J. K., Speech-language pathologists' connotations of stuttering. *J. Speech Hearing Res.*, *25*, 75–80 (1982).

Ragsdale, J. D., and Sisterhen, D. H., Hesitation phenomena in the spontaneous speech of normal and articulatory-defective children. *Lang. Speech*, *27*, 235–44 91984).

Rahman, P., *The Self-concept and Ideal Self-concept of Stutterers as Compared to Nonstutterers*. M. A. Thesis, Brooklyn Coll. (1956).

Ralston, L. D., Stammering: A stress index in Caribbean classrooms. *J. Fluency Dis.*, *6*, 119–33 (1981).

Ramig, P., and Adams, M. R., Rate reduction strategies used by stutterers an dnonstutterers during high- and low-pitched speech. *J. Fluency Dis.*, *5*, 27–41 (1980).

Ramig, P. R., and Adams, M. R., Vocal changes in stutterers and nonstutterers during high- and low-pitched speech. *J. Fluency Dis.*, *6*, 15–33 (1981).

Ramig, P. R., Krieger, S. M., and Adams, M. R., Vocal changes in stutterers and nonstutterers when speaking to children. *J. Fluency Dis.*, *7*, 369–84 (1982).

Randoll, D., Erfahrungen und Ergebnisse bei der Anwendung des Systematic Fluency Training for Young Children (SFTYC) von R. E. Shine. Sprachheilarb., *33*, 227–40 (1988).

Rantalaka, S.-L., and Petri-Larmi, M., Haloperidol (Serenase) in the treatment of stuttering. *Folia Phoniat.*, *28*, 354–61 (1976).

Rapaport, D., *Diagnostic Psychological Testing*. Chicago: The Yearbook Publishers (1946).

Rappaport, B., and Bloodstein, O., The role of random blackout cues in the distribution of moments of stuttering. *J. Speech Hearing Res.*, *14*, 874–79 (1971).

Rastatter, M., and Dell, C. W., Simple motor and phonemic processing reaction times of stutterers. *Percept. Mot. Skills*, *61*, 463–66 (1985).

Rastatter, M. P., and Dell, C. W., Reaction times of moderate and severe stutterers to monaural verbal stimuli: Some implications for neurolinguistic organization. *J. Speech Hearing Res.*, *30*, 21–27 (1987a).

Rastatter, M. P., and Dell, C. W., Simple visual versus lexical decision vocal reaction times of stuttering and normal subjects. *J. Fluency Dis.*, *12*, 63–69 (1987b).

Rastatter, M. P., and Dell, C., Vocal reaction times of stuttering subjects to tachistoscopically presented concrete and abstract words: A closer look at cerebral dominance and language processing. *J. Speech Hearing Res., 30,* 306–10 (1987c).

Rastatter, M. P., and Dell, C. W., Reading reaction times of stuttering and non-stuttering subjects to unilaterally presented concrete and abstract words. *J. Fluency Dis., 13,* 319–29 (1988).

Rastatter, M. P., and Harr, R., Measurements of plasma levels of adrenergic neurotransmitters and primary amino acids in five stuttering subjects: A preliminary report (biochemical aspects of stuttering). *J. Fluency Dis., 13,* 127–39 (1988).

Rastatter, M. P., and Loren, C. A., Visual coding dominance in stuttering: Some evidence from central tachistoscopic stimulation (tachistoscopic viewing and stuttering). *J. Fluency Dis., 13,* 89-95 (1988).

Rastatter, M. P., Loren, C., and Colcord, R., Visual coding strategies and hemispheric dominance characteristics of stutterers. *J. Fluency Dis., 12,* 305–15 (1987).

Rastatter, M. P., McGuire, R. A., and Loren, C., Linguistic encoding dominance in stuttering: Some evidence for temporal and qualitative hemispheric processing differences. *J. Fluency Dis., 13,* 215–24 (1988).

Ratner, N. B., Measurable outcomes of instructions to modify normal parent-child verbal interactions: Implications for indirect stuttering therapy. *J. Speech Hearing Res., 35,* 14–20 (1992).

Ratner, N. B. and Sih, C. C., Effects of gradual increases in sentence length and complexity on children's dysfluency. *J. Speech Hearing Dis., 52,* 278–87 (1987).

Ratusnik, D. L., Kiriluk, E., and Ratusnik, C. M., Relationship among race, social status, and sex of preschoolers' normal dysfluencies: A cross-cultural investigation. *Lang. Speech Hearing Serv. Schools, 10,* 171–77 (1979).

Razdolsky, V. A., O sostoyanii rechi v odinochestve u zaikayushchikhsya. *Zh. Nevropatol. Psikhiat., 65,* 1717–20 (1965).

Records, M. A., Heimbuch, R. C., and Kidd, K. K., Handedness and stuttering: A dead horse? *J. Fluency Dis., 2,* 271–82 (1977).

Redwine, G. W., An experimental study of relationships between self-concepts of fourth and eighth grade stuttering and nonstuttering boys. *Speech Monogr., 26,* 140–41 (1959). Abstract.

Reed, C. G., and Godden, A. L., An experimental treatment using verbal punishment with two preschool stutterers. *J. Fluency Dis., 2,* 225–33 (1977).

Reed, C. G., and Lingwall, J. B., Some relationships between punishment, stuttering, and galvanic skin responses. *J. Speech Hearing Res., 19,* 197–205 (1976).

Reed, C. G., and Lingwall, J. B., Conditioned stimulus effects on stuttering and GSRs. *J. Speech Hearing Res., 23,* 336–43 (1980).

Reich, A., Till, J., and Goldsmith, H., Laryngeal and manual reaction times of stuttering and nonstuttering adults. *J. Speech Hearing Res., 24,* 192–96 (1981).

Reimann, A., Phonetische Untersuchungen über lautabhängige Vokallängen im Sprechen redgestörter Jugendlicher. *Sprachheilarb., 21,* 1–14 (1976).

Reis, R., and Adams, M. R., Comments on "The Adams and Reis Observations Revisited." *J. Fluency Dis., 3*, 299–302 (1978).

Rentschler, G. J., Driver, L. E., and Callaway, E. A., The onset of stuttering following drug overdose. *J. Fluency Dis., 9*, 265–84 (1984).

Resick, P. A., Wendiggensen, P., Ames, S., and Meyer, V., Systematic slowed speech: A new treatment for stuttering. *Behav. Res. Ther., 16*, 161–67 (1978).

Resnick, S., and Tureen, P., Evaluation of fluent and disfluent speech segments by stutters and nonstutterers. *J. Fluency Dis., 15*, 1–8 (1990).

Rheinberger, M. B., Karlin, I. W., and Berman, A. B., Electroencephalographic and laterality studies of stuttering and nonstuttering children. *Nerv. Child, 2*, 117–33 (1943).

Rhodes R., Shames, G., and Egolf, D., "Awareness" in verbal conditoning of language themes during therapy with stutterers. *J. Communic. Dis., 4*, 30–39 (1971).

Richardson, LaV. H., A personality study of stutterers and non-stutterers. *J. Speech Dis., 9*, 152–60 (1944).

Richter, E., Ein Beitrag zur Ätiologie des Stotterns. *Sprachheilarb., 27*, 239–45 (1982).

Rickard, H. C., and Mundy, M. B., Direct manipulation of stuttering behavior: An experimental-clinical approach. In Ullmann, L. P., and Krasner, L. (eds.), *Case Studies in Behavior Modification*. New York: Holt, Rinehart and Winston (1965).

Rieber, R. W., A study in psycholinguistics and communication disorders. *Linguistics, No. 160*, 33–70 (1975).

Rieber, R. W., Breskini, S., and Jaffe, J., Pause time and phonation time in stuttering and cluttering. *J. Psycholinguist. Res., 1*, 149–54 (1972).

Rieber, R. W., Smith, N., and Harris, B., Neuropsychological aspects of stuttering and cluttering. In Rieber, R. W. (ed.), *The Neuropsychology of Language*. New York: Plenum Press (1976).

Rieber, R. W., and Wollock, J., The historical roots of the theory and therapy of stuttering. *J. Communic. Dis., 10*, 3–24 (1977).

Riley, G. D., A stuttering severity instrument for children and adults. *J. Speech Hearing Dis., 37*, 314–20 (1972).

Riley, G. D., and Riley, J., Motoric and linguistic variables among children who stutter: A factor analysis. *J. Speech Hearing Dis., 45*, 504–14 (1980).

Riley, G. D., and Riley, J., A component model for treating stuttering in children. In Peins, M. (ed.), *Contemporary Approaches in Stuttering Therapy*. Boston: Little, Brown (1984).

Riley, G., and Riley, J., Oral motor discoordination among children who stutter. *J. Fluency Dis., 11*, 335–44 (1986).

Riley, G., and Riley, J., Treatment implications of oral motor discoordination. In Peters, H. F. M., Hulstijn. W., and Starkweather, C. W. (eds.), *Speech Motor Control and Stuttering*. Amsterdam: Elsevier (1991).

Riley, J., High self-expectations: Comparing stuttering to dysarticulating children. *Asha, 25*, 160 (1983). Abstract.

Ringel, R. L., and Minifie, F. D., Protensity estimates of stutterers and nonstutterers. *J. Speech Hearing Res., 9*, 289–96 (1966).

Ritterman, S. I., and Reidenbach, J. W., Jr., Inter-digital variability in the palmer sweat indices of adult stutterers. *J. Fluency Dis., 1*, 33–46 (1975).

Ritzman, C. H., A cardiovascular and metabolic study of stutterers and non-stutterers. *J. Speech Dis., 8*, 161–82 (1943).

Robb, M. P., Lybolt, J. T., and Price, H. A., Acoustic measures of stutterers' speech following an intensive therapy program. *J. Fluency Dis., 10*, 269–79 (1985).

Robbins, M. G., *The Effect of Varying Conditions of Rehearsal on the Frequency of Stuttering.* Ph. D. Dissert., City Univ. N.Y. (1971).

Robbins, S. D., A plethysmographic study of shock and stammering in a trephined stammerer. *Amer. J. Physiol., 52*, 168–81 (1920).

Robbins, S. D., The role of rhythm in the correction of stammering. *Quart. J. Speech, 21*, 331–43 (1935).

Robey, R. R., An investigation of the validity of the Iowa Scale of Attitude Toward Stuttering in terms of social desirability and acquiescent response set intrusion. *Asha, 18*, 682 (1976). Abstract.

Roland, B. C., Eye-movements of stutterers and nonstutterers during silent, oral, and choral reading. *Percept. Mot. Skills, 35*, 297–98 (1972).

Roman, K. G., Handwriting and speech. In Barbara, D. A. (ed.), *Psychological Aspects of Speech and Hearing.* Springfield, Ill.: Charles C Thomas (1960).

Ronson, I., Linguistic cues in stuttering: Selected sentence types and the anticipatory struggle hypothesis. *Speech Hearing Rev., 7*, 38–45 (1975).

Ronson, I., Word frequency and stuttering: The relationship to sentence structure. *J. Speech Hearing Res., 19*, 813–19 (1976).

Root, A. R., A survey of speech defectives in the public elementary schools of South Dakota. *Elem. Sch. J., 26*, 531–41 (1926).

Rosenbek, J. C., Stuttering secondary to nervous system damage. In Curlee, R. F., and Perkins, W. H. (eds.), *Nature and Treatment of Stuttering: New Directions.* San Diego: College-Hill Press (1984).

Rosenbek, J., Messert, B., Collins, M., and Wertz, R. T., Stuttering following brain damage. *Brain Lang., 6*, 82–96 (1978).

Rosenberg, S., and Curtiss, J., The effect of stuttering on the behavior of the listener. *J. Abnorm. Soc. Psychol., 49*, 355–61 (1944).

Rosenberger, P. B., Wheelden, J. A., and Kalotkin, M., The effect of Haloperidol on stuttering. *Amer. J. Psychiat., 133*, 331–34 (1976).

Rosenfield, D. B., Stuttering and cerebral ischemia. New Eng. J. Med., 287, 991 (1972).

Rosenfield, D. B., and Freeman, F. J., Stuttering onset after laryngectomy. *J. Fluency Dis., 8*, 265–68 (1983).

Rosenfield, D. B., and Goodglass, H., Dichotic testing of cerebral dominance in stutterers. *Brain, Lang., 11*, 170–80 (1980).

Rosenfield, D. B., Miller, S. D., and Feltovich, M., Brain damage causing stuttering. *Trans. Amer. Neurol. Assoc., 105*, 181–83 (1980).

Rosenfield, D. B., and Nudelman, H. B., Neuropsychological models of speech dysfluency. In Rustin, L., Purser, H., and Rowley, D. (eds.), *Progress in the Treatment of Fluency Disorders.* London: Taylor and Francis (1987).

Rosenfield, D. B., Viswanath, N. S., Callis-Landrun, L., Di Danato, R., and Nudelman, H. B., Patients with acquired dysfluencies: What they tell us about developmental stuttering. In Peters, H. F. M., Hulstijn, W., and Starkweather, C. W. (eds.), *Speech Motor Control and Stuttering.* Amsterdam: Elsevier (1991).

Ross, F. L., A comparative study of stutterers and nonstutterers on a psychomotor discrimination task. In Johnson, W., and Leutenegger, R. R. (eds.), *Stuttering in Children and Adults*. Minneapolis: Univ. Minn. Press (1955).

Rosso, L. J., and Adams, M. R., A study of the relationship between the latency and consistency of stuttering. *J. Speech Hearing Res.*, 12, 389–93 (1969).

Roth, C. R., Aronson, A. E., and Davis, L. J., Jr., Clinical studies in psychogenic stuttering of adult onset. *J. Speech Hearing Dis.*, 54, 634–46 (1989).

Rotter, J. B., Studies in the psychology of stuttering: XI. Stuttering in relation to position in the family. *J. Speech Dis.*, 4, 143–48 (1939).

Rotter, J. B., A study of the motor integration of stutterers and nonstutterers. In Johnson, W., and Leutenegger, R. R. (eds.), *Stuttering in Children and Adults*. Minneapolis: Univ. Minn. Press (1955).

Rouma, G., Enquête scolaire sur les troubles de la parole chez les écoliers Belges. *Int. Arch. Schulhygiene, 2*, 151–89 (1906).

Rousey, C. G., Arjunan, K. N., and Rousey, C. L., Successful treatment of stuttering following closed head injury. *J. Fluency Dis.*, 11, 257–61 (1986).

Rousey, C. L., Stuttering severity during prolonged spontaneous speech. *J. Speech Hearing Res., 1*, 40–47 (1958).

Rousey, C. L., Goetzinger, C. P., and Dirks, D., Sound localization ability of normal, stuttering, neurotic, and hemiplegic subjects. A.M.A. *Arch. Gen. Psychiat., 1*, 640–45 (1959).

Rubin, H., and Culatta, R., A point of view about fluency. *Asha, 13*, 380–84 (1971).

Runyan, C. M., and Adams, M. R., Perceptual study of the speech of "successfully therapeutized" stutterers. *J. Fluency Dis., 3*, 25–39 (1978),.

Runyan, C. M., and Adams, M. R., Unsophisticated judges' perceptual evaluations of the speech of "successfully treated" stutterers. *J. Fluency Dis., 4*, 29–38 (1979).

Runyan, C. M., Bell, J. N., and Prosek, R. A., Speech naturalness ratings of treated stutterers. *J. Speech Hearing Dis., 55*, 434–38 (1990).

Runyan, C. M., and Bonifant, D. C., A perceptual comparison: All-voiced versus typical reading passage by children. *J. Fluency Dis., 6*, 247–55 (1981).

Runyan, C. M., Hames, P. E., and Prosek, R. A., A perceptual comparison between paired stimulus and single stimulus methods of presentation of the fluent utterances of stutterers. *J. Fluency Dis., 7*, 71–77 (1982).

Runyan, C. M., and Runyan, S. E., A fluency rules therapy program for young children in the public schools. *Lang. Speech Hearing Services Schools, 17*, 276–84 (1986).

Russell, J. C., Clark, A. W., and van Sommers, P., Treatment of stammering by reinforcement of fluent speech. *Behav. Res. Ther., 6*, 447–53 (1968).

Rustin, L., Kuhr, A., Cook, P. J., and James, I. M., Controlled trial of speech therapy versus oxprenolol for stammering. *Brit. Med. J., 283*, 517–19 (1981).

Rustin, L., Purser, H., and Rowley, D. (eds.), *Progress in the Treatment of Fluency Disorders*. London: Taylor and Francis (1987).

Rustin, L., Ryan, B. P., and Ryan, B. V., Use of the Monterey Programmed Stuttering Therapy in Great Britain. *Brit. J. Dis., Communic., 22*, 151–62 (1987).

Rutherford, B. R., Speech reeducation for the birth injured. *J. Speech Dis., 3*, 199–206 (1938).

Ryan, B. P., Operant procedures applied to stuttering therapy for children. *J. Speech Hearing Dis., 36*, 264–80 (1971).

Ryan, B. P., *Programmed Therapy for Stuttering in Children and Adults.* Springfield, Ill.: Charles C. Thomas (1974).

Ryan, B., Stuttering therapy in a framework of operant conditioning and programmed learning. In Gregory, H. H. (ed.), *Controversies About Stuttering Therapy.* Baltimore: Univ. Park Press (1979).

Ryan, B. P., Maintenance programs in progress—II. In Boberg, E. (ed.), *Maintenance of Fluency: Proceedings of the Banff Conference.* New York: Elsevier (1981).

Ryan, B. P., Articulation, language, rate, and fluency characteristics of stuttering and nonstuttering preschool children. *J. Speech Hearing Res., 35*, 333–42 (1992).

Ryan, B. P., and Van Kirk, B., The establishment, transfer, and maintenance of fluent speech in 50 stutterers using delayed auditory feedback and operant procedures. *J. Speech Hearing Dis., 39*, 3–10 (1974).

Sacco, P. R., and Metz, D. E., Comparison of period-by-period fundamental frequency of stutterers and nonstutterers over repeated utterances. *J. Speech Hearing Res., 32*, 439–44 (1989).

St. Louis, K. O. (ed.), *The Atypical Stutterer: Principles and Practices of Rehabilitation.* Orlando, Fl.: Academic Press (1986).

St. Louis, K. O., The stuttering/articulation connection. In Peters, H. F. M., Hulstijn, W., and Starkweather, C. W. (eds.), *Speech Motor Control and Stuttering.* Amsterdam: Elsevier (1991).

St. Louis, K. O., and Atkins, C. P., Nonstutterers' perceptions of stuttering and speech difficulty. *J. Fluency Dis., 13*, 375–84 (1988).

St. Louis, K. O., Clausell, P. L., Thompson, J. N., and Rife, C. C., Preliminary investigation of EMG biofeedback induced relaxation with a preschool aged stutterer. *Percept. Mot. Skills, 55*, 195–99 (1982).

St. Louis, K. O., and Hinzman, A. R., A descriptive study of speech, language, and hearing characteristics of school-aged stutterers. *J. Fluency Dis., 13*, 331–55 (1988).

St. Louis, K. O., Hinzman, A. R., and Hull, F. M., Studies of cluttering: Disfluency and language measures in young possible clutterers and stutterers. *J. Fluency Dis., 10*, 151–72 (1985).

St. Louis, K. O., Murray, C. D., and Ashworth, M. S., Coexisting communication disorders in a random sample of school-aged stutterers. *J. Fluency Dis., 16*, 13–23 (1991).

Sakata, R., and Adams, M. R., Comparisons among various forms of individual stutterers' disfluency. *J. Communic. Dis., 5*, 232–39 (1972).

Samar, V. J., Metz, D. E., and Sacco, P. R., Changes in aerodynamic characteristics of stutterers' fluent speech associated with therapy. *J. Speech Hearing Res., 29*, 106–13 (1986).

Samson, C. L., and Cooper, E. B., Motor perseverative behavior in adult stutterers and nonstutterers. *J. Fluency Dis., 5*, 359–72 (1980).

Sander, E. K., Reliability of the Iowa Speech Disfluency Test. *J. Speech Hearing Dis., Monogr. Suppl. 7*, 21–30 (1961).

Sander, E. K., Frequency of syllable repetition and "stutterer" judgments. *J. Speech Hearing Dis., 28,* 19–30 (1963).

Sander, E. K., Interrelations among the responses of mothers to a child's disfluencies. *Speech Monogr., 35,* 187–95 (1968).

Santostefano, S., Anxiety and hostility in stuttering. *J. Speech Hearing Res., 3,* 337–47 (1960).

Sayles, D. G., Cortical excitability, perseveration, and stuttering. *J. Speech Hearing Res., 14,* 462–75 (1971).

Scarbrough, H. E., A quantitative and qualitative analysis of the electroencephalograms of stutterers and non-stutterers. *J. Exper. Psychol., 32,* 156–67 (1943).

Schaef, R. A., The use of questions to elicit stuttering adaptation. *J. Speech Hearing Dis., 20,* 262–65 (1955).

Schaeffer, M., and Shearer, W., A survey of mentally retarded stutterers. *Ment. Retard., 6,* 44–45 (1968).

Schäfersküpper, P., *Pathophysiologie und Therapie des Stotterns.* Berlin: Marhold (1982).

Schäfersküpper, P., and Dames, M., Speech rate and syllable durations in stutterers and nonstutterers. In Peters, H. F. M., and Hulstijn, W. (eds.), *Speech Motor Dynamics in Stuttering.* New York: Springer (1987).

Schäfersküpper, P., and Simon, T., The mean fundamental frequency in stutterers and nonstutterers during reading and spontaneous speech. *J. Fluency Dis., 8,* 125–32 (1983).

Schiavetti, N., Judgments of stuttering severity as a function of type and locus of disfluency. *Folia Phoniat., 27,* 26–37 (1975).

Schiavetti, N., Martin, R. R., Haroldson, S. K., and Metz, D. E., Psychophysical analysis of audiovisual judgments of speech naturalness of nonstutterers and stutterers. *J. Speech Hearing Res., 37,* 46–52 (1994).

Schiavetti, N., Sacco, P. R., Metz, D. E., and Sitler, R. W., Direct magnitude estimation and interval scaling of stuttering severity. *J. Speech Hearing Res., 26,* 568–73 (1983).

Schiller, F., Aphasia studied in patients with missile wounds. *J. Neurol. Neurosurg. Psychiat., 10,* 183–97 (1947).

Schilling, A., Elektronystagmographische Befunde als Hinweis auf zentrale Koordinationsdefekte bei Stotterern. *Arch. Ohr.-Nas.-Kehlk. Heilk., 175,* 457–61 (1959).

Schilling, A., Röntgen-Zwerchfell-Kymogramme bei Stotterern. *Folia Phoniat., 12,* 145–53 (1960).

Schilling, A., Organische Faktoren bei der Entstehung des Stotterns. *HNO, 10,* 149–53 (1962).

Schilling, A., Die medikmamentöse Unterstützung der Therapie des Stotterns. *HNO, 11,* 300–04 (1963).

Schilling, A., asnd Biener, W., Messung der Vibrationsempfindung mittels Audiometer und Ergebnisse dieser Untersuchung bei Stotterern. *Nervenarzt, 30,* 279–81 (1959).

Schilling, A., and Göler, D., Zur Frage der Monotonie-Untersuchung beim Stottern. *Folia Phoniat., 13,* 202–18 (1961).

Schilling, A., and Krüger, W., Untersuchungen über die Motorik sprachgestörter Kinder, *HNO, 8,* 205–09 (1960).

Schindler, M. D., A study of educational adjustments of stuttering and nonstuttering children. In Johnson, W., and Leutenegger, R. R. (eds.), *Stuttering in Children and Adults*. Minneapolis: Univ. Minn. Press (1955).

Schlanger, B. B., Speech examination of a group of institutionalized mentally handicapped children. *J. Speech Hearing Dis., 18*, 339–49 (1953).

Schlanger, B. B., *Mental Retardation*. New York: Bobbs-Merrill (1973).

Schlanger, B. B., and Gottsleben, R. H., Analysis of speech defects among the institutionalized mentally retarded. *J. Speech Hearing Dis., 22*, 98–103 (1957).

Schlesinger, I. M., Forte, M., Fried, B., and Melkman, R., Stuttering, information load, and response strength. *J. Speech Hearing Dis., 30*, 32–36 (1965).

Schlesinger, I. M., Melkman, R., and Levy, R., Word length and frequency as determinants of stuttering. Psychonomic Sci., 6, 255–56 (1966).

Schmitt, L. S., and Cooper, E. B., Fundamental frequencies in the oral reading behavior of stuttering and nonstuttering male children. *J. Communic. Dis., 11*, 17–23 (1978).

Schmoigl, S., and Ladisch, W., EEG investigation in stutterers. *Electroencephalogr. Clin. Neurophysiol. 23*, 184–85 (1967).

Schönhärl, E., Altersbedingte Wandlungen im Strukturbild des Stotterns. *HNO, 12*, 152–54 (1964).

Schroeder, P. L., and Ackerson, L., Relation of personality and behavior difficulties to disorders of speech. In West, R. (ed.), *A Symposium on Stuttering*. Madison, Wis.: College Typing Co. (1931).

Schuell, H., Sex differences in relation to stuttering: Part I. *J. Speech Dis., 11*, 277–98 (1946).

Schuell, H., Sex differences in relation to stuttering: Part II. *J. Speech Dis., 12*, 23–28 (1947).

Schultz, D. A., A study of nondirective counseling as applied to adult stutterers. *J. Speech Dis., 12*, 421–27 (1947).

Schulz, H., Vergleichende Untersuchung von Sprachbehinderten und Nichtsprachbehinderten Schülern des 3. Schuljahres mit dem Rechentest DRE 3 von Samstag, Sander und Scyhmidt. *Sprachheilarb., 22*, 86–95 (1977).

Schulze, H., Time pressure variables in the verbal parent-child interaction patterns of fathers and mothers of stuttering, phonologically disordered and normal preschool children. In Peters, H. F. M., Hulstijn, W., and Starkweather, C. W. (eds.), *Speech Motor Control and Stuttering*. Amsterdam: Elsevier (1991).

Schwartz, D., and Webster, L. M., More on the efficacy of a protracted precision fluency shaping program. *J. Fluency Dis., 2*, 205–15 (1977).

Schwartz, H. D., and Conture, E. G., Subgrouping young stutterers: Preliminary behavioral observations. *J. Speech Hearing Dis., 31*, 62–71 (1988).

Schwartz, H. D., Zebrowski, P. M., and Conture, E., Behaviors at the onset of stuttering. *J. Fluency Dis., 15*, 77–86 (1990).

Schwartz, M., *Stuttering Solved*. New York: Lippencott (1976).

Scripture, E. W., *Stuttering, Lisping, and Correction of the Speech of the Deaf*, 2nd ed. New York: Macmillan (1931).

Scripture, M. K., and Kittredge, W. B., An attempt to determine another etiological factor of stuttering through objective measurement. *J. Educ. Psychol., 14*, 162–73 (1923).

Seaman, R. S., *A Study of the Responses of Stutterers to the Items of the Rosenzweig Picture-Frustration Study*. M. A. Thesis, Brooklyn Coll. (1956).

Sedláček, C., Reactions of the autonomic nervous system in attacks of stuttering. *Folia Phoniat.*, *1*, 97–103 (1948).

Sedláčková, E., Exploration de l'équilibre végétatif dans le bégaiement et le bredouillement. *Folia Phoniat.*, *15*, 68–77 (1963).

Seebach, M. A., and Caruso, A. J., Voice onset time during fluent speech: Young stutterers and nonstutterers. *Asha*, *21*, 764 (1979). Abstract.

Segre, R., Recherches sur l'influence corticale et palido-striale dans les syndromes spasmodiques. *Rev. Laryngol. Otol. Rhinol.*, *72*, 279–81 (1951).

Seidel, A., Weinstein, R. B. and Bloodstein, O., The effect of interposed conditions on the consistency of stuttering. *J. Speech Hearing Res.*, *16*, 62–66 (1973).

Seider, R. A., Gladstien, K. L., and Kidd, K. K., Language onset and concomitant speech and language problems in subgroups of stutterers and their siblings. *J. Speech Hearing Res.*, *25*, 482–86 (1982).

Seider, R. A., Gladstien, K. L., and Kidd, K. K., Recovery and persistence of stuttering among relatives of stutterers. *J. Speech Hearing Dis.*, *48*, 402–09 (1983).

Sermas, C. E., and Cox, M. D., The stutterer and stuttering: Personality correlates. *J. Fluency Dis.*, *7*, 141–58 (1982).

Seth, G., An experimental study of the control of the mechanism of speech, and in particular that of respiration in stuttering subjects. *Brit. J. Psychol.*, *24*, 375–88 (1934).

Seth, G., Psychomotor control in stammering and normal subjects: An experimental study. *Brit. J. Psychol.*, *49*, 139–43 (1958).

Sewell, W., and Mussen, P., The effects of feeding, weaning and scheduling procedures on childhood adjustment and the formation of oral symptoms. *Child Dev.*, *23*, 185–191 (1952).

Shackson, R., An action current study of muscle contraction latency with special reference to latent tetany in stutterers. *Arch. Speech*, *1*, 87–111 (1936).

Shaffer, G. L., Measures of jaw movement and phonation in nonstuttered and stuttered production of voiced and voiceless plosives. *Speech Monogr.*, *7*, 85–92 (1940).

Shames, G. H., The relationship between the attitude toward stuttering of secondary stutterers and several of their personality charcteristics. *Speech Monogr.*, *18*, 241 (1951). Abstract.

Shames, G. H., An investigation of prognosis and evaluation in speech therapy. *J. Speech Hearing Dis.*, *17*, 386–92 (1952).

Shames, G. H., and Beams, H. L., Incidence of stuttering in older age groups. *J. Speech Hearing Dis.*, *21*, 313–16 (1956).

Shames, G. H., Egolf, D. B., and Rhodes, R. C., Experimental programs in stutterering therapy. *J. Speech Hearing Dis.*, *34*, 30–47 (1969).

Shames, G. H., and Florance, C. L., *Stutter-free Speech: A Goal for Therapy*. Columbus: Merrill (1980).

Shames, G. H., and Rubin, H. (eds.), *Stuttering Then and Now*. Columbus, Ohio: Merrill (1986).

Shames, G. H., and Sherrick, C. E., Jr., A discussion of nonfluency and stuttering as operant behavior, *J. Speech Hearing Dis.*, *28*, 3–18 (1963). Reprinted in Barabara, D. A. (ed.), *New Directions in Stuttering*. Springfield, Ill.: Charles C Thomas (1965).

Shane, M. L. S., Effect on stuttering of alteration in auditory feedback. In Johnson, W., and Leutenegger, R. R. (eds.), *Stuttering in Children and Adults*. Minneapolis: Univ. Minn. Press (1955).

Shapiro, A. I., An electromyographic analysis of the fluent and dysfluent utterances of seveal types of stutterers. *J. Fluency Dis., 5*, 203–31 (1980).

Shaw, C. K., and Shrum, W. F., The effects of response-contingent reward on the connected speech of children who stutter. *J. Speech Hearing Dis., 37*, 75–88 (1972).

Shearer, W. M., Speech: Behavior of middle ear muscle during stuttering. *Science, 152*, 1280 (1966).

Shearer, W. M., and Baud, H. E., Adaptation in mentally retarded stutterers and nonstutterers. *J. Communic. Dis., 3*, 118–22 (1970).

Shearer, W. M., and Simmons, F. B., Middle ear activity during speech in normal speakers and stutterers. *J. Speech Hearing Res., 8*, 203–07 (1965).

Shearer, W. M., and Williams, J. D., Self-recovery from stuttering. *J. Speech Hearing Dis., 30*, 288–90 (1965).

Sheehan, J., The modification of stuttering through non-reinforcement. *J. Abnorm. Soc. Psychol., 46*, 51–63 (1951).

Sheehan, J. G., Theory and treatment of stuttering as an approach-avoidance conflict. *J. Psychol., 36*, 27–49 (1953).

Sheehan, J., Conflict theory of stuttering. In Eisenson, J. (ed.), *Stuttering: A Symposium*. New York: Harper & Row (1958a).

Sheehan, J. G., Projective studies of stuttering. *J. Speech Hearing Dis., 23*, 18–25 (1958b).

Sheehan, J. G., *Stuttering: Research and Therapy*. New York: Harper & Row (1970).

Sheehan, J. G., Stuttering behavior: A phonetic analysis. *J. Communic. Dis., 7*, 193–212 (1974).

Sheehan, J. G., Conflict theory and avoidance-reduction therapy. In Eisenson, J. (ed.), *Stuttering: A Second Symposium*. New York: Harper & Row (1975).

Sheehan, J. G., Level of aspiration in female stutterers: Changing times? *J. Speech Hearing Dis., 44*, 479–86 (1979).

Sheehan, J. G., Problems in the evaluation of progress and outcome. In Perkins, W. H. (ed.), *Stuttering Disorders*. New York: Thieme-Stratton (1984).

Sheehan, J. G., Cortese, P. A., and Hadley, R. G., Guilt, shame, and tension in graphic projections of stuuttering. *J. Speech Hearing Dis., 27*, 129–39 (1962).

Sheehan, J. G., Frederick, C. J., Rosevear, W. H., and Spiegelman, M. A., A validity study of the Rorschach prognostic rating scale. *J. Proj. Tech., 18*, 233–39 (1954).

Sheehan, J., Hadley, R., and Gould, E., Impact of authority on stuttering. *J. Abnorm.Psychol., 72*, 290–93 (1967).

Sheehan, J. G., and Lyon, M. A., Role perception in stuttering. *J. Communic. Dis., 7*, 113–25 (1974).

Sheehan, J. G., and Martyn, M. M., Spontaneous recovery form stuttering. *J. Speech Hearing Res., 9*, 121–35 (1966).

Sheehan, J. G., and Martyn, M. M., Stuttering and its disappearance. *J. Speech Hearing Res., 13*, 279–89 (1970).

Sheehan, J., Martyn, M. M., and Kilburn, K. L., Speech disorders in retardation. *Amer. J. Ment. Defic., 73*, 251–56 (1968).

Sheehan, J. G., and Sheehan, V. M., Avoidance-reduction therapy: A response-suppression hypothesis. In Perkins, W. H. (ed.), *Stuttering Disorders*. New York: Thieme-Stratton (1984).

Sheehan, J. G., and Voas, R. B., Tension patterns during stuttering in relation to conflict, anxiety-binding, and reinforcement. *Speech Monogr., 21*, 272–79 (1954).

Sheehan, J. G., and Zelen, S., A level; of aspiration in stutterers and nonstutterers. *J. Abnorm. Soc. Psychol., 51*, 83–86 (1955).

Sheehan, J., and Zussman, C., Rorschachs of stutterers compared with a clinical control. *Amer. Psychol., 6*, 500 (1951). Abstract.

Sheets, B. V., *A Study of the Visual Perseverative Tendencies in Stutterers and Normal Speakers*. M. A. Thesis, Univ. Utah (1941).

Shenker, R. C., and Finn, P., An evaluation of the effects of supplemental "fluency" traniing during maintenance. *J. Fluency Dis., 10*, 257–67 (1985).

Sherman, D., Clinical and experimental use of the Iowa Scale of Severity of Stuttering. *J. Speech Hearing Dis., 17*, 316–20 (1952).

Sherman, D., Reliability and utility of individual ratings of severity of audible characteristics of stuttering. *J. Speech Hearing Dis., 20*, 11–16 (1955).

Sherman, D., and McDermott, R., Individual ratings of severity of moments of stuttering. *J. Speech Hearing Res., 1*, 61–67 (1958).

Sherman, D., and Trotter, W. D., Correlation between two measures of the severity of stuttering. *J. Speech Hearing Dis., 21*, 426–29 (1956).

Sherman, D., Young, M., and Gough, K., Comparison of three measures of stuttering severity. *Proc. Iowa Acad. Sci, 65*, 381–84 (1958).

Sherrard, C. A., Stuttering as "false alarm" responding. *Brit. J. Dis., Communic., 10*, 83–91 (1975).

Shine, R. E., Assessment and fluency training and the young stutterer. In Peins, M. (ed.), *Contemporary Approaches in Stuttering Therapy*. Boston: Little, Brown (1984).

Shipp, T., Izdebski, K., and Morrissey, P., Physiologic stages of vocal reaction time. *J. Speech Hearing Res., 27*, 173–78 (1984).

Shopwin, C. D., An experimental investigation of the passive-dependency component in adult male stutterers. *Speech Monogr., 26*, 143 (1959). Abstract.

Shrum, W. F., A comparison of the effect of masking noise and increased vocal intensity on the frequency of stuttering, *Asha, 4*, 408 (1962). Abstract.

Shtremel, A. Kh., Zaikanie v syndrome levoi temennoi doli. *Zh. Nevropatol. Psikhiat., 63*, 828–32 (1963).

Shulman, E., Factors influencing the variability of stuttering. In Johnson, W., and Leutenegger, R. R. (eds.), *Stuttering in Children and Adults*. Minneapolis: Univ. Minn. Press (1955).

Shumak, I. C., A speech situation rating sheet for stutterers. In Johnson, W., and Leutenegger, R. R. (eds.), *Stuttering in Children and Adults*. Minneapolis: Univ. Minn. Press (1955).

Sichel, R. N., *Initial Phoneme in Relation to Disfluency in the Spontaneous Speech of Nonstuttering Preschool Children*. M. S. Thesis, Brooklyn Coll. (1973).

Siegel, G. M., Punishment, stuttering, and disfluency. *J. Speech Hearing Res., 13*, 677–714 (1970).

Siegel, G. M., and Hanson, B., The effect of response-contingent neutral stimuli on normal speech disfluency. *J. Speech Hearing Res., 15*, 123–33 (1972).

Siegel, G. M., and Haugen, D., Audience size and variations in stuttering behavior. *J. Speech Hearing Res., 7*, 381–88 (1964).

Siegel, G. M., Lenske, J., and Broen, P., Suppression of normal speech disfluencies through response cost. *J. Appl. Behav. Anal., 2*, 265–76 (1969).

Siegel, G. M., and Martin, R. R., Experimental modification of disfluency in normal speakers. *J. Speech Hearing Res., 8*, 235–44 (1965a).

Siegel, G. M., and Martin, R. R., Verbal punishment of disfluencies in normal speakers. *J. Speech Hearing Res., 8*, 245–51 (1965b).

Siegel, G. M., and Martin, R. R. Punishment of disfluencies in normal speakers. *J. Speech Hearing Res., 9*, 208–18 (1966).

Siegel, G. M., and Martin, R. R., Verbal punishment of disfluencies during spontaneous speech. *Lang. Speech, 10*, 244–51 (1967).

Siegel, G. M., and Martin, R. R., The effects of verbal stimuli on disfluencies during spontaneous speech. *J. Speech Hearing Res., 11*, 358–64 (1968).

Silverman, E.-M., Situational variability of preschoolers' disfluency: Preliminary study. *Percept. Mot. Skills, 33*, 1021–22 (1971).

Silverman, E.-M., Generality of disfluency data collected from preschoolers. *J. Speech Hearing Res., 5*, 84–92 (1972a).

Silverman, E.-M., Preschoolers' speech disfluency: Single syllable word repetitoin. *Percept. Mot. Skills, 35*, 1002 (1972b).

Silverman, E.-M., Clustering: A characteristic of preschoolers' speech disfluency. *J. Speech Hearing Res., 16*, 578–83 (1973a).

Silverman, E.-M., The influence of preschoolers' speech usage on their disfluency frequency. *J. Speech Hearing Res., 16*, 474–81 (1973b).

Silverman, E.-M., Word position and grammatical function in relation to preschoolers' speech disfluency. *Percept. Mot. Skills, 39*, 267–72 (1974).

Silverman, E.-M., Effect of selected word attributes on preschoolers' speech disfluency: Initial phoneme and length. *J. Speech Hearing Res., 18*, 430–34 (1975).

Silverman, E.-M., Communication attitudes of women who stutter. *J. Speech Hearing Dis., 45*, 533–39 (1980).

Silverman, E.-M., Speech-language clinicians' and university students' impressions of women and girls who stutter. *J. Fluency Dis., 7*, 469–78 (1982).

Silverman, E.-M., and Van Opens, K., An investigation of sex bias in classroom teachers' speech and language referrals. *Lang. Speech Hearing Serv. Schools, 11*, 169–74 (1980).

Silverman, E.-M., and Williams, D. E., A comparison of stuttering and nonstuttering children in terms of five measures of oral language development. *J. Communic. Dis., 1*, 305–09 (1968).

Silverman, E.-M., and Zimmer, C. H., Women who stutter: Personality and speech characteristics. *J. Speech Hearing Res., 22*, 553–64 (1979).

Silverman, E.-M., and Zimmer, C. H., Demographic characteristics and treatment experiences of women and men who stutter. *J. Fluency Dis., 7*, 273–85 (1982).

Silverman, E.-M., Zimmer, C. H., and Silverman, F. H., Variability of stutterers' speech disfluencies: The menstrual cycle. *Percept. Mot. Skills, 38*, 1037–38 (1974).

Silverman, F. H., Concern of elementary-school stutterers about their stuttering. *J. Speech Hearing Dis., 35*, 361–63 (1970a).

Silverman, F. H., Course of nonstutterers' disfluency adaptation during 15 consecutive oral readings of the same material. *J. Speech Hearing Res., 13*, 382–86 (1970b).

Silverman, F. H., Distribution of instances of disfluency in consecutive readings of different passages by nonstutterers. *J. Speech Hearing Res., 13*, 874–82 (1970c).

Silverman, F. H., A note on the degree of adaptation by stutterers and nonstutterers during oral reading. *J. Speech Hearing Res., 13*, 173–77 (1970d).

Silverman, F. H., The effect of rhythmic auditory stimulation on the disfluency of nonstutterers. *J. Speech Hearing Res., 14*, 350–55 (1971).

Silverman, F. H., Disfluency and word length. *J. Speech Hearing Res., 15*, 788–91 (1972).

Silverman, F. H., Disfluency behavior of elementary-school stutterers and nonstutterers. *Lang. Speech Hearing Serv. Schools, 5*, 32–37 (1974).

Silverman, F. H., How "typical" is a stutterer's stuttering in a clinical environment? *Percept. Mot. Skills, 40*, 458 (1975).

Silverman, F. H., Do elementary-school stutterers talk less than their peers? *Lang. Speech Hearing Serv. Schools, 7*, 90–92 (1976a).

Silverman, F. H., Long-term impact of a miniature metronome on stuttering: An interim report. *Percept. Mot. Skills, 42*, 1322 (1976b).

Silverman, F. H., Dimensions of improvement in stuttering. *J. Speech Hearing Res., 23*, 137–51 (1980a).

Silverman, F. H., The stuttering problem profile: A task that assists both client and clinician in defining therapy goals. *J. Speech Hearing Dis., 45*, 119–23 (1980b).

Silverman, F. H., Are professors likely to report having "beliefs" about the intelligence and competence of students who stutter? *J. Fluency Dis., 15*, 319–21 (1990).

Silverman, F. H., and Bohlman, P., Flute stuttering. *J. Fluency Dis., 13*, 427–28 (1988).

Silverman, F. H., and Bloom, C. M., Spontaneous recovery of nonstutters' disfluency following adaptation. *J. Speech Hearing Res., 16*, 452–55 (1973).

Silverman, F. H., and Goodban, M. T., The effect of auditory masking on the fluency of normal speakers. *J. Speech Hearing Res., 15*, 543–46 (1972).

Silverman, F. H., and Silverman E.-M., Stutter-like behavior in the manual communication of the deaf. *Percept. Mot. Skills, 33*, 45–46 (1971).

Silverman, F. H., and Paynter, K. K., Impact of stuttering on perception of occupational competence. *J. Fluency Dis., 15*, 87–91 (1990).

Silverman, F. H., and Trotter, W. D., Impact of pacing speech with a miniature electronic metronome upon the manner in which a stutterer is perceived. *Behav. Ther., 4*, 414–19 (1973).

Silverman, F. H., and Umberger, F. G., Effect of pacing speech with a miniature electronic metronome on the frequency and duration of selected disfluency behaviors in the spontaneous speech of adult stutterers. *Behav. Ther., 5*, 410–14 (1974).

Silverman, F. H., and Williams, D. E., Loci of disfluencies in the speech of non-stutterers during oral reading. *J. Speech Hearing Res., 10*, 790–94 (1967a).

Silverman, F., and Williams, D., Loci of disfluencies in the speech of stutterers. *Percept. Mot. Skills, 24*, 1085–86 (1967b).

Silverman, F. H., and Williams, D. E., A proportional measure of stuttering adaptation. *J. Speech Hearing Res., 11*, 444–46 (1968).

Silverman, F. H., and Williams, D. E., The adaptation effect for six types of speech disfluency. *J. Speech Hearing Res., 14*, 525–30 (1971).

Silverman, F. H., and Williams, D. E., Performance of stutterers on a single-word adaptation task. *Percept. Mot. Skills, 34*, 565–66 (1972a).

Silverman, F. H., and Williams, D. E., Prediction of stuttering by school-age stutterers. *J. Speech Hearing Res., 15*, 189–93 (1972b).

Silverman, F. H., and Williams, D. E., Use of revision by elementary-school stutterers and nonstutterers. *J. Speech Hearing Res., 16*, 584–85 (1973).Silverman, L. H., Klinger, H., Lustbader, L., Farrel, J., and Martin, A. D., The effects of subliminal drive stimulation on the speech of stutterers. *J. Nerv. Ment. Dis., 155*, 14–21 (1972).

Simon, C. T., Complexity and breakdown in speech situations. *J. Speech Dis., 10*, 199–203 (1945).

Široký, A., Langová, J., Morávek, M., and Šváb, L., The occurrence of the saddle-formed nystagmus in stutterers. *Activitas Nervosa Superior, 20*, 146–48 (1978).

Skalbeck, O. M., The relationship of expectancy of stuttering to certain other designated variables associated with stuttering. *Speech Monogr., 24*, 146 (1957). Abstract.

Slorach, N., and Noehr, B., Dichotic listening in stuttering and dyslalic children. *Cortex, 9*, 295–300 (1973).

Smith, A. M., Treatment of stutterers with carbon dioxide. *Dis. Nerv. System, 14*, 243–44 (1953).

Smith, A., Neural drive to muscles in stuttering. *J. Speech Hearing Res., 32*, 252–64 (1989).

Smith, A., Denny, M., and Wood, J., Instability in speech muscle systems in stuttering. In Peters, H. F. M., Hulstijn, W., and Starkweather, C. W. (eds.), *Speech Motor Control and Stuttering.* Amsterdam: Elsevier (1991).

Smith, A., and Luschei, E. S., Assessment of oral-motor reflexes in stutterers and normal speakers: Preliminary observations. *J. Speech Hearing Res., 26*, 322–28 (1983).

Smith, K. M., Blood, I. M., and Blood, G. W., Auditory brainstem responses of stutterers and nonstutterers during speech production. *J. Fluency Dis., 15*, 211–22 (1990).

Snidecor, J. C., Why the Indian does not stutter. *Quart. J. Speech, 33*, 493–95 (1947).

Snidecor, J. C., Tension and facial appearance in stuttering. In Johnson, W., and Leutenegger, R. R. (eds.), *Stuttering in Children and Adults.* Minneapolis: Univ. Minn. Press (1955).

Snyder, M. A., Stuttering and coordination: An investigation of the relationship between the stutterer's coordination and his speech difficulty. *Logos, 1*, 36–44 (1958).

Soderberg, G. A., A study of the effects of delayed side-tone on four aspects of stutterers' speech during oral reading and spontaneous speech. *Speech Monogr.*, *27*, 252–53 (1960). Abstract.

Soderberg, G. A., Phonetic influences upon stutteringr. *J. Speech Hearing Res.*, *5*, 315–20 (1962a).

Soderberg, G. A., What is "average" stuttering? *J. Speech Hearing Dis.*, *27*, 85–86 (1962b).

Soderberg, G. A., The relations of stuttering to word length and word frequency. *J. Speech Hearing Res.*, *9*, 584–89 (1966).

Soderberg, G. A., Linguistic factors in stuttering. *J. Speech Hearing Res.*, *10*, 801–10 (1967).

Soderberg, G. A., Delayed auditory feedback and stuttering. *J. Speech Hearing Dis.*, *33*, 260–67 (1968).

Soderberg, G. A., A comparison of adaptation trends in the oral reading of stutterers, inferior speakers and superior speakers. *J. Communic. Dis.*, *2*, 99–108 (1969a).

Soderberg, G. A., Delayed auditory feedback and the speech of stutterers: A review of studies. *J. Speech Hearing Dis.*, *34*, 20–29 (1969b).

Soderberg, G. A., Relations of word information and word length to stuttering disfluencies. *J. Communic. Dis.*, *4*, 9–14 (1971).

Solomon, N. D., A comparison of rigidity of behavior manifested by a group of stutterers compared with "fluent" speakers in oral and other performances as measured by the Einstellung-effect. *Speech Monogr.*, *19*, 198 (1952). Abstract.

Sommers, R. K., Brady, W. A., and Moore, W. H., Jr., Dichotic ear preferences of stuttering children and adults. *Percept. Mot. Skills*, *41*, 931–38 (1975).

Sovǎk, M., Das vegetative Nervensystem bei Stotterern. Monatsschr. Ohrenheilk. *Laryngo-Rhinol.*, *69*, 666–80 (1935).

Spadino, E. J., *Writing and Laterality Characteristics of Stuttering Children*. New York: Columbia Univ. Teachers Coll. (1941).

Spencer, G., The status of environmental and group cohesiveness in the treatment of stuttering. *Aust. J. Human Communic. Dis.*, *4*, 140–45 (1976).

Spielberger, C. D., The effects of stuttering behavior and response set on recognition thresholds. *J. Person.*, *25*, 33–45 (1956).

Spriestersbach, D. C., *An Exploratory Study of the Motility of the Peripheral Oral Structures in Relation to Defective and Superior Consonant Articulation*. M. A. Thesis, Univ. Iowa (1940).

Spriestersbach, D. C., An objective approach to the investigation of social adjustment of male stutterers. *J. Speech Hearing Dis.*, *16*, 250–57 (1951).

Stager, S. V., Heterogeneity in stuttering: Results from auditory brainstem response testing. *J. Fluency Dis.*, *15*, 9–19 (1990).

Stang, H., Stationäre mehrdimensionale Verhaltenstherapie bei stotternden Kindern und Jugendlichen—Ein Erfahrungsbericht. *Sprache-Stimme-Gehör*, *8*, 16–19 (1984).

Starbuck, H. B., and Steer, M. D., The adaptation effect in stuttering speech behavior and normal speech behavior. *J. Speech Hearing Dis.*, *18*, 252–55 (1953).

Starbuck, H. B., and Steer, M. D., The adaptation effect in stuttering speech behavior and normal speech behavior. *J. Speech Hearing Dis.*, *18*, 252–55 (1953).

Starbuck, H. B., and Steer, M. D., The adaptation effect in stuttering and its relation to thoracic and abdominal breathing. *J. Speech Hearing Dis., 19,* 440–49 (1954).

Stark, R. E., and Pierce, B. R., The effects of delayed auditory feedback on a speech-related task in stutterers. *J. Speech Hearing Res., 13,* 245–53 (1970).

Starkweather, C. W., The case against base rate comparisons in stuttering experimentation. *J. Communic. Dis., 4,* 247–58 (1971).

Starkweather, C. W., A multiprocess behavioral approach to stuttering therapy. In Perkins, W. H. (ed.), *Stuttering Disorders.* New York: Thieme-Stratton (1984).

Starkweather, C. W., *Fluency and Stuttering.* Englewood Cliffs, N.J.: Prentice-Hall (1987).

Starkweather, C. W., Armson, J. M., and Amster, B. J., An approach to the study of motor speech mechanisms in stuttering. In Rustin, L. Purser, H., and Rowley, D. (eds.), *Progress in the Treatment of Fluency Disorders.* London: Taylor and Francis (1987).

Starkweather, C. W., Franklin, S., and Smigo, T. M., Vocal and finger reaction times in stutterers and nonstutterers: Differences and correlations. *J. Speech Hearing Res., 27,* 193–96 (1984).

Starkweather, C. W., and Gottwald, S. R., The demands and capacities model II: Clinical applications. *J. Fluency Dis., 15,* 143–57 (1990).

Starkweather, C. W., Hirschman, P., and Tannenbaum, R. S., Latency of vocalization onset; Stutterers versus nonstutterers. *J. Speech Hearing Res., 19,* 481–92 (1976).

Starkweather, C. W., and Lucker, J., Tokens for stuttering. *J. Fluency Dis., 3,* 167–80 (1978).

Starkweather, C. W., and Myers, M., Duration of subsegments within the intervocalic interval in stutterers and nonstutterers. *J. Fluency Dis., 4,* 205–14 (1979).

Starr, H. E., The hydrogen ion concentration of the mixed saliva considered as an index of fatigue and of emotional excitation, and applied to a study of the metabolic etiology of stammering. *Amer. J. Psychol., 33,* 394–418 (1922).

Starr, H. E., Psychological concomitants of high alveolar carbon dioxide: A psychobiochemical study of the etiology of stammering. *Psychol. Clin., 17,* 1–12 (1928).

Stassi, E. J., Disfluency of normal speakers and reinforcement. *J. Speech Hearing Res., 4,* 358–61 (1961).

Steer, M. D., A qualitative study of breathing in young stutterers. *Speech Monogr., 2,* 152–56 (1935).

Steer, M. D., The general intelligence of college stutterers. *Sch. Soc., 44,* 862–64 (1936).

Steer, M. D., Symptomatologies of young stutterers. *J. Speech Dis., 2,* 3–13 (1937).

Steer, M. D., and Johnson, W., An objective study of the relationship between psychological factors and the severity of stuttering. *J. Abnorm. Soc. Psychol., 31,* 36–46 (1936).

Stefankiewicz, S. P., and Bloodstein, O., The effect of a four-week interval on the consistency of stuttering. *J. Speech Hearing Res., 17,* 141–45 (1974).

Stephen, S. C. G., and Haggard M. P., Acoustic properties of masking/delayed feedback in the fluency of stutterers and controls. *J. Speech Hearing Res., 23,* 527–38 (1980).

Stephenson-Opsal, D., and Ratner, N. B., Maternal speech rate modification and childhood stuttering. *J. Fluency Dis., 13,* 49–56 (1988).

Stern, E., A preliminary study of bilingualism and stuttering in four Johannesburg schools. *J. Logopaed., 1,* 15–25 (948).

Sternberg, M. L., *Auditory Factors in Stuttering.* M. A., Thesis, Univ. Iowa (1946).

Stewart, C., Evans, W. B., and Fitch, J. L., Oral form perception skills of stuttering and nonstuttering children measured by stereognosis. *J. Fluency Dis., 10,* 311–16 (1985).

Stewart, J. L., The problem of stuttering in certain North American Indian societies. *J. Speech Hear Dis., Monogr. Suppl. 6* (1960).

Still, A. W., and Griggs, S., Changes in the probability of stuttering following a stutter: A test of some recent models. *J. Speech Hearing Res., 22,* 565–71 (1979).

Stock, E., Untersuchungen zur Intonation bei Stotterern. *Folia Phoniat., 18,* 447–61 (1966).

Stocker, B., and Gerstman, L. J., A comparison of the probe technique and conventional therapy for young stutterers. *J. Fluency Dis., 8,* 331–39 (1983).

Stocker, B., and Parker, E., The relationship betwen auditory recall and dysfluency in young stutterers. *J. Fluency Dis., 2,* 177–87 (1977).

Stocker, B., and Usprich, C., Stuttering in young children and level of demand. *J. Childhood Communic. Dis., 1,* 116–31 (1976).

Streifler, M., and Gumpertz, F., Cerebral potentials in stuttering and cluttering. *Confin. Neurol., 15,* 344–59 (1955).

Stromsta, C., A spectrographic study of dysfluencies labeled as stuttering by parents. *De Tehrapia Vocis et Loquelae, Vol. 1,* XIII Congr. Int. Soc. Logoped. Phoniat. (1965).

Stromsta, C., Interaural phase disparity of stutterers and nonstutterers. *J. Speech Hearing Res., 15,* 771–80 (1972).

Stromsta, C., *Elements of Stuttering.* Oshtemo, Mich.: Atsmonts Publishing (1986).

Stromsta, C., Acoustic and electrophysiologic correlates of stuttering and early developmental reactions. In Peters, H. F. M., and Hulstijn, W. (eds.), *Speech Motor Dynamics in Stuttering.* New York: Springer (1987).

Stromsta, C. P., A methodology related to the determination of the phase angle of bone-conducted speech sound energy of stutterers and nonstutterers. *Speech Monogr., 24,* 147–48 (1957). Abstract.

Stromsta, C., and Fibiger, S., Physiological correlates of the core behavior of stuttering. *Proc. 18th Congr. Int. Assoc. Logoped. Phoniat.* Washington, D.C.: Amer. Speech-Lang.-Hearing Assoc. (1981).

Strother, C. R., A study of the extent of dyssynergia occurring during stuttering spasm. *Psychol. Monogr., 49,* 108–27 (1937).

Strother, C. R., and Kriegman, L. S., Diadochokinesis in stutterers and nonstutterers. *J. Speech Dis., 8,* 323–35 (1943).

Strother, C. R., and Kriegman, L. S., Rhythmokinesis in stutterers and nonstutterers. *J. Speech Dis., 9,* 239–44 (1944).

Sussman, H. M., Contrastive patterns of interhemispheric interference to verbal and spatial concurrent tasks in right-handed, left-handed and stuttering populations. *Neuropsychologia, 20*, 675–84 (1982).

Sussman, H. M., and MacNeilage, P. F., Hemispheric specialization for speech production and perception in stutterers. *Neuropsychologia, 13*, 19–26 (1975).

Suter, C. B., Hutchinson, J. M., and Mallard, A. R., Visible correlates of stuttering severity. *Asha, 21*, 733 (1979). Abstract.

Sutton, S., and Chase, R. A., White noise and stuttering. *J. Speech Hearing Res., 4*, 72 (1961).

Sváb, L., Gross, J., and Langová, J., Stuttering and social isolation: Effect of social isolation with different levels of monitoring on stuttering frequency (a pilot study). *J. Nerv. Ment. Dis., 155*, 1–5 (1972).

Swift, W. J., Swift, E. W., and Arellano, M., Haloperidol as a treatment for adult stuttering. *Comprehens. Psychiat., 16*, 61–67 (1975).

Tanberg, M. C., A study of the role of inhibition in the moment of stuttering. In Johnson, W., and Leutenegger, R. R. (eds.), *Stuttering in Children and Adults*. Minneapolis: Univ. Minn. Press (1955).

Tapia, F., Haldol in the treatment of children with tics and stutterers—and an incidental finding. *Psychiat. Quart., 43*, 647–49 (1969).

Tatchell, R. H., Van den Berg, S., and Lerman, J. W., Fluency and eye contact as factors influencing observers' perceptions of stutterers. *J. Fluency Dis., 8*, 221–31 (1983).

Tate, M. W., and Cullinan, W. L., Measurement of consistency of stuttering. *J. Speech Hearing Res., 5*, 272–83 (1962).

Tate, M. W., Cullinan, W. L., and Ahlstrand, A., Measurement of adaptation in stuttering. *J. Speech Hearing Res., 4*, 321–39 (1961).

Tatham, M. A. A., Implications on stuttering of a model of speech production. In Lebrun, Y., and Hoops, R., (eds.), *Neurolinguistic Approaches to Stuttering*. The Hague: Mouton (1973).

Tawadros, S. M., An experiment in the group psychotherpay of stutterers. *Int. J. Sociom. Sociat., 1*, 181–89 (1957).

Taylor, I. K., The properties of stuttered words. *J. Verb. Learn. Verb. Behav., 5*, 112–18 (1966a).

Taylor, I. K., What words are stuttered? *Psychol. Bull., 65*, 233–42 (1966b).

Tyalor, I. K., and Taylor, M. M., Test of predictions from the conflict hypothesis of stuttering. *J. Abnorm, Psychol., 72*, 431–33 (1967).

Taylor, W. L., Lore, J. I., and Waldman, I. N., Latencies of semantic aphasics, stutterers and normal controls to cloze items requiring unique and non-unique oral responses. *Proc. Ann. Conv. Amer. Psychol. Assoc., 78*, 75–76 (1970).

Telser, E. B., An assessment of word finding skills in stuttering and nonstuttering children. *Dissert. Abstr. Int., 32 (6-B)*, 3693–94 (1971).

Ten Cate, M. J., Über die Untersuchung der Atmungsbewegung bei Sprachfehlern. *Monatsschr. Sprachheilk., 12*, 247, 321 (1902).

Thomas, J. D., A psychophysiologic and personality assessment of stutterers as measured by conditionability, extraversion, and neuroticism. *Asha, 18*, 637 (1976). Abstract.

Thompson, A. H., A test of the distraction explanation of disfluency modification in stuttering. *J. Fluency Dis., 10*, 35–50 (1985).

Thorn, K. F., *A Study of the Personality of Stutterers as Measured by the MMPI.* Ph.D. Dissert., Univ. Minn. (1949).

Thümer, St., Thumfart, W., and Kittel, G., Elektromyographische Untersuchungsbefunde bei Stotterern. *Sprache-Stimme-Gehör, 7*, 125–27 (1983).

Tiffany, W. R., Sound mindedness: Studies in the measurement of "phonetic ability." *West. Speech, 27*, 5–15 (1963).

Tiffany, W. R., and Hanley, C. N., Adaptation to delayed sidetone. *J. Speech Hearing Dis., 21*, 164–72 (1956).

Till, J. A., Reich, A., Dickey, S., and Sieber, J., Phonatory and manual reaction times of stuttering and nonstuttering children. *J. Speech Hearing Res., 26*, 171–80 (1983).

Timmons, B. A., and Boudreau, J. P., Delayed auditory feedback and the speech of stuttering and nonstuttering children. *Percept. Mot. Skills, 46*, 551–55 (1978a).

Timmons, B. A., and Boudreau, J. P., Speech disfluencies and delayed auditory feedback reactions of stuttering and nonstuttering children. *Percept. Mot. Skills, 47*, 859–62 (1978b).

Timmons, R. J., A study of adaptation and consistency in a response-contingent punishment situation. *Speech Monogr., 34*, 311–12 (1967). Abstract.

Tippett, D. C., and Siebens, A. A., Distinguishing psychogenic from neurogenic dysfluency when neurologic and psychologic factors coexist. *J. Fluency Dis., 16*, 3–12 (1991).

Toomey, G. L., and Sidman, M., An experimental analogue of the anxiety-stuttering relationship. *J. Speech Hearing Res., 13*, 122–29 (1970).

Tornick, G. B., and Bloodstein, O., Stuttering and sentence length. *J. Speech Hearing Res., 19*, 651–54 (1976).

Toscher, M. M., and Rupp, R. R., A study of the central auditory processes in stutterers using the Synthetic Sentence Identification (SSI) test battery. *J. Speech Hearing Res., 21*, 779–92 (1978).

Travis, L. E., Dysintegration of the breathing movements during stuttering. *Arch. Neurol. Psychiat., 18*, 673–90 (1927a).

Travis, L. E., A phono-photographic study of the stutterer's voice and speech. *Psychol. Monogr., 36*, 109–41 (1927b).

Travis, L. E., A comparative study of the performances of stutterers and normal speakers in mirror tracing. *Psychol. Monogr., 39*, 45–50 (1928a).

Travis, L. E., The influence of the group upon the stutterer's speed in free association. *J. Abnorm. Soc. Psychol., 23*, 45–51 (1928b).

Travis, L. E., Speech Pathology. New York: D. Appleton-Century (1931).

Travis, L. E., Dissociation of the homologous muscle function in stuttering. *Arch. Neurol. Psychiat., 31*, 127–33 (1934).

Travis, L. E., The unspeakable feelings of people, with special reference to stuttering. In Travis, L. E. (ed.), *Handbook of Speech Pathology.* New York: Appleton-Century-Crofts (1957).

Travis, L. E., and Fagan, L. B., Studies in stuttering: III. A study of certain reflexes during stuttering. *Arch. Neurol. Psychiat., 19*, 1006–13 (1928).

Travis, L. E., and Herren, R. Y., Studies in stuttering: V. A study of simultaneous antitropic movements of the hands of stutterers. *Arch. Neurol. Psychiat., 22*, 487–94 (1929).

Travis, L. E., Johnson, W., and Shover, J., The relation of bilingualism to stuttering. *J. Speech Dis.*, 2, 185–89 (1937).

Travis, L. E., and Knott, J. R., Brain potentials from normal speakers and stutterers. *J. Psychol.*, 2, 137–50 (1936).

Travis, L. E., and Knott, J. R., Bilaterally recorded brain potentials from normal speakers and stutterers. *J. Speech Dis.*, 2, 239–41 (1937).

Travis, L. E., and Lindsley, D. B., An action current study of handedness in relation to stuttering. *J. Exper. Psychol.*, 16, 258–70 (1933).

Travis, L. E, and Malamud, W., Brain potentials from normal subjects, stutterers, and schizophrenic patients. *Amer. J. Psychiat.*, 93, 929–36 (1937).

Travis, L. E., Malamud, W., and Thayer, L. R., The relationship between physical habitus and stuttering. *J. Abnorm. Soc. Psychol.*, 29, 132–40 (1934).

Travis, L. E., Tuttle, W. W., and Cowan, D. W., A study of the heart rate during stuttering. *J. Speech Dis.*, 1, 21–26 (1936).

Travis, V., A study of the horizontal dysintegration of breathing during stuttering. *Arch. Speech*, 1, 157–69 (1936).

Treon, M., and Tamayo, F. M. V., The separate and combined effects of GSR biofeedback and delayed auditory feedback on stuttering: A preliminary study. *J. Fluency Dis.*, 1, 3–9 (1975).

Trombly, T., Responses of stutterers and normal speakers to a level of aspiration [inventory]. *Cent. States Speech J.*, 16, 179–81 (1965).

Trombly, T. W., A comparative study of stutterers' levels of aspiration for speech and non-speech performances. *Speech Monogr.*, 26, 143–44 (1959). Abstract.

Trotter, W. D., The severity of stuttering during successive readings of the same material. *J. Speech Hearing Dis.*, 20, 17–25 (1955).

Trotter, W. D., Relationship between severity of stuttering and word conspicuousness. *J. Speech Hearing Dis.*, 21, 198–201 (1956).

Trotter, W. D., and Bergmann, M. F., Stutterers' and nonstutterers' reactions to speech situations. *J. Speech Hearing Dis.*, 22, 40–45 (1957).

Trotter, W. D., and Brown, L., Speaking time behavior of the stutterer before and after speech therapy. *J. Speech Hearing Res.*, 1, 48–51 (1958).

Trotter, W. D., and Lesch, M. M., Personal experiences with a stutter-aid. *J. Speech Hearing Dis.*, 32, 270–72 (1967).

Trotter, W. D., and Silverman, F. H., Experiments with the stutter-aid. *Percept. Mot. Skills*, 36, 1129–30 (1973).

Trotter, W. D., and Silverman, F. H., Does the effect of pacing speech with a miniature metronome on stuttering wear off? *Percept. Mot. Skills*, 39, 429–30 (1974).

Tsunoda, T., and Moriyama, H., Specific pattern of cerebral dominance for various sounds in adult stutterers. *J. Aud. Res.*, 12, 216–27 (1972).

Tuck, A. E., An alaryngeal stutterer: A case history. *J. Fluency Dis.*, 4, 239–43 (1979).

Turnbaugh, K. R., Guitar, B. E., and Hoffman, P. R., Speech clinicians' attribution of personality traits as a function of stuttering severity. *J. Speech Hearing Res.*, 22, 37–45 (1979).

Turnbaugh, K., Guitar, B., and Hoffman, P., The attribution of personality traits: The stutterer and nonstutterer. *J. Speech Hearing Res.*, 24, 288–91 (1981).

Tuthill, C., A quantitative study of extensional meaning with special reference to stuttering. *J. Speech Dis.*, 5, 189–91 (1940).

Tuthill, C., A quantitaqtive study of extensional meaning with special reference to stuttering. *Speech Monogr., 13*, 81–98 (1946).

Twitmyer, E. B., Stammering in relation to hemo-respiratory factors. *Quart. J. Speech, 16*, 278–83 (1930).

Uenishi, S., Mori, T., and Mizumachi, T., Changes of maximum blood pressure in stutterers. *dsh Abstr., 13*, 299 (1973).

Ulliana, L., and Ingham, R. J., Behavioral and nonbehavioral variables in the measurement of stutterers' communication attitudes. *J. Speech Hearing Res., 49*, 83–93 (1984).

Umeda, K., Electroencephalographic study of stutterers. *dsh Abstr., 2*, 356 (1962a).

Umeda, K., A psychophysiological study of stutterers. *dsh Abstr., 2*, 266 (1962b).

Uys, I. C., 'n Ondersoek na sekere biolinguistiese verskynels by hakkel. *J. So. Afr. Logoped. Soc., 17*, 67–78 (1970).

Vaane, E., and Janssen, P., Different types of disfluencies and some phonological factors. *Logoped. Foniat., 50*, 14–20 (1978).

Valyo, R. A., PGSR responses of stutterers and nonstutterers during periods of silence and verbalization. *Asha, 6*, 422 (1964). Abstract.

Van Dusen, C. R., A study of the relation of the relative size of the two hands to speech. *Speech Monogr., 4*, 127–34 (1937).

Van Dusen, C. R., A laterality study of nonstutterers and stutterers. *J. Speech Dis., 4*, 261–65 (1939).

van Lieshout, P. H. H. M., Hulstijn, W., and Peters, H. F. M., Word size and word complexity: Differences in speech reaction time between stutterers and nonstutterers in a picture and word naming task. In Peters, H. F. M., Hulstijn, W., and Starkweather, C. W. (eds.), *Speech Motor Control and Stuttering*. Amsterdam: Elsevier (1991).

van Lieshout, P. H. H. M., Peters, H. F. M., Starkweather, C. W., and Hulstijn, W., Physiological differences between stutterers and nonstutterers in perceptually fluent speech: EMG amplitude and duration. *J. Speech Hearing Res., 36*, 55–63 (1993).

Van Riper, C., A new test of laterality. *J. Exper. Psychol., 17*, 305–13 (1934).

Van Riper, C., The quantitative measurement of laterality. *J. Exper. Psychol., 18*, 372–82 (1935).

Van Riper, C., Study of the thoracic breathing of stutterers during expectancy and occurrence of stuttering spasm. *J. Speech Dis., 1*, 61–72 (1936).

Van Riper, C., The effect of devices for minimizing stuttering on the creation of symptoms. *J. Abnorm. Soc. Psychol., 32*, 185–92 (1937a).

Van Riper, C., The effect of penalty upon frequency of stuttering spasms. *J. Genet. Psychol., 50*, 193–95 (1937b).

Van Riper, C., The influence of empathic response on the frequency of stuttering. *Psychol. Monogr., 49*, 244–46 (1937c).

Van Riper, C., The preparatory set in stuttering. *J. Speech Dis., 2*, 149–54 (1937d).

Van Riper, C., A study of the stutterer's ability to interrupt stuttering spasms. *J. Speech Dis., 3*, 117–19 (1938).

Van Riper, C., *Speech Correction: Principles and Methods*. New York: Prentice-Hall (1939).

Van Riper, C., *Speech Correction: Principles and Methods*, 3rd ed. Englewood Cliffs, N. J.: Prentice-Hall (1954).

Van Riper, C., Experiments in stuttering therapy. In Eisenson, J. (ed.), *Stuttering: A Symposium*. New York: Harper & Row (1958).

Van Riper, C., *Speech Correction: Principles and Methods*, 4th ed. Englewood Cliffs, N. J.: Prentice-Hall (1963).

Van Riper, C., The use of DAF in stuttering therapy. *Brit. J. Dis. Communic.*, *5*, 40–45 (1970).

Van Riper, C., *The Nature of Stuttering*. Englewood Cliffs, N.J.: Prentice-Hall (1971).

Van Riper, C., *Speech Correction: Principles and Methods*, 5th ed. Englewood Cliffs, N.J.: Prentice-Hall (1972).

Van Riper, C. *The Treatment of Stuttering*. Englewood Cliffs, N.J.: Prentice-Hall (1973).

Van Riper, C., *The Nature of Stuttering*, 2nd ed. Englewood Cliffs, N.J.: Prentice-Hall (1982).

Van Riper, C., and Hull, C. J., The quantitative measurement of the effect of certain situations on stuttering. In Johnson, W., and Leutenegger, R. R. (eds.), *Stuttering in Children and Adults*. Minneapolis: Univ. Minn. Press (1955).

Van Riper, C., and Milisen, R. L., A study of the predicted duration of the stutterer's blocks as related to their actual duration. *J. Speech Dis.*, *4*, 339–46 (1939).

Vanryckeghem, M., and Brutten, G., J., The Communication Attitude Test: A test-retest reliability investigation. *J. Fluency Dis.*, *17*, 177–90 (1992).

Van Wyk, M., 'N oudiovisuele analise van woorddeelherhalings by hakkelaars. *So. Afr. J. Communic. Dis.*, *25*, 64–79 (1978).

Vaughn, C.-L. D., and Webster, W. G., Bimanual handedness in adults who stutter. *Percept. Mot. Skills*, *68*, 375–82 (1989).

Venkatagiri, H. S., The relevance of DAF-induced speech disruption to the understanding of stuttering. *J. Fluency Dis.*, *5*, 87–98 (1980).

Venkatagiri, H. S., Reaction time for voiced and whispered /a/ in stutterers and nonstutterers. *J. Fluency Dis.*, *6*, 265–71 (1981).

Venkatagiri, H. S., A comparison of DAF-induced disfluencies with stuttering. *J. Communic. Dis.*, *15*, 385–93 (1982a).

Venkatagiri, H. S., The influence of linguistic stress on stuttering. *Asha*, *24*, 730 (1982b). Abstract.

Venkatagiri, H. S., Reaction time for /s/ and /z/ in stutterers and nonstutterers: A test of discoordination hypothesis. *J. Communic. Dis.*, *15*, 55–62 (1982c).

Victor, C., and Johannsen, H. S., Untersuchung zur zerebralen Dominanz für Sprache bei Stotterer mittels Tachistoskopie. *Sprache-Stimme-Gehör*, *8*, 74–77 (1984).

Villarreal, J. J., The semantic aspects of stuttering in non-stutterers: Additional data. *Quart. J. Speech*, *31*, 477–79 (1945).

Viswanath, N. S., Global- and local-temporal effects of a stuttering event in the context of a clausal utterance. *J. Fluency Dis.*, *14*, 245–69 (1989).

Viswanath, N. S., Temporal structure is reorganized when an utterance contains a stuttering event. In Peters, H. F. M., Hulstijn, W., and Starkweather, C. W. (eds.). *Speech Motor Control and Stuttering*. Amsterdam: Elsevier (1991).

Voelker, C. H., On the semantic aspects of stuttering in nonstutterers. *Quart. J. Speech, 28*, 78–80 (1942).

Walker, S. T., and Walker, J. M., Differences in heart-rate variability between stutterers and nonstutterers following arousal. *Percept. Mot. Skills, 36*, 926 (1973).

Wall, M. J., A comparison of syntax in young stutterers and nonstutterers. *J. Fluency Dis., 5*, 345–52 (1980).

Wall, M. J., Language-based therapies for the young child stutterer. *J. Childhood Communic. Dis., 6*, 40–49 (1982).

Wall, M. J., Starkweather, C. W., and Cairns, H. S., Syntactic influences on stuttering in young child stutterers. *J. Fluency Dis., 6*, 283–98 (1981).

Wall, M. J., Starkweather, C. W., and Harris, K. S., The influence of voicing adjustments on the location of stuttering in the spontaneous speech of young child stutterers. *J. Fluency Dis., 6*, 299–310 (1981).

Walle, E. L., Intracarotid sodium amytal testing on normal, chronic adult stutterers. *J. Speech Hearing Dis., 36*, 561 (1971).

Wallen, V., A Q-technique study of the self-concepts of adolescent stutterers and nonstutterers. *Speech Monogr., 27*, 257–58 (1960). Abstract.

Wallin, J. E. W., A census of speech defectives among 89,057 public-school pupils—a preliminary report. *Sch. Soc., 3*, 213–16 (1916).

Walnut, F., A personality inventory item analysis of individuals who stutter and individuals who have other handicaps. *J. Speech Hearing Dis., 19*, 220–27 (1954).

Walton, D., and Mather, M. D., The relevance of generalization techniques to the treatment of stammering and phobic symptoms. *Behav. Res. Ther., 1*, 121–25 (1963).

Ward, D. G., A study of the responses of listeners to dysfluencies of speech. *Speech Monogr., 34*, 312 (1967). Abstract.

Watson, B. C., and Alfonso, P. J., A comparison of LRT and VOT values between stutterers and nonstutterers. *J. Fluency Dis., 7*, 219–41 (1982).

Watson, B. C., and Alfonso, P. J., Foreperiod and stuttering severity effects on acoustic laryngeal reaction time. *J. Fluency Dis., 8*, 183–205 (1983).

Watson, B. C., and Alfonso, P. J., Physiological bases of acoustic LRT in nonstutterers, mild stutterers, and severe stutterers. *J. Speech Hearing Res., 30*, 434–47 (1987).

Watson, B. C., Freeman, F. J., Chapman, S. B. Miller, S., Finitzo, T., Pool, K. D., and Devous, M. D. Sr., Linguistic performance deficits in stutterers: Relation to laryngeal reaction time profiles. *J. Fluency Dis., 16*, 85–100 (1991).

Watson, B. C., Pool, K. D., Devous, M. D., Sr., Freeman, F. J., and Finitzo, T., Brain blood flow related to acoustic laryngeal reaction time in adult developmental stutterers. *J. Speech Hearing Res., 35*, 555–61 (1992).

Watson, J. B., Profiles of stutterers' and nonstutterers' affective, cognitive, and behavioral communication attitudes. *J. Fluency Dis., 12*, 389– 405 (1987).

Watson, J. B., A comparison of stutterers' and nonstutterers' affective, cognitive, and behavioral self-reports. *J. Speech Hearing Res., 31*, 377–85 (1988).

Watts, F., The treatment of stammering by the intensive practice of fluent speech. *Brit. J. Dis. Communic., 6*, 144–47 (1971).

Weber, C. M., and Smith, A., Autonomic correlates of stuttering and speech assessed in a range of experimental tasks. *J. Speech Hearing Res., 33*, 690–706 (1990).

Webster, L. M., and Brutten, G., An audiovisual behavioral analysis of the stuttering moment. *Behav. Ther., 3*, 555–60 (1972).

Webster, L. M., and Gould, W. J., The effect on stuttering of selectively anesthetizing certain nerve tracts. In Webster, L. M., and Furst, L. C. (eds.), *Vocal Tract Dynamics and Dysfluency.* New York: Speech and Hearing Inst. (1975).

Webster, R. L., Stuttering: A way to eliminate it and a way to explain it. In Ulrich, R., Stachnik, T., and Mabry, J. (eds.), *Control of Human Behavior, Vol. 2.* Glenview, Ill.: Scott, Foresman (1970).

Webster, R. L., A behavioral analysis of stuttering: Treatment and theory. In Calhoun, K. S., Adams, H. E., and Mitchell, K. M. (eds.), *Innovative Treatment Methods in Psychopathology.* New York: Wiley (1974).

Webster, R. L., An operant response shaping program for the establishment of fluency in stutterers. *dsh Abstr., 15*, 136 (1975).

Webster, R. L., Empirical considerations regarding stuttering therapy. In Gregory, H. H. (ed.), *Controversies About Stuttering Therapy.* Baltimore: Univ. Park Press (1979a).

Webster, R. L., Masking influences on speech onset latencies in stutterers and normals. *Asha, 21*, 693 (1979b). Abstract.

Webster, R. L., Evolution of a target-based behavioral therapy for stuttering. *J. Fluency Dis., 5*, 303–20 (1980).

Webster, R. L., Manipulation of vocal tone: Implications for stuttering. In Peters, H. F. M., Hulstijn, W., and Starkweather, C. W. (eds.), *Speech Motor Control and stuttering.* Amsterdam, Elsevier (1991).

Webster, R. L., and Dorman, M. F., Decreases in stuttering frequency as a function of continuous and contingent forms of auditory masking. *J. Speech Hearing Res., 13*, 82–86 (1970).

Webster, R. L., and Dorman, M. F., Changes in reliance on auditory feedback cue as a function of oral practice. *J. Speech Hearing Res., 14*, 307–11 (1971).

Webster, R. L., and Lubker, B. B., Interrelationships among fluency producing variables in stuttered speech. *J. Speech Hearing Res., 11*, 754–66 (1968a).

Webster, R. L., and Lubker, B. B., Masking of auditory feedback in stutterers' speech. *J. Speech Hearing Res., 11*, 221–22 (1968b).

Webster, R. L., Schumacher, S. J., and Lubker, B. B., Changes in stuttering frequency as a function of various intervals of delayed auditory feedback. *J. Abnorm. Psychol., 75*, 45–49 (1970).

Webseter, W. G., Neuropsychological models of stuttering: I. Representation of sequential response mechanisms. *Neuropsychologia 23*, 263–67 (1985).

Webster, W. G., Neuropsychological models of stuttering: II. Interhemispheric interference. *Neuropsychologia, 24*, 737–41 (1986a).

Webster, W. G., Response sequence organization and reproduction by stutterers. *Neuropsychologia, 24*, 813–21 (1986b).

Webster, W. G., Rapid letter transcription performance by stutterers. *Neuropsychologia, 25*, 845–47 (1987).

Webster, W. G., Neural mechanisms underlying stuttering: evidence from bimanual handwriting performance. *Brian Lang., 33,* 226–44 (1988).

Webster, W. G., Sequence initiation performance by stutterers under conditions of response competition. *Brain Lang., 36,* 286–300 (1989a).

Webster, W. G., Sequence reproduction deficits in stutterers tested under non-speeded response conditions. *J. Fluency Dis., 14,* 79–86 (1989b).

Webster, W. G., Concurrent cognitive processing and letter sequence transcription deficits in stutterers. Can. *J. Psychol, 44,* 1–13 (1990a).

Webster, W. G., Evidence in bimanual finger-tapping of an attentional component to stuttering. *Behav. Brain Res., 37,* 93–100 (1990b).

Webster, W. G., and Poulos, M., Handedness distributions among adults who stutter. *Cortex, 23,* 705–08 (1987).

Webster, W. G., and Ryan, C. R. R., Task complexity and manual reaction times in people who stutter. *J. Speech Hearing Res., 34,* 708–14 (1991).

Weinberg, B., Stuttering among blind and partially sighted children. *J. Speech Hearing Dis., 29,* 322–26 (1964).

Weiner, A. E., Patterns of vocal fold movement during stuttering. *J. Fluency Dis., 9,* 31–49 (1984a).

Weiner, A. E., Stuttering and syllable stress. *J. Fluency Dis., 9,* 301–05 (1984b).

Weiner, A. E., Vocal control therapy for stutterers. In Peins, M. (ed.), *Contemporary Approaches in Stuttering Therapy.* Boston: Little, Brown (1984c).

Weisberger, S. E., An analysis of stuttering as a function of the stutterer's response to an array of standard projective stimuli involving themes of sexuality, aggression, and parental authority. *Speech Monogr., 34,* 313 (1967). Abstract.

Weiss, A. L., and Zebrowski, P. M., Patterns of assertiveness and responsiveness in parental interactions with stuttering and fluent children. *J. Disfluency Dis., 16,* 125–41 (1991).

Weiss, A. L., and Zebrowsky, P. M., Disfluencies in the conversations of young children who stutter: Some answers about questions. *J. Speech Hearing Res., 35,* 1230–38 (1992).

Weiss, A. L., and Zebrowski, P. M., The narrative productions of children who stutter: A preliminary view. *J. Fluency Dis., 19,* 39–63 (1994).

Weiss, D. A., *Cluttering.* Englewood Cliffs, N.J.: Prentice-Hall (1964).

Welch, I. L., An investigation of the listening proficiency of stutterers. *Speech Monogr., 28,* 125–26 (1961). Abstract.

Well, C. D., and Terrell, S. L., Attitudes and reactions of preschool and school-age children toward a child speaker with stuttering patterns. *Folia Phoniat., 38,* 369 (1986). Abstract.

Wells, B. G., and Moore, W. H., Jr., EEG alpha asymmetries in stutterers and nonstutterers: effects of linguistic variables on hemispheric processing and fluency. *Neuropsychologia, 28,* 1295–1305 (1990).

Wells, G. B., Effect of sentence structure on stuttering. *J. Fluency Dis., 4,* 123–29 (1979).

Wells, G. B., A feature analysis of stuttered phonemes. *J. Fluency Dis., 8,* 119–24 (1983).

Wells, P. G., and Malcolm, M. T., Controlled trial of the treatment of 36 stutterers. *Brit. J. Psychiat., 119,* 603–04 (1971).

Wendahl, R. W., and Cole, J., Identification of stuttering during relatively fluent speech. *J. Speech Hearing Res.*, 4, 281–86 (1961).

Wepman, J. M., Familial incidence in stammering. *J. Speech Dis.*, 4, 199–204 (1939).

Wertenbroch, W., Die Behandlung von Stotterern mit Haloperidol. *Sprachheilarb.*, 21, 78–82 (1976).

West, R., The phenomenology of stuttering. In West, R., (ed.), *A Symposium on Stuttering*. Madison, Wis.: College Typing Co. (1931).

West, R., An agnostic's speculations about stuttering. In Eisenson, J. (ed.), *Stuttering: A Symposium*. New York: Harper & Row (1958).

West, R., and Ansberry, M., *The Rehabilitation of Speech*, 4th ed. New York: Harper & Row (1968).

West, R., and Ansberry, M., and Carr, A., *The Rehabilitation of Speech*, 3rd ed. New York: Harper & Bros. (1957).

West, R., Kennedy, L., and Carr, A., *The Rehabilitation of Speech*, rev. ed. New York: Harper & Bros. (1947).

West, R., Nelson, S., and Berry, M. F., The heredity of stuttering. *Quart. J. Speech*, 25, 23–30 (1939).

West, R. and Nusbaum, E., A motor test for dysphemia. *Quart. J. Speech*, 15, 469–79 (1929).

Westby, C. E., Language performance of stuttering and nonstuttering children. *J. Communic. Dis.*, 12, 133–45 (1979).

Westphal, G., An experimental study of certain motor abilities of stutterers. *Child Dev.*, 4, 214–21 (1933).

Weuffen, M., Untersuchung der Wortfindung bei normalsprechenden und stotternden Kindern und Jugendlichen im Alter von 8 bis 16 Jahren. *Folia Phoniat.*, 13, 255–68 (1961).

Wexler, K. B., Developmental disfluency in 2-, 4-, and 6-year-old boys in neutral and stress situations. *J. Speech Hearing Res.*, 25, 229–34 (1982).

Wexler, K. B., and Mysak, E. D., Disfluency characteristics of 2-, 4-, and 6-year-old males. *J. Fluency Dis.*, 7, 37–46 (1982).

White, P. A., and Collins, S. R. C., Stereotype formation by inference: A possible explanation for the "stutterer" stereotype. *J. Speech Hearing Res.*, 27, 567–70 (1984).

White House Conference Committee Report on Child Health and Protection, Section III, "Special Education: The Handicapped and the Gifted." New York: D. Appleton Century (1931).

Wiechmann, J., and Richter, E., Die Häufigkeit des Stotterns beim Singen. *Folia Phoniat.*, 18, 435–46 (1966).

Wieneke, G., and Janssen, P., Duration variations in the fluent speech of stutterers and nonstutterers. In Peters, H. F. M., and Hulstijn, W. (eds.), *Speech Motor Dynamics in Stuttering*. New York: Springer (1987)

Wieneke, G., and Janssen, P., Effect of speaking rate on speech timing variability. In Peters, H. F. M., Hulstijn, W., and Starkweather, C. W. (eds.), *Speech Motor Control and Stuttering*. Amsterdam: Elsevier (1991).

Wiener, N., Cybernetics. New York: Wiley (1948).

Wijnen, F., and Boers, I., Phonological priming effects in stutterers. *J. Fluency Dis.*, 19, 1–20 (1994).

Wiener, N., Cybernetics. New York: Wiley (1948).

Wilkins, C., Webster, R. L., and Morgan, B. T., Cerebral lateralization of visual stimulus recognition in stutterers and fluent speakers. *J. Fluency Dis.*, *9*, 131–41 (1984).

Williams, A. M., and Marks, C. J., A comparative analysis of the ITPA and PPVT performance of young stutterers. *J. Speech Hearing Res.*, *15*, 323–29 (1972).

Williams, D. E., Masseter muscle action potentials in stuttered and nonstuttered speech. *J. Speech Hearing Dis.*, *20*, 242–61 (1955).

Williams, D. E., A point of view about "stuttering." *J. Speech Hearing Dis.*, *22*, 390–97 (1957).

Williams, D. E., and Kent, L. R., Listener evaluations of speech interruptions. *J. Speech Hearing Res.*, *1*, 124–31 (1958).

Williams, D. E. Melrose, B. M., and Woods, C. L., The relationship between stuttering and academic achievement in children. *J. Communic. Dis.*, *2*, 87–98 (1969).

Williams, D. E., and Silverman, F. H., Note concerning articulation of school-age stutterers. *Percept. Mot. Skills*, *27*, 713–14 (1968).

Williams, D. E., Silverman, F. H., and Kools, J. A., Disfluency behavior of elementary-school stutterers and nonstutterers: The adaptation effect. *J. Speech Hearing Res.*, *11*, 622–30 (1968).

Williams, D. E., Silverman, F. H., and Kools, J. A., Disfluency behavior of elementary-school stutterers and nonstutterers: The consistency effect. *J. Speech Hearing Res.*, *12*, 301–07 (1969a).

Williams. D. E., Silverman, F. H., and Kools, J. A., Disfluency behavior of elementary-school stutterers and nonstutterers: Loci of instances of disfluency. *J. Speech Hearing Res.*, *12*, 308-18 (1969b).

Williams, D. E., Wark, M., and Minifie, F. D., Ratings of stuttering by audio, visual, and audiovisual cues. *J. Speech Hearing Res.*, *6*, 91–100 (1963).

Williams, H. G., and Bishop, J. H., Speed and consistency of manual movements of stutterers, articulation-disordered children, and children with normal speech. *J. Fluency Dis.*, *17*, 191–203 (1992).

Williams, J. D., and Martin, R. B., Immediate versus delayed consequences of stuttering responses. *J. Speech Hearing Res.*, *17*, 569–75 (1974).

Wilson, D. M. *A study of the Personalities of Stuttering Children and Their Parents As Revealed Through Projection Tests*. Ph.D. Dissert., Univ. S. Calif. (1950).

Wilson, R. G., *A Study of Expressive Movements in Three Groups of Adolescent Boys, Stutterers, Non-stutterers, Maladjusted and Normals, By Means of Three Measures of Personality, Mira's Myokinetic Psychodiagnosis, the Bender-Gestalt, and Figure Drawing*. Ph.D. Dissrt., Western Reserve Univ. (1950).

Wingate, M. E., Calling attention to stuttering. *J. Speech Hearing Res.*, *2*, 326–35 (1959).

Wingate, M. E., Evaluation and stuttering. Part I: Speech characteristics of young children. *J. Speech Hearing Dis.*, *27*, 106–15 (1962a).

Wingate, M. E., Personality needs of stutterers. *Logos*, *5*, 35–37 (1962b).

Wingate, M. E., Recovery from stuttering. *J. Speech Hearing Dis.*, *29*, 312–21 (1964).

Wingate, M. E., Behavioral rigidity in stutterers. *J. Speech Hearing Res.*, *9*, 626–29 (1966a).

Wingate, M. E., Prosody in stuttering adaptation. *J. Speech Hearing Res.*, *9*, 550–56 (1966b).

Wingate, M. E., Slurvian skill of stutterers. *J. Speech Hearing Res.*, *10*, 844–48 (1967a).

Wingate, M. E., Stuttering and word length. *J. Speech Hearing Res.*, *10*, 146–52 (1967b).

Wingate, M. E., Sound and pattern in "artificial" fluency. *J. Speech Hearing Res.*, *12*, 677–86 (1969).

Wingate, M. E., Effect on stuttering of changes in audition. *J. Speech Hearing Res.*, *13*, 861–73 (1970).

Wingate, M. E., Phonetic ability in stuttering. *J. Speech Hearing Res.*, *14*, 189–94 (1971).

Wingate, M. E., Deferring the adaptation effect. *J. Speech Hearing Res.*, *15*, 547–50 (1972).

Wingate, M. E., Expectancy as basically a short-term process. *J. Speech Hearing Res.*, *18*, 31–42 (1975).

Wingate, M. E., *Stuttering: Theory and Treatment*. New York: Irvington (1976).

Wingate, M. E., Criteria for stuttering. *J. Speech Hearing Res.*, *20*, 596–600 (1977).

Wingate, M. E., The first three words. *J. Speech Hearing Res.*, *22*, 604–12 (1979).

Wingate, M. E., Questionnaire study of laryngectomee stutterers. *J. Fluency Dis.*, *6*, 273–81 (1981a).

Wingate, M. E., Sound pattern in artificial fluency: Spectrographic evidence. *J. Fluency Dis.*, *6*, 95–118 (1981b).

Wingate, M. E., Early position and stuttering occurrence. *J. Fluency Dis.*, *7*, 243–58 (1982).

Wingate, M. E., The recurrence ratio. *J. Fluency Dis.*, *9*, 21–29 (1984a).

Wingate, M. E., Stutter events and linguistic stress. *J. Fluency Dis.*, *9*, 295–300 (1984b).

Wingate, M. E., Adaptation, consistency and beyond: I. Limitations and contradictions. *J. Fluency Dis.*, *11*, 1–36 (1986).

Wingate, M. E., and Hamre, C. E., Stutterers' projection of listener reaction. *J. Speech Hearing Res.*, *10*, 339–43 (1967).

Winitz, H., Repetitions in the vocalizations of children in the first two years of life. *J. Speech Hearing Dis.*, *Monogr. Suppl. 7*, 55–62 (1961).

Winkelman, N. W., Jr., Chlorpromazine in the treatment of neuropsychiatric disorders. *J. Amer. Med. Assoc.*, *155*, 18–21 (1954).

Winkler, L. E., and Ramig, P., Temporal characteristics in the fluent speech of child stutterers and nonstutterers. *J. Fluency Dis.*, *11*, 217–29 (1986).

Wischner, G. J., *Stuttering Behavior and Learning: A Program of Research*, Ph.D. Dissert., Univ. Iowa (1947).

Wischner, G. J., Stuttering behavior and learning: A preliminary theoretical formulation. *J. Speech Hearing Dis.*, *15*, 324–35 (1950).

Wischner, G. J., Anxiety-reduction as reinforcement in maladaptive behavior: Evidence in stutterers' representations of the moment of difficulty. *J. Abnorm. Soc. Psychol.*, *47*, 566–71 (1952a).

Wischner, G. J., An experimental approach to expectancy and anxiety in stuttering behavior. *J. Speech Hearing Dis.*, *17*, 139–54 (1952b).

Witt, M. H., Statistische Erhebungen über den Einfluss des Singens und Flüsterns auf das Stottern, *Vox*, *11*, 41–43 (1925).

Wohl, M. T., The incidence of speech defect in the population. *Speech*, *15*, 13–14 (1951).

Wohl, M. T., The electronic metronome—an evaluative study. *Brit. J. Dis. Communic., 3,* 89–98 (1968).

Wohl, M. T., The treatment of non-fluent utterance—a behavioural approach. Brit., *J. Dis. Communic., 5,* 66–76 (1970).

Wolk, L., Vocal tract dynamics in an adult stutterer. *So. Afr. J. Communic. Dis., 28,* 38–52 (1981).

Wolk, L., Edwards, M. L., and Conture, E. G., Coexistence of stuttering and disordered phonology in young children. *J. Speech Hearing Res., 36,* 906–17 (1993).

Wolpe, J., *Psychotherapy by Reciprocal Inhibition.* Stanford, Calif.: Stanford Univ. Press (1958).

Wong, C. Y. Y., and Bloodstein, O., Effect of adjacency on the distribution of new stutterings in two successive readings. *J. Speech Hearing Res., 20,* 35–39 (1977).

Wood, F., Stump, D., McKeehan, A., Sheldon, S., and Proctor, J., Patterns of regional cerebral blood flow during attempted reading aloud by stutterers both on and off haloperidol medication: Evidence for inadequate left frontal activation during stuttering. *Brain Lang., 9,* 141–44 (1980).

Woods, C. L., Social position and speaking competence of stuttering and normally fluent boys. *J. Speech Hearing Res., 17,* 740–47 (1974).

Woods, C. L., Does the stigma shape the stutterer? *J. Communic. Dis., 11,* 483–87 (1978).

Woods, C. L., and Williams, D. E., Speech clinicians' conceptions of boys and men who stutter. *J. Speech Hearing Dis., 36,* 225–34 (1971).

Woods, C. L., and Williams, D. E., Traits attributed to stuttering and normally fluent males. *J. Speech Hearing Res., 19,* 267–78 (1976).

Woolf, G., The assessment of stuttering as struggle, avoidance, and expectancy. *Brit. J. Dis. Communic., 2,* 158–71 (1967).

Wulff, J., Lippen- Kiefer- Zungen- und Handreaktionen auf Reizdarbietungen nach unterschiedlichen Zeitintervallen bei normalsprechenden und bei stotternden Kindern im Alter von etwa 14 Jahren. *Vox, 21,* 40–45 (1935).

Wyatt, G. L., A developmental crisis theory of stuttering. *Lang. Speech, 1,* 250–64 (1958).

Wyatt, G. L., *Language Learning and Communication Disorders in Children.* New York: Free Press (1969).

Wyatt, G. L., and Herzan, H. M., Therapy with stuttering children and their mothers. *Amer. J. Orthopsychiat., 23,* 645–59 (1962).

Wynia, B. L., *The Consistency Effect in the Speech Repetitions of Normal Speaking Young Children,* M. S., Thesis, Penn. State Univ. (1964).

Wynne, M. K., and Boehmler, R. M., Central auditory function in fluent and disfluent normal speakers. *J. Speech Hearing Res., 25,* 54–57 (1982).

Yairi, E., Disfluency rates and patterns of stutterers and nonstutterers. *J. Communic. Dis., 5,* 225–31 (1972).

Yairi, E., Effects of binaural and monaural noise on stuttering. *J. Aud. Res., 16,* 114–19 (1976).

Yairi, E., Disfluencies of normally speaking two-year-old children. *J. Speech Hearing Res., 24,* 490–95 (1981).

Yairi, E., Longitudinal studies of disfluencies in two-year-old children. *J. Speech Hearing Res., 25,* 155–60 (1982).

Yairi, E., The onset of stuttering in two- and three-year-old children: A preliminary report. *J. Speech Hearing Dis., 48,* 171–77 (1983).

Yairi, E., and Ambrose, N., A longitudinal study of stuttering in children: A preliminary report. *J. Speech Hearing Res., 35,* 755–60 (1992a).

Yairi, E., and Ambrose, N., Onset of stuttering in preschool children: Selected factors. *J. Speech and Hearing Res., 35,* 782–88 (1992b).

Yairi, E., Ambrose, N. G., and Niermann, R., The early months of stuttering: A developmental study. *J. Speech Hearing Res., 36,* 521–28 (1993).

Yairi, E., andClifton, N. F., Jr., Disfluent speech behavior of preschool children, high school seniors, and geriatric persons. *J. Speech Hearing Res., 15,* 714–19 (1972).

Yairi, E., and Hall, K. D., Temporal relations within repetitions of preschool children near the onset of stuttering: A preliminary report. *J. Communic. Dis., 26,* 231–44 (1993).

Yairi, E., and Jennings, S. M., Relationship between the disfluent speech behavior of normal speaking preschool boys and their parents. *J. Speech Hearing Res., 17,* 94–98 (1974).

Yairi, E., and Lewis, B., Disfluencies at the onset of stuttering. *J. Speech Hearing Res., 27,* 155–59 (1984).

Yairi, E., and Williams, D. E., Speech clinicians' stereotypes of elementary school boys who stutter. *J. Communic. Dis., 3,* 161–70 (1970).

Yairi, E., and Williams, D. E., Reports of parental attitudes by stuttering and by nonstuttering children. *J. Speech Hearing Res., 14,* 596–604 (1971).

Yannatos, G., L'hydroxyzine dans la thérapeutique des bégaiements. *J. Franc. ORL, 9,* 293–96 (1960).

Yaruss, J. S., and Conture, E. G., F2 transitions during sound/syllable repetitions of children who stutter and predictions of stuttering chronicity. *J. Speech Hearing Res., 36,* 883–96 (1993).

Yates, A. J., Delayed auditory feedback. *Psychol. Bull., 60,* 213–32 (1963).

Yeakle, M. K., and Cooper, E. B., Teacher perceptions of stuttering. *J. Fluency Dis., 11,* 345–59 (1986).

Yeudall, L. T., A neuropsychological theory of stuttering. *Sem. Speech Lang., 6,* 197–223 (1985).

Yonovitz, A., and Shepherd, W. T., Electrophysiological measurement during a time-out procedure in stuttering and normal speakers. *J. Fluency Dis., 2,* 129–39 (1977).

Yoshiyuki, H., Phonatory initiation, termination, and vocal frequency change reaction times of stutterers. *J. Fluency Dis., 9,* 115–24 (1984).

Yoss, K. A., and Darley, F. L., Developmental apraxia of speech in children with defective articulation. *J. Speech Hearing Res., 17,* 399–416 (1974).

Young, M. A., Predicting ratings of severity of stuttering. *J. Speech Hearing Dis., Monogr. Suppl. 7,* 31–54 (1961).

Young, M. A., Identification of stutterers from recorded samples of their fluent speech. *J. Speech Hearing Res., 7,* 302–03 (1964).

Young, M. A., Audience size, perceived situational difficulty, and stuttering frequency. *J. Speech Hearing Res., 8,* 401–07 (1965).

Young, M. A., Observer agreement: Cumulative effects of rating many samples. *J. Speech Hearing Res., 12,* 135–43 (1969a).

Young, M. A., Observer agreement: Cumulative effects of repeated ratings of the same samples and of knowledge of group results. *J. Speech Hearing Res., 12,* 144–55 (1969b).

Young, M. A., Anchoring and sequence effects for the category scaling of stuttering severity. *J. Speech Hearing Res., 13,* 360–68 (1970).

Young, M. A., Stuttering severity and instructions to increase speaking rate. Ill. *Speech Hearing J., 8,* 3–6 (1974).

Young, M. A., Comment on "Stuttering Frequency and the Onset of Phonation." *J. Speech Hearing Res., 18,* 600–02 (1975a).

Young, M. A., Observer agreement for marking moments of stuttering. *J. Speech Hearing Res., 18,* 530–40 (1975b).

Young, M. A., Onset, prevalence, and recovery from stuttering. *J. Speech Hearing Dis., 40,* 49–58 (1975c).

Young, M. A., Comparison of stuttering frequencies during reading and speaking. *J. Speech Hearing Res., 23,* 216–17 (1980).

Young, M. A., A reanalysis of "Stuttering Therapy: The Relation Between Attitude Change and Long-Term Outcome." *J. Speech Hearing Dis., 46,* 221–22 (1981).

Young, M. A., Identification of stuttering and stutterers. In Curlee, R. F., and Perkins, W. H. (eds.), *Nature and Treatment of Stuttering: New Directions.* San Diego: College-Hill Press (1984).

Young, M. A., Evaluating differences between stuttering and nonstuttering speakers: The group difference design. *J. Speech Hearing Res., 37,* 522–34 (1994).

Young, M. A., and Downs, T. D., Testing the significance of the agreement among observers. *J. Speech Hearing Res., 11,* 5–17 (1968).

Young, M. A. and Prather, E. M., Measuring severity of stuttering using short segments of speech. *J. Speech Hearing Res., 5,* 256–62 (1962).

Yovetich, W. S., Message therapy: Language approach to stuttering therapy with children. *J. Fluency Dis., 9,* 11–20 (1984).

Yovetich, W. S., Booth, J. C., and Tyler, R. S., The effect of dysfluencies on attention in stutterers and nonstutterers. *Human Communic., 1,* 29–39 (1977).

Zaleski, T., Rhythmic skills in stuttering children. *De Therapia Vocis et Loquelae, Vol. I.* XIII Congr. Int. Soc. Logoped. Phoniat. (1965).

Zaliouk, D., and Zaliouk, A., Stuttering, a differential approach in diagnosis and therapy. *De Therapia Vocis et Loquelae, Vol. I.* XIII Congr. Int. Soc. Logoped. Phoniat. (1965).

Zaner, A. R., *Speech Defects Noted Among Amputees.* M. A. Thesis, Univ. Wis. (1950).

Zebrowski, P. M., Duration of the speech disfluencies of beginning stutterers. *J. Speech Hearing Res., 34,* 483–91 (1991).

Zebrowski, P. M., and Conture, E. G., Judgments of disfluency by mothers of stuttering and normally disfluent children. *J. Speech Hearing Res., 32,* 625–34 (1989).

Zebrowski, P. M., Conture, E. G., and Cudahy, E. A., Acoustic analysis of young stutterers' fluency: Preliminary observations. *J. Fluency Dis., 10,* 173–92 (1985).

Zelen, S. L., Sheehan, J. G., and Bugental, J. F. T., Self-perceptions in stuttering. *J. Clin. Psychol., 10,* 70–72 (1954).

Zenner, A. A. Ritterman, S. I., Bowen, S. K., and Gronhovd, K. D., Measurement and comparison of anxiety levels of parents of stuttering, articulatory defective, and normal-speaking children. *J. Fluency Dis., 3,* 273–83 (1978).

Zenner, A. A., Webster, L. M., and Fitzgerald, R. G., The consistency of behaviors in stutterers and nonstutterers during massed oral readings of the same material: A difference measure. *Asha, 16,* 567 (1974). Abstract.

Zerneri, L., Tentatives d'application de la voix retardée ("delayed speech feedback") dans la thérapie du bégaiement. *J. Franc. ORL, 15,* 415–18 (1966).

Zimmermann, G., Articulatory behaviors associated with stuttering: Cinefluorographic analysis. *J. Speech Hearing Res., 23,* 108-21 (1980a).

Zimmermann, G., Articulatory dynamics of fluent utterances of stutterers and nonstutterers. *J. Speech Hearing Res., 23,* 95–107 (1980b).

Zimmermann, G., Stuttering: A disorder of movement. *J. Speech Hearing Res., 23,* 122–36 (1980c).

Zimmermann, G. N., and Hanley, J. M., A cinefluorographic investigation of repeated fluent productions of stutterers in an adaptation procedure. *J. Speech Hearing Res., 26,* 35–42 (1983).

Zimmermann, G. N., and Knott, J. R., Slow potentials of the brain related to speech processing in normal speakers and stutters. *Electroencephalogr. Clin. Neurophysiol., 37,* 599–607 (1974).

Zimmermann, G., Liljeblad, S., Frank, A., and Cleeland, C., The Indians have many terms for it: Stuttering among the Bannock-Shoshoni. *J. Speech Hearing Res., 26,* 315–18 (1983).

Zimmermann, G. N., Smith, A., and Hanley, J. M., Stuttering: In need of a unifying conceptual framework. *J. Speech Hearing Res., 24,* 25–31 (1981).

Zsilavecz, U., Cybernetic functioning in stuttering. *So Afr. J. Communic. Dis., 28,* 60–66 (1981).

SUBJECT INDEX